Changing Disease Patterns and Human Behaviour

Changing Disease Patterns and Human Behaviour

Edited by

N. F. Stanley and R. A. Joske

Departments of Microbiology and Medicine
University of Western Australia

1980

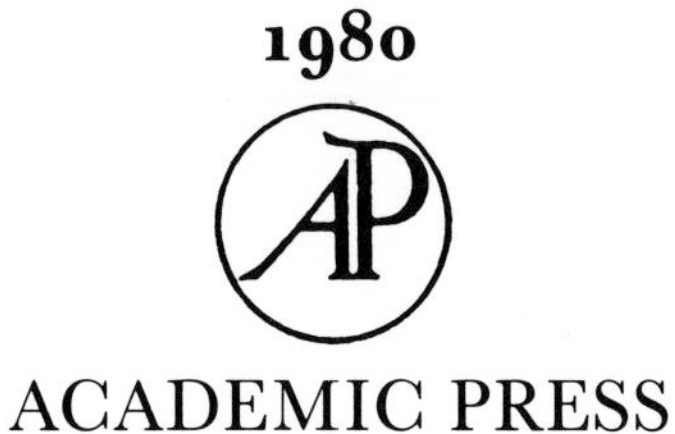

ACADEMIC PRESS

A Subsidiary of Harcourt Brace Jovanovich, Publishers

London · New York · Toronto · Sydney · San Francisco

ACADEMIC PRESS (LONDON) LTD
24/28 Oval Road
London NW1

United States Edition published by
ACADEMIC PRESS INC.
111 Fifth Avenue
New York, New York 10003

British Library Cataloguing in Publication Data
Changing disease patterns and human behaviour.
1. Environmentally induced diseases
2. Medical geography 3. Social medicine
I. Stanley, Neville Fenton II. Joske, R. A.
616.07'1 RB152 80–41082

ISBN 0–12–663560–9

Printed in Great Britain
by Mackays of Chatham

Contributors

R. T. APPLEYARD Department of Economic History, University of Western Australia, Nedlands, Western Australia 6009, Australia

B. K. ARMSTRONG Department of Medicine, University of Western Australia, Nedlands, Western Australia 6009, Australia

FRANCIS L. BLACK Department of Epidemiology and Public Health, Yale University School of Medicine, 60 College Street, New Haven, Connecticut 06510, U.S.A.

STEPHEN BOYDEN, Human Ecology Programme, Centre for Resource and Environmental Studies, Australian National University, Box 4, P.O., Canberra, Australian Capital Territory 2600, Australia

JAMES R. BUSVINE Musca, 26 Braywick Road, Maidenhead, Berks. SL6 1DA, England

JOHN L. FARRANDS Department of Science and the Environment, P.O. Box 449, Woden, Australian Capital Territory 2606, Australia

FRANK FENNER Centre for Resource and Environmental Studies, Australian National University, Box 4, P.O., Canberra, Australian Capital Territory 2600, Australia

MICHAEL GRACEY Gastroenterological Research Unit, Princess Margaret Children's Medical Research Foundation, Subiaco, Western Australia 6008, Australia

DAVID I. GROVE Department of Medicine, University of Western Australia, Nedlands, Western Australia 6009, Australia

IAN GUST Virology Department, Fairfield Hospital, Yarra Bend Road, Fairfield, Victoria 3078, Australia

JOHN HIGGINSON International Agency for Research on Cancer, World Health Organization, 150, Cours Albert-Thomas, 69372, Lyon Cédex 2, France

ANTHONY HORDERN 40 Fullers Road, Chatswood, New South Wales 2067, Australia

NORMAN HOWARD-JONES 28 chemin Colladon, 1209 Geneva, Switzerland

DAISAKU IKEDA The Soka Gakkai, 32 Shinanomachi, Shinjuku-ku, Tokyo 160, Japan

R. A. JOSKE Department of Medicine, University of Western Australia, Nedlands, Western Australia 6009, Australia

MAX KAMIEN Department of Community Practice, University of Western Australia, Claremont Community Health Centre, Claremont 6010, Western Australia, Australia

H. W. de KONING Division of Environmental Health, World Health Organization, 1211 Geneva 27, Switzerland

I. D. LADNYI World Health Organization, 1211 Geneva 27, Switzerland

R. B. LEFROY Department of Medicine, University of Western Australia, Nedlands, Western Australia 6009, Australia

MICHAEL McCALL Department of Medicine, University of Western Australia, Queen Elizabeth II Medical Centre, Nedlands, Western Australia 6009, Australia

JOHN S. MACKENZIE Department of Microbiology, University of Western Australia, Nedlands, Western Australia 6009, Australia

A. J. McMICHAEL Division of Human Nutrition, Commonwealth Scientific and Industrial Research Organization, Kintore Avenue, Adelaide, South Australia 5000, Australia

WILLIAM H. McNEILL Department of History, The University of Chicago, 1126 East 59th Street, Chicago, Illinois 60637, U.S.A.

IAN MADDOCKS 215 Brougham Place, North Adelaide, South Australia 5006, Australia

CEDRIC A. MIMS Department of Microbiology, Guy's Hospital Medical School, London Bridge, London SE1 9RT, England

N. A. MITCHISON Department of Zoology, University College London, Gower Street, London WC1E 6BT, England

DAVID MORLEY Institute of Child Health, 30 Guilford Street, London WC1N 1EH, England

R. S. MORTON 9 Cortworth Road, Ecclesall, Sheffield S11 9LN, England

S. OFOSU-AMAAH Department of Community Health, University of Ghana Medical School, P.O. Box 4236, Accra, Ghana

ANTHONY J. RADFORD Department of Primary Care and Community Medicine, Flinders Medical Centre, Bedford Park, South Australia 5042, Australia

G. ANTHONY RYAN Department of Social and Preventive Medicine, Monash Medical School, Alfred Hospital, Prahran, Victoria 3181, Australia

N. F. STANLEY Department of Microbiology, University of Western Australia, Nedlands, Western Australia 6009, Australia

PETER UNDERWOOD and ZDENKA UNDERWOOD Department of

Community Practice, University of Western Australia, Claremont Community Health Centre, Claremont 6010, Western Australia, Australia
JULIAN de ZULUETA Casa de Mondragón, Ronda (Málaga), Spain

Preface

Professional health workers (such as the editors of this book) are generally too occupied with the daily minutiae of their duties to consider the remote implications of increasing use of a changing and developing medical technology. It is nevertheless salutary periodically to attempt to see where this process is leading us. This book is such an attempt. It tries to present an overall perspective of the evolution of human diseases and man's responses to them, and from this, to look forward to and predict health problems of the coming years.

In this task the editors have received enthusiastic help from a large number of invited collaborators, and from the publishers, Academic Press. Particularly, we would acknowledge the assistance of Mrs. Peta Locke, A.I.P.S., for continued secretarial work far beyond the normal call of duty, Mr. Harry Upenieks, A.R.P.S., R.B.P., for art work, and to our wives for their continuing encouragement and helpful criticism.

N.F.S.

May 1980 R.A.J.

Contents

Part III. Some Patterns of Health Care

Part IV. Problems of Development and Urbanization

Part V. Epilogue

General Introduction

Most physicians and others involved in the study of human disease and the day-to-day practice of medicine rarely have time or opportunity to consider the broader implications of their work in the general context of human evolution and culture. There are nevertheless close and dependent relations between human physical and cultural evolution and the diseases affecting mankind.

These relations have been mentioned in passing by many writers throughout the ages. Much of this work is scattered through monographs, texts and papers in medicine, microbiology, history and sociology, but there has been little recent endeavour to gather these many strands of evidence and conjecture into a single work. The present volume contains a series of essays on this general theme. It is not intended to be complete. We have selected subjects and invited contributions which seem to us to have significant general implications, and where recent thought or laboratory or field studies has provided new insights into a developing field of great importance.

The book may be viewed in a number of ways, each different but valid in itself.

It is in one sense a history of mankind, though not a history of human interaction or achievement, or a history derived from formal documentation. Rather it is concerned with the interaction between the developing and multiplying human species and its environment, more particularly the organisms in the human ecosphere which react with man to cause human disease. It is thus equally a study of the evolutionary history of man and his parasites and pathogens, since the evolution of host and parasite is necessarily interdependent. Much of this history is unwritten and has been inferred from studies of the general biology of disease in man and other species. It is not a history of medicine in the sense of preventive or curative medicine, but of human diseases and their development and consequences, especially the reciprocal relations between human endeavour and human disease.

The book may also be seen in some sense as a study in microbiology. This is because, for most of human existence, the major human diseases have been those caused by infectious agents. It is not, however, in any way devoted to the formal systematic or diagnostic microbiology that is found in texts of microbiology or comprises the daily work of most medical microbiologists. It considers rather the evolutionary relations between man and his pathogens, including the development of diseases and their effects on human development in the past and their possible future consequences.

This general viewpoint implies that the book may also be regarded as a contribution to sociology. The development of human culture, especially the formation and growth of cities, has profoundly altered the ecological environment in which men live. This has itself modified both qualitatively and quantitatively patterns of human life, disease, and death. Urban agglomeration has resulted in an increase in human disease, while increased human mobility has been conditioned by disease, and, conversely, has resulted in spread of diseases to virgin and susceptible populations. These interactions have conditioned life styles and led to new technology with results sometimes tragic and sometimes beneficial.

We regard these sociological implications of the book as particularly important. Those trained in the general disciplines collectively termed sociology are becoming increasingly important in making decisions affecting social policy. But it is our belief that many such persons have little knowledge of or pay little heed to the general principles of biological evolution. We consider that this represents a grave danger and may lead to serious errors, since human capabilities are the result of generations of Darwinian selection. It is our hope that this volume may help to redress this balance.

These wide aims necessarily make the book fragmentary and incomplete. Each chapter has been written as an entity, and there is inevitably some overlap between them; indeed in one or two instances there is frank disagreement. This reflects the state of knowledge in the field, and we have not attempted to modify the views of contributors for the sake of a consistency beyond the bounds of present knowledge.

The book has been designed for an educated but not a strictly professional readership. It should provide a general survey for scientists, especially biologists, anthropologists, sociologists and workers in health fields, as well as background information for politicians and civil servants, and an introduction for educated laymen to an important area of debate in a field of increasing public importance. It might also serve as a text for tertiary courses, such as in the humanities for engineers or in biology for classicists.

The book is in five parts. The first section considers some general aspects of the theme. The second provides a more detailed survey of some important diseases due to microorganisms. The third section describes some of the many methods of provision of health care. The fourth section brings a change of emphasis, and discusses the changing patterns of disease and diseases of the developed society. The first three sections are basically concerned with the past; the fourth section looks equally to the present and future. The essays in the fifth and final section consider some means of reaction to these problems.

This book therefore must be regarded as largely speculative. But it is about a subject upon which we think speculation and debate are essential to the future of our species.

Part I

Evolutionary Aspects

Introduction

The five chapters in this first section discuss the general ecological background of human disease. Dr Frank Fenner and Dr William McNeill discuss the relations between developing human culture and disease, especially the effects of migration and urbanization, while Dr Francis Black attempts to interpret the past by a survey of existing pre-agricultural societies. Dr James Busvine takes a longer view, and explores the possible routes of development of the close and dependent relations between man and microorganisms and insects which may link them in nature. The final chapter by Dr Norman Howard-Jones outlines some aspects of preventive medicine: man's response to the pathogens which share his world.

There are three subjects of great importance which are relevant to, but have not been included in, this section: formal genetics, the evolution of the mind, and the broad field of ethnology.

Human genetics has not been discussed formally since there are a number of good texts in this field, but a genetic approach is implicit in many subsequent chapters, and the reader will find the work more understandable if he reads them with this in mind.

The human brain is undoubtedly the result of Darwinian selection, but the relation between this and the mental make-up and potential of man is not clear. Ethnology—the study of man as an animal species—is closely allied to this problem, but again, despite much recent stimulating work, there seems no consensus opinion. These facets, like genetics, are implicit in subsequent chapters, and this approach will lead the reader to greater understanding. He is nevertheless warned that this field—the evolution of the mind—is a centre of controversy among many biologists and sociologists.

1

Sociocultural Change and Environmental Diseases

Frank Fenner

Centre for Resource and Environmental Studies, Australian National University, Canberra, ACT, Australia

---

The relative importance of different environmental diseases has been undergoing major changes in parallel with the great changes in human society caused by cultural evolution. . . .

The world is now a composite of many stages of sociocultural evolution; environmental diseases occur which are appropriate to each.

I. Introduction

The outstanding feature of man, as distinct from other animals, is the extent to which non-genetic evolutionary change, associated with human culture, has altered man's relationships both with other human beings and to his environment. In this chapter I will examine in a necessarily superficial way what these changes have been over the last million years, and how they have affected the diseases associated with man's environment. We know much more about the changes in human health over the last few hundred and especially the last 50 years than about those that occurred during the first million years, and this book is devoted mostly to changes in the recent past. I will also devote some space to a few diseases that have become important in the recent past and are not dealt with in detail in other chapters.

If one considers animals other than man, four kinds of "environmental" disease can be distinguished:

(a) infections and infestations, by viruses, bacteria, protozoa, helminths and parasitic arthropods;
(b) starvation, usually the result of fluctuations of weather or climate that affect the size of the population dependent upon a particular food resource;
(c) accidental injury and sudden death, often associated with carnivorous predators;
(d) poisoning, from the ingestion of poisonous plants or toxin-containing carrion.

Primitive man was subject to all of these kinds of environmental stress, although it is likely that avoidance of poisonous plants was learnt very early in man's cultural evolution, and one of the earliest results of the controlled use of fire and weapons was to provide some protection against predators. At the other end of the cultural spectrum—modern man in the post-industrial societies of Europe and North America—we find a different range of environmental diseases. Infections, especially with viruses and bacteria, are still common, but are rarely lethal; starvation has been abolished, but a variety of other diseases in which nutrition plays a role (obesity, diabetes, some cancers, cardiovascular disease) have become evident; there are injuries associated with the machines that industrial man invented; and poisoning is due mainly to addictive drugs (including alcohol and tobacco) and the effects of some of the novel chemicals that have resulted from modern chemical research and technology.

Of course, the transition between these extreme situations was not sudden; there were the major intermediate sociocultural stages associated first with the development of agriculture, and then irrigated agriculture, long before the industrial revolution. Nor are these changes yet general for all mankind; there are still the remnants of a few hunter-gatherer societies left, nomadic pastoralists and dry-land farmers still comprise a significant population group occupying the semi-arid regions of the world, and most people in the world still live in villages and are sustained by irrigated agriculture. Likewise with the patterns of disease. Besides the extremes that I have already described, there were important and characteristic changes in the pattern of environmental diseases associated with each of these major sociocultural changes.

In the following pages I shall sketch a broad picture of the sociocultural evolution of man and consider the effects of some of the major changes in his culture on the diseases associated with his environment. It is convenient to consider first the infectious diseases, several of which will be elaborated on in Section II of the book, and then some of the "diseases of progress", which are described in greater detail in Section IV.

II. Sociocultural Evolution of Man

Before considering the behaviour of infectious agents, we must look at the sociocultural changes that man has undergone, in terms of parameters relevant to infectious diseases (Table I). The background against which infectious diseases of man must be viewed is a transition in a relatively few generations (from the point of view of genetic evolution) from small and scattered groups of hunter-gatherers (which has been the cultural state of man for most of his existence), through the neolithic revolution to man the farmer, living in small villages but with a few large towns and cities, and only yesterday, as it were, the power revolution occurred, and with it the increasing aggregation of much greater numbers of human beings in large and very large cities. Infectious diseases by necessity must be transmitted from one host to another of the same or different species. The two most important parameters affecting their nature and frequency are (a) changes in the closeness of contact of man with other animals, either directly or via arthropod vectors, and (b) the alteration in the size of the aggregations of human beings and the communications within and between these aggregations.

The sociocultural changes that have affected the non-infectious

TABLE I. *The Time-Scale of Sociocultural Changes in Man, in Relation to the Number of Generations, World Population and the Size of the Human Communities*

Number of years before present	World population (millions)	Number of generations	Sociocultural state	Size of human communities
500 000	0.1	25 000	Hunter and food-gatherer	Scattered nomadic bands of <100 persons
10 000	5	500	Development of agriculture	Relatively settled villages of <300 persons
6000	50	300	Development of irrigated agriculture	Few cities of ≈ 100 000 persons; mostly villages of <300
250	600	10	Introduction of steam power	Some cities of ≈ 500 000 persons; many cities of ≈ 100 000; many villages of ≈ 1000
140	1000	5	Introduction of sanitary reforms	
0	4000		Modern urbanized man	Some cities of >5 000 000 persons; many cities of >500 000; relatively fewer villages of ≈ 1000

environmental diseases do not fit on the time-scale used in Table I; they are the product of the last few hundred years, mainly, so far, in Europe and North America, and have become particularly evident during the last quarter century.

III. Modes of Transmission of Infectious Diseases

The key to the survival of infectious agents in nature is their transmission from one host to the next. It is impossible to consider in this one chapter the varied and often intricate modes of transmission of many of the agents that infect man (especially the helminths and protozoa). Two important examples of the latter, schistosomiasis and malaria, are discussed in detail in Chapters 10 and 11. Here I shall make some general observations about viral and bacterial infections. Figure 1 represents diagrammatically the major surfaces of the body from which microbes can be released, and across which they may achieve entry to the tissues of the body.

The data presented in Tables II and III show that some viruses and some bacteria exist which take advantage of each ecological "niche", in terms of routes of entry and exit. Much the most common portals of entry are the respiratory and gastrointestinal tracts, since they are exposed to large volumes of potentially contaminated air or food/water, and each offers a large surface area of cells unprotected by the horny

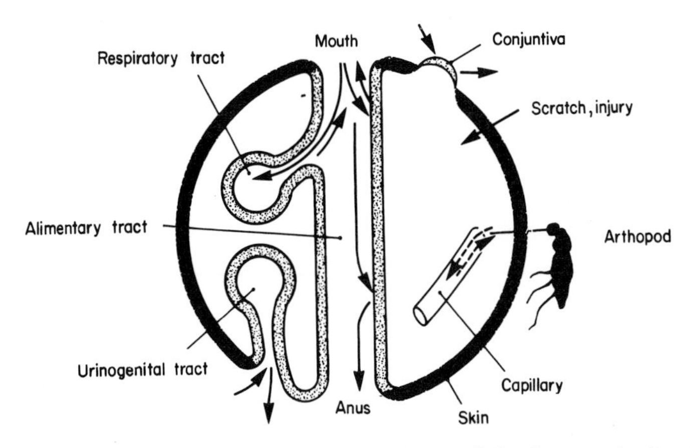

Fig. 1. Diagram illustrating the major surfaces of the human body that are involved in the entry and exit of bacteria, rickettsias and viruses from the tissues of the body. (From Mims, C.A. (1976) "The Pathogenesis of Infectious Diseases", Academic Press, London.)

TABLE II. *The Transmission of Some Viral Infections of Man*

Route of exit	Route of transmission	Examples of infections	Mode/route of entry	Duration of human infectivity	Animal reservoir
Respiratory (mouth and nose)	Aerosol	Smallpox	Inhalation	Short	No
		Measles	Inhalation	Short	No
		Varicella	Inhalation	Short, but recurrent with zoster	No
		Influenza	Inhalation	Short	No
		Rhinovirus	Inhalation	Short	No
Saliva	Bite	Rabies	Skin	Nil	Yes
	Kissing	Mononucleosis (CMV and EBV)	Mouth	Long	No
	via hand/fomites	Herpes simplex type 1	Mouth	Recurrent	No
Faeces	Stool → hand/fomite	Enteroviruses	Mouth	Short	No
		Hepatitis A	Mouth	Short	No
		Rotavirus	Mouth	Short	No
	Stool → water	Hepatitis A	Mouth	Short	Seafood (passive)
		Parvoviruses	Mouth	Short	
		Enteroviruses	Mouth	Short	
Skin	Air	Smallpox	Inhalation	Short	No
	Skin → skin	Warts	Abrasions	Long	No
		Molluscum contagiosum	Abrasions	Long	No
Blood	Mosquitoes and ticks	Arboviruses (several genera, many species)	Bite	Short	Yes
	Injection/transfusion, wounds	Hepatitis B	Injection or abrasions	Long/recurrent	No
Genital	Genital	Herpes simplex type 2	Venereal	Recurrent	No
		Cytomegalovirus	Venereal	Recurrent	No
Placenta	Vertical to fetus	Rubella	Blood	Short/recurrent	No
		Cytomegalovirus	Blood	Short/recurrent	No
		Epstein-Barr virus	Blood	Short/recurrent	No

TABLE III. *The Transmission of Some Bacterial and Rickettsial Infections of Man*

Route of exit	Route of transmission	Examples of infecting agents	Mode/route of entry	Duration of human infectivity	Multiplication outside body	Animal reservoir
Respiratory	Aerosol	Pneumococci	Inhalation	Short	No	No
		Streptococci	Inhalation	Short	No	No
		Mycobacterium tuberculosis	Inhalation	Long	No	Sometimes
		M. leprae	Inhalation	Long	No	No
	Animal dust	*Rickettsia burnetii*	Inhalation	Nil	No	Yes
Faeces	Stool → hand/fomites, water, food	*Shigella*	Ingestion	Short	Yes	No
		Salmonella (most species)	Ingestion	Short	Yes	Yes
		Salmonella typhi	Ingestion	Recurrent	Yes	No
		Vibrio cholerae	Ingestion	Short	Yes	No
		Staphylococci (toxin)	Ingestion	Short	Yes	No
Skin	Lesion	Staphylococci	Abrasions	Long	No	No
		Streptococci	Abrasions	Short	No	No
		Treponema pertenue	Abrasions	Long	No	No
Blood/tissue	Flea	*Pasteurella pestis*	Bite	Short	No	Yes
	Louse	*Rickettsia prowazekii*	Bite	Short (rare recurrent)	No	No
	Mite	*Rickettsia tsutsugamushi*	Bite	Short	No	Yes
Genital	Penis/cervix	*Neisseria gonorrhoeae*	Veneral	Short	No	No
		Treponema pallidum	Veneral	Long	No	No

layer that the skin presents to the outside world. Whether a particular virus or bacterium infects via the gastrointestinal or via the respiratory tract (or both) depends upon the way in which the microbe is introduced (in aerosols or food, for example), on its resistance to various non-specific inhibitors occurring in each system, and on whether suitable cellular receptors are present. But the skin barrier can be transgressed; by bites (arthropod bites are especially important: plague, rickettsial and arboviral infections), injections and abrasions.

Features that are important in determining whether particular infectious diseases will occur in the small isolated bands of human beings characteristic of ancient man and modern hunter-gatherer societies are those listed in the last two columns of Table II and the last three columns of Table III, namely the existence of extrahuman sources of the infectious agent, and the duration (or recurrent nature) of infectivity in the case of bacteria and viruses that have no animal reservoir.

IV. The Influence of Sociocultural Conditions on Infectious Diseases

With this information as a background, we can consider what diseases would be likely to have occurred among human populations at various stages of their sociocultural evolution.

A. Infectious Diseases of Hunter-Gatherer Societies

From the point of view of infectious diseases, the important features of man at the palaeolithic hunter-gatherer stage were the small size of the band and its infrequent close contact with members of other closed bands, and the fact that even in palaeolithic times man was a relatively long-lived animal, once the risks of birth and infancy had been successfully surmounted. Because of their close personal contact and communal habits, the microbial flora characteristic of man under these circumstances was probably shared by all members of the group.

Infections of the hunter-gatherers were as follows.

Present

From animal reservoirs: arbovirus infections, rickettsiosis, rabies, salmonellosis

Chronic and latent: chickenpox-zoster, herpes simplex and other herpesvirus infections, tuberculosis, leprosy, treponematosis

"Saprophytes" which could become pathogens (trauma): staphylococci, streptococci

Absent

"Human" viral diseases: localized—respiratory or enteric diseases; generalized—measles, smallpox

Some "human" bacterial infections: shigellosis, cholera, typhoid fever

Black and Morley (Chapters 3 and 7, respectively) discuss the basic community size needed to maintain measles virus; the same situation holds for all the generalized human viral infections in which there is no animal reservoir and latency and recurrent excretion do not occur. Thus several viral diseases that we now regard as being "characteristically human", such as measles, smallpox and rubella, could not have existed in palaeolithic man. Immunity due to prior infection is not as durable in many of the diseases of mucous surfaces (intestinal and respiratory tracts) as it is in the generalized infections, but such immunity lasts long enough to ensure that the human enteric and respiratory viruses that are so common now could not have survived in man as the sole host in societies of a few hundred individuals. There is ample present-day evidence that respiratory viral diseases "die out" in isolated communities in Arctic and Antarctic regions, in spite of the severe weather conditions that prevail there. The only "specifically human" viral diseases that we could expect to find in primitive man are those marked by latency and recurrent infectivity, like herpes simplex and chickenpox-zoster. Viral diseases were therefore rather uncommon amongst hunter-gatherers; most were not "human" diseases but were caused by viruses of some other animal which "accidentally" infected man, notably the arboviruses and sometimes rabies.

Much the same principles apply to bacterial and rickettsial diseases, although some potentially pathogenic bacteria can survive indefinitely on the surface of the skin or on mucous membranes and invade the body when a breach of the surface is produced by minor or severe trauma. Thus staphylococcal and streptococcal infection of wounds may have occurred from nasal carriers of these bacteria. Tuberculosis, leprosy, and treponematosis, with their characteristic features of chronicity and recurrent excretion, could survive in small communities; and of course primitive man was subject to many bacterial and rickettsial infections acquired from other animals or arthropods, such as salmonellosis, plague, leptospirosis, and flea-borne and mite-borne typhus.

B. Infectious Diseases in Societies Based on Agriculture

The development of agriculture led to a great change in human habits. No longer were men nomads, and no longer was the population size of a group limited by the availability of hunted or collected food. Villages developed, and the close contact between larger numbers of people, allied to their lack of understanding of sanitation, led to accelerated exchange of their gut flora and the development of endemic enteric bacterial infections. It is likely that the generalized viral infections and most of the enteric and respiratory viruses still failed to become established.

Infectious diseases in primitive villagers were as follows.

Present

All those found in hunter-gatherers
Enteric bacterial infections
Some respiratory infections

Absent

Measles, smallpox, rubella
Some "human" respiratory viruses
Some "human" enteric viruses

C. Infectious Diseases in the Cities

When irrigation made large-scale agriculture possible, some men and women started to live in towns and cities. The pattern of viral infections was greatly influenced by the development of these larger societies, for now community size sometimes exceeded the minimum level needed to maintain diseases like smallpox, measles and rubella, and a large close-knit society permitted the ready spread of faecal–oral and respiratory viruses.

Infectious diseases in cities were as follows.

Infections in primitive cities

Maximun likelihood—all disease associated with human-to-human spread; some arthropod-transmitted diseases less common than in villages

Infections in advanced cities:

Present: measles, rubella, respiratory viruses, venereal diseases
Absent or controlled: enteric bacteria (viruses)—"clean" water supplies;
some specific human viral infections—vaccination;
Many bacterial infections—chemotherapy

The neolithic origins of the "human" respiratory viruses remain speculative; the progenitors of the present large range of different serotypes of rhinoviruses, coronaviruses and influenzaviruses must have been acquired from some animal source. Many animals live in large enough groups to sustain such viruses because their turnover rate (that is, their length of life and the rate of accession of new susceptibles) is much more rapid than in man.

Once the "prototype" respiratory and enteric viruses had been successfully established in human communities, they were subjected to natural selection for survival, which operated, as always, at the level of transmission. Since local secretory antibody provides homologous protection for at least a few years, antigenically novel viruses had a better opportunity of becoming established and multiplying to a sufficiently high titre to be transmitted, and this process led in time to the development of a large number of antigenically different enteric and respiratory viruses.

D. Urbanization

Urbanization is a recent phenomenon, dating back only a few hundred years and still increasing, especially in developing countries. It was caused primarily by the recruitment of country folk to the cities. Initially, during the industrial revolution in Europe and North America, and up to the present day in developing countries, urbanization was accompanied by intense squalor and poverty and a greatly increased incidence of the associated infectious diseases. Some of these, like the water-borne bacterial diseases, were controlled by sanitary measures, introduced in Western countries in the middle of the nineteenth century; other diseases, such as tuberculosis, took a terrible toll, especially of adolescent migrants from rural areas. In the early days of urbanization, the hospitals themselves were hotbeds of infection with a variety of agents, notably the enteric organisms, staphylococci, and the streptococci that cause septicaemia and pneumonia. Even today the control of bacterial cross-infection in hospitals calls for continuing vigilance.

Ultimately the combination of wealth, with attendant improvement in dwellings and a decrease in crowding, sanitation in the form of a safe water supply and adequate disposal of excreta, and, finally, the development of effective antibacterial drugs, has diminished the importance of bacterial diseases as causes of death and severe morbidity in the great conurbations that characterize the modern world.

Viral infections of the gastrointestinal tract have not disappeared as rapidly as the enteric bacterial pathogens; polioviruses, rotaviruses, echoviruses, parvoviruses and infectious hepatitis virus still circulate widely. Perhaps this is a reflection of laboratory methods. We take no notice of intestinal bacteria unless they cause disease. Many enteric viruses appear to be non-pathogenic in the vast majority of cases, but because of the sort of laboratory techniques required for viral isolation all positive results are recorded. We know that there has been a great diminution in the circulation of enteric viruses in modern cities of Western man compared with places like Karachi or Calcutta. Indeed, paradoxically, the development of poliomyelitis as a recognizable epidemic disease at the beginning of the twentieth century was due to improvements in hygiene. In "unsewered" cities, infection with polioviruses was universal in infancy (and still is, in the absence of vaccination with oral poliovaccine). However, apart from a few unrecognized deaths, polioviruses usually fail to produce symptoms in infants, but make them immune to infection later in life. When the primary infection was postponed to later childhood by improved sanitation, an age group was exposed in which, for physiological reasons, invasion of the central nervous system by poliovirus became much more common, so that epidemics of "infantile paralysis" occurred. Infectious hepatitis appears to be following an identical pattern, and in affluent societies it now ranks as the most serious endemic viral disease of man (see Chapter 6).

The number and variety of respiratory viral infections of man are probably in a stage of explosive evolutionary expansion at the present time. As outlined earlier, man the hunter lived in aggregations too small to maintain respiratory viruses which produced acute infection without prolonged or recurrent viral excretion. The great increase in the numbers of human beings, their crowding into ever-larger cities, and the increasing travel between these cities are tending to make the "human" world into a single ecological as well as intensely interacting political unit. The respiratory viruses of northern and southern hemispheres, and of east and west, are mingled by air travellers, so that the population of almost any large city in the world today is potentially exposed to human respiratory viruses from all over the world. With this increased exposure there is, of course, increased opportunity for evolutionary radiation, especially in the antigenicity of the viral protein coats.

It is not easy to see how the minor respiratory infections can be controlled. Vaccines are practicable and sensible for only a few relatively serious diseases; the vast majority of viral infections do not justify either the cost or the risk of vaccination. Yet in the aggregate these "minor" infections may be quite important in producing general ill health and potentiating the adverse effects of inspired pollutants. "Air-sanitation" is effective only under very special and local conditions; we can never expect to produce "sanitized" air as we do expect to produce safe drinking water. And if effective specific antiviral drugs are produced their use will carry the risks associated with any drug (and it is sobering to think how much sickness is caused by drugs given for therapeutic purposes), they will be used only in relatively serious diseases and will act for a short time only.

E. European Colonization and the Spread of Infectious Diseases

Until the development of ocean-going ships in Europe during the fourteenth century, urban and rural man was largely confined to the continents in which his progenitors had lived as primitive agriculturists and nomads. When large-scale human movement, usually connected with wars and conquest, did occur between Asia and Europe it was associated with major epidemics, of which the "Black Death" (plague) and smallpox were the most devastating. The explosive period of European colonization of all the other continents had profound effects on the disease patterns, in both the migrants and the indigenes. European man took his endemic diseases to new virgin populations, and there were explosive outbreaks of measles and smallpox, for example, in the native inhabitants of America and Oceania. Smallpox in particular had a major impact on human history, notably in the conquest of the American Indians in North, Central and South America, and in the breakup of the Hottentot tribes in southern Africa (see Chapters 2 and 13).

Conversely European man intruded on situations in which the indigenous inhabitants had acquired, by natural selection, considerable genetic resistance to diseases often lethal to the European, for example, falciparum malaria and yellow fever in Africa. The slave ships of the sixteenth and seventeenth centuries took the vector or urban yellow fever, *Aedes aegypti*, as well as the yellow fever virus itself, to South America, where both rapidly established themselves and the virus became enzootic in jungle primates.

The European colonists also took their domesticated animals with them. Cattle, sheep and horses, in the large herds used for pastoral purposes, encountered environments virtually free of novel pathogenic microbes in Australia, where the native animal population was sparse and zoologically novel; but in Africa they were exposed to a host of viruses and other parasites which had evolved with the great herds of ungulates. Many of the viruses were arthropod-borne, and in the new host animals they caused devastating epizootics of diseases like bluetongue, rinderpest, Rift Valley fever, Nairobi sheep disease, African horse sickness, African swine fever and so on. Having become established in the sheep and cattle of the colonists in Africa, some of these diseases were then transported to other countries, just as yellow fever had been; and in quite recent times bluetongue virus became established in Europe and the United States, African horse sickness spread to India, and African swine fever virus to South America.

The livestock industries of Australia, the last continent colonized and one free from serious indigenous diseases, have been maintained free of the exotic scourges of sheep and cattle only by strict quarantine. Yet with the increased traffic between continents even this protection is breaking down; during the last decade, for example, Newcastle disease virus (albeit a highly attenuated strain) has become enzootic there.

Air travel, vastly increased in volume and operating between continents at speeds within the incubation periods of most diseases, has converted the world of man into a single ecological unit. New influenza viruses now spread with the speed of plane rather than ship or train travel; during the last decade cholera has spread to every continent.

F. The Spread of Cholera, especially since 1961

The first and in many ways most significant manifestation of the altered disease relationships created by industrialization was the global spread of cholera, which had long been endemic in India, being spread periodically around the subcontinent by celebrants at Hindu pilgrimages to the Lower Ganges. Occasionally the disease had reached China, travelling by ship. In 1817 a new factor entered the picture; the Calcutta epidemic was carried to unfamiliar ground by English troops and ships both overland to India's northern frontiers, and by sea to Ceylon, Indonesia, China and Japan, Syria, Anatolia and the Caspian shores. In the 1830s cholera became global, initially spread by military movements, then to Ireland and with Irish immigrants to North America. It also became established in Mecca, thus adding the Moslem pilgrimage to its Hindu pilgrimage dispersal routes, and epidemics initiated in Mecca were recorded about every second year between 1831 and 1912.

Cholera caused many deaths in India, but being thoroughly familiar, excited no special alarm or surprise there. The situation was totally different elsewhere, both in the Moslem world and in Europe, where cholera created widespread panic. The first outbreak in Britain, in 1832, led to the establishment of local boards of health, which were ineffective. More significantly, the reappearance of cholera in 1848 was the direct cause of the establishment by Parliament of the Central Board of Health, which was able to institute far-reaching programmes of public sanitation that had been advocated for a decade or more by reformers, the best-known of whom was Edwin Chadwick. All this occurred years before the classical demonstration by John Snow, in

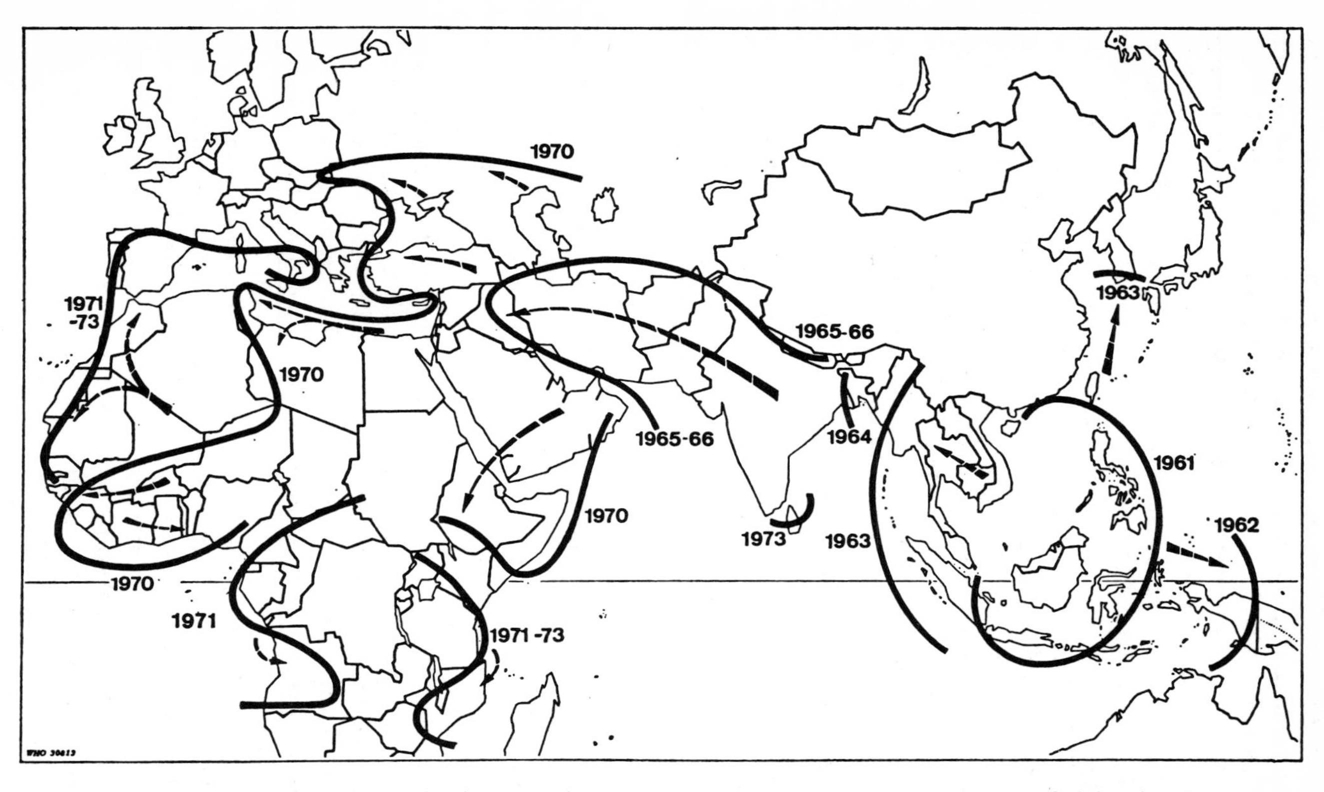

Fig. 2. The global spread of cholera in the seventh pandemic, up to 1973. This began in the Celebes in 1961 and is still in progress; the vibrio concerned is the El Tor biotype. (From *WHO Wkly Epidem. Rec.* No. 27, 1974, 229–231.)

1854, of the spread of cholera from a single contaminated source of drinking water, and almost 40 years before Koch's demonstration in 1883 that *Vibrio cholerae* was the cause of the disease.

Besides the endemic occurrence of cholera in many of the countries in which it had been seeded, and the frequent small epidemics that originated in Mecca, there have been five other pandemics since the second pandemic of 1826–37, in which waves of the disease spread widely from the endemic foci in Asia. The seventh and last pandemic, to which the rest of this section will be devoted, started in the Celebes in 1961. It was caused by a biotype of *Vibrio cholerae* called El Tor, so named after the quarantine camp in Sinai, where in 1905 six peculiar strains of *Vibrio* had been isolated from the dead bodies of returned Mecca pilgrims who had shown no signs of choleraic disease either during life or post mortem. There was continuing controversy among bacteriologists about the significance of this organism, and the next important epidemiological finding was the observation of its association with a disease, then called "paracholera", in the Celebes in 1937. During the next 20 years this organism caused a small number of cases of clinical cholera in surrounding islands of Indonesia, but in 1961 it suddently began to spread widely, and initiated the seventh and so far the most widespread pandemic of cholera, which is still in progress (Fig. 2).

The classical biotype continued to cause most cases of cholera reported on the Indian subcontinent, but it was replaced by El Tor vibrio by 1965 in India and by 1972 in Bangladesh. Elsewhere the El Tor biotype spread from its original focus in Indonesia to countries of South East Asia and then through the Middle East and down the western and eastern sides of Africa and into Europe. In most countries of West Africa, fishermen and traders played a major role in the spread of cholera along rivers and sea routes, thereby affecting coastal towns and fishing villages. Nomads, moving with their cattle in search of water during the dry season, also helped its spread. The introduction of cholera was always followed by explosive outbreaks, particularly in rural areas and in suburbs of metropolitan areas without piped water supplies.

Cholera invaded French West Africa in the fourth pandemic in 1868 and again during the fifth pandemic in 1893–94, but did not then gain a foothold there. The increased traffic and population density, as well as the environmental conditions, have created conditions favourable for its endemic persistence, and both outbreaks and sporadic cases have continued to occur in several African countries up to the present time. Outbreaks also occurred in Italy and Portugal, and in 1978 a small outbreak occurred in the United States, the first since 1911. There was a substantial outbreak in the isolated Gilbert Islands, in the central Pacific Ocean, in 1977–78, and cases were imported into many European countries and Australia.

An event of considerable epidemiological importance were outbreaks associated with the consumption of contaminated food served on board two international aircraft, which led to about forty recognized cases in Australia, three in New Zealand and two in England. Even more bizarre was the suggestion that cholera vibrios from the toilet canisters of high-flying passenger aircraft could serve as a source of the sporadic cholera in Europe (1970–75) in the flight paths of regular air services from Calcutta.

After an initial period of appeals for emergency help and especially for vaccines, by about 1970 the health authorities in many cholera-affected countries were placing greater emphasis on the improvement of water supply and excreta disposal and food hygiene, and had refrained from mass vaccination. Nevertheless, dishonest and irrational behaviour such as concealment of cases, and insistence of vaccination of all incoming travellers, remains all too common a response of government authorities to this disease.

V. Modern Technological Society and Environmental Diseases

The last quarter century has seen a remarkable change in the nature of environmental diseases among the wealthy citizens of advanced industrial societies. Many of the serious infectious diseases are now effectively controlled, but there may be an actual increase in morbidity due to trivial viral infections. A few kinds of infections have become more prevalent because of particular social or technological practices: hepatitis A with injections, both for medical purposes and by drug addicts, cytomegalovirus infections with immunosuppression. Other practices in medical and veterinary technology pose new threats, notably the selection of drug-resistant bacteria, and the spread by plasmids of multiple drug resistance between different species of bacteria.

A. Nutritional Diseases

Nutritional diseases have changed in character. Starvation is virtually unknown in affluent societies and even in the poor countries famines cause far fewer deaths than they did 50 years ago, mainly because of improvements in food distribution networks. But changes in food preferences and the development of food technology now contribute to a variety of new kinds of disease. Gross vitamin deficiency diseases, unknown in hunter-gatherer or village agricultural societies, became rampant in the early cities of the industrial revolution, but have now virtually disappeared in the cities of the modern Western world. On the other hand, the abundance of food, the high proportion of animal fats now consumed, and the high degree of refinement of most cereal foods are believed to be important contributory factors to a number of the "diseases of progress" described in Section V, notably dental caries, diabetes, cardiovascular disease and cancers of the gastrointestinal tract.

B. Trauma

Certainly since early neolithic times, and probably before that, warfare was an important cause of injuries and death, and from the Middle Ages onwards the disruptive effects of warfare greatly exacerbated nutritional and infectious diseases—wars were traditionally associated with famine and pestilence. Modern warfare is conducted on a much wider scale, and is much more expensive than wars of earlier times, but probably causes a relatively lower morbidity and mortality. Widespread nuclear warfare, if ever practised, would introduce death and destruction, especially of non-combatants, of a different order of magnitude from anything yet experienced.

Even during peacetime modern industrial society has introduced machines that greatly increase the risk of injury and death. Especially among young adults, motor vehicle crashes cause proportionately more damage and death than predators ever did to early man. No measures have yet been devised to control this epidemic, although a number of "technological fixes" slow down the rate of increase of car-induced injury and death. Temporary shortages of liquid fuel in 1973–74 led to imposition of speed limits in order to save fuel. In spite of the concomitant decrease in road accidents, speed limits were raised again in most countries as soon as the petrol crisis was over. The eventual disappearance of petroleum-based fuels may be the only way in which the car crash epidemic will be controlled, if indeed alternative fuels are by then too expensive for general use.

C. Poisoning

One of the most pervasive and interesting of the changes that have occurred since the beginning of the industrial revolution, and particularly since the Second World War, is in the poisons that modern man now ingests and inhales. Ancient poisons persist, and occasionally cause widespread illness, as in epidemics of favism. The new poisons differ from the old in their origin, for they are mostly chemical substances produced by modern chemical technology which are truly novel, and thus previously unknown in nature. A few of these have ill-effects on man which are usually chronic, long-term and cumulative rather than acute, and are therefore difficult to recognize. In addition to the novel chemical poisons, some old poisons, like alcohol and morphine derivatives, appear to have increased effects in some segments of modern society because of changes in social behaviour.

Among the poisons that modern man inhales the most important are those associated with cigarette smoking, which contribute not only to lung carcinoma but also to cardiovascular and chronic pulmonary disease. Other important and relatively new poisonous chemicals are the sulphur and nitrogen oxides and other emissions that occur in exhaust gases from motor vehicles and in the discharges of furnaces that burn fossil fuels.

Novel chemicals that may be poisonous are often first recognized among those occupationally exposed, e.g. to vinyl chloride. The carcinogenic effects of asbestos fibres have been suspected for years but solid evidence of the ubiquity of these fibres has only recently become available. Other chemical poisons, for example the heavy metals, have been recognized as such for many years, but changes in chemical technology have greatly changed the scale and sometimes the nature of the material discharged into the environment. Likewise, highly radioactive materials have existed in nature for years. They become poisons only when used in ignorance of their effects, as in the early days of radium treatment and in the production of luminous watch dials, or when the scale of their production and the difficulties of their safe transportation and storage pose risks of a novel kind.

Finally, there are the chemicals whose influence on man's health is not direct or certain, but which may have critically important effects on human well-being. These are characterized by substances like the fluorocarbons and nitrogen oxides, which may react with stratospheric ozone and in the long term have effects both on the opacity of the atmosphere to ultraviolet light and on the climate of the earth. It is even more difficult to gather objective evidence about this kind of change than it is to elucidate the direct health effects of novel chemicals.

VI. Conclusions

Looked at from the perspective of human evolution, environmental diseases have always been important, but the relative importance of different diseases has been undergoing major changes in parallel with the great changes in human society caused by cultural evolution. In a few instances, such as with falciparum malaria, the biological selective effect has been so severe that recognizable genetic changes have occurred in the human population (see Chapter 8); in other instances, as with yellow fever, plague and smallpox, we suspect that some genetic selection has occurred but it cannot be readily demonstrated. For the most part, however, the main impact of environmental diseases has been on non-genetic sociocultural evolution.

The world is now a composite of all stages of sociocultural evolution, with all the kinds of environmental disease appropriate to each stage. However, even though human evolution, both biological and cultural, has occurred very rapidly (compared with other animals, and using a generational time-scale), it seems that the driving forces of modern technology, especially communications technology, will make "modernization" and its attendant advantages and disadvantages all-pervasive. It is important that its dangers are clearly recognized, so that technology becomes and remains the servant and not the master of man.

2

Migration Patterns and Infection in Traditional Societies

William H. McNeill
Department of History, The University of Chicago, Chicago, Illinois, USA

Climate sets up . . . infectious gradients that . . . make it perilous for human beings to migrate into warmer and wetter lands . . . a city [constitutes] an intense local peak in the disease gradient. . . .

Innumerable examples illustrate the disastrous repercussions of new disease encounters for previously inexperienced populations.

I. Climatic Gradients and Disease Patterns

Bands of hunters and gatherers that have been observed by medically competent outsiders seem to exhibit a high level of general health. Varied diet and plenty of walking perhaps contribute to this result, but a more important factor is that the numerical smallness of a band that moves to a new campsite every few days makes it difficult to establish anal–oral and other infectious cycles that are characteristic of settled communities. Village farmers, by contrast, commonly carry a considerable load of infections, though much depends on the wetness and warmth of the climate in which they dwell. Cold weather and dry conditions inhibit many of the insect-borne infections, for example, while warmth and wetness multiply the number and variety of micro-organisms lying in wait to infect a suitable human host.

Climate thus sets up what may be described as infection gradients that used to make it perilous for human beings to migrate into warmer and wetter lands than those from which they came. Innumerable invaders of India were undone by this fact, for example; similarly, several medieval German emperors died in Italy while attempting to make good their control over Rome. The most striking modern example of this phenomenon was illustrated by the fate of Europeans in tropical Africa who, early in the nineteenth century, survived on the average less than a year from the time of their arrival. Migration down a disease gradient into cooler and drier lands was far safer, though encounter with an unfamiliar infection could be dangerous to the migrant.

Such risks were much intensified when it was an army or other dense mass of human beings that moved up or down a climatic disease gradient. Sudden outbreaks of lethal epidemics were always a danger for the intruders, as the fate of King Sennacharib in 701 B.C. illustrates. Armies, indeed, were places where men risked death deliberately, but until the twentieth century more died from infections than from the results of enemy action. Pilgrimage was the other institutional form of behaviour that prepared people for death. Trains of pilgrims, moving to and from holy places, rivalled armies as propagators of infections, as the career of cholera in the nineteenth century shows.

Patterns of infection defined by climate were, however, systematically modified wherever large cities came into existence. Such human agglomerations intensified exposure to infection by increasing the pace of encounter among strangers and multiplying the number of potential hosts so that infectious chains were less likely to be interrupted. A city, in other words, constituted an intense local peak in the disease gradient; and the intensity of its infectious load, in general, increased with its size. Climate could accentuate or diminish urban infectious diseases; indeed in temperate climates infectious disease commonly peaked in the warm months of the year. But cold winters, like those of Peking, or cool summers, like those of London, were no protection against the intensification of infections that arose when large numbers of human beings lived close together without a sanitary water supply, sewage disposal, or any of the other public health measures we take for granted today.

II. Urbanization and New Diseases

Until some time in the nineteenth century cities rivalled armies (and pilgrimages) in provoking death. Urban births did not match deaths; and the world's cities were maintained only by a current of in-migration from the healthier countryside. London in the eighteenth century, for example, required an annual average in-migration of 5000 persons just to maintain itself. The total of 500 000 for the century was considerably larger than the entire population of the city in 1700. Other European cities for which similar calculations have been made show the same pattern in early modern times, and there is every reason to suppose that Asian cities exhibited the same dependence on migrants from the countryside.

A major reason for the unhealthiness of cities was the fact that a new class of distinctively modern diseases could and did establish themselves among massed populations that exceeded a critical size. These diseases pass from host to host by droplet infection, and, if they do not prove lethal, provoke long-lasting antibody reactions. The familiar array of standard childhood diseases of the recent past—measles, mumps, smallpox, whooping cough, and others—are examples of infections distinctive of civilization. They probably established themselves among human populations by transfer from animal herds large enough to maintain a perpetual supply of unexposed individuals so that the chain of infection would not break. Only when human populations became large enough to do the same could these diseases become firmly established among people. Sometimes the required population size was quite large: measles, for example, needed a population of over 450 000 to sustain itself in the twentieth century, before medical prophylaxis began to interfere with its infectious cycle. This meant, of course, that only in relatively large cities or among populations closely connected with cities by steady movement to and fro could the measles virus long survive. Sudden flare-up of infection in remote villages or among wandering tribesmen could occur when some contact with a carrier took place; but in such communities the measles infection would swiftly run out of unexposed hosts and die away. Only where a sufficient number of newborns could be found (in recent times about 7000 uninfected infants were required) could the measles virus survive indefinitely as a human infection. Even then, its survival was precarious. Infection rose to peaks at more or less regular intervals, and then dwindled away almost to the disappearing point until the virus again made contact with a fresh crop of vulnerable children during their early school years and spread swiftly among them, only to subside again and repeat the cycle some two years subsequently (see also page 44).

This pattern of coexistence between human beings and measles as observed and assigned statistical parameters about 20 years ago was, of course, the result of lengthy mutual adaptation, both biological and cultural. The custom of sending children to school at age 5–6 years, for example, defined the age at which they were most likely to get the measles. The fact that few children died of the disease meant that no very strenuous efforts were made to prevent exposure, thus assuring the virus of a continued existence.

Comparably exact data about other childhood infections is unavailable because medical prophylaxis had begun to interfere with the patterns of their propagation before observers knew enough to formulate the question statistically. In their "natural" state the other important diseases of childhood probably did not require populations quite as large as the 450 000 needed by measles, since measles was one of the most explosively infectious of such diseases and was therefore liable to run out of potential hosts more rapidly than other viruses. But smallpox and the rest of the infectious diseases behaved in a similar way, and like measles, could only avoid extinction within relatively large human communities.

Just when such diseases first established themselves among human populations is impossible to say, but they could only flourish securely in civilized societies where numbers were relatively large and where at least a few persons (merchants, soldiers, vagabonds, pilgrims) moved incessantly across considerable distances. In the short term, the effect of each successful transfer of disease from animal herds was to increase the parasitic burden of civilized urban dwellers. In the long term, however, the effect was to confer upon disease-experienced city populations a powerful epidemiological weapon in their subsequent encounters with previously isolated, disease-inexperienced communities.

Before considering briefly this aspect of the disease experience of civilized peoples, however, it would be well to analyse more exactly the consequences of city life for human population movements in times past. If cities could be sustained only by in-migration, this required that rural dwellers somehow produce a surplus of children, as well as a surplus of food with which to satisfy urban requirements. Exact balance between supply and demand could never be sustained for very long. Population deficit (registered by resort to compulsory recruitment into urban and military occupations, e.g. slavery) was almost as troublesome in the historic record as population surplus (registered by peasant uprisings, starvation, and rural epidemics). Yet we can assert that civilizations were successful and enduring only when they enforced a moral code that encouraged fecundity and also restrained the ruthlessness of rent and tax collectors, so as to make life livable for the rural cultivators. Only then could conditions in the countryside sustain the regular current of migration to town which was essential if civilized social structures were to persist indefinitely.

A major difficulty was that contacts with city populations exposed villagers to risk of infections over and above those that could exist locally on a stable basis. Periodic outbreak of such viral diseases as measles and smallpox could be very costly to rural populations, for if the disease in question had not appeared in a village for, say, 30 years, then everyone under age 30 was susceptible. In such a circumstance, deaths among young adults and parents would be far more costly to the community than the deaths of an equal number of small children would be. Yet until communications achieved a suitable intensity, rural populations grouped into comparatively small villages remained liable to this kind of sporadic visitation by the diseases of civilization. As with the urban populations, the more prevalent a given infection became, the less costly to the society, even if an unchanging proportion of those infected died. If an infection became endemic, so that only infants were likely to fall ill and die, replacement became relatively easy. Demographic peaks and valleys, with all the strains upon subsistence such instability entailed, could even out or disappear completely.

Statistical information about disease and population is almost completely lacking for all but the most recent centuries. It is therefore impossible to say just how patterns of epidemic and endemic infection intersected with fluctuating birth and death rates through the centuries to promote regional differentiation of wealth and population density. Yet these parameters of human life obviously lay behind and affected greatly the tangled political and cultural record that is accessible.

Although precision and detail are unattainable, landmarks can be discerned amidst all the fog of uncertainty. One thing to look for is change in patterns of long-distance travel that might introduce unfamiliar diseases to new parts of the earth. Resulting epidemics are likely to attain such severity as to leave perceptible traces in the historical record, at least for historians who have a modicum of epidemiological awareness of how virgin populations react to exposure to new infections.

III. Migration Patterns and New Diseases

In modern times, innumerable examples illustrate the disastrous repercussions of new disease encounters for previously inexperienced populations. When the Spaniards invaded the Aztec and Inca empires in the sixteenth century, for example, Europeans and Africans brought a long array of lethal infections with them across the Atlantic. Consequently, American Indian (Amerindian) populations were exposed to a long series of devastating epidemics, against which they had no established resistances whatever. Heavy death toll resulted, intensified by social and psychological disorganization in the face of unparalleled disaster. Recent studies, though differing as to the absolute number of deaths, agree in recognizing the magnitude of the disaster. Populations shrank to perhaps as little as one-twentieth of the pre-Columbian totals within 130 years of Cortez' arrival in Mexico. Many small communities were completely wiped out.

This encounter was certainly not the first time that a disease-experienced population carried a devastating infection into a human community which had no prior experience of, or exposure to, the infection in question. On the contrary, this kind of encounter became possible from the time when the diseases distinctive of civilization first established themselves in densely populated cities and their hinterlands. In all probability, the disruptive effect upon the disease-inexperienced partner, so apparent in the New World, also occurred in the Old World. Such events, indeed, must have taken place over and over again along the expanding frontiers of each of the major civilizations of Eurasia. Indeed it seems no more than logical to suggest that epidemiologically emptied borderlands regularly facilitated the expansion of civilized people and social structures onto new ground. Such expansion was, assuredly, a persistent feature of times past. Each of the great civilizations of Eurasia, after all, took shape within a relatively small area, and expanded the territory under its sway by converting barbarians to civilized styles of life and/or by settling peasant emigrants on new land.

We may be sure that in all encounters between civilized and previously isolated populations one of the most inescapable demonstrations of civilized superiority was epidemiological. As we have just seen, diseased-experienced populations had adjusted their patterns of life to allow them to survive in the presence of infections that were widely lethal to peoples who lacked experience. We now believe that antibodies mattered more than prayer; but in times past, when lethal infection was ascribed to supernatural causes, prayer and other forms of customary prophylaxis were deemed important in averting death. Since disease-experienced civilized populations could survive better when epidemic struck, their inexperienced fellow sufferers—or those who survived—found it very hard to resist conversion to civilized patterns of belief and conduct. Differential distribution of antibodies in human bloodstreams therefore had the effect, in all probability, of sustaining the expansion of civilized ideas and practices among an ever-widening circle of other peoples who deliberately abandoned divergent cultural heritages in hope of warding off pestilential death.

Nevertheless civilized populations were not always safe from exposure to some new and lethal infection, since initial disease patterns were far from homogeneous. On at least three occasions in Old World history the inauguration of new patterns of travel exposed large and dense civilized populations to new infections for the first time. On these occasions, the afflicted human masses suffered the same sort of disadvantage that smaller communities regularly faced when first encountering disease-bearers. Hence heavy die-off and far-reaching cultural changes analogous to those accompanying the absorption of border isolates into the body politic of an expanding civilization can be seen—sporadically—among Eurasian civilized populations too.

The earliest of these major disease landmarks occurred in the first Christian centuries, when caravans and ships began to link China and India with the Mediterranean coastlines. In course of the second and third centuries A.D., new and lethal diseases arrived in both China and Europe along the new trade routes. Serious depopulation resulted. This was registered politically by the collapse of the Han and Roman empires. Far-reaching cultural changes ensued, e.g. the widespread conversion to Buddhism and Christianity that occurred in China and the Mediterranean lands. Nothing so drastic seems to have happened in India and the Middle East, perhaps because the populations of those regions had less that was new to encounter in the way of infectious diseases than was the case towards the fringes of the civilized world of that age.

The second major landmark in disease diffusion may be associated with the establishment of the Mongol Empire in the thirteenth century. After Genghis Khan and his heirs had united most of northern Eurasia into a single empire, military movements and slower caravans created a ramshackle network of a kind that had never been known before. A probable side effect was the transfer of *Yersinia pestis*, the bacillus of bubonic plague, from an earlier region of endemicity among burrowing rodents in the Burma–Yunnan borderlands to the burrowing rodents of the Eurasian steppe.

New exposures of human populations to the plague resulted, chief among them the dramatic outbreak of the Black Death in Europe and the Middle East that occurred after 1346. However severe the depopulation of Europe may have been—and estimates range between 25 and 33 per cent—the destruction of nomad populations of the steppe was presumably even greater, and so severe that they never really recovered.

Cultural reactions to the Black Death were not inconsiderable but the most remarkable—flagellation, pilgrimage, frenetic dancing and the like—were also suicidal and so did not endure. Medical rituals of quarantine and religious rituals of intercession did become enduring responses to the plague in the parts of Europe exposed to the infection. Really pervasive alterations of Europe's cultural outlook depended on many factors, among which the encounter with lethal infection on a new scale was only one. Nevertheless, the intensification of a secular outlook, associated with the Renaissance, and the contradictory assertion of a more immediate personal dependence on God, associated with Reformation and Counter-reformation, can both be viewed as modulated forms of the extreme and suicidal responses called forth at the time of the first onset of the Black Death.

The third unmistakable landmark in changing patterns of disease and migration was associated with the opening of the oceans to regular commerce through the discoveries of European mariners of the late fifteenth and early sixteenth centuries. The disaster this spelled for American populations has already been referred to. Similar disastrous die-offs occurred in other, less densely inhabited lands where civilized infections had previously been unknown: Australia, southern Africa, New Zealand and all the other islands of Oceania. Overland, too, hunters and gatherers of Siberia suffered the same fate as the Indians of the Canadian north when Europeans began to move among them in pursuit of furs.

The result, globally, was to open much new land to European settlement, increasing the proportion of people of European descent in the world very substantially at the expense of the diverse local inhabitants who had previously occupied the territories in question. Instead of expanding over contiguous land areas, as had happened earlier in civilized history, Europe's modern expansion leaped across ocean distances, relying, however, on the same sort of epidemiological advantage that had always assisted settlement and frontier expansion from the time when civilized forms of infection were first established.

Within the more disease-experienced regions of the globe, however, the intensified contacts sustained and provoked by European shipping meant that epidemics tended to yield to endemic patterns of infection for more and more diseases within wider and wider areas. The greater ease with which a population can survive losses from endemic infection has already been explained. Hence, as this change took place, civilized populations could increase their numbers wherever extra hands could produce extra food to feed the additional mouths. The result was a massive population growth that sustained European overseas expansion for some four centuries, and disease experience lay behind China's almost equally impressive expansion into landward borderlands all the way from Manchuria in the north to Yunnan–Burma and Indo-China in the south. As before, population fluctuations appear to have been most pronounced in China and Europe; the civilized populations of India and the Middle East grew less precipitously, perhaps because an increase in food supplies was less feasible in those lands than in China and Europe, where the establishment of new crops derived from the Americas (maize and potatoes, mainly) went hand in hand with the first phases of modern population explosion.

These three major landmarks of humanity's encounter with infections occurred before anyone had an accurate idea of how the most important infectious diseases were transmitted from host to host. Medical and folk practices often did affect the prevalence of a given disease, sometimes increasing exposure to it but more commonly reducing disastrous encounters. Such traditional adjustments to infectious disease attained new levels of efficiency when doctors began to decipher the ways in which particular infections passed from host to host, and figured out ways to intercept the path of infection or else render it less damaging by artificially provoking the formation of antibodies.

Effective public health measures have become known and generally available only in comparatively very recent times. The first human disease germ was identified under the microscope less than a century ago, in 1882, and efficacious delivery of preventive medicine to most of the world had to wait until after the Second World War. In this short time, nevertheless, long-standing patterns of infection and migration have been profoundly disrupted. New behaviour will, sooner or later, surely adapt to the difference in our ecological situation; but this will take time. In the meanwhile, humanity is confronted with an unparalleled population boom which puts an ever-increasing strain upon medical skills seeking to counterbalance the liability to pestilential infection created by the mere existence of a dense and contiguous population of a single species.

3

Modern Isolated Pre-agricultural Populations as a Source of Information on Prehistoric Epidemic Patterns

Francis L. Black

Department of Epidemiology and Public Health, Yale University School of Medicine, New Haven, Connecticut, USA

Did [pre-agricultural man] have a whole different set of infections which have since disappeared? . . . The prehistoric pre-agricultural world was subject to a . . . limited spectrum of infectious diseases.

In large measure modern advances can do no more than return us to the state of health that mankind enjoyed 10 000 years ago.

I. Introduction

In this chapter modern pre-agricultural populations which have remained isolated from surrounding societies are examined with the aim of reconstructing a picture of the disease problems which pertained universally during the millenia when all mankind subsisted in the pre-agricultural mode. This picture should then exhibit the conditions to which our evolutionary heritage is best fitted. Isolated pre-agricultural societies have persisted into the late nineteenth and twentieth centuries in the tropical forests of South America and South-East Asia, in the Kalahari Desert and in Australia, and in the North American Arctic. Various island populations might also be considered isolated, but, except for the Andaman Islands, their cultures were not pre-agricultural when they first became accessible to study. A number of studies have also been made on incidence of specific diseases in some of the most isolated tribes of tropical Africa, but none was really pre-agricultural and none sufficiently isolated to exclude frequent disease introductions. Isolation is important to the shape of this picture not only because a primitive society in contact with more developed groups will be distorted by exogenous ideas and artifacts, but also because the persistence of individual infectious diseases is dependent on the number of persons in contact with one another.

Those pre-agricultural populations which have survived into this century have done so only in some of the most inhospitable parts of the world and there they attain only very low population densities (Table I). These density estimates must be crude because the definition of territory occupied by primitive cultures can only be defined arbitrarily and estimates of prehistoric cultures are based on indirect evidence. Nevertheless, it is apparent that the population densities of persisting populations span the prehistoric estimate and that both differ from post-agricultural densities by more than two orders of magnitude. Contemporary pre-agricultural societies either live in family groups which may gather once a year into groups of no more than 1000 persons or, where defence against other humans is necessary, they may live in villages which rarely reach 1000 members before splitting. In the latter case, groups which split retain common cultural characteristics but often exhibit hostility toward one another as vigorous as that directed toward totally foreign groups. In either case, the circuit of one man's acquaintances rarely exceeds 1000 persons. There is no reason to think that prehistoric cultures differed in this regard: larger pre-agricultural settlement sites are unknown, and the capacity of even the most

TABLE I. *Population Densities*

Territory	Number of inhabitants per km^2	Reference
Undeveloped area of Amazon	0.02	Black *et al.*, 1978
Yanomama Territory	0.15	Neel and Weiss, 1975
Kalahari	0.09	Harpending, 1976
North Greenland (ice-free area)	0.02	Gilberg, 1948
Canadian Arctic	0.03	Stefansson, 1937
Australia	0.04	White, 1977
World Mesolithic	0.04	Deevey, 1960
India, China and Roman Empire	20.00	Llewellyn-Jones, 1975
World, present	30.00	

appropriate land would be hard pressed to sustain larger populations. A possible exception may have occurred in special locations where marine life brought quantities of food to one location.

II. Non-infectious Diseases

Data on non-infectious diseases in primitive society have been difficult to collect for several reasons. These diseases do not occur in distinct epidemics and often severity of the disease is more important than its simple presence. Non-infectious diseases are often highly age-dependent, but primitive societies do not record ages, and age estimates may entail considerable error when the people are exposed to extremes of weather outside our own range of familiarity. When one does get a set of age estimates one usually finds, in a primitive society, that relatively few people survive into the age group where non-infectious disease is most prevalent. Analyses of the causes of death (Neel and Weiss, 1975; Black *et al.*, 1978) indicate that epidemics of infectious disease imported in the early post-contact period are a major cause of this deficit but that accidents and warfare have also played major roles. In spite of these limitations on the data it is quite clear that the prevalence of several non-infectious diseases in these societies is different from what is encountered in the cosmopolitan world.

A. Cardiovascular Disease

Hypertensive heart disease is rare or absent in these populations (Schaefer, 1959; Truswell *et al.*, 1972; Oliver *et al.*, 1975; R. V. Lee, personal communication). Mean blood pressures are consistently low and do not increase with age (Fig. 1). Blood pressures are especially low in the two tropical rain-forest populations that have been tested. As well as the low averages, individuals with elevated blood pressure are rare. Whereas in a cosmopolitan population the 95th percentile for diastolic pressure is above 100 for both sexes at all ages over 40 years, Schaefer (1959) found only two Eskimo with diastolic pressures over 100 mmHg and both had renal disease; we found that none of 300 Brazilian Indians had pressures this high; Truswell found none of 150 !Kung had a diastolic pressure over 110 mmHg. Truswell *et al.* (1972) and Oliver *et al.* (1975) suggested that the low blood pressures are related to very low salt intake, but salt intake by the Eskimo seems to have been variable and other differences may also be important.

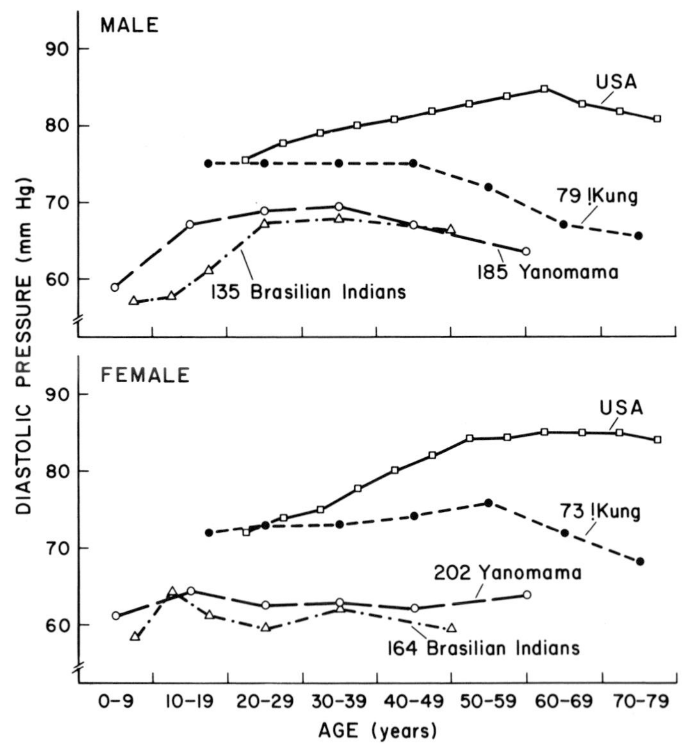

Fig. 1. Mean diastolic pressure by sex and age in a normal USA population as determined by Lasser and Master (1959) and in the !Kung of the Kalahari (Truswell and Hansen, 1976), the Yanomama of Venezuela (Oliver *et al.*, 1975), and in several tribes of Pará state, Brazil (Lee *et al.*, 1979, personal communication).

Other forms of heart disease are also rare. Using an electrocardiogram, Truswell and Hansen (1976) found no evidence of cardiac disease in 97 !Kung adults. Coronary heart disease might go unidentified if it caused rapid death, but sudden death from natural causes was not found except in the elderly in a survey of mortality in the Brazilian Indians (Black *et al.*, 1978). Valvular heart disease has been found in some populations: Truswell and Hansen (1976) found three cases in 152 !Kung examined in the 1960s and Schaefer (1959) noted two cases in 4000 Eskimo. In both studies this disease was thought to be the result of streptococcal infections which may have been an exclusively post-contact malady.

B. Cancer

Bellizzi (1962) reported no cancer in 1200 Brazilian Kayapo Indians whom he examined in 1958. In recent years, since transportation has become available from the area of the Kayapo to a central hospital, the recognized cancer rate has been about one per year for 10 000 Indians. In contrast, Schaefer *et al.* (1975) described 198 cancer cases coming into a similar medical service from the Eskimo of Canada's North West Territories between 1950 and 1974. Only 90 cases would have been expected in a population of the same age structure in the rest of Canada. There was a marked increase in incidence within the period of Schaefer's study, the rate going from 78 per 100 000 in the 1950s to 169 from 1969–72. This increased incidence was largely attributable to cancers of the lung and the cervix. Rates for cancer of the salivary glands and kidney were consistently high and nasopharyngeal cancers were frequent in one district. Schaefer's study was made at a time when Eskimo life had been extensively altered by contact with Caucasians. The lung cancer rate is readily explicable by the increase in smoking. Cervical and nasopharyngeal cancers are two of the forms of this disease most closely associated with virus infections, infections which may also have been recent introductions. The apparently conflicting data from the rain forest and the Arctic might be reconciled if cancer occurs in low incidence only until isolation is broken, but the difficulty in getting good age-specific data in the early post-contact period renders this hypothesis speculative.

C. Allergic Disease

Several authors have reported (*Lancet*, 1976) that asthma and other allergic diseases are relatively rare in little-developed rural communities. The same seems to hold for isolated primitive populations.

Schaefer (1959) saw no bronchial asthma in the Canadian Eskimo, nor have we found it in examining Brazilian Indians. Truswell and Hansen (1976) reported no asthma in the !Kung but did mention six cases of chronic bronchitis in persons over 60 years of age.

We have been able to confirm unusually low levels of hypersensitivity in the Brazilian Indian by experimental test. Persons in cosmopolitan society acquire a temporary local sensitivity to specific allergens when given serum from a sensitive individual intradermally. This is the Prausnitz–Kustner test. When we performed this test on thirty Brazilian Indians using sera from two ragweed-sensitive persons followed by an extract of ragweed pollen, we observed little or no reaction (Kantor *et al.*, 1979). The theory used to explain the test depends on participation of a third component, basophilic leucocytes, which are sensitized to the antigen by combination with a specific kind of antibody in the serum, IgE. The normal immune response to infection with intestinal worms involves the production of large quantities of IgE, and individuals with these parasites are likely to have so much IgE directed against the worms that the combining sites on their cells are fully occupied. These saturated cells are not free to react with the relatively small amounts of antibody produced against pollens. We were able to show that the Indians who failed to react to ragweed carry large amounts of IgE and that they react with a patch of red itchy skin when injected with an antigen prepared from the *Ascaris* worm. Thus they have competent cells and enough antibody to saturate them. This situation represents a particularly striking instance in which a genetic trait, which was beneficial in defending mankind against the parasites that attacked him in a more primitive mode of life, has become a serious source of disease in our modern environment.

III. Infectious Diseases

Infectious diseases are caused by living mutable agents and in considering ancient patterns we must be prepared to find that some diseases are new, that some have disappeared and that some are greatly changed. The life cycle of a micro-organism is so much shorter than that of a mammal that the micro-organism's opportunity for mutation is much greater. In the time taken for one human generation, a poliovirus can pass through as many generations as man has traversed since *Australopithecus* lived. When myxomatosis virus was introduced to Australia, the rabbits of that country were threatened with extinction and, if this had happened, the virus would also have died out (Fenner and Ratcliffe, 1965). Accommodation between virus and host was reached first by mutation of the virus to reduce virulence; only later did a more resistant strain of rabbits arise. In man, measles and smallpox seem to be relatively new diseases and McNeill (1976) has identified historical records which may represent the first epidemics of these diseases in China and the Mediterranean during the second and third centuries A.D. Cockburn (1963) has presented a forceful case for the thesis that the evolution of infectious diseases in man has been determined by social as well as genetic change. It will be my purpose to demonstrate that a most important social change has been the change from small self-contained pre-agricultural communities to our modern interdependent world society.

A. Effect of Population Size on Epidemic Pattern

1 Epidemic Disease

The length of time an infectious agent can survive in one host is limited to the time until the host is killed or to the time it takes the host to develop an effective immune reponse or, if no immunity appears, to the normal life span of the host. Before this time is up, if its strain is to survive, the virus, bacterium or other parasite must find a new susceptible host. Sooner or later, and in cohesive pre-agricultural villages usually soon, all individuals in the community will have become infected, and only new births will provide a continuing source of susceptible individuals. If there are no persistent infections, the disease will die out unless the number of births is enough to provide a continuous sequence of new cases.

Measles is an example. The measles virus can persist in one person for about two weeks, from the time of infection to appearance of neutralizing antibody. This virus must, therefore, move at least 26 times a year and can only survive in a population which produces that number of babies. Of course, the babies are not planned so that they become available at regular intervals. Also, the virus tends to spread more easily in winter and its profligacy, in consumption of susceptibles at that time, may cause difficulty in summer, when its transmission is less efficient. In an urban area where measles spreads quickly, as many as 40 000 births a year may be needed to sustain the virus (Bartlett, 1960). In rural areas where the virus spreads more slowly, a smaller number may suffice, but 10 000 births per year seems to be the lower limit (Black, 1966). This number of births requires a total population of between 200 000 and one million persons. Thus measles cannot persist in a single pre-agricultural community. It can sometimes spread from one community to another and thus extend its stay, but spread between modern pre-agricultural communities has never been adequate to sustain it. The 1951 epidemic in south-western Greenland affected nearly everyone in the Julianahab district but did not spread to neighbouring Frederikshab (Christensen *et al.*, 1953). The 1952 epidemic in the Canadian Arctic crossed Hudson Strait to Baffin Island but did not reach the other Arctic islands nor cross Hudson Bay to its western side (Peart and Nagler, 1954). The 1954 epidemic on the upper Xingu River of Brazil spread to several neighbouring tribes but never moved north to affect Suia or Txukarramae (Nutels, 1968).) Historically, when measles was first introduced to the most populous parts of the New World it caused far-ranging epidemics. However, all the outbreaks in Mexico and Peru in 1531–39, in Canada in 1635, in the Amazon area in 1745, and in Tierra del Fuego in 1884 appear to have been the first experience with the disease in each area, and every epidemic seems to have required a separate introduction from outside (Black *et al.*, 1971). Measles and any other disease with a similar epidemiological pattern could not continue very long in a pre-agricultural world; if these diseases ever appeared, they would soon have become extinct.

2 Endemic Disease

Some viruses and bacteria and a good many larger parasites are not eliminated from the body by the immune response but co-exist with their host, perhaps causing death some years later, perhaps not affecting the host's life expectancy. If the immune response, while failing to eliminate the agent, completely blocks the agent's ability to exit in infectious form, then the epidemiological effect is the same as if the agent were killed. However, if the agent is released, even occasionally, an entirely different picture results.

This is best exemplified by varicella virus. The disease which results from the initial infection with this virus, chickenpox, is terminated by the immune response within a few weeks, just as in measles. During the acute phase virus spreads from one person to another and, as in measles, sharp epidemics may result. Frequently, however, the immune system fails to eliminate all the virus at the end of the acute phase, and live viral genome persists in certain nerve cells particularly in the dorsal root ganglia (Bastian *et al.*, 1974). Many years later, when antibody titres have waned, this latent virus may reactivate and, travelling along the nerve where it is protected from the remaining immunity, it may reach the skin to produce new lesions in the form of shingles and to again release infectious virus. Thus the full cycle of varicella virus in one person may be much more than the usual three or four weeks and close to a full human life span. Instead of having to find a new host every two weeks, this virus needs a new one as seldom as once every 50 years. From this ratio one might estimate that where measles persistence requires a population of 500 000, varicella might persist in a population of only 400, and that is at least approximately true. Hope-Simpson (1954) was the first to study this phenomenon. He was able to show that on the Island of Yell in the Shetlands, where the human population was only 2000, varicella virus was able to persist without fade-outs and reintroduction. Gilberg (1948) noted a chickenpox outbreak in a population of 300 in northern Greenland during the winter when there was no change of introduction from outside. Only children were infected, an indication that there had been a preceding outbreak about a decade earlier. I have seen a similar outbreak in an isolated Amazon tribe affecting youths to about 25 years of age. Although the population was only 80 persons, the varicella virus must have persisted these 25 years. This pattern shows a more effective symbiotic relationship between virus and man than that exhibited by measles. The wide distribution of varicella virus in modern primitive societies suggests that it has had considerable time to spread; there is nothing to suggest that it was not carried to the Americas by the original settlers.

Some disease agents of this class, such as hepatitis and Epstein-Barr (EB) virus, are more likely to cause significant disease when they infect older persons than when they infect young children. A highly endemic situation may therefore cause less morbidity than a situation in which a susceptible individual escapes infection for several years. Infectious mononucleosis, for instance, is unknown in the Brazilian tribes although the causative agent, EB virus, is very prelavent.

3 Zoonoses

A third epidemiological pattern exists which may not only be compatible with, but may sometimes be better adapted to, primitive than modern human society. In this the infective agent has avoided the specialization which would limit it to a single host. It may infect man, but it is not dependent exclusively on man for its persistence and it can find hosts among other species with higher reproductive rates. Staying with the viral examples, one might cite the disease haemorrhagic fever with renal syndrome also known as Korean haemorrhagic fever. Lee *et al.* (1978a) have shown that this disease has a cycle in a wild mouse, *Apodemus*. While the virus may be transmitted from man to man it is not dependent on the human cycle. Outbreaks are most likely to occur when the mouse populations become high and where man comes into close contact with the rodent. Many other infectious agents utilize an arthropod as an intermediate host facilitating transfer from one mammal to another, and arthropods themselves may occasionally act as the reservoir if the agent is transmitted transovarially from one arthropod generation to another (Thompson and Beaty, 1977). Insofar as primitive societies lived in closer contact with wild animal species than more evolved cultures, these diseases may have been more prevalent in the distant past.

B. Reconstruction of Epidemiologic Experience of Isolated Communities

Declining infectious disease mortality rates in much of the world over the last century led to an overgeneralized assumption that advancing civilization was accompanied by diminished disease prevalence. While it had long been recognized that isolated Arctic communities were free of many diseases (Paul and Freeze, 1933), it was Polunin (1953) who showed that this was also true of isolated communities even when they had a simple culture and lived in a tropical environment. He pointed out that "diseases which conferred lasting immunity" did not persist in aboriginal Malayan villages, and he related this to community size (Polunin, 1967).

It is difficult, however, to obtain direct data on disease incidence in isolated communities, because continued surveillance destroys their isolation. J. R. Paul and his colleagues (1951) demonstrated the value of serological techniques in providing information on disease epidemics which had occurred many years earlier when isolation was relatively intact. They studied sera collected in 1949 from north Alaskan Eskimo and found type 2 poliovirus neutralizing antibody in 90% of persons over 19 years of age but in few who were younger, type 1 antibody in 50% of persons over 30 years of age but in few who were younger, and type 3 antibody only in persons over 40 years of age. By inquiry and old records, they were able to identify epidemics of paralytic disease in 1930 and about 1915. They suggested that the 1930 epidemic was caused by type 2 virus and the earlier one by type 1. They were not able to relate the type 3 antibodies to an epidemic, but this must have been still earlier and because type 3 virus generally causes the least morbidity the epidemic may have been mild. An important aspect of this study is the finding that persons born after the epidemic were not infected, as shown by their lack of antibody. Clearly the viruses did not remain active in the community once they had infected most of the population living at the time.

A virus which cannot persist in small communities may or may not have been introduced to a particular community prior to the time the community is studied. If the virus has not been present within one life span, no one in the community will have antibody and in this case one cannot say that the virus could not have persisted. However, very often when a virus is absent from one community, a sharp age-specific cut-off of antibody prevalence is found in other isolated communities and this is clear evidence of failure to persist, unless the critical age coincides with some regular life event.

Alternatively, if there is evidence of infection in a high proportion of all age groups, one knows that the agent has been in the community recently. If this pattern is found regularly in several communities, one can presume that the agent is widely distributed and, unless recent events have been unusual in all the communities, the agent must have been widely distributed in time as well as space. In other words, this agent is endemic.

Again, if the prevalence of specific antibodies is proportional to age, but low in younger age groups, the causative agent must have been present recently and must have affected only a small part of the population. Increasing prevalence with age suggests the cumulative effect of many low intensity epidemics. This pattern occurs with an agent which does not spread readily among humans but which is introduced frequently to the human community from some persistent source. These agents which have a cycle in a non-human reservoir and only occasionally infect man are zoonotic or saprophytic.

C. Data on Individual Infectious Diseases

Using the methods described above, my colleagues and I have collected data from Brazilian Indian tribes which indicate that most of the diseases we have investigated can be grouped into three categories, as in Table II (Black *et al.*, 1970, 1974; Black, 1975). Similar data from Australasian and Oceanic populations from the work of Adels and Gajdusek (1963), Brown and Gajdusek (1971), Brown *et al.* (1975, 1976) and Lang *et al.* (1977) are amenable to this classification. The hepatitis A entry is based on the study of Skinhøf *et al.* (1977) which showed that this virus swept Greenland in 1947–48 and then died out. To these serological data we have added information garnered from studying other persistent manifestations of past infections. Dick and Shick skin tests done by Heinbecker and Irvine-Jones (1928) on Baffin Island Eskimos in 1927 provided evidence that *Corynebacterium diphtheriae* and *Streptococcus pyogenes* fall into the first epidemiological group. No one tested in that community showed evidence of infection with *C. diphtheriae* and there was a sharp cut-off in sensitivity to *S. pyogenes* (Dick

TABLE II. *Epidemiological Classification of Infectious Agents*

	Group I: Epidemic	Group II: Endemic	Group III: Zoonosis
	Absent or occurring in sharp temporally limited outbreaks	Most persons in small communities infected at early age	Infection dependent on contact with extra-human reservoir
Viruses	Measles Mumps Respiratory syncytial Parainfluenzae 1, 2 and 3 Influenza A and B Poliomyelitis 1, 2 and 3 Smallpox Dengue Hepatitis A	Herpes simplex type 1 Epstein-Barr virus (infectious mononucleosis) Cytomegalovirus Varicella-zoster Hepatitis B	Yellow Fever Mayaro
Bacteria	*Streptococcus pneumoniae* 1, 2, 3, 6, 12, 14, 19 and 23 *Corynebacterium diphtheriae* *S. pyogenes* A	*Escherichia coli* (toxigenic)	*Clostridium tetani*
Parasites		*Ascaris lumbricoides* Hookworm Whipworm	*Toxoplasma gondii* *Trichenella spiralia* Tapeworm

test) in persons under 12 years of age. The absence of any smallpox scars on the Indians we have studied indicates that variola virus has been excluded from their areas. The epidemiological classification in Table II of enteric parasites is based on presence of parasitic forms in stools studied in Malaya by Polunin (1953) and in Brazil in 1979 by R. B. Whitaker and C. L. Patton (personal communication).

There are some agents which do not give consistent patterns in all areas studied. The BK virus, a human agent related to certain animal tumour viruses, was found in all the Australasian populations studied by Brown *et al*. (1975) but not in South American Indian populations (see also Candeias *et al*., 1977). Here the geographic differentiation is consistent enough for it to appear that the agent was not endemic in any isolated American population. The virus may either have evolved after the original migrants to the New World had left the Old World population centres, or it may have been lost by the migrants at some point where their numbers were small. The work of Polunin (1953) also indicated that tinea, ringworm, was endemic in Malay tribes, but we have not seen it in South American tribes and we are not sure whether it belongs in group II or III. Again, the pattern of antibodies against *Entamoeba histolytica* in the South American tribes is variable and amoebic dysentery seems to be endemic in some tribes but excluded from others. This may depend on historic accident or reflect the distribution of extra human reservoirs.

Thus the position of a few agents varies with local circumstance or history. This may blur our view of the line between groups II and III, but, in general, we can be quite sure that the agents in group I do not have, in their present form, the characteristics which would permit them to exist in primitive societies. These agents and their diseases must have been excluded from the pre-agricultural world. This group includes most of the virus diseases and some of the bacterial infections most prominent in cosmopolitan communities. Agents in group II are well adapted to persist in small population groups but they are responsible for relatively little serious disease. Their ability to coexist at this high level of symbiotic adaptation suggests a long period of coexistence with man. Agents in group III are largely dependent on non-human hosts and their presence in prehistoric human communities probably depended on local faunal characteristics.

D. Chronic Infections With High Mortality

Although the above techniques have proven versatile, they do not provide information on three important microorganisms which cause chronic, seriously debilitating diseases. These diseases, tuberculosis, malaria and syphilis, are the subjects of other chapters of this book, but some mention of them in the context of the pre-agricultural societies seems necessary. The causal agents exhibit long periods of infectiousness but, unlike group II agents, they are very damaging to the human host and may create an unstable situation threatening the continuance of the human population. Perhaps the most important disease is tuberculosis. A history of this infection in living people can be accurately determined by tuberculin testing. Evidence of tuberculosis has been found in most primitive communities at the time when they first become available for study. Nutels (1968) found positive reactors in several Xingu tribes at the time when they had had very little contact with outsiders, but he also found some tribes that appeared to be free of the disease. He, clearly, believed that where he found tuberculosis, it had been introduced. A major reason for believing this was evidence from serial surveys of the rapid pace at which the disease could spread within a tribe. The Txukahamae showed 5% positive in 1962, 12% in 1966 and 32% in 1967 (Nutels *et al.*, 1967). Arctic studies (Hall, 1865; Heinbecker and Irvine-Jones, 1928; Gilberg, 1948) also indicated that tuberculosis was an exogenous infection and very high mortality rates were reported. Hall stated that "consumption" caused more deaths than all other diseases together in southern Baffin Island, and Gilberg reported that 35% of all deaths in northern Greenland were due to tuberculosis. If the disease was originally endemic in pre-agricultural societies it seems not to have been nearly as widespread as it is now. Tuberculosis is one of the few diseases for which there is good evidence, from studies of twins, that genetically determined differences influence susceptibility (Comstock, 1978). It seems probable that these differences, if differentially expressed in various populations, would affect selective pressures.

The second important disease for which our techniques are inappropriate is malaria. Here there is more specific evidence of genetic differences affecting susceptibility in man. Distribution patterns of these genetic traits have been useful indicators of past patterns of malaria distribution. None of the resistance traits have been found in an appreciable proportion of any American Indian group. This, coupled with historic evidence, provides convincing reason to believe that malaria did not occur in the Western Hemisphere prior to 1492 (Dunn, 1965). The two most important resistance traits, Duffy negative, which confers resistance to *Plasmodium vivax* malaria, and haemoglobin S, which reduces the impact of *P. falciparum*, both seem to have originated in Africa. The Duffy negative trait is widely dispersed in Africa, suggesting a long history of *P. vivax*, but haemoglobin S is unevenly distributed, and Livingstone (1958) has suggested that *P. falciparum* only became a serious problem with the introduction of more intensive agriculture. Wiesenfeld (1967) has calculated on the basis of prevalence of the S gene that this occurred in Africa about 2000 years ago. Again, while we cannot presume that malaria in man is an altogether new disease, it is clear that it was much less prevalent in prehistoric times than in recent centuries.

Much has been said about the origin of syphilis and the theory that it was endogenous only to the Western Hemisphere before 1490 (Crosby, 1972). We found evidence of highly endemic, but apparently innocuous, treponemal infection in the Kayapa Indians (Lee *et al.*, 1978b). This is essentially the kind of stable relationship which one would expect to find where there is long-term endemicity. If, however, one tries to fit this finding to the theory of transport to the Eastern Hemisphere by Columbus' men, one must presume either that Caucasians were much more susceptible than the Indians to the effect of infection, or that the organism mutated rapidly to much greater pathogenicity. Then, in the next 150 years, the *Treponema* must either have effected a selection of its new host population for greater resistance or the organism must have spontaneously reversed its evolution, regressing to reduced virulence. Neither of these latter hypotheses is very attractive.

E. Extrapolations

If the generalizations which the data suggest were always valid, that is, if acute infections of limited duration were excluded from primitive society unless they had a non-human reservoir, and if persistent infections were always well-adapted to these cultures, then we could predict which infections would be found in these societies without making a survey for each. On this basis the common cold viruses would be excluded but the adenoviruses would be widely distributed, and the agent of whooping cough, *Bordetella pertussis*, would not be found, but *Staphylococcus aureus* would. While the work has been in progress we have inevitably tended to anticipate, in this way, what to expect. Quite often these preconceptions proved to be wrong when we expected endemicity: poliomyelitis cases may excrete virus for six months and the resultant immunity does not prevent reinfection, yet in a variety of situations the virus has failed to persist; herpes simplex type 2, the genital form, can be as persistent as type 1, yet we have failed to find evidence of it in the South American tribes; *Corynebacterium diphtheriae* may find chronic carriers, but the Arctic data indicates its exclusion. On the other hand, we have found no instance of an agent which does not enter some long-term relationship with man persisting in the tribes we have studied.

If we postulate that the diseases in group I are new to mankind since the development of agriculture, we must consider the sources from which they have arisen. They may have come from older human diseases since displaced, as old strains of influenza are periodically displaced by new strains; but influenza is a special case because, with its segmented genome, it can generate new genetic combinations with unusual rapidity. It seems too, that the old influenza genomes do not really become extinct but persist in other animals (Webster and Laver, 1972). More likely, the new diseases have arisen by adaptation to man of pathogens from other species. Each of the agents in this group has taxonomic relatives infecting other species: canine distemper for measles, the group A arboviruses for rubella, and Newcastle disease of chickens for mumps, etc. Adaptation of viruses and other parasites to new hosts is achieved frequently in the laboratory. There is no reason why it would not occur in nature.

If pre-agricultural man was spared so many of our afflictions, did he have a whole different set of infections which have since disappeared?

We have seen the disappearance of diseases in modern times either after a deliberate campaign, as with smallpox, or for undetermined reasons, as with the more severe form of scarlet fever. We have not, however, found any disease in the South American tribes that was not already known in the larger community; nor do I know of any infectious disease confined to primitive populations of other parts of the world. A few diseases in group II or III may attain unusual prevalence rates, as Kuru among the New Guinea Fore (Gajdusek, 1977) or Jorge Lobo's blastomycosis among the Kaiabi Indians (Lacaz *et al.*, 1972), but these diseases were known elsewhere, albeit by another name. The diseases in group II may attain high prevalence rates in primitive populations, but morbidity, if different, is unusually low. Presumably there existed in the past disease agents which we do not know now how to test for, but if so, they do not seem to cause problems in modern isolated populations. The pre-agricultural societies, until their isolation is broken, have fewer infectious diseases to contend with than more civilized people around them. Very probably the prehistoric pre-agricultural world was subject to a similarly limited spectrum of infectious diseases.

IV. Conclusion

Other chapters in this book emphasize the great reduction in infectious disease that has followed modern medical developments and still others discuss the reduction in non-infectious diseases that may be achieved by environmental control. In large measure, however, it seems that these modern advances can do no more than return us to the state of health that mankind enjoyed 10 000 years ago. Our chief modern killers, cancer and cardiovascular disease, seem to have been relatively rare at that time. Smallpox, which we have now eliminated with such effort, and many other infectious diseases were probably non-existent. Allergic diseases seem to have been a lesser problem. Set against this, a number of parasitic diseases were more prevalent than in advanced societies but possibly no more so than in modern underdeveloped societies. Other infections like those of the Herpesvirus group may have been more prevalent but have actually caused less morbidity. We have brought this increase in disease upon ourselves by changes in our life style: by eating more salt, by inhaling more tobacco smoke, by ridding our guts of worms and by associating together in large communities. Of course, early peoples died too: the great counterbalancing force seems to have been violent death: by abortion, infanticide, accident and war.

References

Adels, B. R. and Gajdusek, D. C. (1963). *Am. J. Hyg.* **77**, 317–343.
Bartlett, M. S. (1960). *Jl R. Statist Soc. A* **123**, 27–44.
Bastian, F. O., Rabson, A. S., Yee, C. L. and Trolka, T. S. (1974). *Archs Path.* **97**, 331–333.
Bellizzi, A. M. (1962). *Rev. Brasil Ciurgia* **44**, 170–178.
Black, F. L. (1966). *J. theor. Biol.* **11**, 207–211.
Black, F. L. (1975). *Science, N.Y.* **187**, 515–518.
Black, F. L., Woodall, J. P., Evans, A. S., Liebhaber, H. and Henle, G. (1970). *Am. J. Epidem.* **91**, 430–438.
Black, F. L., Hierholzer, W. J., Woodall, J. P. and Pinheiro, F. de P. (1971). *J. infect. Dis.* **124**, 306–317.
Black, F. L., Hierholzer, W. J., Pinheiro, F. de P., Evans, A. S., Woodall, J. P., Opton, E. M., Emmons, J. E. and West, B. S. (1974). *Am. J. Epid.* **100**, 230–250.
Black, F. L., Pinheiro, F. de P., Oliva, O., Hierholzer, W. J., Lee, R. V., Briller, J. E. and Richards, V. A. (1978). *Med. Anthrop.* **2**, 95–127.
Brown, P. and Gajdusek, D. C. (1971). *Am. J. trop. Med. Hyg.* **19**, 170–175.
Brown, P., Tsai, T. and Gajdusek, D. C. (1975). *Am. J. Epidem.* **102**, 331–340.
Brown, P., Collins, W. E., Gajdusek, D. C. and Miller, L. H. (1976). *Am. J. trop. Med. Hyg.* **25**, 775–776.
Candeias, J. A. N., Baruzzi, R. G., Pripas, S. and Iunes, M. (1977). *Rev. Saude Publ. São Paulo* **11**, 510–514.
Christensen, P. V., Schmidt, H., Bang, H. O., Andersen, V., Jordal, B. and Jensen, O. (1953). *Acta med. scand.* **144**, 430–449.
Cockburn, T. A. (1963). "The Evolution and Eradication of Infectious Diseases". Johns Hopkins Press, Baltimore.
Comstock, G. W. (1978) *Am. Rev. resp. Dis.* **117**, 621–622.
Crosby, A. W. (1972) "The Columbian Exchange". Greenwood, Westport, Conn.
Deevey, E. S. Jr (1960). *Scient. Am.* **203**, 194–204.
Dunn, F. L. (1965). *Hum. Biol.* **37**, 385–393.
Fenner, F. J. and Ratcliffe, F. N. (1965). "Myxomatosis". Cambridge Univ. Press, Cambridge, England.
Gajdusek, D. C. (1977). *Science, N.Y.* **197**, 943–960.
Gilberg, A. (1948). "Eskimo Doctor". Norton, New York.
Hall, C. F. (1865). "Life among the Esquimaux". Low Son and Marston, London.
Harpending, H. (1976). *In* "Kalahari Hunter-Gatherers" (R. B. Lee and I. deVore, Eds). Harvard Univ. Press, Cambridge, Mass.
Heinbecker, P. and Irvine-Jones, E. (1928). *J. Immun.* **15**, 395–406.
Hope-Simpson, R. E. (1954). *Lancet* ii, 1299–1302.
Kantor, F. S., Black, F. L., Lee, R. V. and Pinheiro, F. P. (1979). *Fedn Proc. Fedn Am. Socs exp. Biol.* **38**, 931.

Lacaz, C. S., Baruzzi, R. G. and Siqueira, W. Jr (1972). Introducão a georgrafia Medica do Brasil". Edgard Blucher, São Paulo.
Lancet (1976). Editorial i, 894.
Lang, D. J., Garruto, R. M. and Gajdusek, D. C. (1977). *Am. J. Epidem.* **106**, 480–487.
Lasser, R. P. and Master, A. M. (1959). *Geriatrics* **14**, 345–360.
Lee, H. W., Lee P. W. and Johnson, K. M. (1978a). *J. infect. Dis.* **137**, 298–308.
Lee, R. V., Black, F. L., Hierholzer, W. J. and West, B. L. (1978b). *Am. J. Epidem.* **107**, 46–53.
Livingstone, F. B. (1958). *Am. Anthrop.* **60**, 533–588.
Llewellyn-Jones, D. (1975). "People Populating", 24. Faber, London.
McNeill, W. H. (1976). "Plagues and Peoples". Doubleday, London.
Neel, J. V. and Weiss, K. M. (1975). *Am. J. phys. Anthrop.* **42**, 25–51.
Nutels, N. (1968). *PAHO Sci. Pub.* 165.
Nutels, N., Ayres, M. and Salzano, F. M. (1967). *Tubercle* **48**, 195–200.
Oliver, W. J., Cohen, E. L. and Neel, J. V. (1975). *Circulation* **52**, 146–151.
Paul, J. H. and Freeze, H. L. (1933). *Am. J. Hyg.* **17**, 517–535.
Paul, J. R., Riordon, J. T. and Melnick, J. L. (1951). *Am. J. Hyg.* **54**, 275–285.
Peart, A. F. W. and Nagler, F. P. (1954). *Can. J. publ. Hlth* **45**, 146–157.
Polunin, I. V. (1953). *Med. J. Malaya* **8**, 55–114.
Polunin, I. V. (1967). *In* "Diseases of Antiquity" (D. Brothwell and A. T. Sandison, Eds), 69–97. Thomas, Springfield, Ill.
Schaefer, O. (1959). *Can. med. Ass. J.* **81**, 386–393.
Schaefer, O., Hildes, J. A., Medd, L. M. and Cameron, D. C. (1975). *Can. med. Ass. J.* **112**, 1399–1404.
Skinhølf, P., Mikkelsen, F. and Hollinger, F. B. (1977). Am. J. Epidem. **105**, 140–147.
Stefansson, V. (1937). "Encyclopedia Britannica", Vol. 8, 708–710.
Thompson, W. H. and Beaty, B. J. (1977). *Science, N.Y.* **196**, 530–531.
Truswell, A. S. and Hansen, J. D. L. (1976). *In* "Kalahari Hunter-Gatherers" (R. B. Lee and I. deVore, Eds). Harvard Univ. Press, Cambridge, Mass.
Truswell, A. S., Kennelly, B. M., Hansen, J. D. L. and Lee, R. B. (1972). *Am. Heart J.* **84**, 5–12.
Webster, R. G. and Laver, W. G. (1972). *Virology* **48**, 433–444.
White, I. M. (1977). *In* "Health and Disease in Tribal Societies". Ciba Symposium 49. Elsevier, Amsterdam.
Wiesenfeld, S. L. (1967). *Science, N.Y.* **157**, 1134–1140.

4

The Evolution and Mutual Adaptation of Insects, Microorganisms and Man

James R. Busvine*
Maidenhead, England

In the course of evolution a remarkable series of adaptations occurred, involving the alternation of parasitism between a large animal (or plant) and a small creature such as an arthropod (commonly an insect). This arrangement was found to be beneficial to organisms originally parasitic on the smaller host, as well as those on the larger ones. . . .

Only a relatively few exceptional [insects] are serious pests . . . a few thousand species of insects have become adapted to feeding on vertebrate blood.

---

* Emeritus Professor of Entomology, London School of Hygiene and Tropical Medicine.

I. Insect Pests and Disease Vectors

When insects are very troublesome, it is difficult to realize that only a relatively few exceptional forms are serious pests. Chapman (1973) gives a figure of 4500, which is about 0.6% of known species. Most of them damage plants or plant products, as shown by the fact that agriculture claims about 97% of insecticidal usage (Hamon, 1976). Among pests of public health importance, the most serious are the bloodsucking forms, which include important disease vectors.

The mouthparts of primitive insects were adapted for chewing and biting their food, so that substantial modifications were necessary to enable them to pierce tissues and suck blood. These changes evolved several times, in various groups, and in different ways. Probably the earliest adaptation was by the bugs, or Hemiptera, which very early specialized in sucking the sap of plants. They have become a large and successful group, which includes many plant pests. A small proportion turned their attention to attacking other insects and sucking their juices; and from these a few adapted to attacking vertebrates, and some of them will feed on human blood.

The ectoparasitic lice and fleas probably developed from scavenging forms, feeding on debris in burrows and nests, then on skin products among fur and feathers, and finally on blood. Somewhat more puzzling is the widespread habit of bloodsucking in the order Diptera, which includes mosquitoes, biting midges, sandflies and blackflies. In these groups, the males feed only on nectar; but the females, needing protein for egg production, take blood meals. It is not easy to guess how this came about.

The more advanced families of Diptera nearly all lick up liquid food, having lost the piercing stylets used by the more primitive types for bloodsucking. In some of them, however, the habit redeveloped in a different way, as follows. Many flies and blowflies associate with large mammals, such as cattle, and drink up their sweat, lachrymal fluid and the blood from small scratches. A few of these insects have developed rasps on their tongue-like mouthparts, to abrade scabs; and thence, the change to a spine-tipped spike was the next step. This is the mechanism used by both sexes of tsetse flies, stable flies and some others.

In these various ways, a few thousand species of insects have become adapted to feeding on vertebrate blood, mainly of warm-blooded mammals and birds. These emerged about 150 million years ago, but relatively late in the evolution of insects, which probably extend back 300 million years (see Fig. 1). Most of the blood sucking forms are fairly

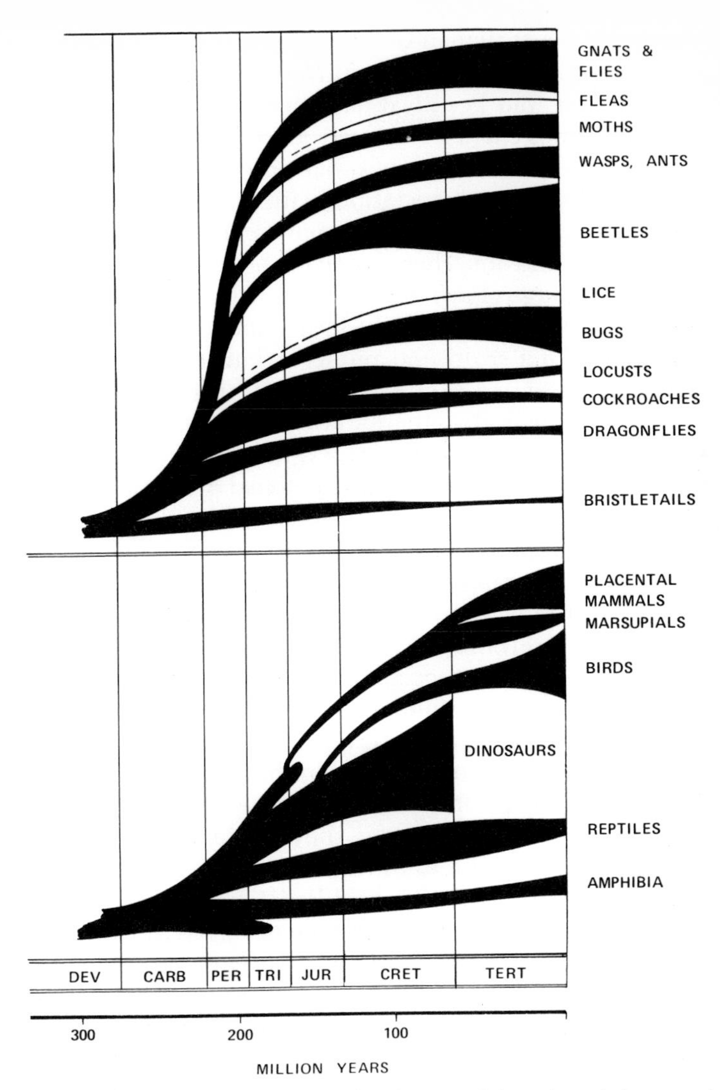

Fig. 1. Simplified evolutionary trees of the insects (above) and the vertebrates (below). Key to geological eras: Dev, Devonian; Carb, Carboniferous; Per, Permian; Tri, Triassic; Jur, Jurassic; Cret, Cretaceous; Tert, Tertiary.

catholic in taste, but some have become adapted to one or a few closely related host species. Man appeared on the scene so late that he has attracted the undivided attention of only a very few parasitic insects; in short, three kinds of lice, which infest his head, his underclothes or his pubic hair. Sucking lice tend to be more closely associated with a particular host species than most other blood feeders. While some of the latter have probably been accidental transfers from animals sharing a shelter or dwelling, our lice must have been inherited from subhuman stock, because the genera concerned are restricted to primates and widely separated from the lice of other animals (Ferris, 1951). Their further development in association with man has interesting and important practical aspects. First, since speciation is now thought to require spatial separation, there is the problem of the evolution on the same host, of closely related species adapted to different parts of the body. Presumably when our ancestors lost most of their hair except for the widely separated scalp and pubic region, the sites of infestation were sufficiently isolated to prevent the interbreeding which inhibits speciation. It happens that the hairs of the head differ considerably from those of the pubic region, which are thicker and more widely spaced. Hence, the two forms of lice developed quite different morphology and habits, the claws of the pubic louse being adapted to the coarse widely separated pubic hairs and the insect itself settling to a sedentary life, which keeps it confined largely to that region.

The exact status of the other two forms of lice has caused controversy. They are certainly closely related in the genus *Pediculus*, and their separation must have occurred in relatively recent times, when adoption of clothing by early man offered a new environmental niche for the body louse. Isolation is not very complete; but recent evidence involving people with double infestations has shown that opportunities for interbreeding do not blur the distinct identity of the two forms (Busvine, 1978). For this reason, they could be regarded as good species. A possible solution to the separation question has been proposed for a similar problem with bird lice. Clay (1957) suggested that specialization to a particular body region occurred in widely separated groups of the hosts, which subsequently became united and infested with two distinct species of parasite. A tentative hypothesis to account for the human case might be as follows. *Homo sapiens*, with rather sparse body hair, probably originated in a warm or tropical environment. As a result of competition (? with other hominoids) he ventured into colder regions and began to use skins and other clothing. Eventually, his body hair almost vanished and his lice retreated to the scalp in one region and to the clothing in another. Subsequently, mixing of the two groups of men allowed infestation with two species of lice.

So much for the theoretical aspect. Of practical importance is the fact that, though biologically closely related, head lice and body lice present two very different public health problems. Body lice are only prevalent among people who do not change their underwear at all regularly, and are consequently being eliminated from all but unhygienic communities. Head lice, however, are not necessarily killed by the mildly warm water used to wash hair, and they persist in most civilized countries. Crab lice are widely prevalent in a small proportion of most populations.

It has been shown that head lice, as well as body lice, can transmit relapsing fever in the laboratory; and both, as well as crab lice, could act as vectors of typhus (evidence summarized by Weyer, 1978). But body lice are by far the most important in actual epidemics. Therefore these diseases, though once prevalent in Europe, are now restricted to areas of widespread lousiness in Central Africa and parts of South America. After the First World War some 30 million cases occurred in Eastern Europe, with about 10% deaths (Zinsser, 1935); now the global total is about 15 000 cases annually, with a few hundred deaths (WHO, 1974).

Since these lice are restricted to man, they can only transmit human diseases. Other bloodsucking insects, more catholic in taste, may bring infections from reservoirs of pathogens in wild or domestic animals; alternatively, they too can transmit a strictly human disease, such as malaria. In either case, their willingness to bite man is critical; some will do so very reluctantly, others eagerly and those are the dangerous vectors. The factors responsible for choice of host are complex and not fully understood. Some are quite simple components, such as the warmth, humidity and carbon dioxide emitted by all warm-blooded animals. More specific factors are the body odour, size, shape and colour of the host. These are the criteria used by insects which feed in open country; i.e. many culicine mosquitoes, blackflies, tsetse flies and horseflies.

Apart from the characteristics of the host, however, the actual environment of the encounter may be important. Human dwellings, for example, are attractive to many insects with a predilection for caves and shelters. It is very likely that the common bedbug began its association with man during a cave-living period in human pre-history, since all of its relatives in the highly specialized bedbug family feed on cave-haunting creatures—either bats, or swallows and swifts. Unlike the lice, which have been with us since primordial times, the bedbug only became cosmopolitan during the historical era. The first record of this pest in England was in the sixteenth century (Mouffet, 1634). The other bloodsucking group of bugs, the South and Central American Triatominae, or conenose bugs, are less specialized and degenerate. Primarily adapted to living in the nests and lairs of birds and beasts, some species find ill-constructed rural hovels a convenient alternative.

Fleas constitute a small peculiar group of insects, of uncertain origin, possibly an offshoot from primitive Diptera. Even within the order, there are phylogenetic puzzles due to convergent evolution; that is, modifications to suit a similar habitat, rather than inherited from a common ancestor (Traub, 1971). The larvae are non-parasitic and live on debris in the nest or lair of the adult's host. For this reason, fleas do not parasitize nomadic animals, like ungulates or wandering monkeys (Hopkins, 1957). The so-called human flea, *Pulex irritans*, can infest a considerable number of wild and domestic animals. Farmers will confirm the liability of pigs to be heavily infested. Perhaps this is how the association with man began; as Holland (1969) has pointed out, the primitive human dwelling is not unlike a pigsty and man and pig share several other parasites. The most dangerous disease-transmitting species of mosquitoes are also those which associate with human dwellings. Thus of nearly 500 species of *Anopheles*, only a score or so are important malaria vectors, because of their willingness to bite man, usually indoors. The more numerous culicine species (perhaps 1500) include many tiresome biting pests which attack us in open country. However, two of the most dangerous disease vectors linger near dwellings: *Aedes aegypti*, vector of both urban yellow fever and dengue, and *Culex fatigans*, which transmits filariasis. Sometimes, too, human activities provide convenient breeding sites for particular mosquitoes. Species which naturally tend to breed in polluted water adapt easily to drains and cesspits (for example, *C. fatigans*). Other forms, which prefer small rock pools, find convenient sites in water-filled tins, gutters and miscellaneous debris around dwellings, as does *A. aegypti*.

Apart from bloodsucking insects, there are others which have become pests because human habitations and their contents supply their natural needs. Food stores, of course, are ideal for species of beetles and moths which breed in seeds and dry vegetable matter. Their depredations are serious; but, because of the sedentary habit of the food-destroying grubs, they present no danger to health. The more mobile houseflies and cockroaches, however, may be involved in disease transmission (Roth and Willis, 1957). Not only do they visit and soil human foodstuffs, but they are prone to visit drains and privies in search of water and (in the case of flies) breeding sites; from these, they can import disease germs. This method of pathogens passing to new hosts, however, is not very reliable and generally no more than an alternative to other means of transmission. The involvement of bloodsucking arthropods produced a more efficient system, and it may be of interest to speculate on how this came about.

II. Transmission of Parasitic Microorganism by Biting Insects

In discussing this subject, it is useful to consider the problems which parasitic microorganisms have to overcome (Busvine, 1975). The microorganisms concerned comprise viruses, rickettsiae, bacteria, protozoa and parasitic nematodes. All of them are very small, the largest of the single-celled forms being about 10 to 50 μm long, and the filarial nematodes about 300 μm long by 6 μm thick. Such tiny creatures are, to a large extent "in passive slavery to forces of the environment" (Huxley, 1941); flagella or cilia may transport them a metre or so in an aqueous medium, but generally they are dependent on chance forces of wind and water. This does not matter so much for the great majority, which are saprophytes in soil or some such extensive habitat; but the parasitic forms must sooner or later make the journey to a new host. This is certainly imperative for the pathogenic forms, whose host may sicken and die.

There are various solutions to this problem. If the host is an animal, parasitic microorganisms may colonize another one during social, familial or sexual contacts. Alternatively, they can invade the gut and be passed out with the faeces, with the chance of contaminating food or water of the host. Or they can be coughed or sneezed out in droplets, to be inhaled by another potential host.

In the course of evolution, however, a remarkable series of adaptations occurred, involving the alternation of parasitism between a large animal (or plant) and a small creature such as an arthropod (commonly, an insect). This arrangement was found to be beneficial to organisms originally parasitic on the smaller host, as well as those on the larger ones. For the former, a large animal like a vertebrate represented a big and long-lived reservoir, capable of infecting many of the small creatures over a long period. The parasites of vertebrates, on the other hand, found a new long-range method of transmission. Where human or animal diseases are concerned, the arthropod involved is usually described as the "vector" and the vertebrate as the "reservoir". In some circumstances, however, the roles may not be so obvious. Thus some arthropods, such as ticks, are quite long-lived and may also pass on the pathogen to their progeny (by transovarial transmission), so that they virtually constitute reservoirs. On the other hand, a man infected with malaria or yellow fever and whisked to another continent by air, could certainly spread the disease, though he would normally be called a "carrier". Dengue was recently introduced into the Pacific Islands in this way and imported malaria is increasing in several countries (see Chapter 9).

The arthropods, especially the insects, have proved to be important vectors, because many of them habitually associate with vertebrates; this is particularly true of the bloodsucking ones. The simplest transmission system consists merely in contamination of the mouthparts with blood pathogens. This mechanical method of infection, by various biting flies, is responsible for spreading surra among horses and camels. It may also account for some cases of human sleeping sickness (Buxton, 1955), though most are due to a complex cycle exclusive to tsetse flies, as mentioned below. The virulent rabbit disease myxomatosis is also dependent on mechanical inoculation by biting insects. In Australia the main vectors were mosquitoes (Fenner *et al.*, 1952), whereas in England rabbit fleas were principally responsible (Lockley, 1954).

The method of mechanical transmission, however, is not very efficient, since the very small traces of blood on the mouthparts may not contain enough pathogens to infect a new host. Also, they would soon dry up, which would harm many microorganisms. Therefore, mechanical transmission is only likely to succeed when an insect, disturbed during feeding, immediately resumes on another animal. In subsequent evolution there was more and more radical infection of the vector, and a progression from casual involvement of various bloodsuckers to association with a particular genus of vectors. Probably the first step was for the pathogen to proliferate in the foregut of the vector, thus increasing the chances of infection. This occurs in tsetse flies carrying nagana, a trypanosomal disease lethal to imported horses and cattle in Africa; and also in the human diseases kala-azar and oriental sore, carried by sandflies. Somewhat more efficient is plague transmission by fleas, in which the bacilli multiply to such an extent that they often block the gut, so that some of them are regurgitated when the hungry fleas try to feed again.

Pathogens which multiply in the gut of the vector can also be passed out with its faeces in an infective state. Examples are louse-borne typhus and Chagas' disease. The infective faeces may enter abrasions in the skin, following scratching by the host, or they can dry to a fine powder and become inhaled or enter a mucous membrane.

In a further stage of parasitizing the vector, the pathogens may penetrate the gut wall and invade its tissues, though this complicates the matter of escaping to enter the next host. A simple solution is for the arthropod to be eaten, which must often happen when an animal grooms itself. An example is the transmission of the dog tapeworm, *Dipylidium caninum*, one stage of which occurs in a flea and is released when the dog swallows it. A human disease transmitted in this way is louse-borne relapsing fever, the spirochaetes of which are confined in the insect's body cavity. Infection can occur when primitive people "pop" lice between their teeth.

There are obvious limitations to a transmission system which involves the death of the vector, which can thus only infect one new host. A better arrangement is for infection to occur during subsequent bites of the vector. A simple example is provided by the forms of filariasis, in which the tiny worms make their way to the insect's proboscis and burst out during the next blood meal. This method of infection occurs with mosquitoes transmitting urban filariasis and the blackflies which carry onchocerciasis. In the final and most efficient system, the pathogens in the arthropod's body make their way to the salivary glands and are injected into one or more new hosts with the saliva. Several widespread and important diseases are spread like this, including malaria, yellow fever, dengue, sleeping sickness, mosquito-borne encephalitis and some forms of tick-borne relapsing fever (see also Chapter 9).

III. The Origin of Two-Host Pathogens

Presumably, microorganisms alternatively parasitic on arthropods and vertebrates began as parasites of one of them and extended their range to the other host. It is not always easy to guess which was the original host. Obviously there is no fossil evidence to trace their evolution, but something can be learnt from the biology of their existing relatives. Thus the Rickettsiae responsible for louse-borne and other forms of typhus belong to a group virtually all of which are parasitic on arthropods at some stage; so these were probably the original hosts. Other parasites which probably began as parasites of invertebrates are the trypanosomes, which cause sleeping sickness, transmitted by tsetse flies, and Chagas' disease, spread by trypanosomal bugs (Hoare, 1967). Other trypanosomes not involving man are carried by leeches to frogs or fishes; and in contrast to the variety of invertebrate hosts involved, there is only one species which passes directly between vertebrates (it causes a venereal infection of equines, almost certainly a secondary adaptation).

At one time it was considered that insects were the primary hosts of malarial parasites, since they are all spread by mosquitoes to a variety of tree-living animals (birds, bats, monkeys and man—who may have once been arborial) (Christophers, 1934). However, further consideration of related parasitic protozoa suggests that the remote ancestors were parasites of vertebrates, perhaps gut parasites. Later, invasion of the bloodstream allowed the use of blood-suckers as intermediate hosts, and finally, only mosquitoes were involved (Mattingly, 1969).

The relapsing fevers, transmitted by lice and ticks, belong to spirochaetes of the genus *Borrelia*. Both types of arthropod vector are unaffected by their presence and the ticks can pass them on to their progeny; these facts point to a long association with the arthropods (Walton, 1973). If, however, these were the original hosts, *Borrelia* must be an anomalous kind of spirochaete, since other genera are associated with ulcers of the mouth or genitalia or lung abscesses. Furthermore, distant relatives are the treponemes, responsible for the tropical skin diseases yaws and pinta. Still others are free-living and are found in mud, sewage and polluted water, while some occur in oysters and other molluscs. In short, the affinities of *Borrelia* are obscure.

A similar uncertainty prevails in the origin of the plague bacillus, *Yersinia pestis*. Little can be deduced from the characteristics of related bacteria. Only one of these, *Francisella tularensis*, is involved in a disease transmitted by arthropods (tularaemia) and this species differs substantially in morphology and immunology.

IV. Infectivity and Virulence

Whatever the origin of a two-host parasite, the extension to a new host must have involved adaptations analogous to the initiation of the original parasitism. Apart from the mechanical arrangements for transfer, there would need to be development of new enzyme systems to assimilate nutrients from a different type of tissue and also adaptation to neutralize the protective immunological reactions of the new host. These developments must involve complex biochemical changes to meet the particular characteristics of the new animal. Such adaptations are often rather specific, so that many pathogens will only thrive in a limited range of vectors and hosts. Thus the species of *Plasmodium* responsible for human malaria will only develop in man and must be transmitted by anopheline mosquitoes. Sleeping sickness trypanosomes will only develop fully in tsetse flies, though other biting flies may transfer them mechanically.

After the major step of establishing a system of alternating hosts, the microorganisms may extend its range to yet more species. Though not as radical as the original change to an entirely different organism, extension to a new vector or host must involve some adjustments. In the early imperfect stages, this may result in harm to either host or vector; in other words, virulence. In the course of time, however, diseases tend to evolve to a benign state, with improved chances of survival for both host and parasite; and this condition is generally regarded as evidence of a long-established association between a microorganism and its host.

Many human diseases transmitted by arthropods are almost certainly extensions from cycles in wild animals and their arthropod parasites, which have reached the stage of natural immunity. Examples are scrub typhus, Rocky Mountain spotted fever, Chagas' disease and Rhodesian sleeping sickness. There are, however, other vector-borne diseases carried over from wild animals, in which the latter suffer to various degrees. Thus jungle yellow fever kills many American forest monkeys and "sylvatic" plague periodically decimates wild rodents.

Extension of vector-borne infections of wild animals to man would depend on opportunities for frequent human feeds by the vectors concerned. Occasional infections would be unlikely to establish themselves in the alien tissues. If, however, a change in human habits or the environment allowed the vectors frequent opportunities to feed on man, there would be a chance for a mutant capable of developing in man to establish itself. Human defences would be unprepared and severe virulence could result. In some cases, a further environmental change (or dependence on a new vector associated with man) might isolate the pathogen, so that an exclusively human disease resulted; for example, malaria, typhus or louse-borne relapsing fever. Some of the changes mentioned could have occurred in relatively recent times, corresponding to the environmental changes wrought by emerging human urbanization. Not only would this involve vectors ready to take advantage of the shelter of human dwellings (as mentioned earlier) but also other mammalian reservoirs, in the form of domestic animals or commensal pests, like rats and mice. Examples are typhus and plague.

The pathogen of typhus, *Rickettsia prowazekii*, is closely related to another pathogen, *R. typhi*, which occurs in wild rodent populations and is transmitted among them by various ectoparasites, including fleas. Sometimes a rodent flea bites man and transfers the infection, which is ill-adapted and causes only a mild disease, murine typhus. It is possible, however, that a mutant form of the Rickettsia began to be spread through human populations by the body louse, causing epidemic typhus. It could be that this innovation occurred in relatively recent times, since the Rickettsiae are lethal to lice as well as being dangerous to man; perhaps in historical times, since there is no mention of a disease which can be identified as typhus earlier than the fifteenth century (Zinsser, 1935). Plague records extend back much further; but this may be because that disease is more easily recognized and described.

So far as plague is concerned, there seems to be no evidence of a change in the nature of the pathogen during the course of human history; but there have been profound changes in its distribution and importance (Hirst, 1953). As is generally known, plague is a disease of wild rodents, transmitted among them by their fleas. These do not readily bite man, so that sylvatic plague foci are not dangerous, except to fur trappers. Plague epidemics are begun by the transference of the infection from wild rodents to scavenging rodents on the periphery of human settlements; and from them, urban pest rats acquire the disease, to which they are very susceptible. The presence of numerous dead town rats is a dire warning of impending plague. In temperate climates, the common rat flea, *Nosopsyllus fasciatus*, is reluctant to bite man; but the tropical rat flea, *Xenopsylla cheopis*, will often feed on man, especially if desperately hungry after the death of its rat host, with the possible result of plague developing. Human cases are not infectious to rats, because the plague bacilli are concentrated in the buboes, or swellings in the armpit and groin. Sometimes, however, intense lung infections develop and these pneumonic cases can spread plague by droplet inhalation (see Chapter 14).

The original home of bubonic plague may have been Central Africa or perhaps Central Asia; certainly the latter part of the world was an early source of plague, which travelled with rats and fleas in caravans to cause the epidemics which were recorded throughout history. Camel trains, however, are slow and restricted; but with the great expansion of ocean trade in the nineteenth century, plague was spread all round the world, from a source in China. The first result was a series of urban epidemics in seaports; but from these, new foci were set up in the hinterlands of various continents. There they remain today, among wild rodents in California, South America and South Africa. The chances of their spreading into modern cities, however, is remote, except in some ill-kept tropical towns. This is because the likelihood of a rat flea attacking man depends on the location of the dying rat. The rat common in modern cities, *Rattus norwegicus*, lives underground in sewers, with little or no contact with humans. Whereas the dangerous plague rat *R. rattus*, is a climbing type, which readily invades wooden buildings and was common in medieval towns. This rat is now rare in modern cities except, to some extent, in warehouses.

The great changes in human populations over the past 10 000 years, with the growth of agriculture and later, urbanization, have affected the importance and distribution of many diseases (McNeill, 1977, and this volume) including those transmitted by vectors. Malaria, for example, is well known to have waxed and waned as past civilizations emerged and declined. To some extent, this could be due to the increased opportunities for breeding of the mosquito vectors, when the destruction and disorganization of war interrupted careful agricultural drainage schemes. This would have brought extra disease to augment the ill-effects of the war and hasten the decline of a civilization.

In recent times, we have seen a marginally successful attempt to eradicate malaria from the world, by attacking the vectors with insecticides, especially DDT. Though effective in eliminating the disease from very large peripheral areas, the attempt failed in the hyperendemic tropical zone, largely because the mosquitoes developed resistance to the insecticide (Harrison, 1978) (see also Chapter 10).

Another mosquito-borne disease where the incidence is changing because of human development is urban filariasis. Nelson (1977) has pointed out that, with about 400 million people at risk, there are probably more infected cases now than 100 years ago, when Patrick Manson incriminated mosquitoes as the vectors. This is largely due to population growth in the tropics, combined with the enormous growth of unhygienic slums around tropical cities, which have provided a vast increase in breeding sites for the urban vector, in drains and cesspits. This insect, too, has become largely immune to chemical pesticides.

At one time, the new potent synthetic insecticides seemed to promise an easy solution to vector-borne disease. In the last 10 to 15 years, however, their use has been hampered by increasing concern about environmental pollution and by pest resistance. The first difficulty can be overcome by using less persistent and more specific insecticides (though they are more expensive); but resistance remains as a severe handicap. Nevertheless, insecticides are likely to play a valuable role for a decade or two, if carefully used in combination with other measures (Busvine, 1977). The optimum solution for many diseases is a general improvement in living standards. So far as vector-borne diseases are concerned, this should eliminate ectoparasites such as lice and fleas, as well as many house pests like bugs and triatomids. Better sanitation (especially water-borne sewage) should greatly reduce *Culex fatigans* and many flies and blowflies. Raising living standards, alas, is an enormous task. Moreover, there are some vectors which originate beyond the effects of personal or urban hygiene, such as blackflies, tsetse flies and many anopheline mosquitoes. These present a challenge to physicians, entomologists and chemists, to find suitable drugs and pesticides. Much, too, depends on the importance accorded to these diseases by politicians and, indeed, the people they represent. One sometimes wonders what progress could have been made if they had attracted the money and effort expended on atomic weapons or even on rockets to explore space.

References

Busvine, J. R. (1975). "Arthropod Vectors of Disease". Arnold, London.
Busvine, J. R. (1977). *In* "Medical Entomology Centenary Symposium Papers", 106–110. Royal Society of Tropical Medicine and Hygiene, London.
Busvine, J. R. (1978). *Syst. Ent.* **3**, 1–8.
Buxton, P. A. (1955). "The Natural History of Tsetse Flies", p. 644. Lewis, London.
Chapman, T. (1973). *S.P.A.N.* **16**, 51.
Christophers, R. (1934). *Proc. R. Soc. Med.* **27**, 991–1000.
Clay, T. (1957). Symposium: "Host Specificity among Parasites of Vertebrates". Univ. Neuchatel.
Fenner, F., Woodroofe, G. M. and Day, M. F. (1952). *Aust. J. exp. Biol. med. Sci.* **30**, 139–152.
Ferris, G. F. (1951). The sucking lice. *Mem. Pacific Coast Ent. Soc., San Francisco.*
Hamon, J. (1976). "Proc. Workshop on Implications of Pesticide Use". Centre for Overseas Pest Research, London.
Harrison, G. (1978). "Mosquitoes, Malaria and Man". Dutton, New York.
Hirst, L. F. (1953). "The Conquest of Plague". Clarendon Press, Oxford.
Hoare, C. A. (1967). *Adv. Parasit.* **5**, 47.
Holland, G. P. (1969). *Mem. ent. Soc. Can.* No. 61.
Hopkins, G. H. E. (1957). Symposium: "Host Specificity among Parasites of Vertebrates". Univ. Neuchatel.
Huxley, J. (1941). "Uniqueness of Man". Chatto and Windus, London.
Lockley, R. M. (1954). *Vet. Rec.* **66**, 434.
McNeill, W. H. (1977). "Plagues and Peoples". Blackwell, Oxford.
Mattingly, P. F. (1969). "The Biology of Mosquito-borne Disease". Allen and Unwin, London.
Mouffet, T. (1634). "Insectorum sive minimorum Animalium Theatrum". London.
Nelson, G. S. (1977). *In* "Medical Entomology Centenary Symposium Papers". Royal Society of Tropical Medicine and Hygiene, London.
Roth, M. and Willis, E. R. (1957). *Smithson. misc. Collns* **134**, No. 10.
Traub, R. (1971). *Bull. Br. Mus. nat. Hist. (Zool.)* **22**, (12).
Walton, G. A. (1973). "Proceedings of the International Symposium on the Control of Lice and Louse-borne Diseases". PAHO/WHO, Washington.
Weyer, F. (1978). *Z. angew. Zool.* **65**, 87–112.
World Health Organization (1974). *Wld Hlth Org. Chronicle* **28**, 427.
Zinsser, H. (1935). "Rats, Lice and History". Routledge, London.

5
Prelude to Modern Preventive Medicine

Norman Howard-Jones*
Geneva Switzerland

. . . The most ancient form of preventive medicine was adherence to a regimen supposedly conducive to health. . . . A key element . . . was . . . epidemiological surveillance . . . quarantine was powerless to affect the spread of cholera. . . . The total eradication of smallpox constitutes the greatest triumph of man over disease that the world has ever seen.

* Formerly Director, Division of Editorial and Reference Services, World Health Organization.

I. Introduction

Apart from various superstitious practices, the most ancient form of preventive medicine was adherence to a regimen supposedly conducive to health. Prescriptions for health and longevity have abounded at all times, and they continue to be addressed to the public, whether by health authorities, individual physicians, or health faddists. A typical physician's recipe is George Cheyne's *An Essay of Health and Long Life*, published in 1725 and warmly recommended to James Boswell by Samuel Johnson.[1] Cheyne wrote:

> Most men know when they are ill, but very few when they are well. And yet it is most certain that 'tis easier to *preserve* health than to *recover* it, and to *prevent* Diseases than to *cure* them.

Cheyne relied on observations made "on my own crazy carcase and the Infirmities of others I have treated". For him, the road to good health was the choice of a place of residence by reference to its atmospheric conditions, its altitude, and the nature of its soil, as also to diet, sleep, exercise, and the passions. Cheyne's recipe for the preservation of health, like those of so many before and after him, referred only to individual physical fitness—supposedly a shield against disease—and was devoid of any notion of specific pathogens or of community action directed to the prevention of disease.

The first organized community measures of preventive medicine were the quarantine restrictions against plague that are generally thought to have had their origin in Venice in the fifteenth century. Plague continued to be a scourge in Europe until the seventeenth century, the last epidemic in Britain breaking out in 1665.[2] In the rest of Europe the disease died out a few years later—a notable relapse being the epidemic of 1720 in Marseilles. While it was plague that gave rise to the elaborate system of maritime quarantine and *cordons sanitaires* on land, the system persisted until well into the nineteenth century because of the ever-present threat from the Levant and, later, the successive pandemics of cholera. This system represented the assertion of the superior claim of the public good over private property and personal liberty. In the public interest, supposedly contaminated goods were ruthlessly destroyed, and cases and contacts were sequestered from the outside world for days and sometimes weeks.

Papon has provided a contemporary account of maritime quarantine procedures in force in France in the year 1800.[3] Masters of plague-infected or suspect ships were required to stand before the iron gate of a lazaret, swear to tell the truth, and throw the ship's bill of health into a basin of vinegar. An official would then, after ensuring with the aid of iron tongs that the bill was well immersed, place it on the end of a plank and present it to a *conservateur de la santé*, who would read it without touching it. Regulations promulgated by the French Minister of Commerce in 1835 prescribed similar precautions, and ordained that surgeons could operate on infected patients if clad from head to foot in oilskins and carrying a brazier filled with burning aromatic herbs.[4] In Britain, violation of quarantine regulations by a master of a ship or a quarantine officer entailed the death penalty, but the laws imposing this and some other penalties were repealed in response to pressure from anticontagionists and commercial interests.[5]

II. Epidemiological Surveillance in the Levant

A key element in the European quarantine structure was the system of epidemiological surveillance operated in the Levant by the Higher Council of Health of Constantinople (*Conseil Supérieur de Santé de Constantinople*), which came into being in 1839 as a result of a formal note addressed to the diplomatic representatives of foreign powers in Constantinople by the Sultan of the Ottoman Empire, Mahmoud II, in the previous year. According to a report presented to the first International Sanitary Conference in 1851, the Council at first consisted of twelve members, of whom seven were Christian or Moslem physicians and five representatives of foreign diplomatic missions.[6] By 1848, the members had increased to seventeen, of whom nine represented respectively Austria, Belgium, Britain, France, Greece, Prussia, Russia, Sardinia, and Tuscany. The remaining eight were appointed by Turkey, but four of these were graduates of European medical faculties.

Directly responsible to the Council were local health administrations designated *offices de santé*, each headed by a Moslem director and a physician from a European medical faculty, with a varying number of subordinate staff. These *offices* were located at strategic points, coastal or inland, throughout the Ottoman Empire, and by 1851 their number had attained 63. Each *office* addressed weekly epidemiological reports and mortality returns to the Council, and in the district for which it was reponsible employed agents (*préposés*)—usually old soldiers—to report on new arrivals at their subdistricts and on any deaths. Burials were not allowed until authorized by the local *office*, often after autopsy. Originally each *office* had its own lazaret, but as plague receded five main lazarets were established.

In Egypt a sanitary administration was established in Alexandria in 1831, and twelve years later its scope was enlarged by the participation of seven European Powers. Many years later it became—by a Khedival decree of 3 January 1818[7]—the Sanitary, Maritime and Quarantine Council (*Conseil Sanitaire, Maritime et Quarantenaire*), which continued until it was dissolved by the fourteenth International Sanitary Conference in 1938.[8]

The Constantinople Council can truly be said to represent the first example of concerted intergovernmental action in the field of preventive medicine, and it was responsible for the most elaborate system of epidemiological surveillance that ever existed *sui generis*, without a pre-existing public health infrastructure. There is little room for doubt that the Council was highly effective in reducing the prevalence of plague in the Levant, and thus of limiting at source its importation into an insanitary and rat-ridden Europe. It was dissolved in 1923 by Article 114 of the Treaty of Lausanne of the League of Nations.

III. Cholera—the Plague of the Nineteenth Century

By 1830 plague, while still felt to be a constant threat, had for over a century ceased to be a European health problem. But in that year Europe was for the first time invaded by another epidemic disease from the East—Asiatic cholera—which was to cause a devastating loss of lives and to become for the nineteenth century the scourge that plague had been in earlier times. In the case of plague, while there had been a fanatical anticontagionist minority, the majority in favour of the contagion theory was overwhelming. With cholera it was quite otherwise. Opinions on its communicability were equally divided, both within and between the different European countries. Some believed that cholera was a "purely epidemic" disease in the sense that it resulted from a combination of certain conditions of the atmosphere, soil, noxious emanations from decaying organic matter, and individual predisposition. Others were equally convinced that the disease was conveyed by man and therefore susceptible to quarantine measures.

For the first three decades of the nineteenth century, such knowledge of cholera as was available in Europe was derived from British India, and especially from the official reports from Bombay (1819),[9] Calcutta (1820),[10] and Madras (1824).[11] These reports reflected such contradictory judgments that they provided no adequate guidance for the authorities of countries threatened by the westerly spread of the disease, especially as the authorities received equally contradictory advice from their own medical advisers. Central and local governments decided, therefore, to play for safety by imposing maritime quarantine, establishing *cordons sanitaires*, isolating infected persons, and destroying clothing and other supposedly infected material. However, actual experience of the disease was to lead to the conclusion in some countries, notably Britain, that quarantine was powerless to affect the spread of cholera.

IV. The First European Cholera Epidemics

The first major European city to be invaded by cholera was Moscow. In the late summer of 1830 there was a serious outbreak during the annual fair at Nizhni-Novgorod—now known as Gorki and about 260 miles east of Moscow. As a precautionary measure, the Governor of Moscow Prince Dimitri Vladimirovich Galitzin, established quarantine stations at the entries to the city and required all incoming visitors to be fumigated.[12] In each of the twenty administrative districts of the city—whose population then numbered about 300 000—a medical inspector was appointed and a temporary hospital was established. Galitzin also appointed a Temporary Medical Committee of 24 members, with himself as Chairman.

These careful preventive measures proved to be of no avail, and the first case of cholera occurred in a male domestic servant on 14 September.[13] Before the epidemic subsided, 3% of the population had been affected, with a case mortality of over 50%. The complete failure of rigorous quarantine measures was such as to discourage belief in the contagiousness of cholera, and of the twenty-four members of the Temporary Medical Committee only three believed the disease to be communicable.[14]

From Russia cholera spread to Poland, then in a state of armed insurrection against the Tsar, and thence to Germany, Austria, Hungary, and Bulgaria. In June 1831 it broke out in St Petersburg. By then the whole of Europe was in a state of trepidation and bewilderment at the sudden insurgence of this new and mysterious disease. It struck so suddenly, and with such dramatic effect—and preventive measures against it seemed to be futile. Was it indeed a new disease? Or a new manifestation of an old disease? Was its seat in the circulatory or nervous system or in the alimentary canal? Was it contagious or "purely epidemic"? These were the speculations that preoccupied both the medical profession and the public authorities and that resulted in an unprecedented outpouring of articles, pamphlets, and books.

In an attempt to find answers to these crucial questions, governments of countries not yet affected sent medical missions to countries that had already been invaded by cholera. Among these was a two-man British mission to St Petersburg.[15] But only a few weeks later cholera was imported into north-east England by a ship from Hamburg. Thereupon France, which had previously sent missions to Russia, Poland, and Prussia, dispatched several medical investigators to England, including no less a person than François Magendie.[16] When France was infected from England in March 1832, Belgium and Italy sent missions to Paris, as Prussia and Sweden had earlier done to Russia. These international field investigations were an eloquent indication of the consternation aroused in all European countries by the appearance of this new and terrifying disease and of the will to take all measures to find ways of preventing it from encroaching upon their territories.

Medical opinions, however, were so discordant that they offered no sure basis for preventive measures. While there had been a 21 to 3 majority of the Temporary Medical Council of Moscow against the idea of the communicability of cholera, the British Medical Mission to St Petersburg—in the persons of Dr W. Russell and Dr D. Barry—was convinced that the disease was transmitted from man to man. François Magendie, on the other hand, ridiculed the idea that cholera was communicable.[17]

Faced with the lack of any constructive alternative, the public authorities assimilated cholera prophylaxis to the long-standing quarantine measures that seemed to have been effective in ridding Europe of plague. But the failure of quarantine left personal regimens as the last line of defence, and in numerous tracts issued by governments, academies of medicine, and leading physicians, advice was proffered such as might have been given by George Cheyne over a century before.

In 1831 the Paris Academy of Medicine advised that the abuse of wine or spirits "almost invariably" caused cholera,[18] and similar advice was tendered by the Central Board of Health in London, as also by the medical authorities elsewhere in Europe. Avoidance of dietary or sexual excesses, of cold drinks after hot baths, or of certain (and varying) articles of diet, were also important preventive measures.

When one of the Rothschilds wrote to the eminent Baron Guillaume Dupuytren to ask what advice he would give to the doctors of Berlin and Vienna on the most effective means of preventing cholera, he recommended wearing flannel next to the skin "from head to foot" and the avoidance of irritating food and drink. Desirous that such valuable advice should be made more widely available, Dupuytren had his letter reproduced as a printed pamphlet.[19] In June 1832 cholera was imported into the Western Hemisphere by Irish immigrants. As was to be expected, medical opinions in the New World were echoes of those that had already been expressed in the Old World. In Europe, cholera lingered sporadically until the winter of 1837–38, when it died out and did not reappear for another decade.

In 1848–49 cholera again broke out in Germany, Britain, France, and other European countries. Official medicine in Britain—always leaning towards anticontagionism—was by then firmly convinced that cholera was not communicable, and ever more impatient of the restraints imposed on merchant shipping by irksome quarantine requirements. Entirely rejecting the idea of a specific and communicable cause of cholera, the British saw the prevention of the disease as a sanitary environment in terms of adequate ventilation, sanitary disposal of human wastes, clean piped water, and the abolition of "nuisances" in the form of any malodorous organic matter.

V. The International Sanitary Conferences

The proceedings of the series of fourteen International Sanitary Conferences that started in 1851 constitute a unique but little known record of the conflict of ideas on the nature of epidemic diseases and of measures appropriate for their prevention that was to rage for many years in all the countries of what was then the civilized world. The three diseases on the agenda of the first of these conferences, which was held in Paris and which lasted for no less than 6 months, were cholera, plague and yellow fever.[20] The last of these had made an ephemeral appearance on the Mediterranean littoral some three decades before, but this was its first and last visit to Europe. Plague had not appeared in Europe in epidemic form within living memory, but was still regarded as an ever-present threat. The third disease—cholera—had caused millions of deaths in Europe in the twenty years before the conference, including over a million in the Russian Empire alone. Yet the conference took over ten weeks to decide whether it was appropriate to include this disease as an item of the agenda.

Very early in the discussions an Austrian delegate declared that he was under instructions from his government not to discuss cholera, which was "purely epidemic" and made "more frightening and more fatal" by quarantine measures. He was supported by a British delegate, who also affirmed that cholera was "purely epidemic". The conference had been convened by the French Government, one of whose representatives explained apologetically that cholera had been included in the proposed agenda "as a satisfaction given by France to an opinion that still prevails elsewhere". "Elsewhere" included principally the Papal States, Tuscany, the Kingdom of the Two Sicilies, Russia, and Spain, and it was largely due to them that other participants reluctantly agreed that quarantine regulations against cholera should be discussed.

The second conference was held in 1859, also in Paris, and was largely a repetition of the first.[21] The British delegate again pleaded that cholera should be exempt from preventive measures that he considered futile, and asserted that experience since the first conference had "more and more shown that this disease is not contagious at all". However, as at the first conference, a draft International Sanitary Convention was adopted but never entered into force.

VI. The Unacceptable Truth about Cholera

During the interval between the first two International Sanitary Conferences, two men had simultaneously, independently, and using entirely different approaches, revealed the true nature of cholera—only to be entirely disbelieved by their contemporaries.

In London, John Snow published in 1849 a preliminary account of his conclusions and in 1855 appeared the definitive report of his classical epidemiological investigation of the London cholera epidemic of 1854. In retrospect, Snow's findings and deductions seem so conclusive that it is difficult to understand how his contemporaries could have failed to be convinced by them. But in 1858 John Simon, Medical Officer of the Privy Council, dismissed his conclusions as a "peculiar doctrine", and it took more than 30 years for it to be generally accepted that cholera was primarily a water-borne disease. One of the most persistent and influential opponents of what he derisively called the "drinking-water theory" was the eminent Munich hygienist Max von Pettenkofer, who from 1855 until his death in 1901 continued to expound his "soil theory" (*Bodentheorie*), according to which the cholera pathogen—whatever it was—was harmless until it had undergone a process of maturation in the soil under certain conditions of the level of the ground-water.

In Florence, Filippo Pacini published in 1854 the first of a series of observations on the cholera vibrio, incriminating it as the cholera pathogen and the cause of the dehydration characteristic of the disease.[22] Formal recognition of the crucial importance of Pacini's observations and conclusions had to await over a century, when the International Committee on Bacteriological Nomenclature ruled in 1965 that the vibrio should be known as "*Vibrio cholerae* Pacini 1854".[23]

The contemporaries of Snow and Pacini were so preoccupied by their preconceived notions—and especially by that of the aerial transmission of noxious miasms—that they were blind to the plain truths that had been revealed by accurate observations, both epidemiological and microscopical. At the fourth International Sanitary Conference in 1874 participants voted unanimously that "the ambient air is the principal vehicle of the generative agent of cholera".[24] It was not until the seventh of these conferences in 1892 that there was sufficient international agreement on the aetiology of cholera to make it possible to conclude the first International Sanitary Convention, which contained principally quarantine regulations against cholera for westbound shipping traversing the Suez Canal.[25]

VII. Smallpox

It was long recognized universally that smallpox was transmissible from man to man and that one attack conferred immunity, but it was not until the thirteenth International Sanitary Conference in 1926 that the disease became subject to international sanitary legislation.[26] The reason for this is that smallpox was considered to be endemic in all the countries concerned. Because of this, there was opposition to its receiving international status, but the compromise was reached that only "epidemics", as opposed to first cases, should be internationally notifiable. How many cases constituted an epidemic was left an open question.

For most of the eighteenth century variolation was sporadically practised. It was not, properly speaking, a preventive method, but the artificial induction of the disease in the hope that the attack would be mild yet confer immunity. Such a method presupposed the virtual inevitability of contracting the disease at some stage of life. It never won general acceptance, for it probably caused as many, if not more, outbreaks as it prevented. Moreover, it transmitted not only smallpox, but sometimes also syphilis.

When Edward Jenner published his observations on smallpox vaccination in 1798 the international response was, apart from the inevitable dissenters, remarkably positive. The first government to introduce legislation requiring vaccination was the Grand Duchy of Hesse, which in 1807 enacted a law that made vaccination compulsory for all children and at the same time prohibited variolation.[27] Paradoxically, Britain—the home of vaccination—long remained almost alone among European countries in not having legislation making it compulsory. The first such British law was enacted in 1841, but this was full of loopholes and several further laws tightening its provisions were introduced during the nineteenth century. In other countries, vaccination was enforced with varying degrees of efficacy. Thus during the Franco-Prussian War only 49 out of one-and-a-half million German soldiers died of smallpox, while the disease cost the French Army 23 400 lives.[28]

VIII. Discussion and Reflections

The combination of sequestration of plague victims and the elaborate system of epidemiological surveillance in the Levant was effective in preventing serious outbreaks of the disease in Europe, and belief that it was in some way communicable from man to man was thus reinforced. Against cholera the same preventive measures were adopted but proved to be quite ineffective. This failure contributed to the persistence of entirely erroneous theories as to the cause and mode of transmission of the disease. However, by the time of the third International Sanitary Conference in 1866 all participants agreed that cholera pandemics always started in India.

After the opening of the Suez Canal in 1869, Britain was criticized, especially by the French, as the purveyor of cholera to the rest of the world. However, the British stubbornly resisted the idea that cholera could be conveyed by man, believing the disease to be the product of a generally insanitary environment rather than of a specific pathogen. Paradoxically this conviction, by providing a strong incentive to the great sanitary reforms of the nineteenth century, was instrumental in freeing Britain from cholera some three decades before continental Europe was freed. In fact, no European epidemic was ever imported directly from India by sea. All the cholera pandemics of the nineteenth century, with one exception, travelled slowly westward from India by land. The exception was the fourth pandemic, which started in 1865 when ships from Egypt infected several European mediterranean ports, Egypt itself having become infected by returning Mecca pilgrims.

It was in 1865 that the last epidemic of cholera occurred in Britain. Further outbreaks were prevented by isolation of incoming cases, detention of suspects for 48 hours, and the requirement that all other passengers should give their exact destinations and report any illness to the local medical officer of health. Robert Koch's definitive incrimination of the cholera pathogen in 1884 was greeted with the utmost scepticism by official medicine in Britain—which remained free from cholera, whereas in Germany the Hamburg epidemic of 1892 claimed 8605 lives.[29] In fact, the identification of the pathogen has contributed very little to the control of the disease, the only real protection remaining a sanitary environment.

Smallpox may be regarded as the opposite extreme of cholera in the sense that the only method of prevention is entirely specific, entirely independent of the sanitary environment, and has been available for almost two centuries. As early as 1801, US President Thomas Jefferson foretold that smallpox vaccination would "finally extirpate" the disease from the face of the earth.[30] That it has taken so long for this prophecy to be realized is doubtless due to a combination of circumstances, including legislative loopholes, lack of the means for quality control of the vaccines, and other adventitious reasons. The total eradication of smallpox by the World Health Organization constitutes the greatest triumph of man over disease that the world has ever seen, and will probably so remain for many years to come (see Chapter 13).

References

1. Cheyne, George. "An Essay of Health and Long Life", 2nd edn. Strahan, London, 1725.
2. Hirsch, August. "Handbook of Geographical and Historical Pathology", Vol. 1. New Sydenham Society, London, 1883.
3. Papon, J. P. "De la peste ou les époques de ce fléau et les moyens de s'en préserver", Vol. 2. Paris, 1800.
4. Toy, J. "La réglementation de la défense sanitaire contre la peste, le choléra et la fièvre jaune d'après la Convention de Paris 1903. Paris, 1905.
5. Mullet, C. F. A century of English quarrantine (1709–1825). *Bull. Hist. Med.* 1949, **23**, 527–545.
6. "Proces-verbaux de la conférence sanitaire internationale ouverte à Paris le 27 Juillet 1851". Imprimerie nationale, Paris, 1852. (The "27" in the title is a misprint for 23. The report on the Levant is annexed to the minutes of the 29th session.)
7. Proust, A. "La défense de l'Europe contre le choléra". Masson, Paris, 1892.
8. "Conférence sanitaire international de Paris. 28–31 Octobre 1938. Procès-verbaux". Imprimerie nationale, Paris, 1939.

9. "Reports on the Epidemic Cholera which has Raged Throughout Hindostan and the Peninsula of India Since August 1817". Published under the authority of government, Bombay, 1819.
10. Jameson, J. "Report on the Epidemic Cholera Morbus as It Visited the Territories Subject to the Presidency of Bengal in the Years 1817, 1818 and 1819". Calcutta, 1820.
11. Scot, W. "Report on the Epidemic Cholera as It has Appeared in the Territories Subject to the Presidency of Fort St George". Madras, 1824.
12. Jaehnichen, –. "Quelques réflexions sur le choléra-morbus", Moscow, 1831.
13. Markus, F. C. M. "Rapport sur le choléra-morbus de Moscou". Moscow, 1832.
14. Jachnichen (sic), –. Mémoire sur le choléra-morbus qui règne en Russie, *Gaz. méd. Paris*, 1831, **2**, 85–88.
15. Great Britain. Privy Council. Board of Health. "Official Reports made to Government by Drs Russell and Barry on the Disease Called Cholera Spasmodica, as Observed by Them During Their Mission to Russia in 1831". London, 1832.
16. Magendie, F. *Gaz. méd. Paris*, 1831, **2**, 444. (Text of a letter sent by Magendie from England to the Académie des Sciences, Paris, on 3 December 1831.)
17. Magendie, F. "Leçons sur le choléra-morbus faites au collège de France". Paris, 1832.
18. Académie Royale de Médecine. "Rapport de l'Académie Royale de Médecine sur le choléra-morbus". Paris, 1831.
19. Dupuytren, G. Lettre de M. Le Baron Dupuytren sur le choléra-morbus. A monsieur J. de Rothschild, à Paris, 27/9/31.
20. Reference 6.
21. "Protocoles de la conférence sanitaire internationale ouverte à Paris le 9 avril 1859, Imprimerie nationale, Paris, 1859.
22. Pacini, Filippo. Osservazioni Microscopiche e Deduzioni Patologiche sul Cholera Asiatico. *Gazz. Med. ital. tosc.* 2nd ser. 1854, **6**, 397–405.
23. *Int. Bull. bact. Nomencl.* 1965, **15**, 185.
24. "Procès-verbaux de la conférence sanitaire internationale ouverte à Vienne le 1er Juillet 1874". Imprimerie impériale et royale, Vienne, 1874.
25. "Protocoles et procès-verbaux de la conférence sanitaire internationale de Venise inaugurée le 5 Janvier 1892", Imprimerie nationale de J. Bertero, Rome, 1892.
26. "Conférence sanitaire internationale de Paris, 10 mai–21 juin 1926". Imprimerie nationale, Paris, 1927.
27. Rupp, J.-P. Die hundertjährige Geschichte des deutschen Impfgesetzes. *Die gelben Hefte* 1974, **14**, 23–30.
28. *British Medical Journal* 1897, **i**, 1642–1644.
29. Koch, R. *Arbeiten aus dem Kaiserlichen Gesundheitsamt* 1896, **10**, Anl.2, 26.
30. Stearn, E. Wagner and Stearn, Allen E. "The Effect of Smallpox on the Destiny of the Amerindian", Bruce Humphries Inc., Boston, 1945.

Part II

Human Activity and Some Infectious Diseases

Introduction

The general survey in Part I showed that for much of human history, diseases caused by microorganisms have been the major cause of disability and death. The chapters in this section consider this group of diseases. They fall into two groups. The first group surveys some of these diseases in greater detail and the second more general aspects of the theme. The choice of illustrative diseases has been somewhat arbitrary. They include four conditions of viral origin, one due to a single-celled organism (protozoon) and one to a multicellular organism. They have been selected for several reasons: they include a wide biological spectrum of pathogens and are diseases of importance in their distribution, the numbers of persons affected and the disability, and economic consequences, and have been modified or affected by human action.

These chapters should ideally be read twice, the first study comprising an initial straightforward reading and the second time with the reader trying to put himself in the place of the microorganisms in order to appreciate their mechanisms of survival and spread. These are clearly much more complex than might be thought before study.

The four chapters by Gust, Morley, Mackenzie and Stanley, on virus infections representative of current major challenges, reflect the basically different host–parasite relationships that have evolved through prolonged, short-term or spasmodic association with man.

Hepatitis A may usefully be compared with poliomyelitis. Both are enteroviruses with the faecal-oral route as the major one for transmission of virus between humans. Poliomyelitis has been controlled by vaccination as a result of the development of the technology of cell culture. Hepatitis A control will probably stem from a similar approach. Hepatitis B represents a different problem. The virus causing it is unique among viruses and we still do not understand its pathogenesis, ecology or epidemiology. Rapid diagnosis of the disease is still an urgent requirement as is the production of a vaccine. Perhaps, as Dr Gust suggests, recombinant DNA technology will provide a possible solution to the problems of effective immunization against hepatitis B.

Measles has played both a subtle and dramatic role in the history of empires (see McNeill, Chapter 2) and continues in some parts of the planet to take its severe toll. As this book goes to press, it is likely that measles, through effective vaccination, may well come under control in the USA. Morley examines this interesting natural history and describes the present serious problems of measles and malnutrition in developing countries.

Influenza A represents a problem for man, not only because of antigenic drift and shift, but also because of its rapid transmission and movement throughout the planet. Perhaps the influenza viruses A, B and C represent different stages of adaptation of an ancestral virus to the human host. If this is so, influenza B and C could have had as long an association with man as influenza A, with the viruses being initially derived from some non-human vertebrate host with influenza A possibly remaining zoonotic. Dr Mackenzie discusses how the virus may change in its patterns of transmission and pathogenicity.

The arboviruses will always be with us while there are vertebrates and arthropods in which they can replicate. More than a third (of the 400 arboviruses) cause disease in man and animals. It is most unlikely that the natural virus source can ever be eliminated, so that any control by vaccine or by arthropod is limited and could not result in the elimination of the virus or the disease as is the case with smallpox. The basic difference is that arboviruses are zoonotic diseases while smallpox and poliomyelitis, for example, are peculiar to man. Stanley points out how arbovirus evolution in vertebrates and arthropods has been and continues to be modified by human activity.

With malaria and schistosomiasis we have the ever-present problems of widespread tropical diseases being moved throughout the planet by carriers, as well as our inability to control these diseases effectively in the tropical areas where they are endemic. Imported malaria has increased in many countries over the last decade and this is attributed to the increased movement of humans by air. The stories of both malaria and schistosomiasis are still in the early stages of their writing and both relate to many human activities, particularly those associated with tropical irrigated agriculture and man's use of water.

Modern concepts and technologies of immunology and parasitology are being applied to the problems of both diseases in addition to some other tropical diseases. It is hoped that better understanding and hence diagnosis and control will be forthcoming.

The final three chapters in this section have a different emphasis. The chapter on sexually transmitted disease focuses on a mode of spread of disease utilized by organisms of otherwise different taxonomy, but which is obviously related to human activity and mores. This is followed by two chapters in sharp contrast. The eradication of smallpox is one of the greatest human triumphs in the struggle against disease, but the final chapter leaves us little doubt that this is an isolated event. Infectious diseases are still with us, and will remain so in the foreseeable future.

Dr Morton has attempted to explain the paradox of sexually transmitted diseases where their prevalence has increased in spite of specific cures for gonorrhoea and syphilis. We still know little about the origins and natural histories of this fascinating group of microorganisms whose transmission in man is primarily by the sexual route. A study of terrestrial and marine mammalian venereal diseases could yield interesting comparative data. But Professor Morton, as requested, has confined his essay to a consideration of the social determinants in venereal disease. He carefully examines the data associated with changing patterns of sexual freedon and concludes that these infections will continue indefinitely.

Professor Fenner's account of the eradication of smallpox, an historic event, needs little further comment except to re-emphasize the effectiveness of an international application of existing knowledge. This is a great practical achievement. In spite of this success we still have "new" problems with "new" infectious diseases such as those Professor Cedric Mims discusses in the last chapter of this section. This represents a well-balanced assessment of the current situation and lends some mystery to the future associations of man with exotic disease agents. His main message in health control is a plea for more effective research, understanding and an eternal vigilance.

Present pathogens are adapting to changes in the human situation, which include changes in human life styles, living conditions and mobility, the development of antibiotics and interference with the frequently complex life cycles involving many species.

This section, then, is written somewhat from the point of view of the pathogens. The human response to these organisms (and other diseases) is the theme of the third section.

6

Acute Viral Hepatitis

Ian Gust*

Virology Department, Fairfield Hospital, Melbourne, Australia

---

Viral hepatitis . . . is one of the most common and most widespread infections of man and has been recognized as a clinical entity since the time of Hippocrates.

---

* Director, WHO Collaborating Centre for Virus Reference and Research.

I. Introduction

Although many viral infections may involve the liver "viral hepatitis" is a term restricted by convention to a primary infection of the liver caused by one of at least three agents. It is one of the most common and most widespread infections of man and has been recognized as a clinical entity since the time of Hippocrates. In the 1940s and 1950s two major forms of the disease were defined (Havens *et al.*, 1944; MacCallum and Bradley, 1944; Paul *et al.*, 1945; Stokes *et al.*, 1954) which are now referred to as hepatitis type A and hepatitis type B. Epidemiological studies in patients who acquired the disease naturally and in experimentally infected volunteers have demonstrated that hepatitis A has a relatively short incubation period (15–40 days), is usually transmitted by the faecal–oral route and is highly infectious for close contacts. On the other hand hepatitis B has a long incubation period (30–180 days) is usually transmitted by inoculation of infected blood and has a relatively low rate of person-to-person spread (Murray, 1955; Ward *et al.*, 1958; Krugman *et al.*, 1959, 1962, 1967).

In recent years major advances have occurred in the study of viral hepatitis. Both hepatitis A and B have been transmitted to laboratory animals, the viruses responsible for each disease have been identified and characterized and the first attempts have been made to produce vaccines against them. In addition, serological tests have been developed which make it possible to detect virtually all infections with these agents. Interestingly the development of specific tests has revealed the existence of a third form of hepatitis which is neither hepatitis A nor hepatitis B. The agent or agents responsible for this disease, generally referred to as non-A non-B hepatitis, have not yet been identified.

II. Hepatitis A

While Hippocrates described epidemics of jaundice, its contagious nature does not appear to have been recognized until the eighth century A.D. (Cockayne, 1912). Numerous accounts of the disease appear in the later literature, particularly in association with military campaigns, and epidemics of hepatitis A were a major cause of morbidity among civilians and troops during both the First and Second World Wars. Although a viral aetiology of the disease was first postulated by Bergstrand in 1930, it was not confirmed until the early 1940s and the virus was not identified for another 30 years.

A. The Virus

In 1973 Feinstone and his colleagues at the National Institutes of Health reported the detection of 27 nm virus-like particles in the faeces of several volunteers who had been experimentally infected with hepatitis A (see Fig. 1). Morphologically and serologically identical particles were soon identified in the faeces of patients with naturally acquired infections (Locarnini *et al.*, 1974; Dienstag *et al.*, 1975c; Gravelle *et al.*, 1975) and in the hepatocytes, faeces, serum or bile of

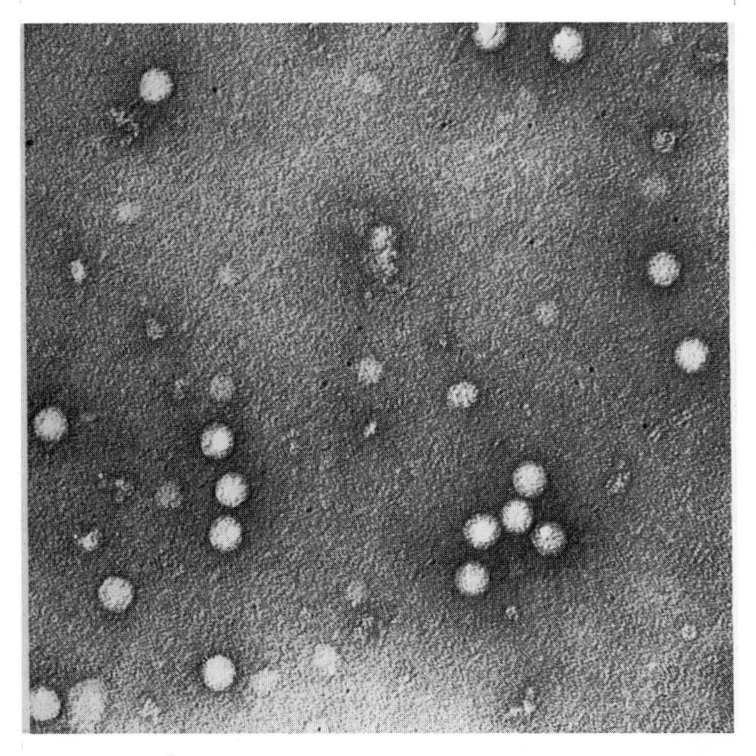

Fig. 1. Hepatitis A virus particles purified from the faeces of a patient with acute hepatitis A. (Photograph kindly supplied by Dr Stephen Locarnini.)

experimentally infected marmosets (Mascoli *et al.*, 1973; Provost *et al.*, 1975a, b) and chimpanzees (Dienstag *et al.*, 1975b; Schulman *et al.*, 1976). While hepatitis A virus (HAV) resembles members of the Picornaviridae and the Parvoviridae, its relative stability to heat, acid and ether, its intracytoplasmic localization (Provost *et al.*, 1975b), the polypeptide composition of its coat (Coulepis *et al.*, 1978) and evidence that its genetic material is single-stranded RNA (Siegl and Frösner, 1978) strongly suggest that it will eventually be classified as an enterovirus within the family Picornaviridae.

B. Pathogenesis.

While HAV does not grow readily in cell culture, the infection has been transmitted to several species of monkeys including marmosets (Provost *et al.*, 1973; Mascoli *et al.*, 1973) and chimpanzees (Purcell *et al.*, 1975). These studies plus a few which were carried out in human volunteers many years ago provide the only available data on the pathogenesis of the disease. It appears that following ingestion of the virus, primary multiplication occurs in the gut, after which HAV spreads to the liver via the blood or the lymphatic system. While faecal shedding has been demonstrated for as long as two to three weeks prior to the onset of jaundice (Krugman *et al.*, 1967), the disease appears to be most communicable late in the incubation period probably because virus titres are at their peak (Fig. 2). Faecal shedding declines rapidly and virus may no longer be detectable at the time the patient seeks medical attention (Dienstag *et al.*, 1975a; Locarnini *et al.*, 1976; Coulepis *et al.*, 1980).

There is no convincing evidence for the existence of a carrier state and what evidence there is suggests that, if carriers do exist, they are of little epidemiological importance.

Relatively little is known about the mechanism of cell damage in hepatitis A. The virus appears to be relatively non-cytocidal, although some direct liver damage has been reported when large doses are administerd intravenously (I. D. Gust, S. M. Feinstone and R. H. Purcell, unpublished observations). Virus particles and specific viral antigen can be detected in the hepatocytes of infected marmosets or chimpanzees days or weeks prior to the onset of hepatitis. Acute liver damage usually begins about the time circulating antibody becomes detectable, suggesting that cellular destruction may be immunologically determined. Such an explanation would help to explain the increasing severity of the infection with age and its tendency to be mild in the immunosuppressed. While a handful of infections with HAV are severe and even fatal, the majority resolve without long-term sequelae.

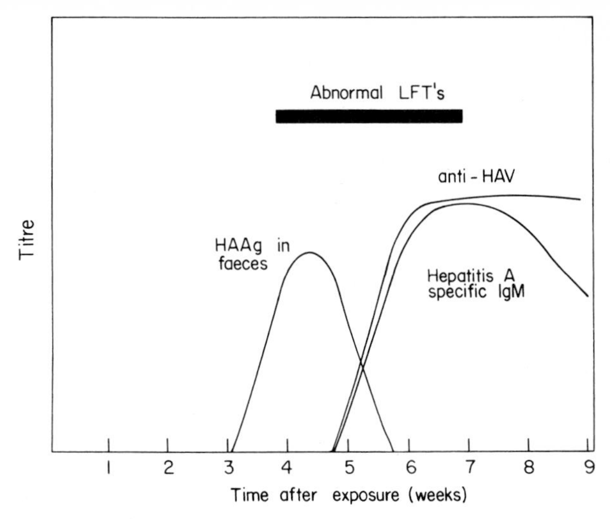

Fig. 2. The serological events in a patient with acute hepatitis A.

There is no evidence that infection with HAV leads to the development of chronic hepatitis or cirrhosis.

C. Laboratory Diagnosis

Currently there are two methods of confirming a diagnosis of hepatitis A, either by detecting the virus (or specific viral antigen) in the patient's faeces or liver during the acute phase of the illness or demonstrating a specific antibody response (Fig. 2). The first method is not widely used because many patients have ceased shedding the virus before they seek medical attention and liver biopsies are rarely performed on patients with acute hepatitis.

The simplest method of confirming the diagnosis is to demonstrate a significant rise in antibody titre in two sera collected during the acute and convalescent phases of the illness. Unfortunately anti-HAV is produced relatively early in the disease and may have reached peak titre by the time the patient is first seen. To overcome this problem several techniques have been developed for detecting hepatitis A specific IgM (Bradley *et al.*, 1977, 1979b; Locarnini *et al.*, 1977, 1979; Frösner *et al.*, 1979). This class of antibody appears to persist for up to 120 days after the onset of symptoms and its presence constitutes strong evidence of recent infection with HAV.

D. Epidemiology

Until recently no accurate data was available on the prevalence of infection with HAV because not all infections are associated with disease and only a small proportion of symptomatic cases are notified to public health authorities. The development of specific tests for detecting current or past infection with the virus has changed this picture. It is now possible to define accurately the rate of infection in any community from which serum specimens can be collected and by examining stored sera to study the pattern of infection over a number of years.

Antibodies to HAV have been detected in every population studied to date. The virus appears to be endemic in developing countries producing largely subclinical infections. While it rarely produces overt disease in the local population, hepatitis A is frequently a problem amongst visitors such as tourists, missionaries, members of the military services and Peace Corps workers (Kendrick, 1972, 1974). Recent data from several groups shows that in developing countries most children become infected before the age of ten years (Villarejos *et al.*, 1976; Vitarana *et al.*, 1978; Gust *et al.*, 1979b). HAV has been shown to be endemic in a number of extremely isolated islands, although how it persists in remote populations with relatively low birth rates is uncertain (Gust *et al.*, 1979a).

The pattern of hepatitis A infection in developed countries differs greatly from that described above and has been affected considerably by improving standards of hygiene and sanitation. Until recently in Australia and America and other wealthy developed countries hepatitis was mainly a disease of children under the age of fifteen years. Moderate rates occurred amongst young adults but relatively few cases were seen among the older population, presumably because the majority were already immune. In the past five to ten years this situation has altered appreciably. In both countries the incidence of hepatitis A has declined and this has been accompanied by an increase in the age at which infections occur and a decline in the prevalence of specific antibody in the population (CDC Report, 1978; Gust *et al.*, 1978). In the USA the incidence of hepatitis A has fallen from a peak of 28·9 per 100 000 in 1971 to 15·5 per 100 000 in 1976 and is calculated to be continuing to decline at 8% per annum.

It is paradoxical that the rising standard of living enjoyed by most Western countries after the Second World War has been accompanied by a rising incidence of hepatitis A. The reason appears to be improvements in the standards of hygiene and sanitation which resulted in many people escaping infection in childhood, a time when the disease would almost certainly have been subclinical. When these children were exposed to the virus later in life, infection was usually associated with jaundice. Hence, although the overall infection rate in the community was declining, the number of cases of hepatitis increased. This trend continued until the early 1970s but as the infection rate continued to fall so the number of cases eventually began to decline as well.

E. Mode of Spread

As far as is known there is no carrier state or animal reservoir in hepatitis A so that the virus is presumably maintained by serial transfer. As infection requires transmission of virus from the bowel contents of one person to the mouth of another, children with anicteric infections play an important part in spreading the disease. Transmission occurs readily under conditions of overcrowding where there is poor hygiene and inadequate sanitation. It is a particular problem during wars and may follow in the aftermath of natural disasters such as earthquakes or typhoons when sanitation services are destroyed and water supplies become contaminated. Water- and food-borne epidemics have been described on many occasions (Melnick, 1957; Mosely, 1959; Chalmers *et al.*, 1967; Dienstag *et al.*, 1975c), when water supplies have become contaminated with human excreta or uncooked food has been prepared by an infected person whose personal hygiene was poor. Most of these outbreaks have been reported from developed countries where a large number of consumers of the food or water can be expected to be susceptible to infection.

Eating clams, mussels and oysters harvested from waters which are subject to faecal contamination is associated with an increased risk to acquiring hepatitis A (Dienstag *et al.*, 1976). Shellfish are able to concentrate HAV from large volumes of water, and while there is no suggestion that the virus is able to replicate in them it may remain viable for several days. If the shellfish are cooked, the mode of preparation is important, as frying will destroy the virus whereas steaming will not (Koff and Sear, 1967).

Although hepatitis A virus can be detected in the blood and urine (Havens *et al.*, 1944; Krugman *et al.*, 1965) of patients incubating the disease, there is no evidence that infection is transmitted by these routes other than in exceptional circumstances. Similarly there is no evidence that the virus can cross the placenta during pregnancy.

F. Isolation

After many years of frustration and disappointment the hepatitis A virus has finally been isolated in cell culture. At the Merck Institute, Hilleman and his co-workers have infected fetal rhesus monkey kidney cells with a strain of HAV which has been passaged over thirty times in marmosets (Provost and Hilleman 1979). When liver extracts from infected marmosets were inoculated into these cells, characteristic intracytoplasmic fluorescence developed and viral particles were released into the supernatant fluid. It has proved possible to passage this strain and to increase its yield considerably. Cell culture now provides a potential source of virus for serological tests and for the production of killed or live vaccines.

G. Prevention and Control

1 General

As with other enteric infections the key to control of hepatitis A is good personal hygiene and proper disposal of faeces. The single most important factor is probably hand washing after going to the toilet and before eating.

2 Immunization

(a) *Passive* Numerous field trials have documented the protection against hepatitis A conferred by immune serum globulin administered prior to exposure or during the incubation period of the disease (Yarrow, 1964; O'Donnell and Cowley, 1966; Wallace, 1966; Reid, 1971). When given in appropriate dose before or within 1–2 weeks of exposure, it prevents illness in 80–90% of those exposed. Also, because it may not suppress infection, long-lasting natural immunity may occur.
(b) *Active* An experimental batch of killed vaccine has been produced from formalin-treated livers obtained from marmosets infected with HAV. This vaccine has proved to be safe and antigenic in marmosets and to protect the animals against challenge with live virus (Provost *et al.*, 1978). The successful adaptation of strains of HAV to growth in cell culture should rapidly result in the development of both killed and live vaccines for use in man.

H. Future Developments

Given reasonable prosperity, freedom from war and a relatively low population growth, one can predict that the current downward trend of hepatitis A in developed countries will continue. The development of an essentially non-immune population makes occasional large epidemics possible and may create problems in the selection of donors from whom batches of immune serum globulin can be prepared. In developing countries, although infection rates will decline, the incidence of illness is likely to increase as living conditions improve and an increasing proportion of infections are delayed until adult life. If a cheap, effective, easily administered vaccine (preferably live attenuated) becomes available it should be possible to control hepatitis A as readily as poliomyelitis.

III. Hepatitis B

Although hepatitis B has been recognized for less than a century, it is one of the most widespread and probably one of the oldest infections of man. The first outbreak was observed in 1883 among shipyard workers (Lürman, 1885) who were vaccinated against smallpox with batches of vaccine containing human serum. Subsequently outbreaks were recorded in situations such as VD clinics and diabetes clinics, where the same syringe was used on several patients. The common factor in each situation appears to be accidental inoculation of blood from a patient or carrier of the virus into a number of susceptible people.

A. The Virus

The hepatitis B virus (HBV) was first detected by Blumberg *et al.* (1965) in the serum of a healthy Australian aboriginal, although its relevance was not appreciated for some years (Okochi and Murakami, 1968; Prince 1968). The virus is morphologically distinct from HAV and much more easily detected. When the serum of an acutely or chronically infected subject is examined under the electron microscope, three morphologically distinct particles can be visualized (Fig. 3)—spherical paricles approximately 22 nm in diameter, tubules of a similar diameter but of variable length (Bayer *et al.*, 1968), and 42 nm double-shelled structures known as the Dane particles (Dane *et al.*, 1970) which are the mature hepatitis B virions. The Dane particle has an outer coat, approximately 7 nm thick, which can be disrupted to release a central core (Almeida *et al.*, 1971). The core of the Dane particle possesses an antigen, the hepatitis B core antigen (HBcAg), which elicits a specific antibody response (Hoofnagle *et al.*, 1973). This antigen is normally not found free in the blood but has been demonstrated in the nucleus of infected hepatocytes by immunofluorescence (Barker *et al.*, 1973) and thin-section electron microscopy (Barker *et al.*,

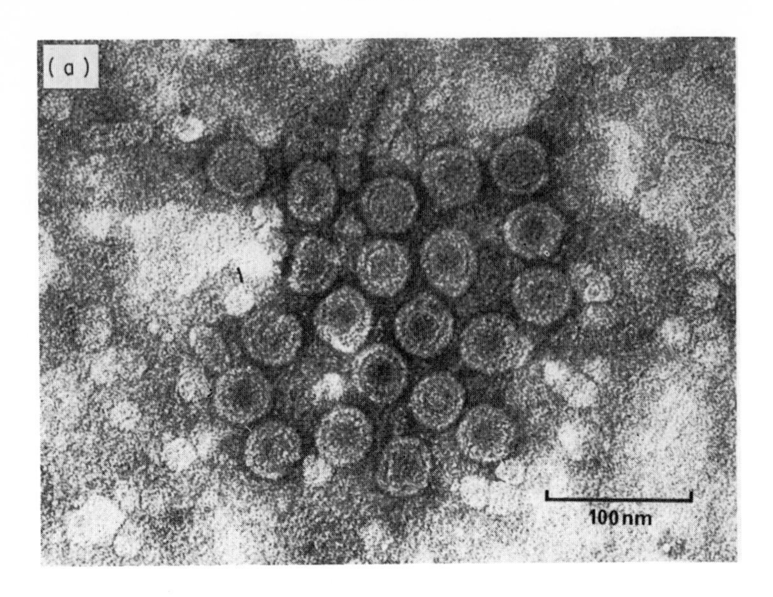

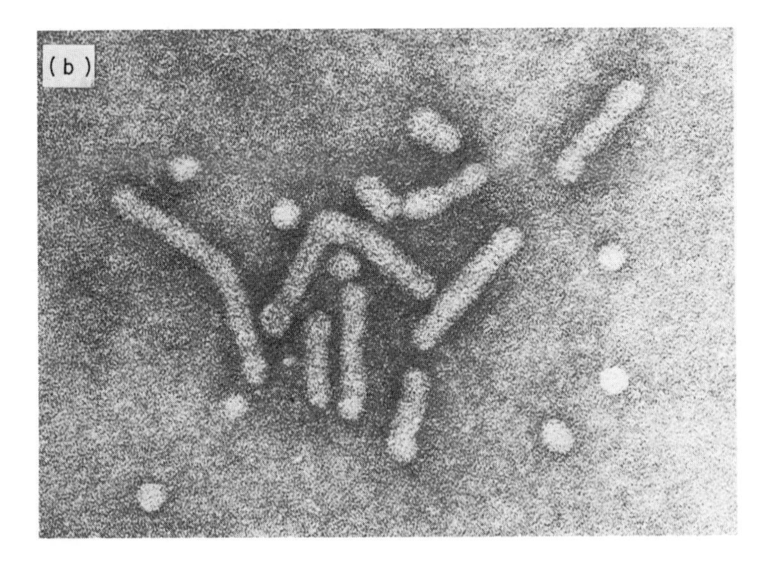

Fig 3. Two electron micrographs of sera from patients with acute hepatitis B demonstrating the three different morphological forms which can be detected. (a) An aggregate of "Dane" particles with occasional tubules. (b) Tubules and spherical forms. (Photographs kindly supplied by Dr John Marshall.)

1974). Intact cores contain an HBV-specific DNA-dependent, DNA polymerase (Kaplan *et al.*, 1973), a double-stranded circular molecule of DNA with a molecular weight of approximately 1·6 million (Robinson *et al.*, 1974) and an additional antigen known as the hepatitis B "e" antigen (HBeAg) (Magnius and Espmark, 1972). The precise role and structure of HBeAg is not known; however, it has been shown to be an excellent marker of the infectivity of sera containing HBsAg (see below).

The 22-nm spherical forms and tubules are normally present in great excess and probably represent coat material which is produced during a relatively inefficient replicative cycle and never assembled. These structures contain no internal components and are hence non-infectious. The surface of all three morphological forms possesses a group of antigens—the hepatitis B surface antigens (HBsAg)—which can be detected serologically and which elicit their own antibody response. Because they react with antigens present on the surface of the virus, antibodies to HBsAg are responsible for protection against reinfection. HBsAgs are remarkably heterogeneous and can be used to divide hepatitis B viruses into a number of major subtypes. These subtypes represent the phenotypic expression of distinct genotypes of the virus and although they are useful epidemiological markers have little clinical relevance. Cross reactivity exists between the different subtypes so that infection with one type appears to result in immunity to each of the others (Purcell *et al.*, 1975).

The hepatitis B virus is currently unclassified and was thought to be unique until Summers *et al.* (1978) discovered a morphologically identical and serologically related particle in the blood of some woodchucks. Reference reagents for detecting this virus are being prepared as it is hoped that the woodchuck will provide a suitable model for studying the pathogenesis of infections with this group of viruses and for evaluating methods of terminating the carrier state.

B. Pathogenesis

While HBV has not been isolated in cell culture, the disease has been transmitted to colony-raised chimpanzees (Maynard *et al.*, 1972; Barker *et al.*, 1973) and rhesus monkeys (London *et al.*, 1972). The precise fate of HBV after it is inoculated into susceptible human or laboratory animal is not known. HBsAg disappears rapidly from the circulation and does not reappear for several weeks (Fig. 4). Levels of HBsAg rise rapidly over the next 2–3 weeks and reach their peak about the time that evidence of liver cell damage appears. As the infection

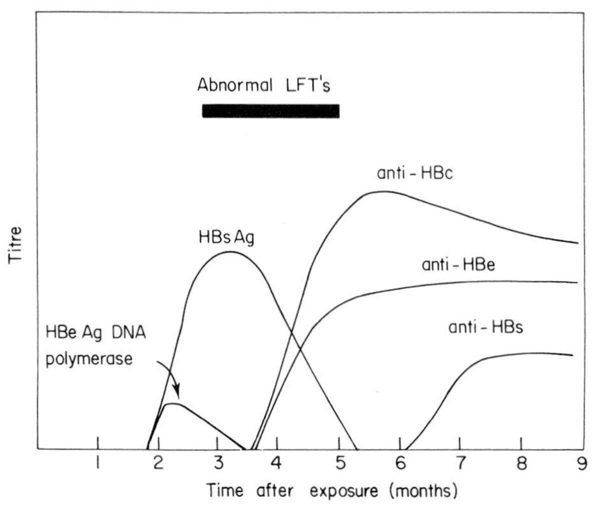

Fig. 4. The serological events in a patient with acute hepatitis B whose illness resolved normally.

progresses, more cells are destroyed, the patient's serum aminotransferase levels rise and he becomes jaundiced. In the majority of patients the HBsAg titre declines over the next few weeks becoming undetectable about or shortly after the liver function tests return to normal (Holland and Alter, 1975). Surprisingly, in view of the magnitude of antigen production, anti-HBs does not develop until late in the patient's convalescence (London *et al.*, 1972). Its appearance is related to the duration of antigenaemia in that if the antigenaemia has been brief antibody will appear early; however, if the antigenaemia has been prolonged antibody may not appear for months or even years. Anti-HBs is responsible for protection against reinfection and persists for many years. Anti-HBc usually appears while HBsAg is still circulating, reaches peak levels in a month or so and persists for life (Hoofnagle *et al.*, 1973). This antibody is the single best marker of active or past infection with the virus.

If sensitive methods are used, HBeAg can be detected briefly in the serum of every patient acutely infected with HBV. Its disappearance is followed by the development of anti-HBe.

HBV differs from HAV in that following infection a proportion of people fail to eliminate the virus from their body and become chronic carriers. Under these circumstances HBsAg persists in the patient's blood for many years, anti-HBs fails to develop and anti-HBc levels tend to be higher than are found after an uncomplicated infection. The reason why some people become carriers and others do not is unknown; however, several predisposing factors are recognized. These include the patient's age, sex and immunological state. In general the earlier in life infection occurs, the more likely a person is to become a chronic carrier. In most population studies the carrier rate has been higher in males than females. Whether this represents a difference in the risk of becoming a carrier or differences in the duration of antigenaemia is not known. Deficiencies in immunological function whether genetic, produced by disease or induced as a result of treatment with certain drugs, predispose towards development of the carrier state. A variety of genetic hypotheses have been put forward to explain the high carrier rates and family clustering observed in many populations. At present there is no convincing evidence to explain this phenomenon which could equally be due to environmental factors. While the majority of chronic carriers remain perfectly well, a proportion develop chronic active hepatitis and cirrhosis. In some parts of the world such as Japan and China chronic carriage of HBsAg is associated with an increased risk of developing hepatocellular carcinoma.

While the mechanism of liver cell damage in patients infected with HBV is unknown, it is almost certainly not due to the direct cytopathic effect of the virus. The most comprehensive hypothesis is that of Chisari *et al.* (1978), who suggest that infection of susceptible liver cells is followed by the production of specific viral proteins and a disturbance of cellular metabolism which results in the production of abnormal immunoregulatory molecules. These molecules have a variety of effects, including removal of the normal inhibition of antibody production to actin- and liver-specific proteins, and the release of cellular attack mechanisms specific for hepatocyte surface membrane antigens and expressed viral antigens. As a result, cellular damage may occur with the leak of cellular constituents which produce cell death. Natural variation in the concentration of these constituents from person to person may account for differences in the severity of infection. The group also suggest that recovery from infection is associated with development of antibody which masks HBsAg on the surface of the hepatocyte and interferes with cellular anti-viral attack systems allowing the normal synthesis of immunoregulatory molecules. An inadequate antibody response may lead to persistent expression of the HBV genome (i.e. induction of the carrier state), persistent synthesis of immunoregulatory molecules, progressive cellular attack on hepatocyte auto-antigens and viral antigens and the development of chronic hepatitis.

The role of immune complexes in HBV infection has been studied extensively but it has not been possible to show that they are responsible for liver cell damage (Gocke, 1978). Immune complexes appear to be involved in the pathogenesis of several extrahepatic manifestations such as the arthritis-dermatitis syndrome (Gocke and MacIntosh, 1973), arthritis associated with chronic active hepatitis (Wands *et al.*, 1975), a form of polyarteritis nodosa (Gocke *et al.*, 1971) and a type of glomerulonephritis (Ozawa, 1976).

C. Laboratory Diagnosis

The most common means of confirming a clinical diagnosis of hepatitis B is to detect HBsAg in the serum during the acute phase of the disease. Although most people do not seek medical attention until either their urine becomes dark or they are recognized to be jaundiced, HBsAg can usually be detected. If the patient is retested at weekly intervals the titre of HBsAg will be found to decline and eventually disappear. If the patient is seen relatively early it may be possible to detect a rising titre of anti-HBc in specimens collected 7–10 days apart. Tests for anti-HBc specific IgM are under development.

A wide variety of techniques are available for detecting HBsAg, anti-HBs and anti-HBc. For the detection of HBsAg the most sensitive specific methods at present are solid-phase radioimmunoassay (Ling and Overby, 1972) and enzyme-linked immunosorbent assay (Wolters *et al.*, 1977). Anti-HBs can be detected by passive haemagglutination (Vyas and Schulman, 1970), radioimmunoprecipitation (Lander *et al.*, 1971), radioimmunoassay (Hollinger *et al.*, 1971) and immune adherence haemagglutination (Mayumi *et al.*, 1971), while the best means of detecting anti-HBc appear to be radioimmunoassay (Purcell *et al.*, 1974) and immune adherence haemagglutination (Tsuda *et al.*, 1975).

D. Epidemiology

Until recently hepatitis B was thought to be a modern disease associated with techniques such as immunization and blood transfusion. However, the detection of high rates of infection amongst isolated population groups who have been largely insulated from contact with western civilization (Woodfield *et al.*, 1972) suggest that the disease is an ancient one. See also Black, this volume. Evidence of infection with HBV has been detected in every population studied to date but the prevalence varies widely. In some countries, e.g. Australia, Great

Britain and Scandinavia, infection is uncommon, whereas in others, e.g. Japan and Thailand, almost every person shows serological evidence of current or past infection (Szmuness, 1975). The prevalence of infection depends upon a complex mix of behavioural, environmental and host factors: in general it is low in developed countries and high in developing countries, particularly those with tropical or subtropical climates. In every population survival of the virus is ensured by the existence of a reservoir of chronic carriers estimated to total between 120–150 million (Szmuness, 1975). Carrier rates vary widely and are generally low in developed countries but may be as high as 15% or more in certain developing countries (Cossart, 1977).

In some developing countries, HBV is hyperendemic and virtually every person is infected early in life. Under these circumstances the carrier rate is usually highest amongst children and young adults and declines with increasing age, suggesting that a proportion of chronic carriers eventually clear the virus from their body.

Considerable differences may exist in the infection rate and carrier rate amongst ethnic groups living in the same area. The most striking differences are found amongst the Melanesian and Indian populations in Fiji (Gust *et al.*, 1979b). Among the former, more than 50% show evidence of infection and the carrier rate is in excess of 12%. By contrast only 10% of the Indian population show serological evidence of infection and the carrier rate is less than 1%. Whether these differences represent genetic differences in susceptibility to infection or environmental and behavioural differences which affect the rate of exposure to the virus is uncertain. Similar differences exist in developed countries; e.g.in Australia while the infection rate in the general population is extremely low, higher rates exist amongst migrants, Aborigines and drug users (Gust and Dimitrakakis, 1978).

In countries in which infection with HBV is relatively uncommon, the highest prevalence of HBsAg is found among the 20–40 year age group and the prevalence of anti-HBs and anti-HBc rises gradually with age. In many developed countries the incidence of hepatitis B is increasing steadily, e.g. in the United States the number of cases reported per year rose from 1497 in 1966 to 14 973 in 1976, representing an increase in incidence from 1·79 to 7·14 per 100 000 population (CDC Report, 1978). Similar trends have been reported in Australia (Gust *et al.*, 1980) and in Sweden (Magnius *et al.*, 1973) and appear to be largely due to the increase in illicit intravenous drug use in these countries.

E. Mode of Spread

The precise mode of acquisition of most infections with HBV is unknown. In most cases infection probably results from blood-borne virus being inoculated through the skin or mucous membrane, although the way in which this occurs varies from country to country and from group to group.

In developed countries hepatitis B has traditionally been a hazard of blood transfusion, the use of shared syringes and exposure to large amounts of potentially infected blood. For these reasons high rates of infection occur in certain occupational groups such as dentists (Feldmann and Schiff, 1973), staff and patients in dialysis units (Drucker *et al.*, 1968), biochemists and haematologists (Lo Grippo and Hayashi, 1973). There is good evidence that the majority of infections with HBV are subclinical and that the severity of the symptoms produced is related to the age of the subject and the infectious dose.

Transmission can occur in the family setting and tends to be related to the degree of crowding of the household and the intimacy of each person to the case or carrier. The way in which transmission occurs is not known. It has been suggested that it may involve accidental percutaneous inoculation following the use of shared razors, tooth brushes, bath brushes or towels. On the other hand contact infection is clearly also important. HBV has been detected in a variety of body secretions and excretions, including saliva (Ward *et al.*, 1972), semen (Goldberg *et al.*, 1974) and vaginal fluid (Mazzur, 1973), so that infection may be transmitted by kissing or by sexual intercourse. The possibility of venereal transmission is strengthened by the observation that persons with a wide range of sexual contacts, such as prostitutes (Papaevangelou *et al.*, 1974) and male homosexuals (Vahrmann, 1973) have a higher than expected rate of seropositivity.

Hepatitis B does not appear to be transmitted faecal-orally and urine is probably not infectious unless contaminated with blood. Droplet spread of the disease has also been postulated, and while HBsAg has been detected in some sneeze samples there is currently no convincing evidence that air borne infections occur.

By far the most important factor in determining infectivity is the presence or absence of HBeAg: patients whose blood contains HBeAg have a much higher chance of infecting their close contacts (Okada *et al.*, 1976; Shikata *et al.*, 1977) than do those in whom HBeAg cannot be detected.

The high prevalence of hepatitis B infection in many tropical countries led to the suggestion that mosquitoes and other bloodsucking insects, such as bedbugs, might be important in transmission of the disease. HBsAg has been detected in several species of insects (Brotman *et al.*, 1973) but there is no convincing evidence that replication occurs (Prince *et al.*, 1972). While the possibility of mechanical transmission exists, several studies have failed to demonstrate an association between mosquito activity and prevalence of HBsAg or anti-HBs (Hawkes *et al.*, 1972) and vastly different rates of infection have been observed between different ethnic groups living in areas of comparable mosquito activity (Simons *et al.*, 1972; Gust *et al.*, 1979b).

Transmission of HBV from chronic carrier mothers to their babies appears to be the single most important factor in determining the prevalence of HBV infection in some areas. The risk of infection depends upon the proportion of HBeAg-positive carrier mothers, and while low in some countries may be as high as 40 % in others (Stevens *et al.*, 1975). Infection of the baby is usually anicteric (Schweitzer *et al.*, 1973) and is recognized by the appearance of HBsAg 60–120 days after birth. Most children infected in this way become chronic carriers of the virus.

The mechanism of infection is uncertain: although HBV can infect the fetus *in utero*, this rarely happens and most infections appear to occur at birth either due to a leak of maternal blood into the baby's circulation, ingestion or accidental inoculation. Studies are in progress to determine whether administration of immune globulin shortly after birth will protect the baby from infection (Kohler *et al.*, 1974; Beasley and Stevens, 1978).

F. Isolation

Despite earlier claims (Jenson *et al.*, 1970; Brighton *et al.*, 1971; Carver and Seto, 1971; Watanabe *et al.*, 1976) the hepatitis B virus has not been successfully isolated in cell culture, although a chronically infected cell line has been derived which produces limited amounts of HBsAg *in vitro* (MacNab *et al.*, 1976).

Recently a major advance occurred with the insertion of DNA extracted from Dane particles into *Escherichia coli* plasmid PBR 322 (Burrell *et al.*, 1979). It has proved possible to clone the DNA and to identify cells which are synthesizing HBcAg and HBsAg. This work may make it possible to develop vaccines against HBV without the traditional need to grow the virus in cell culture.

G. Prevention and Control

1 General
In developed countries the incidence of infection with HBV can be greatly reduced by avoiding exposure to potentially contaminated blood. The rate of post-transfusion hepatitis has been reduced dramatically by assaying all blood intended for transfusion for HBsAg (Koretz *et al.*, 1975; Tateda *et al.*, 1979) and this procedure coupled with regular screening of patients and staff and improved attention to general hygiene has reduced the incidence of hepatitis B in dialysis units (PHLS Survey, 1976).

2 Immunization
(a) *Passive* Passive immunization, using immune serum globulin prepared in developed countries, has been used for the prevention of hepatitis B but the results have been disappointing, presumably because many preparations contained low titres of antibody (Duncan *et al.*, 1947; Holland *et al.*, 1966).

A number of batches of hyperimmune hepatitis B globulin have been produced which contain high titres of anti-HBs. These preparations, which are expensive and in relatively short supply, have been evaluated for both pre- and post-exposure prophylaxis of HBV with conflicting results (CDC Report, 1978). At present their major use is in the management of medical or paramedical personnel who have been accidentally contaminated or inoculated with infectious blood.

(b) *Active* Despite the fact that HBV has not been isolated in cell culture, several vaccines have been produced utilizing the serum of chronic carriers of the disease as a source of antigen. At present three different approaches are being used by workers in several countries.

(i) *Subunit Vaccines.* Subunit vaccines take advantage of the fact that the serum of chronic carriers of HBV may contain from 10^{10}–10^{12} 22 nm particles per ml and that these particles, while non-infectious, carry HBsAg on their surface and can be purified by a variety of biophysical and biochemical techniques. Vaccines produced in this way are usually treated with heat and/or formalin to destroy any residual virus and tested in chimpanzees.

Several batches of vaccine have been produced in the United States and France and these have been shown to be safe, antigenic and effective in chimpanzees (Dreesman *et al.*, 1975; Hilleman *et al.*, 1975; Purcell *et al.*, 1975; Maupas *et al.*, 1976; Reesink *et al.*, 1976). Once the safety of these vaccines has been established in man efficacy studies will be carried out in high risk populations in whom greatest potential benefit can be anticipated, e.g. haemodialysis patients and staff, medical and health care personnel, contacts of patients with acute viral hepatitis or chronic carriers. One study has been in progress for two years (Maupas *et al.*, 1978) and the results are encouraging.

(ii) *Polypeptide Vaccines.* HBsAg is composed of a number of proteins and glycoproteins of which only two are antigenic. Purified preparations of these components have been produced which are safe, antigenic and effective in protecting chimpanzees from infection (Dreesman *et al.*, 1975; Hollinger *et al.*, 1978a). It is currently difficult to see how such a vaccine could be made in commercial quantities, as the yield of vaccine per unit of blood is extremely low and its antigenicity poor.

Despite the pace of development of HBV vaccines, certain problems still remain unresolved. These include the current inability to ensure that vaccines made from the blood of chronic carriers does not also contain the agent or agents of non-A non-B hepatitis, limits to the quantity of high titre antigen positive blood from which to make vaccine, and uncertainty as to the best method of removing residual infectivity. Recombinant DNA technology provides a possible solution to these problems and has opened the door to the possibility of developing synthetic vaccines.

(c) *Antiviral Chemotherapy* In the past two or three years there has been considerable interest in the use of interferon and antiviral substances to treat chronic carriers of HBV, particularly those with unremitting liver disease.

It has been demonstrated that high doses of human lymphocyte and human fibroblast interferon can reduce and occasionally eradicate all evidence of infection (Desmyter *et al.*, 1976; Greenberg *et al.*, 1976) although in some patients these changes were reversed once treatment ceased. Because interferon has side effects such as bone marrow depression, some workers advocate large doses in short bursts to provide intervals for bone marrow recovery to take place.

Recently several groups have been investigating the use of adenine-arabinoside, an antiviral agent which interferes with DNA synthesis, with promising results (Bassendine *et al.*, 1978; Pollard *et al.*, 1978). The recent detection of a virus closely related to HBV which causes a natural infection in woodchucks may provide a system in which such agents can be screened.

H. Future Developments

The major unresolved areas in the study of hepatitis B are the precise mode of transmission of the disease and the optimal way of interrupting it. As HBV appears to be exclusively an infection of man, it is theoretically possible to eradicate provided it proves possible to produce large quantities of a safe, stable, cheap, effective vaccine and to devise a method of interrupting transmission from carrier mothers to their babies.

As chronic infection with HBV appears to be an important factor in the development of hepatocellular carcinoma in some countries it should be possible to reduce considerably the incidence of this disease by mass immunization, although the results may take many years to become apparent.

IV. Non-A Non-B Hepatitis

The idea that human hepatitis exists in only two forms stems from a series of studies carried out in human volunteers more that 20 years ago. While these studies clearly defined two forms of the disease, evidence of the existence of other forms was suggested by the observation of three distinct attacks of hepatitis in the same patient (Havens, 1956; Mosely *et al.*, 1977) and the unimodal distribution of incubation periods in patients who developed post-transfusion hepatitis (Mosely, 1975).

The development of sensitive tests which will detect virtually all infections with HAV and HBV has confirmed the existence of another form of the disease which is currently known as non-A and non-B hepatitis.

A. The Virus

The agent or agents responsible for non-A and non-B hepatitis have not been identified although there have been a number of encouraging reports. Recently Bradley *et al.* (1979a) transmitted the disease to colony-born chimpanzees with three different inocula and identified 25–35 nm virus-like particles in the liver of one animal and similar particles in one of the inocula. These results have not been confirmed nor has convincing evidence been obtained that patients develop antibody to the particles when they recover from the disease. Particles of differing size and shape have been visualized in the serum of patients with non-B hepatitis (Cossart *et al.*, 1975) but none satisfies the rigid criteria required for declaring it an aetiological agent. The consistent failure of the best laboratories in the world to identify the non-A non-B agent has led our group and others to re-examine the assumptions upon which most of the current studies rely. The suggestion has been made that the agent or agents involved may not be conventional viruses but subviral transmissible agents (? viroids) comprised of a short strand of low molecular weight nucleic acid which would not be detected by conventional virological and immunological techniques.

B. Pathogenesis

What little information is available on the pathogenesis of non-A non-B hepatitis has been obtained from prospective studies of transfusion-associated hepatitis (Aach *et al.*, 1978; Alter *et al.*, 1978a; Seef *et al.*, 1978) and limited studies in experimentally infected chimpanzees (Alter *et al.*, 1978b; Hollinger *et al.*, 1978b; Tabor *et al.*, 1978; Bradley *et al.*,1979a) The agent appears to be present in the blood prior to the onset of symptoms and for some weeks later. There is also evidence to suggest that a proportion of infections are followed by development of a carrier state and that a significant number of those infected develop prolonged abnormalities of liver function and disturbances of liver histology consistent with chronic active hepatitis (Berman *et al.*, 1979).

C. Laboratory Diagnosis

As no specific laboratory tests exist, the diagnosis of non-A non-B hepatitis is one of exclusion. A patient is regarded as having this disease if he has no serological evidence of recent infection with hepatitis A, hepatitis B, cytomegalovirus or Epstein-Barr virus.

Several non-specific markers of infection have been described, including elevated levels of antibody to single-stranded DNA (Villarejos *et al.*, 1978) or serum alanine aminotransferase (Aach *et al.*, 1978) or the presence of characteristic antigens in the serum (Shirachi *et al.*, 1978) or liver (Kabiri *et al.*, 1979). To date, none of these methods has proved capable of detecting all non-A non-B infections.

D. Epidemiology

Quite a lot is known of the epidemiology of non-A non-B hepatitis (Purcell *et al.*, 1976) through studies of patients developing post-transfusion hepatitis. The disease was first recognized in this setting (Prince *et al.*, 1974; Feinstone *et al.*, 1975) and is now the major cause of post-transfusion hepatitis in countries which exclude HBsAg-positive donors. In both the United States and Japan more than 85% of episodes of post-transfusion hepatitis are currently non-A non-B, although the disease is usually so mild that most cases would be missed in the absence of prospective studies (Aach *et al.*, 1978; Alter *et al.*, 1978a; Seef *et al.*, 1978; Tateda *et al.*, 1979). Chronic carriers of non-A non-B hepatitis have been identified and there is some evidence to suggest that they are more numerous than carriers of HBV.

Outbreaks of non-A non-B hepatitis have been reported after administration of certain clotting factors (Craske *et al.*, 1975; Wyke *et al.*, 1979) prepared from pooled human plasma and amongst intravenous drug users. The disease is a particular problem in this group and may account for 50% of all episodes of hepatitis (Gust *et al.*, 1978c).

In addition, non-A non-B hepatitis has been shown to be responsible for from 6% up to 25% of sporadic hepatitis in every population which has been studied, although the way in which the disease is acquired is not known.

The incubation period of non-A non-B hepatitis ranges from 2–25 weeks (Aach *et al.*, 1978; Alter *et al.*, 1978a; Hruby and Schauf 1978; Seef *et al.*, 1978) with a mean of about 8 weeks: at least one study has demonstrated a bimodal distribution suggesting that two different aetiological agents may be involved.

E. Mode of Spread

Little is known about the mode of spread of the disease other than the blood of cases or carriers is highly infectious and that clinical infection appears to be uncommon among close contacts.

F. Isolation

Non-A non-B hepatitis has been transmitted to colony-born chimpanzees with a variety of inocula, including blood from acutely and chronically infected individuals and batches of factor VIII and factor IX concentrate (Alter *et al.*, 1978b; Hollinger *et al.*, 1978a; Tabor *et al.*, 1978; Bradley *et al.*, 1979a; Wyke *et al.*, 1979). In general the disease in chimpanzees is extremely mild, often biphasic and has a slightly longer incubation period than in man. Among chimpanzees infected at the National Institutes of Health, two patterns of liver cell damage have been detected by electron microscopy, which may be the manifestations of two different aetiological agents (Shimizu, 1979). There are reports that the disease can also be transmitted to marmosets but these are as yet unconfirmed.

G. Prevention and Control

Control of non-A non-B hepatitis remains a problem. The frequency of post-transfusion hepatitis can be reduced by eliminating commercial blood donors and donors with elevated levels of alanine aminotransferase; however, in some countries this would severely compromise the supply of fresh blood. Immune serum globulin has been used with equivocal results. It would seem certain that no major progress will be made in controlling non-A non-B hepatitis until specific laboratory tests are developed for the aetiological agents.

References

Aach, R. D., Lander, J. J., Sherman, L. A., Miller, W. Y., Kahn, R. A., Gitnick, G. L., Hollinger, F. B., Werch, J., Szmuness, W., Stevens, C. E., Kellner, A., Weiner, J. M. and Mosely, J. W. (1978). *In* "Viral Hepatitis" (G. N., Vyas, S. N. Cohen, and R. Schmid, Eds), 383–396. Franklin Institute Press, Philadelphia.

Almeida, J. D., Rubenstein, D. and Stott, E. J. (1971). *Lancet* ii, 1225–1227.

Alter, H. J., Purcell, R. H., Feinstone, S. M., Holland, P. V. and Morrow, A. G. (1978a). *In* "Viral Hepatitis" (G. N. Cohen, S. N. Cohen, and R. Schmid, Eds), 359–369. Franklin Institute Press, Philadelphia.

Alter, H. J., Purcell, R. H., Holland, P. V. and Popper, H. (1978b). *Lancet* i, 459–463.

Barker, L. F., Chisari, F. V., McGrath, P. P., Dalgard, D. W., Kirchstein, R. L., Almeida, J. D., Edgington, T. S., Sharp, D. G. and Peterson, M. R. (1973). *J. infect. Dis.* **127**, 648–662.

Barker, L. F., Almeida, J. D., Hoofnagle, J. H., Gerety, R. J., Jackson, D. R. and McGrath, P. P. (1974). *J. Virol.* **14**, 1552–1558.

Bassendine, M. F., Chadwick, R. G., Crawford, E. M., Thomas, H. C. and Sherlock, S. (1978). *In* "Viral Hepatitis" (G. N. Vyas, R. N. Cohen and R. Schmid, Eds), 728. Franklin Institute Press, Philadelphia.

Bayer, M. E., Blumberg, B. S. and Werner, B. G. (1968). *Nature, Lond.* **218**, 1057–1059.

Beasley, R. P. and Stevens, C. E. (1978). *In* "Viral Hepatitis" (G. N. Vyas, R. N. Cohen and R. Schmid, Eds), 333–345. Franklin Institute Press, Philadelphia.

Bergstrand, H. (1930). "Uber die Akute und Chronische Gelbe Lebartrophie". Thieme, Leipzig.

Berman, M., Alter, H. J., Ishak, K. G., Purcell, R. H. and Jones, E. A. (1979). *Ann. intern. Med.* **91**, 1–6.

Blumberg, B. S., Alter, H. J. and Visnich, S. (1965). *J. Am. med. Ass.* **191**, 541–546.

Bradley, D. W., Maynard, J. M., Hindman, S. H., Hornbeck, C. L., Fields, H. A., McCaustland, K. A. and Cook, E. J. (1977). *J. clin. Microbiol.* **5**, 521–530.
Bradley, D. W., Cook, E. H., Maynard, J. E., McCaustland, K. A., Ebert, J. W., Dolana, G. H., Petyel, R. A., Kenton, R. J., Heilbrun, A., Fields, H. A. and Murphy, B. L. (1979a). *J. med. Virol.* **3**, 253–269.
Bradley, D. W., Fields, H. A., McCaustland, K. A., Maynard, J. E., Becker, R. H., Whittington, R. and Overby, L. R. (1979b). *J. clin. Microbiol.* **9**, 120–127.
Brighton, W. D., Taylor, P. E. and Zuckerman, A. J. (1971). *Nature, Lond.* 232, 57–58.
Brotman, B., Prince, A. M. and Godfrey, H. R. (1973). *Lancet* i, 1305–1308.
Burrell, C. J., MacKay, P., Greenaway, P. J., Hofschneider, P. H. and Murray, K. (1979). *Nature, Lond.* 279, 43–47.
Carver, D. H. and Seto, D. S. Y. (1971). *Science, N.Y.* **172**, 1265–1267.
Centre for Disease Control. (1978). *Hepatitis Surveillance Report* No. 42, 1–44.
Chalmers, T. C., Grady, G., Koff, R. S., Peterson, J. L. and Muench, H. M. (1967). *In* "The Liver" (A. E. Read.), 155, Butterworth, London.
Chisari, F. V., Routenberg, J. A., Anderson, D. S. and Edgington, T. S. (1978). *In* "Viral Hepatitis" (G. W. Vyas, R. N. Cohen and R. Schmid, Eds), 245–263. Franklin Institute Press, Philadelphia.
Cockayne, E. A. (1912). Q. Jl Med. **6**, 1.
Coulepis, A. G., Locarnini, S. A., Ferris, A. A., Lehmann, N. I. and Gust, I. D. (1978). *Intervirology* **10**, 24–31.
Coulepis, A. G., Locarnini, S. A., Lehmann, N. I. and Gust, I. D. (1980). *J. infect. Dis* **141**, 151–156.
Cossart, Y. E., Field, A. M., Cant, B. and Widdows, D. (1975). *Lancet* i, 72–73.
Cossart, Y. E. (1977). *In* "Viral Hepatitis and Its Control", 106–118. Baillière Tindall, London.
Craske, J., Dilling, N. and Stern, D. (1975). *Lancet* ii, 221–223.
Dane, D. S., Cameron, C. H. and Briggs, M. (1970). *Lancet* i, 695–698.
Desmyter, J., Ray, M. B., De Groote, J., Bradburne, A. F., Desmet, V. J., Edy, V. G., Billian, A., De-Somer, P. and Mortelmans, J. (1976). *Lancet* ii, 645–647.
Dienstag, J. L., Feinstone, S. M., Kapikian, A. Z., Purcell, R. H., Boggs, J. D. and Conrad, M. E. (1975a). *Lancet* i, 765–767.
Dienstag, J. J., Feinstone, S. M., Purcell, R. H., Hoofnagle, J. H., Barker, L. F., London, W. T., Poppper, H., Peterson, J. M. and Kapikian, A. Z. (1975b). *J. infect. Dis.* **132**, 532–545.
Dienstag, J. L., Routenberg, J. A., Purcell, R. H., Hasper, R. R. and Harrison, W. O. (1975c). *Ann. intern. Med.* **83**, 647–650.
Dienstag, J. L., Gust, I. D., Lucas, C. R., Wong, D. C. and Pucell, R. H. (1976). *Lancet* i, 561–564.
Dreesman, G. R., Chariez, R., Saurez, M., Hollinger, F. B., Coutney, R. J. and Melnick, J. L. (1975). *J. Virol.* **16**, 508–515.
Drucker, W., Jungerius, N. A. and Alberts, C. (1968). "Proceedings of the

European Dialysis and Transplant Association, IV International Congress Series", 131, 90. Excerpta Medica, Amsterdam.
Duncan, G. G., Christian, H. A., Stokes, J., Rexer, W. F., Nicholson, J. T. and Edgar, A. (1947). *Am. J. med. Sci.* **213**, 53–57.
Feinstone, S. M., Kapikian, A. Z., Purcell, R. H. (1973). *Science, N.Y.* 1026–1028.
Feinstone, S. M., Kapikian, A. Z., Purcell, R. H., Alter, H. J. and Holland, P. V. (1975), *New Engl. J. Med.* **292**, 767–770.
Feldmann, R. G. and Schiff, E. R. (1973). *Gastroenterology* **65**, 515–539.
Frösner, G. G., Scheid, R., Wolf, H. and Deinhardt, F. (1979). *J. clin. Microbiol.* **9**, 476–478.
Gocke, D. J., Hsu, K., Morgan, C., Bombardieri, S., Lockshin, M., Christian, C. L. (1971). *J. exp. Med.* **134**, 330–336.
Gocke, D. J. and MacIntosh, R. M. (1973). *Gastroenterology* **65**, 542.
Gocke, D. J. (1978). *In* "Viral Hepatitis" (G. N. Vyas, R. N. Cohen, and R. Schmid, Eds), 277–283. Franklin Institute Press Philadelphia.
Goldberg, S. J., Linnaman, C. L. and Connell, A. M. (1974). *Gastroenterology* **66**, 702.
Gravelle, C. R., Hornbeck, C. L., Maynard, J. E., Schable, C. A., Cook, E. A. and Bradley, D. W. (1975). *J. infect. Dis.* **131**, 167–171.
Greenberg, H. B., Pollard, R. B., Lutwick, L. I., Gregory, P. B., Robinson, W. S. and Merrigan, T. C. (1976). *New Engl. J. Med.* **295**, 517–528.
Gust, I. D. and Dimitrakakis, M. (1978). *Med. J. Aust.* **1**, 39–40.
Gust, I. D., Lehmann, N. I. and Lucas, C. R. (1978). *J. infect. Inf. Dis.* **138**, 425–426.
Gust, I. D., Lehmann, N. I., Lucas, C. R., Ferris, A. A. and Locarnini, S. A. (1978c). *In* "Viral Hepatitis" (G. N. Vyas, S. N. Cohen and R. Schmid, Eds), 105–112. Franklin Institute Press, Philadelphia.
Gust, I. D., Lehmann, N. I., Dimitrakakis, M. and Zimmet, P. (1979a). *J. infect. Dis.* **139**, 559–563.
Gust, I. E., Lehmann, N. I. and Dimitrakakis, M. (1979b). *Am. J. Epidemiol.* **110**, 237–242.
Gust, I. D., Dimitrakakis, M. and Lucas, C. R. (1980). *Vox Sang.* **38**, 81–86.
Havens, W. P. Jr., Ward, R., Drill, V. A. and Paul, J. R. (1944). *Proc. Soc. exp. Biol. Med.* **57**, 206–208.
Havens, W. P. Jr (1956). *Ann. intern. Med.* **44**, 199–205.
Hawkes, R. A., Vale, T. G., Marshall, I. D. and MacLennan, R. (1972). *Am. J. Epidemiol.* **95**, 228–237.
Hilleman, M. R., Buynak, E. B., Rochm, R. R., Tytell, A. A., Bertland, A. V. and Lampson, G. P. (1975). *Am. J. med. Sci.* **270**. 401–404.
Holland, P. V., Rubinson, R. M., Morrow, A. G. and Schmidt, P. J. (1966). *J. Am. med. Ass.* **196**, 471–474.
Holland, P. V. and Alter, H. J. (1975). *Med. Clins N. Am.* **59**, 849–855.
Hollinger, F. B., Worndam, V. and Dreesman, G. R. (1971). *J. Immunol.* **107**, 1099–1111.
Hollinger, F. B., Dreesman, G. R., Sanchez, Y., Cabral, G. A. and Melnick, J.

L. (1978a). *In* "Viral Hepatitis' (G. N. Vyas, R. N. Cohen and R. Schmid, Eds), 557–567. Franklin Institute Press, Philadelphia.
Hollinger, F. B., Gitnick, G. L., Aach, R. D., Szmuness, W., Mosley, J. W., Stevens, C. E., Peters, R. L., Weiner, J. M., Werch, J. B. and Lander, J. J. (1978b). *Intervirology* **10**, 60–68.
Hoofnagle, J. H., Gerety, R. J. and Barker, L. F. (1973). *Lancet* ii, 869–873.
Hruby, M. A. and Schauf, V. (1978). *J. Am. med. Ass.* **240**, 1355–1357.
Jenson, A. B., McCombs, R. M., Sakurada, N. and Melnick, J. L. (1970). *Exptl molec. Path.* **13**, 217–230.
Kabiri, M., Tabor, E. and Gerety, R. J. (1979). *Lancet* ii, 221–224.
Kaplan, P. M., Greeman, R. L., Gerin, J. L., Purcell, R. H. and Robinson, W. S. (1973). *J. Virol.* **12**, 995–1005.
Kendrick, M. A. (1972). *J. infect. Dis.* **126**, 684–685.
Kendrick, M. A. (1974). *J. infect. Dis.* **129**, 227–229.
Koff, R. S. and Sear, H. S. (1967). *New Engl. J. Med.* **276**, 737–739.
Kohler, P. F., Dubois, R. S., Merrill, D. A. and Bowes, W. A. (1974). *New Engl. J. Med.* **291**, 1378–1380.
Koretz, R. L., Gitnick, G. L., Mitchell, J. G., Damus, H., Ritman, S. G., Golub, L. and Kash, P. L. (1975). *Am. J. Med.* **59**, 754–760.
Krugman, S., Ward, R., Giles, J. P., Bodansky, O., Milton Jacobs, A. (1959). *New Engl. J. Med.* **261**, 729–734.
Krugman, S., Ward, R. and Giles, J. P. (1962). *Am. J. Med.* **32**, 717–728.
Krugman, S., Ward, R. and Giles, J. P. (1965). *In* "Perspectives in Virology III" (M. Pollard, Ed.), 159. Harper and Row, New York.
Krugman, S., Giles, J. P. and Hammond, J. (1967). *J. Am. med. Ass.* **200**, 365–373.
Lander, J. J., Alter, J. H. and Purcell, R. H. (1971). *J. Immunol.* **106**, 1166–1171.
Lander, J. J., Holland, P. V., Alter, H. J., Chanock, R. M. and Purcell, R. H. (1972). *J. Am med. Ass.* **220**, 1079–1082.
Ling, C. M. and Overby, C. R. (1972). *J. Immunol.* **109**, 234–841.
Locarnini, S. A., Ferris, A. A., Stott, A. C. and Gust, I. D. (1974). *Intervirology* **4**, 110–118.
Locarnini, S. A., Gust, I. D., Ferris, A. A., Stott, A. C. and Wong, M. L. (1976). *Bull. Wld Hlth Org.* **54**, 199–206.
Locarnini, S. A., Ferris, A. A., Lehmann, N. I. and Gust, I. D. (1977). *Intervirology* **8**, 309–318.
Locarnini, S. A., Coulepis, A. G., Stratton, A. M., Kaldor, J. and Gust, I. D. (1979). *J. clin. Microbiol.* **9**, 459–465.
Lo Grippo, G. A. and Hayashi, H. (1973). *Health Lab. Sci.* **10**, 157.
London, W. T., Alter, H. J., Lander, J. J. and Purcell, R. H. (1972). *J. infect. Dis.* **125**, 382–389.
Lürman, A. (1885). *Berl. Klin. Wschr.* **22**, 20–23.
MacCallum, F. O. and Bradley, W. G. (1944). *Lancet* ii, 228.
MacNab, G. M., Alexander, J. J., Lacatsas, G., Bey, E. M. and Urbanowicz, J. M. (1976). *Br. J. Cancer* **34**, 509–515.

Magnius, L. O. and Espmark, J. A. (1972). *Acta Path. microbiol. scan.* (B) **80**, 335–337.
Magnius, L., Berg, R., Bjorvatn, B. and Svedmyr, A. (1973). *Scand. J. infect. Dis.* **5**, 81–83.
Mascoli, C. C., Ittensohn, D. L., Villarejos, V. M., Arquedas, J. A., Provost, P. J. and Hilleman, M. R. (1973). *Proc. Soc. exp. Biol. Med.* **142**, 276–282.
Maupas, P., Goudeau, A., Coursaget, P., Drucker, J. and Bagros, P. (1976). *Lancet* i, 1367–1370.
Maupas, P., Goudeau, A., Coursaget, P. Drucker, J. and Bagros, P. (1978). *Intervirology* **10**, 196–208.
Maynard, J. E., Berquist, K. R., Druishak, D. H. and Purcell, R. H. (1972). *Nature, Lond.* **237**, 514–515.
Mayumi, M., Okochi, K. and Nishioka, K. (1971). *Vox Sang.* **20**, 178–181.
Mazzur, S. (1973). *Lancet* i, 789.
Melnick, J. L. (1957). *In* "Hepatitis Frontiers". Little Brown, Boston, Mass.
Mosely, J. W. (1959). *New Engl. J. Med.* **261**, 748–753.
Mosely, J. W. (1975). *Amer. J. med. Sci.* **270**, 253–270.
Mosely, J. W., Redecker, A. G., Feinstone, S. M. and Purcell, R. H. (1977). *New Engl. J. Med.* **296**, 75–78.
Murray, R. (1955). *Bull N.Y. Acad. Med.* **31**, 341–358.
O'Donnell, B. and Cowley, W. J. (1966). *Med. Offr* **115**, 291.
Okada, K., Kamiyama, I., Inomata, M., Imai, M., Miyakawa, Y. and Mayumi, M. (1976). *New Engl. J. Med.* **294**, 746–749.
Okochi, K. and Murakami, S. (1968). *Vox Sang.* **15**, 374–385.
Ozawa, T., Levinsohn, P., Orsini, E. and McIntosh, R. M. (1976). *Archs Path. lab. Med.* **100**, 484–486.
Papaevangelou, G., Trichopoulas, D., Kremastinou, T. and Papoutsakis, G. (1974). *Br. med. J.* **2**, 256–258.
Paul, J. R., Havens, W. P. Jr., Sabin, A. B. and Phillip, C. B. (1945). *J. Am. med. Ass.* **128**, 911–915.
Pollard, R. B., Smith, J. C., Neal, E. A., Gregory, F. B., Merrigan, T. C. and Robinson, W. S. (1978). *J. Am. med. Ass.* **239**, 1648–1650.
Prince, A. M. (1968). *Proc. natn. Acad. Sci.* U.S.A. **60**, 814–821.
Prince, A. M., Metselaar, D., Kafuko, G. W., Mukwaya, L. G., Ling, C. M. and Overby, L. R. (1972). *Lancet* ii, 247–250.
Prince, A. M., Brotman, B., Grady, G. F., Kuhns, W. J., Hazzi, C., Levine, R. W. and Millian, S. J. (1974). *Lancet* ii, 241–246.
Provost, P. J., Ittensohn, O. L., Villarejos, V. M., Arquedas, J. A. and Hilleman, M. R. (1973). *Proc. Soc. exp. Biol. Med.* **142**, 1257–1267.
Provost, P. J., Ittensohn, D. L., Villarejos, V. M. and Hilleman, M. R. (1975a). *Proc. Soc. exp. Biol. Med.* **148**, 962–969.
Provost, P. J., Wolenski, B. S., Miller, W. J., Ittensohn, O. L., McAleer, W. J. and Hilleman, M. R. (1975b). *Proc. Soc. exp. Biol. Med.* **148**, 532–539.
Provost, P. J. and Hilleman, M. R. (1978). *Proc. Soc. exp. Biol. Med.* **159**, 201–203.

Provost, P. J. and Hilleman, M. R. (1979). *Proc. Soc. exp. Biol. Med.* **160**, 213–221.
Public Health Laboratory Service Survey (1976). *Br. med. J.* i, 1579–1581.
Purcell, R. H., Gerin, J. L., Almeida, J. B. and Holland, P. V. (1974). *Intervirology.* **2**, 231–243.
Purcell, R. H., Dienstag, J. L., Feinstone, S. M. and Kapikian, A. Z. (1975). *Am. J. med. Sci.* **270**, 60–71.
Purcell, R. H. and Gerin, J. L. (1975). *Am. J. med. Sci.* **270**, 395–399.
Purcell, R. H., Alter, H. J. and Deinstag, J. L. (1976). *Yale, J. Biol. Med.* **49**, 243–250.
Reesink, H. W., Van Elven, E. H., Brummelhuis, H. J. G. (1976). "17th Congress of the German Society for Blood Transfusion and Immunohaematology", Vol 3, 119–139.
Reid, D. (1971). *Post. Grad. Med. J.* **47**, 488–489.
Robinson, W. S., Clayton, D. A. and Greeman, R. L. (1974). *J. Virol.* **14**, 384–391.
Schulman, A. N., Deinstag, J. L., Jackson, D. R., Hoofnagle, J. H., Gerety, R. J., Purcell, R. H. and Barker, L. F. (1976). *J. infect. Dis.* **134**, 80–84.
Schweitzer, I. L., Dunn, A. E. G., Peters, R. L. and Spears, R. L. (1973). *Am. J. Med.* **55**, 762–771.
Seef, L. B., Wright, E. C., Zimmerman, H. J., Hoofnagle, J. H., Dietz, A. A., Felsher, B. F., Garcia-Pont, P. H., Gerety, R. J., Greenlee, H. B., Kernan, T., Leevy, C. M., Nath, N., Schiff, E. R., Schwartz, C., Tabor, E., Tambuno, C., Vlahcevic, Z., Zemel, R. and Zimmon, D. S. (1978). *In* "Viral Hepatitis" (G. N. Vyas, S. N. Cohen, and R. Schmid, Eds), 371–381. Franklin Institute Press, Philadelphia.
Shikata, T., Karasawa, T., Abe, K., Uzawa, T., Sunzuki, H., Oda, T., Imai, M., Mayumi, M. and Moritsigu, Y. (1977). *J. infect. Dis.* **136**, 571–576.
Shimizu, Y., Feinstone, S. M., Purcell, R. H., Alter, H. J. and Condon, W. T. (1979). *Science, N.Y.* **205**, 197–199.
Shirachi, R., Shiraishi, H., Tateda, A., Kikuchi, H. and Ishida, N. (1978). *Lancet* ii, 853–856.
Siegl, G. and Frösner, G. G. (1978). *J. Virol.* **26**, 48–53.
Simons, M. J., Yap, E. H., Ong, Y. W., Okochi, K., Mayumi, M. and Nishioka, K. (1972). *Am. J. Dis. Child.* **123**, 405–407.
Stevens, C. E., Beasley, R. P., Tsui, J. and Lee, W. C. (1975). *New Engl. J. Med.* **292**, 771–774.
Stokes, J., Berk, J. E. and Leonard, L. (1954). *J. Am. Med. Ass.* **154**, 1059–1065.
Summers, J. *et al.* Reported by London, W. T. (1978). *In* "Viral Hepatitis" (G. N. Vyas, S. N. Cohen and R. Schmid, Eds), 455–458. Franklin Institute Press, Philadelphia.
Szmuness, W. J. (1975). *Amer. J. Path.* **81**, 629–649.
Tabor, E., Gerety, R. J., Drucker, J. A., Seef, L. B., Hoofnagle, J. H., Jackson, D. R., April, M., Barker, L. F. and Pineda-Tamoudong, G. (1978). *Lancet* i, 463–566.

Tateda, A., Kikuchi, K., Numazaki, Y., Shirachi, R. and Ishida, N. (1979). *J. infect. Dis.* **139**, 511–518.
Tsuda, F., Takahashi, T., Takahashi, K., Miyakawa, Y. and Mayumi, M. (1975). *J. Immunol.* **115**, 834–838.
Vahrmann, J. (1973). *Lancet* **ii**, 157.
Villarejos, V. M., Provost, P. J., Ittensohn, O. L., McLean, A. A. and Hilleman, M. R. (1976). *Proc. Soc. exp. Biol. Med.* **452**, 524–528.
Villarejos, V. M., Arquembourg, P. C., Visona, K. Agnol. Outierrez (1978). *J. med. Virol.* **2**, 359–367.
Vitarana, T., Kanapathipillai, M., Gunasekera, H. D. N., Lehmann, N. I., Dimitrakakis, M. and Gust, I. D. (1978). *Asian J. infect. Dis.* **2**, 247–252.
Vyas, G. N. and Schulman, N. R. (1970). *Science, N.Y.* **170**, 332–333.
Wallace, J. M. (1966). *Med. Offr* **116**, 282.
Wands, J. R., Alpert, E. and Issenbacher, K. J. (1975). *Gastroenterology* **69**, 1286–1291.
Ward, R., Krugman, S., Giles, J. P., Bodansky, O., Milton Jacobs, A. (1958). *New Engl. J. Med.* **258**, 407–416.
Ward, R., Berchert, P., Wright, A. and Kline, E. (1972). *Lancet* ii, 726–727.
Watanabe, M., Umenai, T., Ohori, H. and Ishida, N. (1976). *Br. J. exp. Path.* **57**, 211–216.
Wolters, G., Knijfers, L. P. C., Kacaki, J. and Schuurs, A. H. W. M. (1977). *J. infect. Dis.* **136**, S311–S317.
Woodfield, D. G., Oraka, R. E. and Nelson, M. (1972). *Med. J. Aust.* **2**, 469–472.
Wyke, R. J., Tsiguaye, K. N., Thornton, A., White, Y., Portmann, B., Das, P. K., Zuckerman, A. J. and Williams, R. (1979). *Lancet* i, 520–524.
Yarrow, A. (1964). *Lancet* i, 485–487.

7

Severe Measles

David Morley
Institute of Child Health, London, England

Only recently have we learned why measles has become a mild disease in the Western world. We now realize that the change in fatality from the disease came about due to improved nutrition among children. This improvement was largely due to the changes in diet which allowed small children to receive an adequate intake of energy. In the past in Europe and currently in developing countries, children could not receive sufficient energy because of the bulky nature of their diet.

I. Introduction

With few exceptions almost every person born on our planet this century has experienced measles unless immunized against the disease. For most Western-trained doctors and lay people measles is now a mild disease of childhood. For health workers from developing countries measles is the severest of the so-called immunizing diseases of childhood. For the historian, severe measles may come first among the diseases of childhood which did so much to limit population growth until the eighteenth and nineteenth centuries. The nutrition scientist will point to measles as the disease that has declined most rapidly in severity with improved child nutrition. He may go on to suggest that measles vaccination is the most effective public health measure in improving the nutrition of children in the developing world.

II. History of Measles

Illnesses such as the plague are recognized as altering the course of European history. In Europe the effect of measles was subtle in the part it played in the mortality of small children. With our experience from developing countries we can now support earlier writers such as Creighton (1894), who produced evidence that the loss of weight and emaciation associated with measles might be an important cause of mortality. He wrote: "We shall not correctly understand the part played by measles among the infective maladies of children unless we keep the grand character of it in mind—that is, its effect upon the mortality of infancy and childhood are only in part expressed by the deaths actually occurring under its name."

We do not know the early history of measles. Rhazes, born in Khorasan, Persia in A.D. 860, was one of the first writers satisfactorily to separate measles from smallpox. Unfortunately, this confusion continued and among European physicians Thomas Sydenham, an English physician born in 1624, again made the distinction and provided a satisfactory description of the course of illness. Confusion of this nature still exists; for example, in India the goddess responsible for smallpox is Great Mata while that for measles is Little Mata. In the larger populations of Europe, Africa and Asia, measles probably has existed for tens of thousands, if not millions of years. However, in the more isolated communities, new births may not be sufficient to maintain the disease. When introduced to communities where the disease was not endemic, the results were catastrophic. Brinkner (1938) described severe epidemics when measles was introduced to the people of the Amazon (1749), to Estonia (1829), to the Indians of Hudson Bay Territory (1846), to the Hottentot community of the Cape (1852) and to Tasmania (1854). Apparently the population of Tierra del Fuego was almost wiped out by measles (Hirsch, 1883).

A. Measles in Fiji

The first introduction of measles into Fiji in 1875 is well documented. Thirty per cent of the population died within the space of 3 months. This experience of the severity of measles in isolated communities led to the belief that the high mortality was due to the population having no previous experience of the disease. Such populations were considered to have a low genetic or herd immunity. We now believe this not to be the case, and a study of the history of the epidemic in Fiji suggests other reasons for the high mortality. In this epidemic whole families were affected but due to the state of panic in the population there was nobody to bring them food or water, so in addition to the illness, starvation and the resulting weakness led to an appalling mortality.

As a result of this measles epidemic in Fiji indentured Indian labour was introduced to work on the plantations and the whole history of the island altered. Now the offspring of those labourers compete in approximately equal numbers with the original Fijian population. Although these populations attempt to live harmoniously the presence of people with such a diverse tradition and way of life on one island will continue to creat many difficulties.

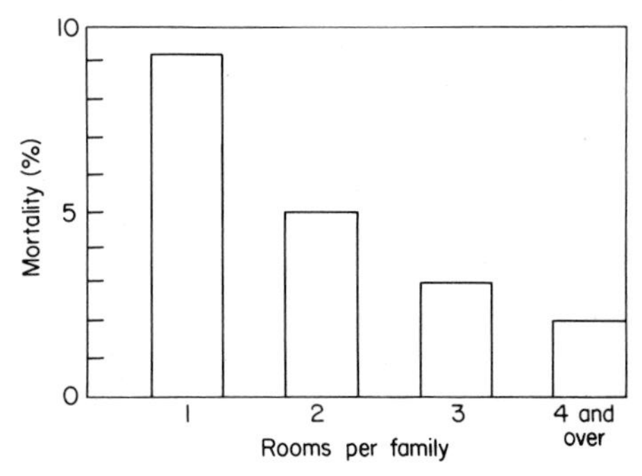

Fig. 1. The relationship between mortality and socioeconomic circumstances in 22 000 cases of measles in Glasgow for the year 1908.

B. Measles in Glasgow

Chalmers (1930) undertook a detailed study of measles in Glasgow in 1908. In that year the mortality from measles in the orphanages exceeded 10%. While mortality was not so high in the rest of the population, Chalmers was able to show a striking difference between social classes. In those days the distinction between socioeconomic groups was made on the number of rooms used by a family. As will be seen in Fig. 1, mortality in those confined to one room was six times greater than in those wealthy enough to be able to afford four rooms or more. Probably no other study has so clearly distinguished the effects of socioeconomic factors expressed as the nutrition available to the children living under the different conditions.

III. Beliefs about Measles

A major failing of medicine has been the inadequate study of beliefs and attitudes to disease. In Europe and America bacteria and viruses are now widely accepted as the cause of infection by the majority of the population. This is not true in the vast rural populations of developing countries where the diseases that all children get are accepted as the presentation of a goddess or some other spirit being. Where, however, diseases are not recognized as affecting all members of the population, they are seen as the result of some failing, frequently sexual, of the child or his parents. In a disease such as measles where the whole appearance of the skin is altered, as well as obvious symptoms such as the running eyes and cough, local attitudes and beliefs are likely to be particularly strong. For example, in the Fiji situation, if whole families went down with measles it was apparent that the neighbours would see this as evidence of a particular evil spirit and their fears of equally being affected leading to their being unwilling to help those afflicted.

In Europe, for a 1000 years, measles was thought to arise from the "bad blood of menstruation". Because menstruation disappeared during pregnancy it was believed that the "bad blood" entered the fetus and reappeared some time after birth as the measles. Laymen and doctors shared this belief, which is found in the writings of Willis (1695). In Africa measles is responsible for restrictions on the diet and even the fluid intake of children during and immediately after the disease. Parents are likely to be worried if a young patient with measles is given an injection. This is because of the very widely held view that the rash must be encouraged to come out and if it does not come out this will be fatal for the child. As mentioned already, in India measles is considered to be due to the goddess Little Mata and the parents of a child with measles will conceal the child at the back of their hut. Doctors working in rural India rarely see the disease. However, in India and most of Asia, doctors will see measles in their more wealthy private patients in whom the disease is likely to be mild. This has led to an inadequate understanding of the severity of the disease and so far no attempts in that country have been made to undertake widespread immunization or to produce the vaccine locally. Elsewhere in Asia the severity of the disease and the awe with which it is held is perhaps brought out in the following proverbs:

A child that gets out of measles is a child that is reborn. (Arabic)

Count your children after the measles has passed. (Arabic)

Smallpox will make your child blind; measles will send him to his grave. (Farsee)

(Morley, 1973)

In South America many of the old customs brought from Europe can be found. There are reports of children being beaten with nettles to bring out the rash. Not infrequently the child may be wrapped in a red blanket and kept in the dark with perhaps a red light.

IV. Distribution of Severe Measles

During a long-term study of children growing up in a West African village the author had an opportunity to make day-to-day observations of the disease and recognize its severity in a way that is impossible in a hospital situation. As well as working in the village, there was an opportunity to see measles in a hospital and during a three-year period measles accounted for 16% of 4475 admissions to the children's ward at the hospital and 22% of the 849 deaths. The severity of measles in West Africa is now well documented. An overall case mortality of 5% has been suggested, although in children admitted to hospital the average mortality from a number of hospitals was found to be 12% (Morley *et al.*, 1966). The highest mortality recorded in West Africa is from the records of an epidemic in Mali (P. J. Imperato, personal communication 1968), where there were 78 deaths amongst 213 cases of measles, a 38% mortality rate. This high mortality was in part due to local beliefs which led to both food and fluid being withheld from those with measles.

In the rest of Africa there are a wide range of reports showing different severities of measles. For example, in a similar hospital study in East Africa the mortality was found to be only 5·5% (Morley *et al.*, 1967). However, this relatively lower mortality may have arisen because apparently all children with measles are admitted to these hospitals. In an excellent epidemiological study of measles in Kenya, Voorhoeve (1978), studying a large rural population, found a 6·5% fatality.

As mentioned already, satisfactory reports of the severity of measles from community studies are infrequent from Asia. However, in a study amongst rural tribal people in Maharashtra, Shah and Junnarkar (1977) found that measles was the number one cause of death between the end of the first month of life and the fifth birthday. Similarly, in Afghanistan, Wakeham (1978) described an appalling mortality of over 40% in some villages which were isolated during winter months.

In South America the severity of measles has been well documented. In the past, Chile documented a 6·5% fatality and considered that this was the most severe infectious disease of children in that country. In an outstanding multi-centre study which included centres in the Caribbean area and North America, Puffer *et al.* (1971) demonstrated a great range in severity of measles. For example, in Recife in the poverty-stricken north-east part of Brazil, measles accounted for almost half the deaths in children and of the children dying with measles nearly three-quarters had evidence of nutritional deficiencies. In other areas of Brazil measles accounted for one-fifth of child deaths; these figures for Brazil and other South American countries were compared with areas in the Caribbean and in North America where during the study there had been no deaths from measles.

V. Description of Severe Measles

For a health worker who has grown up and been trained in the West one of the great surprises in the developing world is the severity of measles. Not only is it more severe but it also develops at a younger age. The age incidence of measles in England and Wales and Nigeria is compared in Fig. 2. Almost one-third of Nigerian children had had measles before they were one year old and three-quarters before they were three years old, whereas in England the majority of children develop measles only after they have attended school. There are several reasons for this marked difference. In West Africa the young child is carried around and is more open to droplet infection perched on its mother's back. This

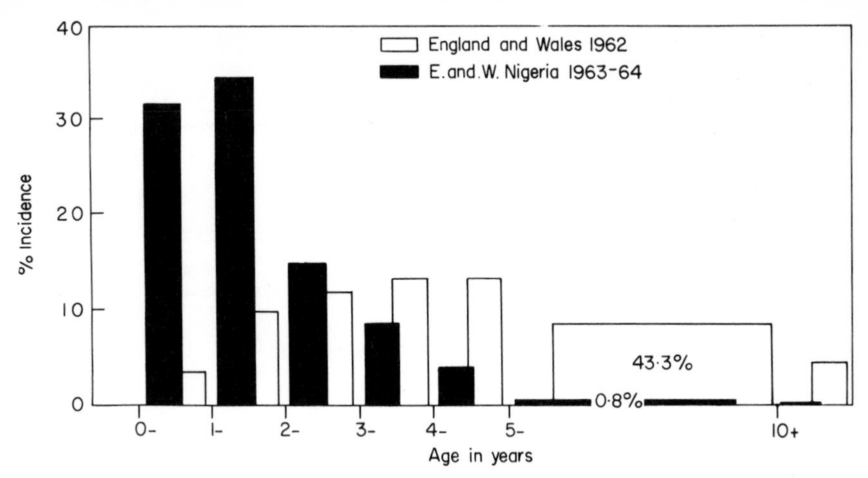

Fig. 2. Comparison of age distribution in England and Nigeria. In Nigeria most children develop measles before the age of 3 years; in England many escape measles until after the age of 5 years.

method of carrying children around has great advantages from the point of view of child development but it does allow the child to become infected by droplets from other children. Secondly, due to the extended family in which the children live with cousins and other young children, it has been shown that infection usually develops from one pre-school child to another rather than from the school child. A third, and possibly most important reason, is that measles in malnourished children may well continue to be infective for very much longer than in well-nourished children.

As well as appearing at a younger age the rash—although it starts similarly—develops in a different way among less well-nourished children. The pink, slightly raised rash which will fade when pressed, is similar to that found in Europe. However, the rash alters in that there is more loss of blood into the tissues and this leads to a darkening of the rash which will not fade when it is pressed. In his description of measles in the ninth century, Rhazes recognized this difference and in his original writings in Arabic when translated into English, the descriptive term "deep red and violet colour" was used. These patches of rash which have darkened tend to peel and this peeling is characteristic of children who are developing the severe form of the disease. In all measles there is some loss of the skin but it is only in the severe form that it is so very noticeable. We of course recognize the rash on the skin.

However, as West Africa mothers continually used to remind the author, the mouth of her child was also very sore at this time, in fact all the epithelial surfaces of the body, including those of the respiratory and gastrointestinal tracts are affected by these changes (Fig. 3). We

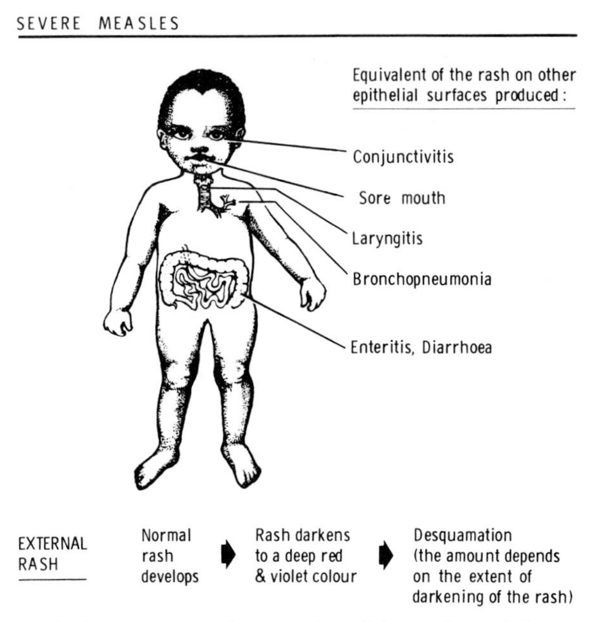

Fig. 3. The association between the severity of the rash and the manifestations of the rash in other epithelial surfaces.

now believe that it is the severity of the rash on these other surfaces which leads to what in the past we have called the "complications" of measles. For example, in the young child the smaller tubes (bronchi) of the lungs are very narrow, perhaps no larger than the lead of a pencil, compared with the size of the pencil in the adult. The epithelial disruption produced by the measles rash on this surface may block the tube and rapidly present as a bronchial pneumonia. Similarly, the disruptive effect of the rash on the mucosa of the bowel presents as diarrhoea which can develop, both in the early stages of the disease and also during the time following the loss of the superficial layers of skin which seem on the outside of the body. This relationship between the changes on the skin and on other epithelial surfaces of the body is shown in Fig. 3.

VI. The Eye

The transparent epithelium of the cornea which covers our eye is highly specialized but does not escape from the measles rash and biopsy of the cornea will demonstrate the microscopic appearance of the measles rash. Unfortunately, the rash on this surface may lead to disruption of the eye and permanent blindness. In a study in Kenya, Sauter (1976) suggested that probably somewhere in the order of half the blindness in Kenya developed following measles. Various reasons for this have been suggested, the most feasible may be that measles precipitates an acute lack of vitamin A; associated with this vitamin A lack is the loss of mucus-secreting cells which act as lubricants and maintain the moisture of the cornea which is essential for its survival. Perhaps the increased tears that are seen in measles may be an attempt to keep the cornea moist in the absence of these mucus-secreting cells. Fortunately, even one massive dose of vitamin A will bring the cells back within a matter of days. The routine use of vitamin A fairly early in the disease in countries where blindness is associated with measles may be an important step. The process by which the eyes are involved ending only too frequently in blindness, may be even more complex. Evidence suggests that the herpesvirus responsible for the "cold spot" may be activated and infect the eye of a child debilitated from measles (Whittle, 1979).

VII. Diarrhoea in Measles

Bronchial pneumonia associated with measles is still well remembered and occasionally seen in Europe and the USA. However, the importance of diarrhoea as a part of measles is only found in earlier textbooks of paediatrics written around the start of this century. An early account of measles in West Africa was given by Daniel in 1852. He was working as a naval surgeon in Ghana (then called the Gold Coast) and reported that dysentery and diarrhoea were then more serious and fatal than pneumonia among the young African children. Mucosal biopsies have been taken unwittingly in children incubating measles and these show cellular changes typical of measles. For a number of reasons diarrhoea plays a major part in the precipation of children into malnutrition and so it is particularly significant in children with severe measles who are already poorly nourished. In some parts of the world one-third or a half of children presenting with the severe forms of malnutrition give a history of measles in the preceding weeks. Almost certainly it is the diarrhoea, associated with measles, that have done much to precipitate this malnutrition.

VIII. Interaction of Measles and Infection

In the past, various reasons have been given for the severity of measles in some communities. For example, it has been suggested that the severe measles in Africa might be a different virus. However, it is difficult to maintain this theory in the face of the large number of children now flying regularly between Africa, Europe and the US. If there were severer forms of the virus severe outbreaks would be expected in other countries. Similarly, the theory was held at one time that there might be a variation in host or herd immunity. Again, this view is now difficult to support. For example, the population in the US comes partly from Africa and partly from Europe. Measles in these two groups is similar and only slight differences in mortality have been present over the last fifty years. Many other studies show that the difference in genetic resistance must be minimal, e.g. the study in Glasgow referred to in Fig 1 and many more recent studies such as one which involved the elite and slum dwellers in Lagos. All these studies emphasize the importance of socioeconomic factors and amongst these nutrition is outstanding.

The two separate forces working to the detriment of the child who is both malnourished and suffering from an infection such as measles are brought out in Fig. 4. It is this cycle of malnutrition and infection that is responsible for the difference in the severity of the disease, with a mortality which may vary as much as 400-fold.

In a study in a West African village the weights of children were recorded before, during and after measles. It was found that around a quarter of the children lost 10% of their weight. This will mean that a child of 10 kg will lose 1 kg in weight. No other common acute infection of childhood was found to have such a dramatic effect on the children's growth curves recorded on a weight chart.

IX. Why Malnutrition Makes Measles More Severe

The full answer to this riddle should be discovered in the next two decades. We do know that the cellular defences of the body are heavily involved in the control of the disease; for example, during measles the normal reaction to tuberculin which identifies children that have

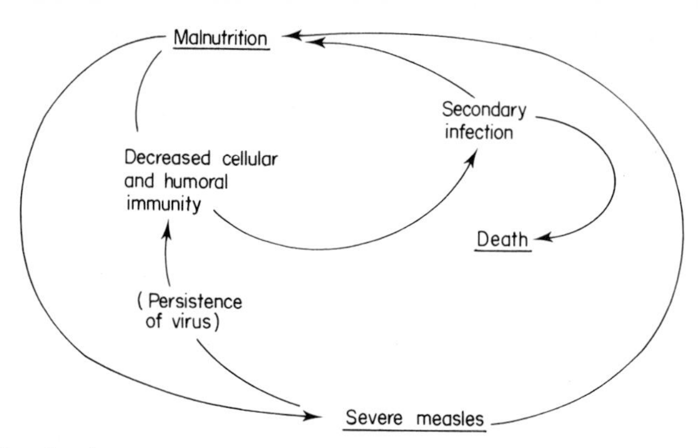

Fig. 4. Measles demonstrates the complexity of the interaction between nutrition and infection better than any other disease.

experienced tuberculosis is no longer present. We also know that the multinucleate cells, which probably arise from several cells that are being destroyed by measles, can be found for a very much longer time in the skin of the mouth and elsewhere in children with severe measles. Particularly significant is the finding of a virus-like material in these cells. Just how long this virus remains viable is unknown but there is now reason to believe that children who are malnourished go on secreting the virus and are therefore infective for a much longer period than well-nourished children. This explains why the infection occurs at a younger age in the poorly nourished children found in developing countries now and in Europe in the past. Measles tends to be more severe in younger children, probably in part because they are more liable to be undernourished, and even if well nourished at the start of the illness their nutritional state is much more labile and within a week of the start of the illness their nutrition may be deteriorating so that they enter the cycle already shown in Fig. 4. In a study in Durban (Coovadia *et al.*, 1978), three-quarters of those children presenting with measles and lymphopenia died or developed chronic lung infections; this is further confirmation that it is the cellular immune response which is particularly damaged by undernutrition in measles.

X. Man's Response to Measles

Only recently have we learned why measles has become a mild disease in the Western world. We now realize that the change in fatality from the disease came about due to improved nutrition among children. This improvement was largely due to the changes in diet which allowed small children to receive an adequate intake of energy. In the past in Europe and currently in developing countries, children could not receive sufficient energy because of the bulky nature of their diet. The characteristics of bulk have been removed from the Western diet by the fine milling of cereals, removal of dietary fibres and the enormous increase in refined sugar and fats and oils (Dearden *et al.*, 1980).

A. Measles Vaccine

The measles virus was first isolated by Enders in 1956 in the USA. Thanks to an intensive effort a vaccine was rapidly produced and a number of trials were undertaken in 1959 and 1960 and measles vaccine was first used in Africa in 1961. The measles vaccine has been widely and successfully used in America and only slightly less in Europe. Measles had now become a rare disease in the US (Fig. 5) and there are plans to eradicate it from the USA by 1982. Unfortunately, this success has not been reflected in the developing countries. A massive campaign for smallpox eradication and measles containment in West Africa was highly successful in controlling smallpox, but only fleetingly affected

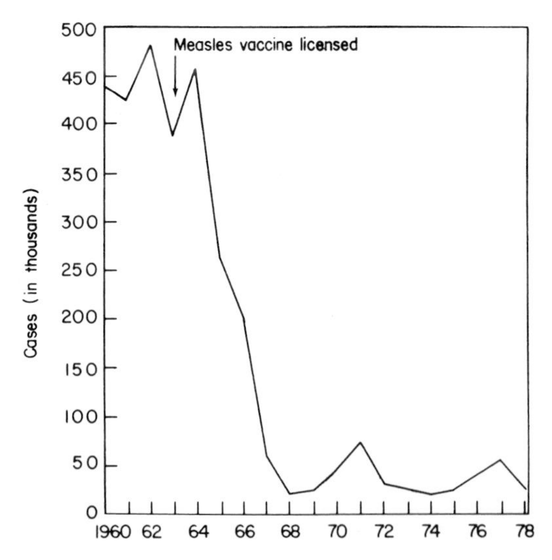

Fig. 5. Experience of measles in the USA. If planned eradication by 1982 is achieved, this will be a model for other countries to follow.

the incidence of measles. Perhaps only in the Gambia was eradication over a period successful. The reasons for this failure were in part financial and in part logistic.

The financial problems arose, not only due to the limited resources available but even more important to the maldistribution of these resources. In almost every developing country the largest slice of health expenditure has been absorbed to an increasing extent by tertiary hospitals. These are teaching and large hospitals which are expensive in skills and personnel and make services available to an elite minority. Figures of this maldistribution of resources are not readily available but an extreme example is that of the expenditure in Maharashtra State in India, 80% of which goes to three cities and only just over 4% to the vast rural population, resulting in a per capita expenditure of only US 2 cents each year. Similarly, only 15% of the Ghanaian budget is spent on primary care and yet for 90% of the population this is the only care they are likely to be able to obtain (Morley and Woodland, 1979). Measles vaccination for the large populations of developing countries will clearly have to wait until political change can lead to a more appropriate distribution of resources. In a country such as Tanzania where the political change has taken place, measles vaccine has become widely available.

The logistic problems are largely those of the cold chain. Unfortunately, measles vaccine is sensitive to both changes in temperature and to sunlight. Even in areas where refrigerators are available, their design is more appropriate for storing milk and eggs in Europe than a living virus vaccine in a tropical climate. As part of their expanded programme for immunization, the World Health Organization has undertaken a detailed study of the problem of keeping measles vaccine in a viable state. As a result, more appropriate top-opening refrigerators are being developed along with cold boxes which will maintain the vaccine in an appropriate state during transport.

Another difficulty arises in finding an appropriate age for vaccination. Unfortunately, vaccine given to an infant that still has protection from maternal antibodies received through the placenta is ineffective. For this reason immunization with measles vaccine in Europe and America is delayed until the fourteenth month. In a developing country at this stage well over a third of children will have suffered from measles. No practical solution to this problem has yet been developed; one possibility is to give the child two doses of vaccine. This is harmless and would improve the chances of protecting a high proportion of children. However, such an approach will make an expensive operation even more costly.

References

Brinkner, J. A. H. (1938). *Proc. R. soc. Med.* **31**, 807.

Chalmers, A. K. (1930). "The Health of Glasgow, 1818–1925". Bell and Bain, Glasgow.

Coovadia, H. M., Wesley, A. and Brain, P. (1978). Immunological events in acute measles influencing outcome. *Archs Dis. Child.* **53**, 861–867.

Creighton. (1894). "A History of Epidemics in Britain", Vol. 2. Cambridge Univ. Press.

Dearden, C., Harman, P., Morley, D. (1980). Eating more fats and oils as a step towards overcoming malnutrition. *Trop. Doc.* **10**, 137–142.

Hirsch, A. (1883). "Handbook of Graphical and Historical Pathology" (C. Creighton, Trans.). The New Sydenham Society, London.

Morley, D. (1973). "Paediatric Priorities in the Developing World", 212. Butterworth, London.

Morley, D. and Woodland, M. (1979). "See How They Grow". Macmillan, London.

Morley, D. C., Martin, W. J. and Allen, I. (1966). Measles in West Africa. *W. Afr. med. J.* **16**, 24.

Morley, D. C., Martin, W. J. and Allen, I. (1967). Measles in East and Central Africa. *E. Afr. med. J.* **44**, 12.

Puffer, R. R., Serrano, C. V. and Dillon, A. (1971). "The Inter-American Investigation of Mortality in Childhood". Interim report of Pan-American Health Organization reproduced from Assignm. Child UNICEF, Paris.

Sauter, J. J. M. (1976). "Xerophthalmia and Measles in Kenya". Drukkerij and van Denderen, Groningen, The Netherlands.

Shah, P. M. and Junnarkar, A. R. (1977). Weight-age of the various "at risk" factors and practicability of management. *In* "'At-risk' Factors and Health of Young Children" (D. B. Jelliffe, Ed.). Cairo.

Voorhoeve, J. (1978). Epidemiology of measles in Kenya. *Trop. geogr. Med.* **29**, 428.

Wakeham, P. F. (1978). Severe measles in Afghanistan. *J. trop. Paediat, env. Child Hlth* **24**, 87.

Whittle, H. (1979). Measles and herpes. *Trans. R. Soc. trop. Med. Hyg.* **73**, 66.

Willis, T. (1695). "The London Practice of Physick". London.

8

Possible Future Changes in the Epidemiology and Pathogenesis of Human Influenza A Virus Infections

John S. Mackenzie

Department of Microbiology, University of Western Australia, Perth, Australia

---

Influenza A virus, its antigenic drift and shift, its ability to spread at a speed equivalent to human travel, its changing patterns of pathogenesis and transmission associated with urbanization, overcrowding, increasing travel, air pollution, cigarette smoking and malnutrition, all suggest that its potential as a producer of great plagues should neither be forgotten nor underestimated.

I. Introduction

Pestilences have brought misery and death to mankind ever since primitive (Neolithic) man first congregated in groups to form villages. Indeed, during the ensuing millenia and with the development of urbanization, infectious diseases such as plague, cholera, diphtheria, smallpox, typhoid and influenza to name but a few, provided the principal form of population control in both cities and highly populated rural communities (Fenner, 1976; McNeill, this volume). Most of these diseases have been brought under control over the past 100 years, with the notable exception of influenza which continued to flourish unchecked causing periodic, explosive pandemics. This continuing lack of restraint prompted Beveridge (1977) to refer to influenza as the last of the great plagues.

Influenza is an acute viral disease of the respiratory tract. It occurs as small, localized outbreaks, as epidemics, or as worldwide pandemics. The viruses belong to the family Orthomyxoviridae which comprises three morphologically similar but antigenically distinct groups, influenza A, B and C.

Influenza A viruses infect man, pigs, horses and a wide variety of domestic and wild birds. Antigenic variation is well documented and is of two types; antigenic drift and antigenic shift. In man, new epidemic strains appear every 1 to 3 years associated with minor changes in the envelope glycoproteins of the virus, the haemagglutinin and neuraminidase, by a process of point mutation and selection; a phenomenon described as antigenic drift. Every 10 to 40 years, however, a new pandemic strain arises in man in which one or both of the envelope glycoproteins are completely different antigenically to those of the preceding strain and to which the population has no prior experience. Such a major change in antigenic profile is described as antigenic shift.

Influenza B and C viruses cause disease in man, but have not been shown to occur naturally, or to cause overt disease, in animals or birds. The type B viruses are responsible for small localized outbreaks or for epidemics, but less frequently than influenza A viruses. Influenza C viruses cause mild upper respiratory tract infections, more akin to the common cold. Both types B and C exhibit antigenic drift but not antigenic shift.

By virtue of their mode of transmission, influenza and other respiratory viruses, can be assumed to have evolved as a consequence of, and parallel to, increasing population density. The genealogy of influenza the virus and the birthplace of influenza the disease are unknown but some information can be gleaned from references to diseases and epidemics which exist in the writings and commentaries of historians and chroniclers living in different ages and cultures. However, this kind of viral archaelogy only provides, at best, an accumulation of suppositions, since most accounts give insufficient details of symptoms or of epidemiological patterns for us to impute an aetiological agent consistent with present-day diseases. Even when detailed descriptions are given, they are frequently compatible with more than one disease. Nevertheless, in a few instances it has been possible to deduce the identity of specific diseases which were similar, if not the same, as those prevalent today. Thus we can be reasonably confident that outbreaks of pandemic and epidemic influenza occurred in the sixteenth century and at frequent intervals thereafter (Beveridge, 1977). It is also tempting to implicate influenza in earlier epidemics, even as far back as the classical era, but the descriptions are too vague for anything more than speculation, and the identities of the causative agents must remain as tantalizing enigmas.

Despite this relatively recent documented history, it is possible that influenza and other respiratory virus diseases have been associated with mankind for several thousand years. However, the origin of the wide variation in structure and antigenicity which is now found among respiratory viruses may be much more recent. Indeed, the current explosion in the world population, together with man's new-found mobility may be highly conducive to the evolution of new respiratory viruses. Similarly, the effects of industrial and social innovations on the quality of the environment may be reflected in changing patterns of specific disease syndromes. It is this potential for changes that forms the underlying theme of this chapter, with particular reference to influenza A viruses. It must be stressed, however, that although influenza A was the first human respiratory virus to be isolated in the laboratory nearly 50 years ago in 1933, the intervening period has been too brief to indicate changes in either the pathogenesis or the epidemiology of the virus. Thus any factors which may induce changes in the accepted ecology of the virus, either singly or collectively, can only be inferred from indirect and circumstantial evidence.

II. Influenza—the Virus

The morphology and composition of influenza A virus has been recently reviewed by Wrigley (1979). Although the shape of virus

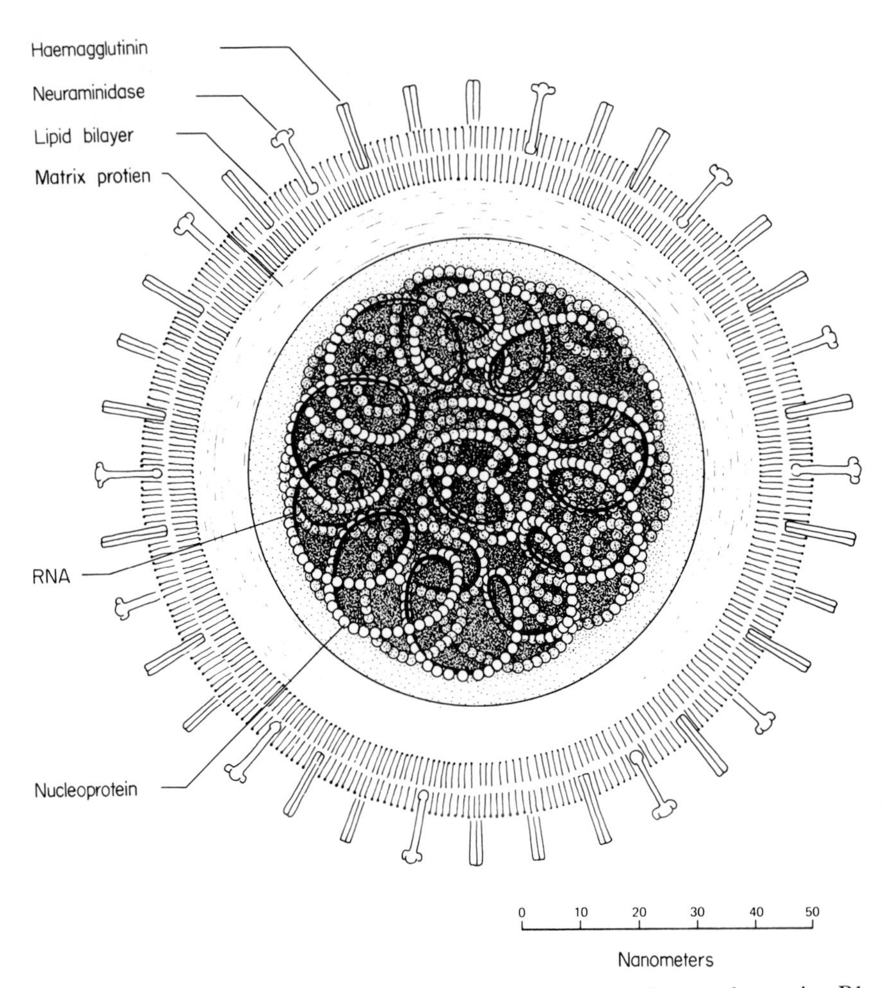

Fig. 1. A schematic cross-section of an influenza A virus. Internal proteins P1, P2 and P3 have not been included. The antigenic profiles of new isolates are described on the basis of their external haemagglutinin and neuraminidase glycoproteins. Thus the current Hong Kong antigenic series are all shown as H3N2.

particles isolated from human infections may vary considerably from pleomorphic spherical forms to long filamentous forms, after being subjected to several laboratory passages they tend to assume a rounded morphology with diameters of about 100–120 nm. The structure of the virion is shown schematically in Fig. 1 and an electron micrograph of the virus is shown in Fig. 2. The virus particles contain seven different

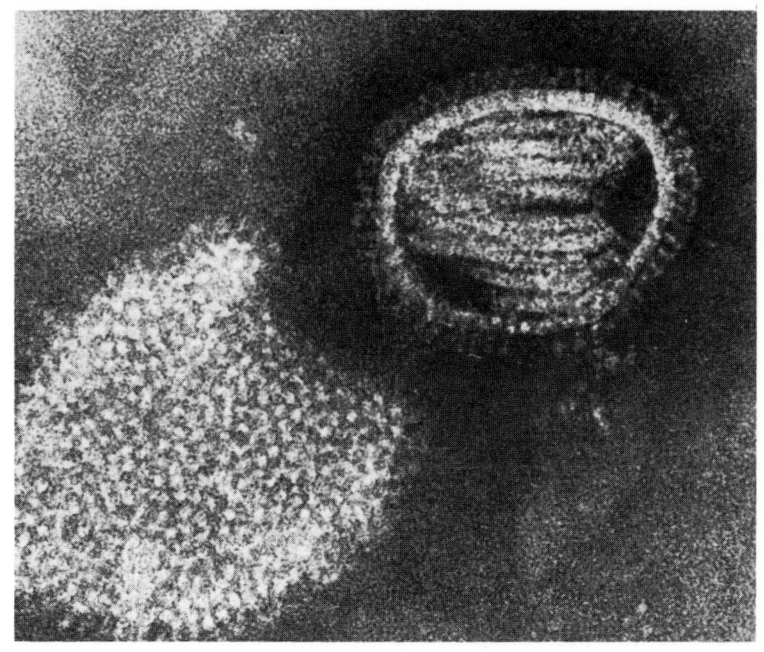

Fig. 2. An electron micrograph of influenza A/Singapore (H2N2) negatively stained with phosphotungstic acid. Magnification × 250 000. The micrograph shows a rounded virus particle with a coiled internal nucleocapsid, and virus envelope bearing haemagglutinin and neuraminidase spikes. (Photograph by courtesy of Dr John Armstrong.)

structural proteins: two external glycoproteins and, within a lipid-containing envelope, five internal proteins. The external glycoproteins, haemagglutinin (HA) and neuraminidase (NA), are responsible for the characteristic surface spikes which project radially from the virus surface. There are believed to be some 700–900 spikes on each spherical virion, the majority of which are HA in an approximate proportion of 5:1. The HA spikes are short triangular rods 18 nm long and 5 nm wide, whereas the NA spikes are mushroom-shaped with square heads 8 × 8 nm and 4 nm thick.

The HA accounts for 25–35% of the total virus protein. It is responsible for virus attachment to susceptible cells and for the ability of the virus to agglutinate erythrocytes. It is the product of a single gene (or genomic fragment) and is generally cleaved during maturation into a heavy and light chain with molecular weights of 45 000–50 000 and 25 000–30 000 respectively (Waterfield *et al.*, 1979).

The two cleaved chains remain associated by means of disulphide bonds to form a subunit, and three subunits comprise the actual HA spike. The HA contains multiple antigenic determinants, some of which are common to all viruses of the same antigenic drift series, whereas others are specific to each individual strain. All the determinants are located on the side of the HA spike just below its tip (Wrigley *et al.*, 1977).

Humoral and local immune reactions concerned with neutralization and protection are mediated principally through antibodies directed against the HA.

The NA is also the product of a single genomic fragment, each spike being a tetramer of four identical glycopeptides with a total molecular weight of about 240 000. The function of the NA is unknown. It is able to hydrolyse sialic acid from the HA receptors on the cell surface, and is believed to play a role in the release of progeny viruses from infected cells (Klenk *et al.*, 1970). Antibody directed against the NA does not neutralize viral infectivity but appears to inhibit the release of progeny virus, thereby reducing the spread of infection (Webster and Laver, 1967).

The glycoprotein spikes possess hydrophobic portions which are inserted into the viral envelope. The envelope is a lipid bilayer derived from cellular cytoplasmic membrane and is acquired as progeny viruses leave the infected cells by a process of budding through the membrane.The cytoplasmic membrane is probably modified prior to virus budding. Beneath the envelope is a layer or matrix of protein about 6 nm thick (Apostolov and Flewett, 1969). This matrix (M) protein is the smallest of the structural proteins, with a molecular weight of about 25 000 and the most abundant, comprising 40% of the total virion protein, but its structure and function are unknown. M protein exhibits type-specific antigenic activity, and although antibody directed against it does not neutralize infectivity, there is some evidence to suggest that antibody might reduce the severity of infection.

The virus core is composed of the nucleoprotein (NP), proteins P1, P2 and P3, and the segmented, single-stranded RNA genome. The NP, which has a molecular weight of about 60 000 has type-specific antigenic activity and is intimately associated with the RNA genome. There are over 1000 molecules of NP per virion. The P1, P2 and P3 proteins, which have molecular weights of between 80 000 and 100 000 are also intimately associated with the genome, but there are very few molecules of each per virion. One or more of these larger proteins is believed to have RNA nucleotidyltransferase activity. The genome consists of eight segments with a combined molecular weight of between 4×10^6 and 5×10^6 (reviewed by Scholtissek, 1978). Each segment is probably a monocistronic message. Thus seven of the eight RNA segments code for the seven virion proteins (P1, P2, P3, HA, NA, NP and M) and the eighth segment codes for two non-structural (NS) proteins, on two different reading frames. The segments may or may not be joined in some way to form coils, but evidence suggests that they replicate independently. It is believed that the RNA replication occurs solely in the nucleus.

III. Influenza—the Disease

Influenza infections may be commonly asymptomatic, may cause only a slight fever, or may result in the typical prostrating illness which is characteristic of major epidemics. The disease and its complications have been reviewed in detail by Mulder and Hers (1972) and by Douglas (1975) and the pathogenesis has been discussed by Mims (1976). After an incubation period of 1–2 days, the typical acute disease has an abrupt onset with a rapid rise in body temperature to 38–40°C. The early symptoms usually include a dry unproductive cough, a severe generalized or frontal headache, malaise and shiveriness, and these are rapidly followed by aching muscles in the limbs and back, joint pains, anorexia and nausea. Respiratory symptoms may be entirely lacking, or if present, most prominent after the systemic symptoms and fever are complete, usually 3 days after infection, although in some instances they may last as long as 7 days. A rather more productive cough may persist for up to 1 to 2 weeks. Most patients are usually able to return to work within 7 to 10 days of the onset of symptoms, but convalescence may be prolonged by lassitude, malaise and depression.

Influenza tends to be milder in children, and although the symptoms are generally similar to those found in adults there is a lower incidence of myalgia, nausea and vomiting are more frequent, and maximal temperatures may be higher (Jordan *et al.*, 1958). A wide range of respiratory and neurological symptoms, however, have been reported among infants and young children admitted to hospital (Price *et al.*, 1976; Paisley *et al.*, 1978). Febrile convulsions, vomiting, coughing, diarrhoea and anorexia were the most common presenting features, with gastrointestinal symptoms prominent in young infants.

The main complications of influenza involve the lower respiratory tract and the cardiovascular and central nervous systems. The most common complications arise from secondary bacterial infections of the ear, paranasal sinuses, bronchi and lungs. Bronchitis, bronchiolitis, laryngotracheobronchitis (croup) and pneumonitis may result from secondary infection with streptococci, staphlococci, pneumococci or *Haemophilus influenzae*. Patients with chronic pulmonary or cardiac disorders are at high risk of developing bronchitis, particularly the elderly, leading to hypoxia and central cyanosis. Such cases undoubtedly contribute to the mortality from influenza. Secondary bacterial pneumonia may develop with bubbling râles, consolidation, dyspnoea and radiological opacity either after the acute viral episode, in which case there is usually a biphasic fever pattern, or as a concomitant infection. *Pneumococcus* has been the most commonly isolated pathogen, but staphlococcal influenzal pneumonia has often been encountered during epidemics. The latter tends to run a fulminating and often fatal course; the patients may die within one or two days after onset, and previously healthy and even young adults may succumb.

Primary influenza pneumonia was first described during the 1958 pandemic, although it undoubtedly occurred in the 1918–19 pandemic. It may account for up to 20% of all cases of influenza-associated pneumonia. The pathological features include epithelial necrosis in the mucosa of the respiratory bronchioles, damage to alveolar cells, necrosis of the capillary walls and thrombosis, with oedema and haemorrhage into the alveoli (Hers *et al.*, 1958). Clinically there is a relentless course of continued fever, leucocytosis, dyspnoea, hypoxia and cyanosis. Patients with pre-existing cardiac disease are particularly susceptible to primary viral pneumonia and account for the majority of fatal cases. There is also evidence which suggests that patients in their third trimester of pregnancy may be at risk (Mackenzie and Houghton, 1974).

Neurological and cardiac complications are less frequent and not so well documented as those of the respiratory tract. Although influenza A has been implicated in myocarditis, encephalitis and the Guillain–Barré syndrome, the virus has seldom been isolated from heart muscle or brain. Nevertheless, viral antigens have been detected in periventricular areas, ependyma and in cells of the hypothalamus and substantia nigra by immunofluorescence.

A number of studies of case fatalities have been reported in patients hospitalized with pneumonia or other complications in which influenza has been confirmed by laboratory diagnosis. Some of these studies have been discussed by Douglas (1975) and Stuart-Harris and Schild (1976). However, influenza is not a notifiable disease, and case fatality rates in the population during epidemic periods have been calculated as excess pneumonia-associated deaths (or influenza-associated if influenza is included on the death certificate) over seasonally adjusted, expected mortality rates. Thus in the vast majority of fatal cases the cause of death was not confirmed by virus isolation. Of the pandemics in modern history, that of 1918–19 stands alone as judged by the total influenza-associated mortality, and although the pandemic took place some 15 years before the virus was first isolated it has been estimated that 20 million people died in excess of the usual expectancy, or 1·17% of the total world population. This pandemic was also unique in that the highest mortality occurred in young adults. Since the abnormally high rate of 1918–19, mortality rates have declined substantially, and in all pandemics and major epidemics most case fatalities have been in the very old, the very young and in those which chronic debilitating disease. Indeed a major change in the pattern of mortality over the past 30 years has undoubtedly come from the advent of chemotherapeutic agents in the treatment of secondary bacterial infection. A number of other factors influence influenza-associated mortality, such as viral virulence and host determinants. These factors have been described by Kilbourne (1975).

IV. Transmission

Influenza is transmitted directly from person to person through aerosols formed by expulsion of the virus from the respiratory tract, and by direct contact. Virus can be detected in nasopharyngeal secretions before the onset of symptoms and for at least 5 days after the illness has developed, with virus titres commonly exceeding 1 million infectious particles per millilitre at the height of illness (Davenport, 1976). Little is known, however, of the minimum virus dose or sites of infection within the respiratory tract; the larger droplets expelled by coughing and sneezing infect the upper respiratory tract, or smaller droplet-nuclei of 1–5 μm, which remain suspended in the atmosphere for longer periods, may infect the pulmonary alveoli. Experimental infection of volunteers by nasal instillation and by small-particle aerosols suggest that both sites of deposition may by involved, and that as little as three infectious virus particles may be sufficient to initiate infection if given by aerosol (Knight and Kasel, 1973). A low relative humidity and a low environmental temperature have been shown to favour the survival of virus in aerosols (Harper, 1963), and studies on the decay of aerosols have indicated that appreciable amounts of virus can remain viable for over an hour. Thus small droplet nuclei could be a mechanism of transmission remote from a source of infection in terms of both distance and time.

Transmission of influenza in the general community varies greatly in different epidemics, probably reflecting the relative proportion of susceptible and resistant subjects present at any one time. However, even in the face of a new pandemic strain when the vast majority of the population is wholly susceptible, virulence and attack rates tend to be inconsistent in different countries. Attack rates seldom exceed 20%, except in closed communities, with the epidemic subsiding before all susceptible persons in the community have become infected. Indeed, a feature of pandemics and larger epidemics is the occurrence of distinct waves of infection, often with higher levels of morbidity in the second wave.

The spread of virus within the community during pandemic and epidemic influenza is not well understood. Children generally have a higher incidence of infection, and may be an important source of spread. It has been suggested that selective immunization of school children may markedly reduce the spread of infection (Monto *et al.*, 1969). Hirst (1947) also suggested the concept of the "dangerous spreader"; that some subjects yield higher titres of virus in nasopharyngeal secretions than others, and are therefore more infectious.

V. Factors which May Alter the Pattern of Transmission and Pathogenesis

A. Poverty, Overcrowding and Urbanization

Increasing urbanization has been a feature of the nineteenth and twentieth centuries in developed countries, with high-density population growth becoming particularly prevalent during the past five decades. A similar influx of people into urban environments has also had a notable impact in many underdeveloped countries. Overcrowding has become an inherent aspect among the impoverished, which can be expected to enhance the incidence of influenza. Indeed, a study by Assaad and Reid (1971) in Glasgow indicated that poverty itself contributes an added environmental burden and increases the risk of mortality. They found that although the occurrence of mortality was equal in various socioeconomic groups, 74% of the deaths among persons in the higher social class who were over 65 years of age were ascribed to influenza together with a pre-existing chronic condition, whereas in only 48% of elderly people in the lower social class was such a condition found.

Crowding is, of course, synonymous with urbanization. Population density must be a major factor in promoting transmission, particularly during cultural pursuits in auditoriums or whenever members of the community are gathered together in close proximity. Schulman (in Fox and Kilbourne, 1973) has commented that cold weather results in the greater indoor congregation of people, and that indoor temperatures in winter reflect warming up of air from outside with little moisture added, thus giving the low humidity that favours survival of virus. Similarly, the low temperature and low humidity of air-conditioning, particularly in commercial buildings, which has become an accepted and common practice in many countries during the past two decades, must surely facilitate virus survival and spread in droplet nuclei and thereby increase the probability of transmission. Although Miller (in Fox and Kilbourne, 1973) has suggested that the occurrence of influenza may be unrelated to commuter transport (buses, trains and private cars), the close proximity of travellers would tend to refute this suggestion. Thus increasing urbanization must undoubtedly serve to increase the ease and frequency of transmission.

B. Increasing Travel and Population Mobility

It has been well-established from retrospective epidemiological studies that influenza can spread at a speed equivalent to human travel (Parsons, cited by Burnet and Clarke, 1942; Hoyle, 1968). Until relatively recently, the movement of viruses between continents was accomplished by ship. This mode of travel may still be important for isolated island communities (Mantle and Tyrrell, 1973) and even between populations in developed countries (Gregg, in Fox and Kilbourne, 1973; Reid, in Fox and Kilbourne, 1973). However, the rapid escalation of international air travel, which for example rose from less than 30 million passengers in 1962 to nearly 400 million in 1972, has enabled a number of viruses and other infectious diseases to be rapidly and effectively disseminated over long distances (Stanley, 1977; Stanley, this volume; Zulueta, this volume).

It is certain that this greatly increased population mobility has played a significant role in facilitating the transmission and seeding of influenza. Indeed, the importation of influenza to US airbases in South-East Asia by aircraft from Taiwan or Hong Kong has been clearly documented by Buescher (in Fox and Kilbourne, 1973), and an outbreak of influenza has been reported among passengers who remained on board a jet airliner delayed by engine failure in Alaska (Moser *et al.*, 1979). The importance of rapid population mobility in the spread of pandemic influenza, however, may not always be apparent. Careful virological and serological studies in 1957 and 1968 showed clearly that early seeding of the virus resulted in small focal or sporadic outbreaks, often over several months, before the epidemic exploded. It is not understood why importation and early seeding does not lead immediately to an epidemic, but a combination of factors are probably involved including the intrinsic virulence and transmissibility of the virus, and environmental conditions.

C. Air Pollution, Occupational Risk and Tobacco Smoke

Epidemiological studies have consistently shown an association between respiratory infection and air pollution. Not only are air contaminants damaging to the tissues of the nasal mucosa and the tracheobronchial tree *per se*, allowing invasion by a number of pathogenic microorganisms, but with long-term exposure they can be immunosuppressive (Holt and Keast, 1977). There is also a considerable body of evidence to indicate that air pollutants, possibly in combination with infection, may be involved in the aetiology of chronic bronchitis and other chronic pulmonary conditions (Crofton and Douglas, 1969) which have been included in the "high-risk" categories for influenza infection. It should be emphasized, in considering the effect and lung clearance of pollutants, that influenza destroys the ciliated epithelium down to the basement membrane (Hers, 1966), that influenza may have a ciliastatic effect (Ballenger *et al.*, 1968), and that influenza infection impairs the inactivation of inhaled bacteria by retarding their ingestion by alveolar macrophages and by allowing bacteria to proliferate within macrophages (Warshauer *et al.*, 1977). Three types of atmospheric contaminants will be briefly considered: environmental gaseous and particulate pollutants, occupational hazards from mineral dusts, and tobacco smoke.

There has been an enormous increase during the past few decades in the amount of gaseous and particulate pollutants which have been disgorged into the atmosphere from sources such as industry, vehicle exhaust emissions and burning of fossil fuels. Most studies examining the effects of air pollutants on influenza infection have concentrated on sulphur dioxide, nitrogen dioxide, photochemical oxidants and particulates. Sulphur dioxide was first associated with an increased incidence of influenza during the 1957 Asian pandemic (Dohan, 1961). A higher incidence of illness was also reported during the 1968–69 Hong Kong pandemic among families in Chattanooga exposed to high levels of nitrogen dioxide and particulates (Shy *et al.*, 1970). Chronic oxidant exposure, however, had no discernible effect on the morbidity of Hong Kong influenza among schoolchildren in various South Californian communities (Pearlman *et al.*, 1971). The influence of nitric oxides, sulphur dioxide, oxidants and formaldehyde on an influenza epidemic in Sophia, Bulgaria, indicated that all four pollutants, in medium quantities, increased the number of influenza cases (Kalpazanov *et al.*, 1976). The effect of nitric oxides and formaldehyde were relatively slow, taking one or two days to become manifest, whereas the effect of sulphur dioxide and oxidants appears to be comparatively faster. Animal models have tended to give conflicting results. Exposure of mice to moderate concentrations of sulphur dioxide (2·5–5·0 ppm) reduced the amount of pneumonia after infection with influenza, but a higher incidence of pneumonia was observed in mice exposed to sulphur dioxide at concentrations of 20 ppm or greater (Fairchild *et al.*, 1972). However, an increased severity of influenza infection was reported in mice which had been continually exposed to 0·03–0·1 ppm of sulphur dioxide for 4 weeks (Ukai, 1977). Post-infection exposure to 6 ppm of sulphur dioxide for 7 days was shown to partially inhibit the growth of influenza in the nose of mice, but not in the lungs (Fairchild, 1977). A similar finding was observed after exposure to 0·6 ppm of ozone for 3 hours after infection, except that the inhibition of viral growth in the nose was more pronounced (Fairchild, 1977). Mice exposed to nitrogen dioxide for moderate periods (37 ppm for 30 days) exhibited markedly increased resistance to aerosol challenge with influenza (Buckley and Loosli, 1969), and squirrel monkeys exposed to nitrogen dioxide for several months did not differ from controls in their susceptibility to influenza (Fenters *et al.*, 1973). However, in an earlier study, nitrogen dioxide inhalation was shown to increase the severity of influenzal pneumonia (Henry *et al.*, 1970). The conflicting results described in animal studies have undoubtedly been due in part to differences in length of exposure, concentration of gases and methods of exposure. It has been shown that short-term exposure (about 7 weeks) to nitrogen dioxide or tobacco smoke may enhance the immune responsiveness of mice, whereas long-term exposure caused a significant degree of immunosuppression (Holt and Keast, 1977; Holt *et al.*, 1979).

Atmospheric pollution may also act in a less direct manner, by causing a depletion in the concentration of small air ions. Ion depleted air is a common product of urbanization. Unipolar low densities of positive or negative ions, or unipolar high densities of positive ions, have been shown to markedly increase the mortality of mice infected with influenza, whereas unipolar high densities of negative ions or low concentrations of mixed ions reduced the death rate (Krueger and Reid, 1972).

It is well established that a number of mineral dusts cause pulmonary functional abnormalities and disease of varying severity (Crofton and Douglas, 1969). Thus it might be expected that the occupational hazard of chronic exposure to mineral dusts could lead to increased risks from influenza infection, both directly and from secondary bacterial invasion, and to a higher incidence of infection. However, little or no epidemiological or experimental investigations have been undertaken. In one study, mice infected with influenza and then subjected 24 or 48 hours later to single or multiple three-hour-long exposures of manganese dioxide aerosols were found to exhibit increased mortality rates, reduced survival times, and increased pulmonary lesions (Maigetter *et al.*, 1976). An enhanced mortality rate has also been reported in mice infected with influenza and then exposed to nickle oxide aerosols (Port *et al.*, 1974).

Considerably more evidence is available on the effects of a self-induced air pollutant, tobacco smoke. Cigarette smokers have been shown to be more susceptible to infection with epidemic influenza than non-smokers (Finklea *et al.*, 1969; Mackenzie *et al.*, 1976), providing they had little or no pre-epidemic humoral antibody titres (Mackenzie *et al.*, 1976). Humoral antibody levels to influenza were significantly increased among smokers who remained well and minimally increased among smokers who were sick, compared with non-smokers (Finklea *et al.*, 1971), which suggested that smokers were also more susceptible to subclinical infections. Furthermore, the longevity of the immune response to a killed subunit influenza vaccine was severely depressed 50 weeks after vaccination in those smokers who had no immunity prior to vaccination (Mackenzie *et al.*, 1976).

It has been established in a murine system that tobacco smoke significantly depresses both humoral and cell-mediated immune mechanisms (Holt and Keast, 1977). Prolonged exposure of mice to tobacco smoke has been shown to depress a primary immune response to influenza infection and to decrease the frequency of seroconversion (Mackenzie, 1976), and although the mice were able to mount a normal secondary immune response, it was less specific than the response elicited in control mice with the production of high titres of cross-reacting antibody (Mackenzie and Flower, 1979a). Moreover, long-term exposure to tobacco smoke has been found to act synergistically with influenza infection to increase the susceptibility of mice to secondary bacterial invasion (Mackenzie and Flower, 1979b).

Thus air quality may be an important factor in potentially altering the pattern of epidemic influenza, with increasing urbanization and industrialization, together with the self-induced pollution caused by cigarette smoking, all serving to influence the incidence and severity of infection.

D. Malnutrition

Protein-energy malnutrition and infectious diseases have been shown to interact synergistically, each augmenting the severity of the other (Scrimshaw *et al.*, 1968). The role of virus infections in precipitating protein-energy malnutrition in the undernourished, and in increasing the morbidity and mortality of those already suffering severe forms of protein-energy malnutrition, has been recently reviewed (Mackenzie, 1978). It was observed that anorexia, vomiting, diarrhoea, urinary nitrogen loss, intestinal malabsorption and increased catabolism caused by virus infections may all contribute to significant weight loss, and the impaired immunocompetence associated with severe forms of protein-energy malnutrition may permit greater viral invasiveness and unrestricted multiplication.

The effect of influenza A infections in the severely malnourished, however, has not been investigated in detail, and indeed influenza has not generally been regarded as a serious epidemic disease in terms of mortality in underdeveloped countries. Nevertheless, it should be remembered that vomiting, diarrhoea and anorexia are common symptoms of influenza infections in infants and young children. It has been reported that, following the severe drought of 1973–74 in the Sahelian countries when marasmus was a common condition, a high mortality occurred from influenza in people of all ages (Chizea, 1974). Similarly, the high morbidity and mortality caused by epidemic influenza in Papua New Guinea (Mackenzie, 1978), and the high morbidity from influenza in children in the Philippines with the concomitant high mortality from pneumonia (Santos-Ocampo and Caspellan, 1977), might both be asociated with the frequent occurrence of protein-energy malnutrition in those countries. It is interesting to note that although measles is one of the most important viral diseases of the malnourished in many parts of the world, often complicated with bronchopneumonia, and a major contributor to severe forms of malnutrition, it is a relatively minor disease in New Guinea (M. P. Alpers, personal communication). A reduced longevity of antibodies to influenza was observed in Gambia (McGregor *et al.*, 1979) but its association with malnutrition was not ascertained, and a reduced immune responsiveness has also been reported after influenza vaccination in Australian Aboriginal children who had medical history suggestive of protein-energy malnutrition in infancy (Jose *et al*., 1970).

In a murine model, protein deprivation was found to enhance markedly the susceptibility to a lethal infection with both mouse virulent and avirulent strains of influenza virus. Viraemia was observed more frequently in protein-deprived mice, and virus persisted longer in the lungs. The humoral immune response was depressed with normal levels of IgG antibody but reduced levels of IgM antibody. Pre-immunization of protein-deprived mice did not affect the virus titres observed in the lungs after homologous challenge, nor did it prevent the spread of virus to the thymus and brain (Pollett *et al*., 1979).

If influenza does present a hazard to the undernourished, the rank poverty found surrounding urban areas in developing countries and the problems of food supplies to a rapidly increasing world population may be reflected in a change in the pattern of influenza epidemiology, and a threat to the well-being of millions. Meanwhile, increasing poverty exacerbated by rising inflation and leading to malnutrition is also a feature, particularly among the elderly, of urban areas in developed countries.

VI. Antigenic Drift in an Immune Population

There is a strong evidence to indicate that the ability of influenza to undergo antigenic drift is the result of selection of mutant virus particles with altered antigenicity of their surface glycoproteins and, therefore, with a growth advantage in the presence of antibody (Webster and Laver 1975). However, not all mutant isolates with novel antigenic characteristics go on to become the next epidemic virus strain. Often several potential strains are isolated immediately prior to an epidemic, of which one succeeds in establishing itself for unknown reasons. With the increased population mobility and the concomitant speed with which influenza can spread, together with the rapidly expanding urbanization facilitating transmission, it is possible that most people in the community are exposed more frequently to influenza than they had been in the past. If this is so, it might then be assumed that the general levels of immunity within the population would also be higher than in the past, and consequently that the selective pressures would be comparatively greater on the virus itself to undergo antigenic drifting. There is no evidence available to substantiate the former contention, that the levels and incidence of immunity are any higher than in previous decades, but the frequency of successful antigenic drift variants has been slightly higher in the last 10 years within the H3N2 antigenic drift series than had been observed in the H0N1, H1N1 or H2N2 series. This may, of course, be a chance occurrence rather than a direct result of increased selective pressure. It is also unknown whether the degree of difference between each of the successive H3N2 variants is any greater than the sequential differences between variants in the previous antigenic drift series, which might be expected under increased selective pressure. Answers to these kinds of questions, however, must await future epidemiological developments.

An increase in the level of immunity may be compounded by the large scale use of influenza vaccines. The annual vaccination of military personnel has been undertaken in some countries for a number of years, and there has recently been increased usage in industry (Walker, 1971; Smith and Pollard, 1979). It has also been suggested that annual vaccination may be justified in the elderly (Mackenzie, 1977). However, it is probable that the amount of vaccine used (and its availability) is of little consequence at present in terms of the overall population immunity, but this may change in the future with the introduction and potential large-scale usage of live vaccines.

VII. Antigenic Shift

The origin of new pandemic strains of influenza A with novel antigenicity is still uncertain. Recent evidence, however, has stongly indicated that antigenic shift might be the result of recombination, or reassortment of genomic fragments, between an avian or animal influenza virus and the human strain prevalent at that time (Webster and Laver, 1975). Thus the new pandemic strain would have one or both of the external antigens from the avian or animal virus, and certain internal antigens from the human strain. Recent pandemic viruses appear to have arisen in South-East Asia and China, and it was therefore suggested that the close proximity with which the inhabitants of these areas live with their domestic animals and birds might have facilitated the chance of the human double infection necessary for reassortment to take place. If this is indeed the mechanism of antigenic shift, it is plausible to imagine that the rapidly increasing population in China and parts of Asia could result in an amplication of the chance of double infections, and thereby, of potential pandemic strains.

A remarkable feature of pandemic influenza is the rapid disappearance of the preceding strain as soon as the new "shift" strain has become established. However, although this has been the rule in 1947,

1957 and 1968 with the emergence of H1N1, H2N2 and H3N2 viruses respectively, recent events have seen a change in this expected pattern. Firstly, during an epidemic of an H3N2 variant in 1976, a pig influenza virus, Hsw1N1, which is believed to be closely related antigenically to the 1918–19 human pandemic strain, briefly occurred in man in Fort Dix, Maryland. However, despite considerable concern that it might signal a return of Spanish influenza, it did not develop further but rapidly disappeared. The second event was even more unexpected; the re-emergence of an H1N1 virus in 1977 in Russia, 20 years after it had been superseded by H2N2 strains. This virus, Russian influenza, has since caused epidemics throughout the world, but it has not been accompanied by the disappearance of the prevalent H3N2 virus; both subtypes have continued to circulate during the past few years, even being isolated from the same epidemics. Indeed, there has been evidence to indicate that a reassortment of antigens has occurred from double infections, with the H1N1 virus gaining certain internal antigens from the H3N2 strain (R. W. Compans, personal communication). Where the H1N1 virus emerged from is unknown, since unlike the Hsw1N1 virus it is not endemic in animals, although cross-reacting glycoproteins have been isolated from birds. Nevertheless, it is unlikely that it has come from an avian source. Whether the H1N1 virus will replace the H3N2 series remains to be seen, but perhaps the incidence of residual immunity, the apparently decreased virulence of strains during the past decade, and the size of the world population, are now sufficient to allow two distinct subtypes to circulate concurrently.

It should also be mentioned that previous variants within a subtype can occasionally re-emerge and cause sporadic cases. A recent example was the isolation in 1979 of an H3N2 virus antigenically similar to one of earliest H3N2 strains that had occurred 11 years previously (Australian Communicable Diseases Intelligence, 1979). Where this virus appeared from, and how it existed in the intervening period, is not known.

VIII. Postscript

The purpose of this chapter has been to briefly present certain environmental factors which could have the potential to alter some of the traditional patterns of human influenza A virus infections. As such, the possible effects exerted by these factors can only be considered as speculative. Many aspects of the ecology, biology and pathogenesis of influenza could not be covered, nor was it realistic to cite all the relevant references. Therefore, to enable the interested reader to gain more information on this remarkable and changeable virus, a number of review papers were chosen for citation in the text.

As a final word on the future and on the potential threat to mankind that a change in the pattern of influenza could pose, it is worth recalling a comment made by Fenner (1976) in his address on "The options for man's future", which was delivered at the thirteenth Pacific Science Congress. In terms of the great plagues of history and their effects on human populations, the most severe epidemic that he could imagine in the future would be ". . . a form of influenza that had the capacity to cause a severe generalized disease, rather than localized respiratory symptoms, with as high a mortality as fowl plague, one of the influenza viruses of birds". Although such a pandemic is most unlikely, perhaps the concept should not be forgotten.

References

Apostolov, K. and Flewett, T. H. (1969). *J. gen. Virol.* **4**, 365–370.
Assaad, F. A. and Reid, D. (1971). *Bull. Wld Hlth Org.* **45**, 113–117.
Australian Communicable Disease Intelligence (1979). No. 79/25. Department of Health, Canberra.
Ballenger, J. J., McFarland, C. R., Harding, H. B. and Koll, M. (1968). *Aspen Emphysema Conference* **11**, 91–102.
Beveridge, W. I. B. (1977). "Influenza: the Last Great Plague". Heinemann, London.
Buckley, R. D. and Loosli, C. G. (1969). *Archs environ. Hlth* **18**, 588–595.
Burnet, F. M. and Clarke, E. (1942). "Influenza: A Survey of the Last 50 years in the Light of Modern Work on the Virus of Epidemic Influenza". Monograph No. 4. Walter and Eliza Hall Institute, Melbourne.
Chizea, D. O. (1974). *J. Am. med. Wom. Ass.* **29**, 499–505.
Crofton, J. and Douglas, A. (1969). "Respiratory Disease". Blackwell, Oxford.
Davenport, F. M. (1976). *In* "Viral Infections of Humans" (A. S. Evans, Ed.) 273–296. Plenum, New York.
Dohan, F. C. (1961). *Archs environ. Hlth* **3**, 387–395.
Douglas, R. G. (1975). *In* "The Influenza Viruses and Influenza" (E. D. Kilbourne, Ed.), 395–447. Academic Press, London and New York.
Fairchild, G. A. (1977). *Archs environ. Hlth* **32**, 28–33.
Fairchild, G. A., Roan, J. and McCarroll, J. M. (1972). *Archs environ. Hlth* **25**, 174–182.
Fenner, F. J. (1976). *In* "Mankind's Future in the Pacific" (R. F. Scagel, Ed.), 140–160. Univ. British Columbia Press, Vancouver.

Fenters, J. D., Findlay, J. C., Port, C. D., Ehrlich, R. and Coffin, D. L. (1973). *Archs environ. Hlth* **27**, 85–89.
Finklea, J. F., Sandifer, S. H. and Smith, D. D. (1969). *Am. J. Epidemiol.* **90**, 390–399.
Finklea, J. F., Hasselblad, V., Riggan, W. B., Nelson, W. C., Hammer, D. I. and Newill, V. A. (1971). *Am. Rev. resp. Dis.* **104**, 368–376.
Fox, J. P. and Kilbourne, E. D. (1973). *J. infect. Dis.* **128**, 361–386.
Harper, G. J. (1963). *Arch. ges. Virusforsche.* **13**, 64–71.
Henry, M. C., Findlay, J., Spangler, J. and Ehrlich, R. (1970). *Archs environ. Hlth* **20**, 566–570.
Hers, J. F. P. (1966). *Am. Rev. resp. Dis.* **93**, 162–171.
Hers, J. F. P., Masurel, N. and Mulder, J. (1958). *Lancet* ii, 1141–1143.
Hirst, G. K. (1947). *J. exp. Med.* **86**, 367–381.
Holt, P. G. and Keast, D. (1977). *Bact. Rev.* **41**, 205–216.
Holt, P. G., Finlay-Jones, L. M., Keast, D. and Papadimitriou, J. M. (1979). *Environ. Res.* **19**, 154–162.
Hoyle, L. (1968). "The Influenza Viruses". Virology Monographs No. 4. Springer-Verlag, Vienna.
Jordan, W. S., Denny, F. W., Badger, G. F., Curtiss, C., Dingle, J. H., Oseasohn, R. and Stevens, D. A. (1958). *Am. J. Hyg.* **68**, 190–212.
Jose, D. G., Welch, J. S. and Doherty, R. L. (1970). *Aust. paediat. J.* **6**, 192–202.
Kalpazanov, Y., Stamenova, M. and Kurchatova, G. (1976). *Environ. Res.* **12**, 1–8.
Kilbourne, E. D. (1975). *In* "The Influenza Viruses and Influenza" (E. D. Kilbourne, Ed.), 483–538. Academic Press, New York and London.
Klenk, H. D., Compans, R. W. and Choppin, P. W. (1970). *Virology* **42**, 1158–1162.
Knight, V. and Kasel, J. A. (1973). *In* "Viral and Mycoplasmal Infections of the Respiratory Tract" (V. Knight, Ed.), 87–123. Lea and Febiger, Philadelphia.
Krueger, A. P. and Reid, E. J. (1972). *Int. J. Biometeor.* **16**, 209–232.
Mackenzie, J. S. (1976). *Life Sci.* **19**, 409–412.
Mackenzie, J. S. (1977). *Br. med. J.* i, 200–202.
Mackenzie, J. S. (1978). *Papua New Guinea med. J.* **21**, 134–151.
Mackenzie, J. S. and Flower, R. L. P. (1979a). *J. Hyg.* **83**, 135–141.
Mackenzie, J. S. and Flower, R. L. P. (1979b). *FEMS Microbiol. Lett.* **5**, 77–79.
Mackenzie, J. S. and Houghton, M. (1974). *Bact. Rev.* **38**, 356–370.
Mackenzie, J. S., Mackenzie, I. H. and Holt, P. G. (1976). *J. Hyg.* **77**, 409–417.
Maigetter, R. Z., Ehrlich, R., Fenters, J. D. and Gardner, D. E. (1976). *Environ. Res.* **11**, 386–391.
Mantle, J. and Tyrrell, D. A. J. (1973). *J. Hyg.* **71**, 89–95.
McGregor, I. A., Schild, G. C., Billewicz, W. Z. and Williams, K. (1979). *Br. med. Bull.* **35**, 15–22.
Mims, C. A. (1976). *In* "Influenza: Virus, Vaccines, and Strategy" (P. Selby

Ed.), 95–105. Sandoz Institute Publication No. 5. Academic Press, London and New York.

Monto, A. S., Davenport, F. M., Napier, J. A. and Francis, T. (1969). *Bull. Wld Hlth Org.* **41**, 537–542.

Moser, M. R., Bender, T. R., Margolis, H. S., Noble, G. R., Kendal, A. P. and Ritter, D. G. (1979). *Am. J. Epidemiol.* **110**, 1–6.

Mulder, J. and Hers, J. F. P. (1972). "Influenza". Wolters-Noordhoff, Gröningen, The Netherlands.

Paisley, J. W., Bruhn, F. W., Lauer, B. A. and McIntosh, K. (1978). *Am. J. Dis. Child.* **132**, 34–36.

Pearlman, M. E., Finklea, J. F., Shy, C. M., Van Bruggen, J. and Newill, V. A. (1971). *Environ. Res.* **4**, 129–140.

Pollett, M., Mackenzie, J. S. and Turner, K. J. (1979). *Aust. J. exp. Biol. med. Sci.* **57**, 151–160.

Port, C. D., Fenters, J. D., Ehrlich, R., Coffin, D. L. and Gardner, D. E. 1974). "Second Conference on Heavy Metals in the Environment". Research Triangle Park, North Carolina.

Price, D. A., Postlethwaite, R. J. and Longson, M. (1976). *Clin. Pediat.* **15**, 361–367.

Santos-Ocampo, P. D. and Caspellan, A. O. (1977). *Ind. Pediat.* **14**, 779–790.

Scholtissek, C. (1978). *Curr. Top. Microbiol. Immun.* **80**, 139–169.

Scrimshaw, N. S., Taylor, C. E. and Gordon, J. E. (1968). "Interactions of Nutrition and Infection". WHO Monograph Series, No. 57.

Shy, C. M., Creason, J. P., Pearlman, M. E., McClain, K. E., Benson, F. B. and Young, M. M. (1970). *J. air Pollut. Contr. Ass.* **20**, 582–588.

Smith, J. W. G. and Pollard, R. (1979). *J. Hyg.* **83**, 157–170.

Stanley, N. F. (1977). *In* "Progress in Immunology III", 701–705. Proceedings of the Third International Congress of Immunology. Australian Academy of Science, Canberra.

Stuart-Harris, C. H. and Schild, G. C. (1976). "Influenza: the Virus and the Disease". Edward Arnold, London.

Ukai, K. (1977). *Proc. Soc. exp. Biol. Med.* **154**, 591–596.

Walker, D. D. (1971). *Trans. Soc. occup. Med.* **21**, 87–92.

Warshauer, D., Goldstein, E., Akers, T., Lippert, W. and Kim, M. (1977). *Am. Rev. resp. Dis.* **115**, 269–277.

Waterfield, M. D., Espelie, K., Elder, K. and Skehel, J. J. (1979). *Br. med. Bull.* **35**, 57–63.

Webster, R. G. and Laver, W. G. (1967). *J. Immun.* **99**, 49–55.

Webster, R. G. and Laver, W. G. (1975). *In* "The Influenza Viruses and Influenza" (E. D. Kilbourne, Ed.), 269–314. Academic Press, New York and London.

Wrigley, N. G. (1979). *Br. med. Bull.* **35**, 35–38.

Wrigley, N. G., Laver, W. G. and Downie, J. C. (1977). *J. molec. Biol.* **109**, 405–421.

9

Man's Role in Changing Patterns of Arbovirus Infections

N. F. Stanley

Department of Microbiology, University of Western Australia, Perth, Australia

The arthropod-borne viruses . . . have been known to have their natural ecology and transmission changed by human intervention.

I. Nature and Characterization of Arboviruses

Arboviruses (*ar*thropod-*bo*rne) are being considered because human activity, deliberate or unintentional, has modified their geographic distribution and their opportunity to infect man and animals of economic importance. Moreover, the diseases they produce have a profound influence on human history.

Arboviruses are functionally defined as viruses which replicate in both a vertebrate host and an arthropod vector, with the arthropod being the natural means of transmission between vertebrate hosts. (Viruses which are mechanically transferred by an arthropod in which they do not multiply are not included in this category, e.g. myxomatosis of rabbits.) Usually there is not detectable illness in either vector or host as a result of this parasitism which has evolved over many thousands of years and in which we can observe both an equilibrium

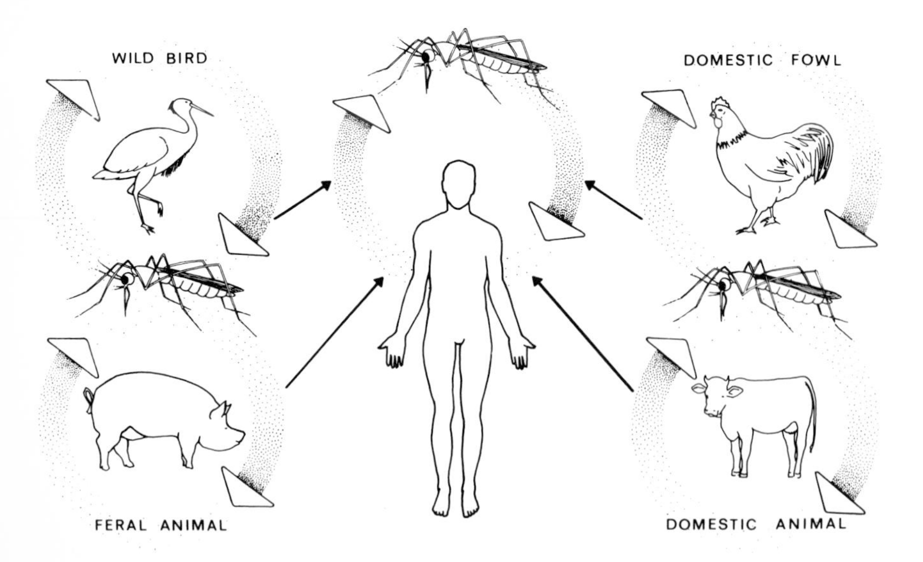

Fig. 1. An outline of virus–vertebrate host–human relationships for an arbovirus such as Murray Valley encephalitis.

FAMILY	Genus	Size (NM)	Diagrammatic Morphology
TOGAVIRIDAE	Alphavirus	50-70	
	Flavivirus	40-50	
REOVIRIDAE	Orbivirus		
	Phytoreovirus	70-80	
	Fijivirus		
BUNYAVIRIDAE	Bunyavirus	90-100	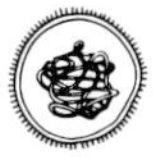
RHABDOVIRIDAE	Rhabdovirus	60 x 170	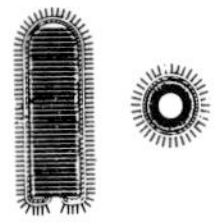

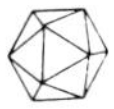

Fig. 2. Seven genera of arboviruses showing approximate size and morphology. *Phytoreovirus* and *Fijivirus* are plant–insect viruses and will not be further considered.

and a marked specificity in spite of the remarkable ability of the virus to replicate in both an arthropod vector and a vertebrate host.*

In the first instance, human infection is accidental and man, as a host, has not been necessary for the survival of the virus in its natural biocenose. However, once a human is infected, it is sometimes possible for arthropod transmission between humans to occur, as in the cases of yellow fever and dengue. It is very easy to see the different ways in which man can disturb this basic survival cycle of the arboviruses (see Fig. 1) and this interference will be discussed later in relation to specific diseases. Activities important in this regard include: (1) human movement and population density; (2) use and control of water (irrigated agriculture and man-made lakes); (3) development and use of insecticides; and (4) interference with the movements and concentrations of vertebrate hosts. Such activities have resulted in the control of a few

* The arthropods of greatest significance are mosquitoes, sandflies (*Phlebotomus* and *Culicoides*) and ixodid and argasid ticks.

TABLE I. *Association of Arboviruses with Clinical Disease*

Syndrome—Fever, headache, plus		Agent: Name	Agent: Status	Vector	Vertebrate source	Geographic distribution
Sore throat, general and local pain, prostration, haemorrhagic signs, shock	Often severe	Yellow fever	Flavivirus	Urban *Aedes aegypti*	Urban *Homo sapiens*	Tropical Central and South America, tropical Africa
		Dengue 1, 2, 3, 4	Flavivirus	*Ae. aegypt*		Philippines, India, South-East Asia, Pacific Islands, Caribbean
		Kyasanur Forest disease	Flavivirus	Ticks	Monkeys	Mysore, India
		Rift Valley fever	Bunyavirus	Culicine mosquitoes	Wild mammals	Africa
Associated with CNS involvement ranging from meningo-encephalitis to severe encephalitis with sequelae	Neurological	Japanese B	Flavivirus	Culex mosquitoes	Wild birds, pigs	Japan, India, China, South-East Asia
		Murray Valley encephalitis	Flavivirus	Culex mosquitoes	Wild birds, mammals	Australia, Papua New Guinea
		St Louis encephalitis	Flavivirus	Culex mosquitoes	Wild birds	USA, Mexico, Panama, Brazil, Argentina
		West Nile	Flavivirus	Culex mosquitoes	Wild birds	Africa, France, Israel, USSR, Pakistan, India
		Equine encephalitis	Alphavirus	Culicine and Anopheline mosquitoes	Rodents, equines, arboreal mammals, wild birds	Canada, USA, Mexico, South America
Malaise, arthralgia, rash. general and localized pains, lymphadenopathy	Usually mild	Ross River	Alphavirus	Culicine	Wild birds, marsupials	Australasia, Papua New Guinea, Pacific Islands
		Chikungunya	Alphavirus	Culcine	Wild birds, bats, domestic animals	South-East Asia, South-East and West Africa
		Dengue 1, 2, 3, 4	Flavivirus	*Ae. aegypti* and *albopictus*	Wild primates	Equatorial, following distribution of *Ae. aegypti*
		West Nile	Flavivirus	*Culex* sp. and ticks	Wild birds, rodents domestic animals	Africa, Europe, Israel, India, South-East Asia
		Changuinola	Orbivirus	*Phlebotomus* sp.	Arboreal mammals, marsupials	Panama

arbovirus diseases as well as in an increased dissemination of some of them.

The functional description of arthropod-borne viruses permits the inclusion of 408 different viruses of 51 antigenic groups in seven genera within four families, as shown in Fig. 2. The plant–insect viruses will not be considered and are not classified as true arboviruses. Approximately one-quarter of the 408 viruses produce disease in man and about 50% have been isolated from mosquitoes and 23% from ticks. Four of those that are mosquito-transmitted and infect humans will form the basis for further discussion in this chapter. The four families listed in Fig. 2 have markedly different morphology and size. The Reoviridae have a double-stranded RNA core and the others a single-stranded RNA core. Figure 3 shows the increase in the numbers of reconized arboviruses resulting from new technology and greater scientific interest, and Table I illustrates the associations of a few of the well-known arboviruses that produce disease in man and/or animals. The greatest numbers of viruses have been isolated in tropical equatorial areas of the planet, especially Africa; but a few have also been located as far south as Macquarie Island and as far north as the Arctic Circle.

Although it appears that man has been incidental to the survival and evolution of arboviruses, it is not correct to assume that his activities

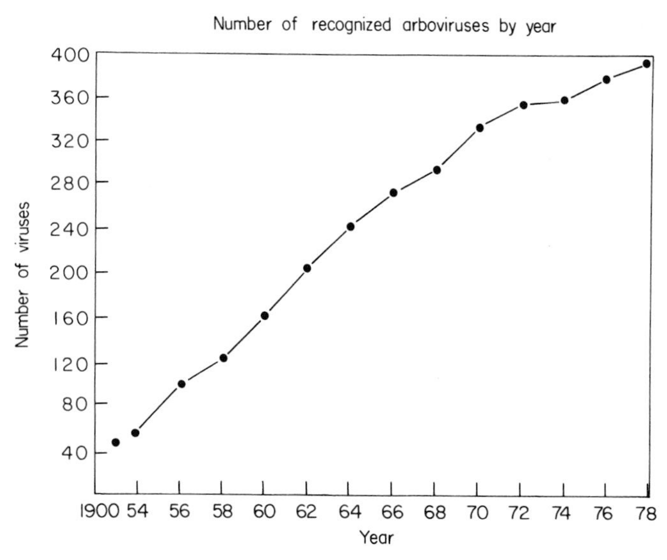

Fig. 3. Numbers of arboviruses characterized by year. The increase reflects the techniques and activities of virologists.

have not significantly altered their natural histories. This chapter examines this question.

Man may be infected in the following ways:

(a) by a person moving into the enzootic areas of virus activity and being bitten by an infected arthropod;
(b) by a person infected as in (a) introducing the virus into an urban situation where arthropod transmission of the virus between humans becomes possible;
(c) by infected arthropods being wind-blown from their natural enzootic geographic location;
(d) by infected vertebrates (e.g. migrating birds) moving to another distant environment which permits the establishment of a new and sometimes transient virus–arthropod–vertebrate cycle;
(e) by laboratory or field-acquired infections of investigators.

Once a human is infected he may carry the virus in his body to another geographically distant environment and the virus may spread to other humans if the appropriate arthropod is present (e.g. dengue, Ross River infection, yellow fever). The survival of the virus depends on adequate viraemia in the vertebrate host, the persistence of virus in the arthropod and sometimes variations which permit the virus to survive in winter or dry seasons—an event sometimes called "overwintering". This may involve transovarial transmission in the arthropod or persistence in a poikilothermic vertebrate such as a snake or lizard. The complexities of these situations are obvious and the establishment of a "new" urban human environment with other arthropods and amplifier hosts such as feral and domestic animals frequently occurs. It is therefore essential to select a particular virus for "in depth" examination if we are to understand the basic ecology which can result in clinically recognizable disease in man.

Arbovirus infections cover a wide disease spectrum from a severe acute infection with a high mortality or serious sequelae to subclinical infection (see Table I). In the latter case the extent of virus infection is estimated by testing for specific serum antibody to the virus. When applied to population groups this is known as "serological epidemiology". It is also necessary to appreciate that we find two different clinical syndromes and a wide spectrum of clinicopathological disease being caused by one virus, as well as one clinical syndrome being produced by a large number of different viruses (see Table I).

Before illustrating these often subtle complexities with specific diseases, an appreciation of the difficulties of studying arboviruses in the field, in the laboratory, in the ward, and at international levels is necessary. Some of the viruses that will be considered have been initially isolated by the intracerebral inoculation of newborn mice with infected blood or tissues or suspensions prepared from ground-up pre-frozen mosquitoes. As an adjunct to mice, fertile chick embryos and mammalian cell or mosquito cell cultures may be used as well as the intrathoracic inoculation of live mosquitoes. The viruses recovered in this way may be characterized morphologically by electron microscopy, by their physical and chemical properties and by their antigenic structure. A specific immune serum for each antigenic type is required. Before acceptance of a virus as a recognized arbovirus or as a "new" type, its properties are checked by reference laboratories and by the Yale Arbovirus Research Unit. Out of necessity has grown an information exchange, an international catalogue and a subcommittee on arbovirus laboratory safety. The International Catalogue of Arboviruses serves as a register of data on the occurrence and characteristics of approved arboviruses. The Information Exchange includes the activities of about 160 laboratories covering all parts of the world. The techniques of virus isolation, characterization and antibody estimation are described by Work and Jozan (1977) and Stanley (1979), and readers are referred to those reviews for specific details of complement-fixation, haemagglutination-inhibition and neutralization tests, and some difficulties of interpretation.

II. An Examination of Selected Arboviruses and their Ecology

In a brief chapter of this kind it is only necessary to select a few representative diseases to illustrate the points of significance. I have chosen three examples from the Flaviviruses and one from the Alphaviruses (see Table I and Fig 2). They are the Flaviviruses, yellow fever, dengue and Murray Valley encephalitis, and the Alphavirus, Ross River virus. With each I will examine the past and present situations, the geographic distribution, the vectors, the vertebrate hosts, the clinical disease and how human activity has modified the situation both intentionally and unintentionally.

A. Yellow Fever

This disease has probably existed in equatorial Africa for many thousands of years. This persistent endemicity has resulted in the local inhabitants developing some resistance to the damaging effects of the virus. Some of the Africans have also developed a specific natural immunity by childhood exposure to the virus when infections have been relatively mild or subclinical. European man's first welcome to West and Central Africa was to endure a severe attack of yellow fever and/or malignant malaria. The death toll was high and the area soon became known as the "white man's grave" (see also Ofosu-Amaah, this volume). Yellow fever presented with early symptoms (like dengue) of high fever, vomiting and severe pains (see Table I). This was frequently followed by jaundice, black vomit, delirium and death.

From this original West African source, yellow fever was introduced (by sailing ships) to Spain, Portugal, South Wales, Central America, the Caribbean, the eastern points of the USA (New York, Boston, Baltimore) and the Mississippi valley. It is believed that yellow fever became widespread in the Caribbean during the seventeenth century. In 1857 6000 people died of yellow fever in Lisbon, and some years later about 13 000 died in the Mississippi valley. To understand this movement and to formulate some control or protection from the disease it was necessary to obtain knowledge of the natural history of the infection.

We now know that in both Africa and America there are two distinct ecological niches for yellow fever virus—one in the jungle and the other urban and associated with man. In both countries tree-top monkeys are involved and in both countries the mosquito *Aedes aegypti* is the one mainly responsible for transmission between humans. But there are significant differences between the African and New World ecologies.

In Africa the virus appears to be transmitted between monkeys by the mosquito *Ae. africanus*, a nocturnal treetop mosquito that bites monkeys while they are sleeping. Almost all species of African monkeys are involved. In the dry season the virus may persist by transovarial transmission in the mosquito or perhaps in an as yet undetermined host. But the main question was how did the virus get from the treetop monkeys and mosquitoes to man? It is known that the monkeys come down from the trees to raid (the human-controlled) plantations and when they are at this lower level, another mosquito, *Ae. simpsoni*, bites them. This mosquito also bites man and thus serves as an effective link between jungle and house. In addition, *Ae. aegypti* is commonly found throughout the world in villages and towns and thus can transmit the virus between people and establish an outbreak. But even if the outbreak is controlled by various means, there is always the jungle yellow fever lurking in the background as the enzootic focus which is not subject to effective control by man.

In South and Central America, a jungle yellow fever pattern has also become established in monkeys. In this situation the virus is transmitted by a *Haemogogus* species of treetop mosquito. These can bite and

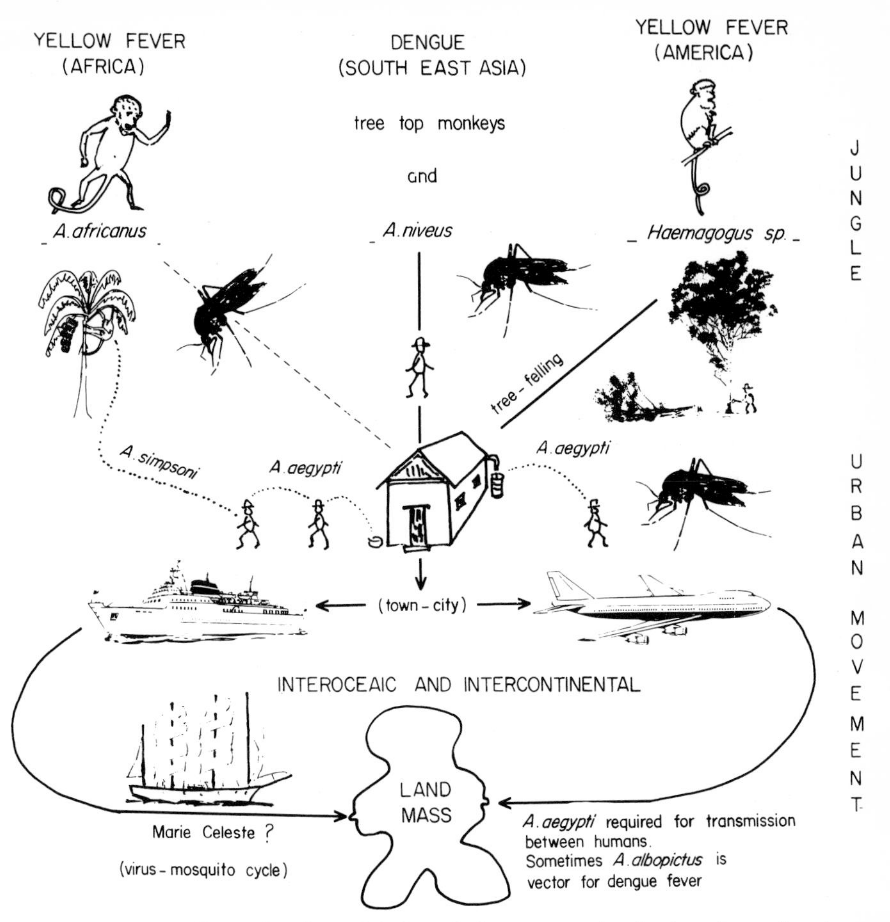

Fig. 4. An outline of yellow fever and dengue cycles in jungle and urban environments.

infect man when the forest trees he is felling fall to the ground. The infected woodcutter returns to his village where *Ae. aegypti* breeds and where transmission occurs between humans. In America this disease has been clinically more severe, both in humans and monkeys, than in Africa. Some of the red-howler monkeys were found dead during intense virus activity. The differences between the African and American situations are given pictorially in Fig. 4, where they are compared with the jungle and urban dengue fever of South-East Asia.

We still know very little about yellow fever, but have had some small success in its prevention in a few places by mosquito (*Ae. aegypti*) control or by massive vaccination campaigns with a live attenuated vaccine; there are still mysterious ecological features that remain unanswered. For example, Port and Wilkes (1979) describe a yellow fever outbreak in The Gambia which occurred in the absence of *Ae. aegypti*, although another mosquito species, *Ae. furcifer/taylori*, was almost certainly the vector for this outbreak. Furthermore, several species of monkey may be involved in the maintenance of yellow fever in West Africa. The classical example of *Ae. aegypti* control was in the construction of the Panama Canal. Yellow fever and malaria prevented de Lesseps from completing the construction, which was achieved only when Major Gorgas instituted effective mosquito control.

If we accept that *Ae. aegypti* and the virus were transported by sailing ships from Africa to America, why has the disease not become established in South-East Asia? And why is the East Coast of Africa relatively free from yellow fever compared with the West Coast and Central Africa? Other viruses (such as Chikungunya) have moved from Africa to South-East Asia but not to Australia or the Pacific Islands. *Aedes aegypti* and monkeys plus an apparently highly susceptible human population exist in millions in South-East Asia. We do not know the answer to these questions, but it is tempting to speculate on the existence of biological barriers. One type of barrier could result from the presence of dengue virus in an ecological niche which would have been suitable for yellow fever virus if it could get established. This could be an interference at the monkey–mosquito–forest level as well as at the human—*Ae. aegypti*—urban level. Another biological barrier may relate to the specific biting habits of some mosquitoes. This can be checked by determining the vertebrate source of blood found in the mosquito after it has fed. These points are relevant when we examine, a little later, the very interesting geographic differences within the Flavivirus complex–Japanese B, West Nile, Murray Valley and St Louis. All are antigenically related and have similar basic ecologies, but territorial overlap is rare.

As a result of trade with Africa via sailing ships carrying slaves and water casks containing *Ae. aegypti* and yellow fever virus, there were continuous outbreaks of yellow fever for more than 250 years. For example:

Yellow fever destroyed Admiral Wheeler's fleet in 1695 before it could attack Martinique

Yellow fever invaded the USA on twenty-six occasions in the eighteenth century

It caused >50% mortality in the forces of the Earl of Albemarle in Cuba in 1762

Yellow fever epidemics occurred in fifty-six different years and on thirty-seven occasions in North America in the nineteenth century

It wiped out the French Army of 25 000 sent by Napoleon Bonaparte to Santo Domingo (Theiler and Downs, 1973)

Following this disastrous Caribbean history, yellow fever virus still remains endemic in equatorial Africa, but it has spared South-East Asia. But what about dengue, whose early home may have been, and still is, South-East Asia?

B. Dengue

The changing pattern of dengue infection is still a mystery and continues to be a most serious health problem in spite of all efforts of microbiologists and intensive national and international activity.

Infection with one of the four dengue viruses may result in an acute febrile illness with severe generalized pains, sweating, and a typical rash. Virus is found in high concentration in the blood (primarily cell-associated) at the height of this acute disease (as many as 10^9 infectious particles per ml blood). In the last twenty-five years a more severe form of dengue (known as dengue haemorrhagic fever—DHF—with or without shock) has been recognized widely in South-East Asia and more rarely elsewhere (Caribbean and Pacific Islands).

Like yellow fever, transmission between humans is mainly by the mosquito *Aedes aegypti*, although, more recently, *Ae. albopictus* has also been implicated (see Fig. 4). Unlike yellow fever, we do not know the original home of dengue and the disease patterns and distributions are currently changing. It has a fascinating history with yellow fever-like drama and associations, so it is appropriate to record the following observations in order to appreciate the alarming picture that now exists.

Outbreaks of dengue were first clinically recognized in the latter part of the eighteenth century, in Cairo and Alexandria (1779), in Batavia (1780), in Cadiz and Seville (1784–86), and in Granada. A short time thereafter a severe epidemic occurred at Lima. During the nineteenth century there were many outbreaks and epidemics severely affecting hundreds of thousands of people, notably in India, the West Indies, North and South America, and these were followed by extensive equatorial outbreaks around the world. It spread with remarkable speed and invaded northern Australia and some Pacific Islands at this time. Of the serious epidemics this century, that occurring in Athens (1927–28) is notable in that it followed a great influx of refugees whose sanitary conditions were poor and *Aedes* sp. breeding habitats were widespread. It is estimated that 90% of the population of Athens and Piraeus were infected (Scott, 1939). Miami, Florida, was affected in 1934 and major epidemics occurred during the 1939–45 World War in South-East Asia and throughout the Pacific Islands (dengue type 1). Subsequently the Pacific Islands were free from dengue for 20 years. But recently (1964–76) the disease has been reintroduced by rapid international travel and it has again spread throughout the Pacific, where it remains endemic in many islands (1971—type 2; 1976—type 1).

Dengue fever is usually a mild disease in children but may present as a more severe disease in adults. On the other hand, the haemorrhagic form (DHF) is a very severe disease of children and affects the indigenous population of endemic areas. It was first clearly recognized in the early 1950s in the Philippines and Thailand. Shock may develop with a mortality rate of up to 10%, and it has been observed since this time outside of South-East Asia, in the Pacific Islands, and in the West Indies. Epidemic dengue was absent from the South Pacific in 1977 and 1978, although sporadic cases occurred. Dengue type 1 virus was introduced into the Caribbean in 1977 (probably from Africa) and this is the first known occurrence of this serotype in the Western hemisphere for 50 years. Theiler and Downs (1973) suggest that, in the interesting Caribbean situation, where both dengue and yellow fever occur, the dengue type 2 virus may have conferred some protection against the yellow fever virus with which there is an antigenic relationship.

How can we explain this fascinating epidemiology and ecology and the two types of clinical disease associated with the one virus? Recent advances in our knowledge that are relevant are:

1. There are four distinct antigenic types of dengue fever virus which share antigens—these are referred to as types 1, 2, 3 or 4.
2. A jungle cycle of dengue fever exists in South-East Asia and this has some similar patterns to jungle yellow fever (see Fig. 4).
3. The demonstration of transovarial transmission of dengue viruses by mosquitoes in the laboratory (not yet proven in nature).
4. The role of vectors in addition to *Ae. aegypti*, e.g. *Ae. albopictus* certainly, and possibly a number of other *Stegomyia* mosquitoes.

The dengue scene at the moment is briefly as follows. The virus is persistently transmitted in the Malaysian jungles between wild monkeys by a jungle mosquito (*Ae. niveus*) in the high canopy of virgin forest, free from man and his domestic mosquitoes (Rudnick, 1977). The combined studies of the Institute for Medical Research at Kuala Lumpur and the G. W. Hooper Foundation at San Francisco have shown that dengue infects man in the jungle and rural environments as well as in urban areas (see Fig 4). Although *Ae. aegypti* is the main vector between humans, *Ae. albopictus* has frequently been the proven vector in Malaysia, Guam and elsewhere.

There is now little doubt that the rapid movement of large numbers of humans by aircraft from South-East Asia to the Pacific Islands has been responsible for the recent introduction of dengue and its spread throughout the South Pacific, which had been free from the disease for 20 years. This was achieved by humans incubating the disease and becoming viraemic after landing. Dengue type 1 virus was probably responsible for the outbreaks of the 1890s, the 1930s and during the Second World War. In 1964 in Polynesia several thousand adults had type 3 infection. In 1971, dengue hit Fiji and Tahiti and then spread through the Pacific. The first was seen at Nandi International Airport and within three months 3000 cases had been notified. In 1971–72 there were in excess of 1000 cases of type 2 infection in Rabaul. In 1972, on Niue Island, 790 of 4600 people were infected and this included 23 cases with severe haemorrhagic disease, of which twelve died; seven children also died of dengue shock syndrome. In 1974, 3671 cases of DHF with 190 deaths were recorded in Indonesia. *Aedes aegypti* appeared to be the main vector in all situations except on the island of Rotuma in the Ellice Island group, where *Ae. rotuma* was the vector. In peninsular Malaysia in 1976, there were 67 cases (mainly type 3) as well as 15 cases of Japanese B encephalitis. Epidemics of DHF are becoming more widespread throughout Indonesia, where all four types of virus exist. Here *Ae. albopictus* was the principal vector for a recent type 3 outbreak in which some patients also developed encephalitis (Gubler, 1977).

Although mosquitoes and other arthropods are being transmitted by aircraft around the world there has yet been no proven virus outbreak associated with the arthropod movement. Wind-blown mosquitoes have not been implicated in the Pacific Islands or South-East Asia, but it has been suggested that when short distances (<100 km) are involved, both yellow fever and dengue could spread this way. This factor cannot be ignored especially when other arboviruses such as bluetongue and African horse sickness survive in their *Culicoides* vectors, being blown by winds for at least 1000 km (Stanley, 1979). This is one way these viruses could have reached Spain and Portugal from Africa.

Humans are only viraemic for a short time, and the direct transmission of dengue virus by *Aedes* sp. between humans cannot adequately explain the interepidemic survival of the virus. The demonstration of transovarial transmission of all four dengue types in one strain of *Ae.*

aegypti by Rosen and his co-workers in Honolulu (Rosen, 1978) suggests an obvious way of virus survival without the intervention of monkey or man as a vertebrate host. This has not yet been shown to occur in nature. If it does, then current strategies for dengue control would have to be modified. In any case, adequate vector control is not possible in many countries, so dengue remains a serious threat to our health and the jet aircraft the major vehicle for its transoceanic movement.

The vastly varying clinical disease produced by dengue virus remains inadequately explained. One view is that the haemorrhagic fever-shock syndrome could result from a hypersensitivity response following a second attack with a different antigenic type of dengue. There will therefore be some reluctance to use the vaccine against type 2 which is being tested in humans and has been shown to protect. Another view is that the vector mosquito could modify the dengue virus. Further pathogenesis studies are clearly needed.

C. Murray Valley Encephalitis

Murray Valley encephalitis (MVE) is one of a complex of antigenically and ecologically similar viruses comprising Japanese B encephalitis (JBE), MVE, St Louis encephalitis (SLE), and West Nile virus (WN). These, like yellow fever and dengue, are Flaviviruses.

The reason for grouping these four arboviruses together is that they are close relatives who are now not on speaking terms with each other. By this I mean they all share antigens, they have similar transmission by *Culex* sp. of mosquitoes (see Tables I and II), they all produce encephalitis and subclinical infection in man, but they have distinctly different geographic localities (see Fig. 5). In India, JBE and WN viruses approximate each other, and also in Borneo there is a close

TABLE II. *Major Arthropod Vectors for MVE, JBE, SLE and WN Viruses*

Virus	Major arthropod vectors
MVE	*Culex annulirostris*, widely distributed over Australia and Papua New Guinea
JBE	*C. tritaeniorhynchus*, widely distributed in South-East Asia; *C. vishnui* in India, and *C. gelidus* in Sarawak
SLE	*C. tarsalis*, *C. pipiens*, *C. quinquefasciatus* and *C. nigripalpis*, depending on geographic site
WN	*C. univittatus* and *C. pipiens*; ticks may be involved

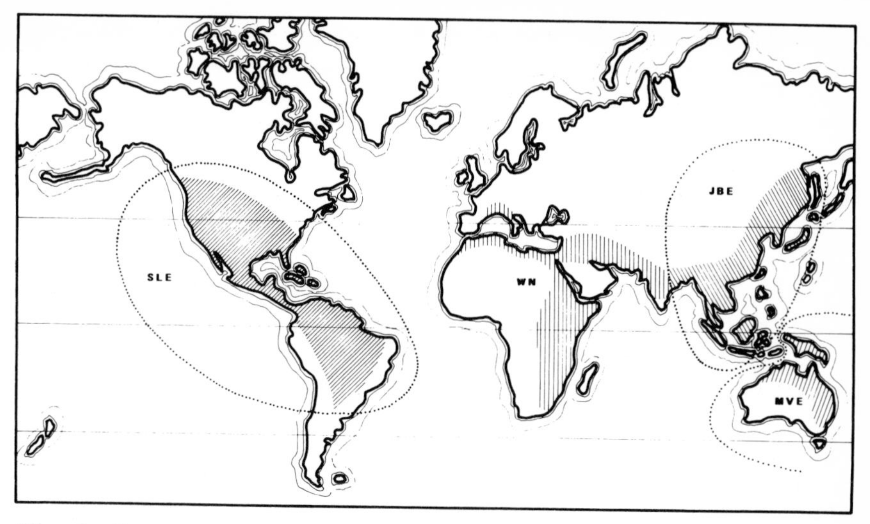

Fig. 5. Geographic distribution of four Flaviviruses: JBE—Japanese B encephalitis; SLE—St Louis encephalitis; MVE—Murray Valley encephalitis; WN—West Nile.

association. In South-East Asia, two that approach each other are JBE and MVE, where the apparent demarcation is associated with Wallace's and Weber's line (see Fig. 6). Studies need to be carried out in this geographic location to see if the known vector of MVE (*C. annulirostris*) and the known major vector for JBE (*C. tritaeniorhinchus*) overlap.

What are the effects of human activities on this group of viruses and on individual members of the group? It is undoubtedly man's use and control of water. This affects the breeding of some *Culex* sp. of mosquitoes and the breeding and feeding habitat and the movement of birds. Relevant activities are the creation of lakes, irrigated agriculture and man's many associations with water and the nature and numbers of feral animals. This is true with SLE in North America, JBE in South-East Asia, and WN infections, and it appears to be happening with MVE in Australia. In view of current research in Australia, I shall present some of the recent findings with MVE, as these are both illustrative and less well-known than the findings with SLE and JBE.

Human outbreaks of encephalitis caused by MVE (the disease is now called Australian encephalitis) have, until 1978, occurred primarily in southern and eastern Australia. Outbreaks in the summers of 1917, 1918, 1922, 1925, 1951, 1956 and 1974 involved about 335 cases with 192 deaths. Since 1974 there has been no clinical MVE and no MVE virus isolations from mosquitoes or vertebrates in eastern and

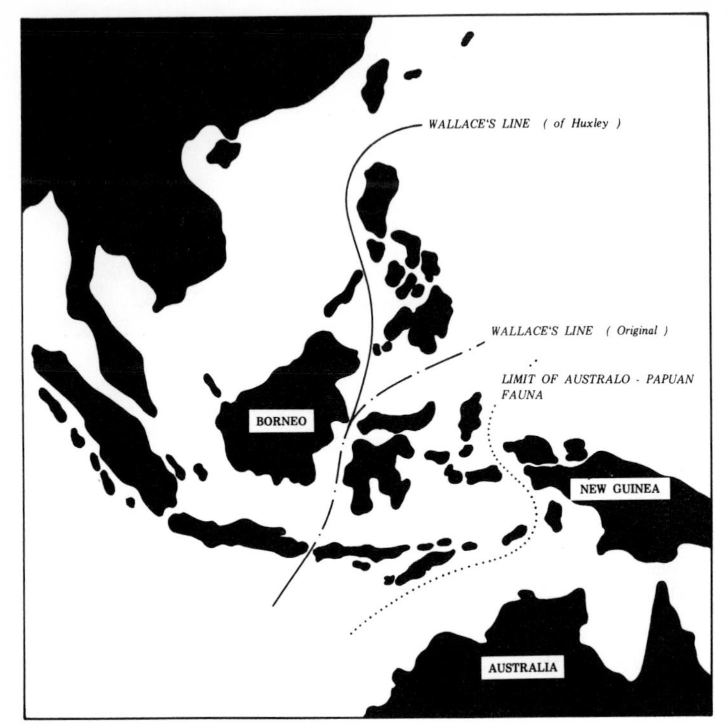

Fig. 6. The possible meeting place for MVE and JBE in South-East Asia.

southern Australia. In 1978 and 1979, however, Australian encephalitis appeared in north-west Australia and since 1972, MVE and the closely related Kunjin virus have been consistently isolated from *C. annulirostris* captured in the north-west. One of the 1978 cases was shown to be due to a Kunjin virus infection.

All available evidence points to MVE being enzootic in northern tropical Australia where *C. annulirostris* and wild birds maintain the virus. Movement of the virus to the south has frequently been associated with heavy rain in the north and the southerly movement of water birds. This hypothesis of a southern epidemic excursion is currently the most acceptable one and Australian virologists have been unable to isolate virus in south-east Australia during interepidemic periods, although there is some serological evidence suggesting virus activity as well as that of the closely related Kunjin virus (Marshall and Woodroofe, 1978).

Our studies in western and northern Australia are being undertaken at a time of dramatic environmental change associated with the use and

TABLE III. *Enzootic Focus*

Virus consistently isolated from mosquito (in all seasons, annually)
Sentinel animals rapidly convert to antibody +ve (weeks)
Aboriginal populations develop antibody at an early age until >90% +ve
Local amplifier hosts are usually antibody +ve
(MVE and Kunjin)

control of water. One of the objectives of our investigation was an attempt to determine the effects of these changes on the virus–mosquito–vertebrate host biocenose. The major changes are:

1. The creation of a large man-made lake (Stanley, 1972).
2. The development of associated irrigated agriculture (plus pesticide spraying) (Stanley, 1975; Liehne *et al.*, 1976a, b, c).
3. The development of an extensive iron ore industry in the Pilbara immediately to the south of the tropical north-west area of Australia (see Fig. 7).
4. A significant increase in tourism.
5. The presence of armed forces in this strategic area.
6. Movement of birds and humans plus the feral animal population.
7. The future development of hydroelectric power requiring the raising of the level of water in Lake Argyle.

We have shown that MVE activity is continuous in the Kimberley as the virus has been isolated each year from *C. annulirostris* captured there. In addition, sentinel animals and humans rapidly acquire antibodies and humans who have lived in the area for more than three years

TABLE IV. *Virus Isolations*[a] *from Mosquitoes Captured in North West Australia (1972–77)*

Mosquito species	No. pools tested	No isolates	%
Culex annulirostris	944	209	22·2
Aedeomyia catasticta	112	37	33·0
Aedes normanensis	18	3	16·7
Ae. tremulus	9	1	11·1
C. fatigans	96	1	1·0
Total	1179	251	21·3

[a] By the intracerebral inoculation of newborn mice

TABLE V. *Virus Isolations from W.A. Mosquitoes: Characterization of 251 Isolates from five Vectors*

Family	Genus	Virus	Mosquito species[a]					
			C. ann.	*Aed. cat.*	*Ae. trem.*	*Ae. norm.*	*C. fat.*	Total
Togaviridae	Flavivirus	Murray Valley	55				1	56
		Kunjin	21		1			22
		Kokobera	2					2
	Alphavirus	Sindbis	15			2		17
		Ross River	1					1
Bunyaviridae	Bunyavirus	Koongol	4					4
		Wongal	29					29
		Non-HA	64					64
Reoviridae	Orbivirus	Corriparta	1	32				33
Rhabdoviridae	Undefined	Kununurra[b] (OR 194)		1				1
		Parry's Creek[b] (OR 189)	3					3
		Kimberley[b] (OR 250)	1					1
Undefined		Wongorr	3			1		4
		OR 540[c]	6					6
		OR 379[c]	2					2
		OR 512[c]	2					2
		OR 869[c]		4				4
Total			209	37	1	3	1	251

[a] Abbreviations as follows: *Culex annulirostris (C. ann.)*; *Aedeomyia catasticta (Aed. cat.)*; *Aedes tremulus (Ae. trem.)*; *Ae. normanensis (Ae. norm.)*; *C. fatigans = quinquefasciatus (C. fat.)*
[b] Now recognized as new.
[c] OR 540 reacts with polyvalent *Anopheles* A immune fluid, reactive to several members of *Anopheles* A, *Anopheles* B and Turlok groups; other isolates tested and found non-reacting to Australian and world group antisera

TABLE VI. *Totals of Mosquitoes Collected during the Arbovirus Monitoring Programme* [a, b]

The 10 Most Common Species[c]

Species		Total caught	% catch[d]
Culex (Culex) annulirostris		98 227	71·80
Anopheles (Cellia) annulipes		12 162	8·89
C. (Culex) fatigans		8 043	5·88
Aedeomyia catasticta		6 694	4·89
A. (Cellia) amictus		5 480	4·00
Aedes (Ochlerotatus) vigilax		1 369	1·00
Ae. (Ochlerotatus) normanensis		1 123	0·82
A. (Anopheles) bancroftii		799	0·58
Coquillettidia xanthogaster		743	0·54
C. (Culex) australicus		405	0·30
Remainder (39 species)		1 750	1·30
Total identified:			136 795
Total unidentified unsorted material:		approximately	46 000
Total captures:		approximately	182 800

[a] These collections include all sites—Kimberley and Pilbara
[b] The collections cover 1972 to June 1979 (16 field trips).
[c] A total of 49 species have been collected
[d] % of total identified catch

usually become immune through subclinical naturally acquired infection. These observations have suggested the presence of enzootic foci (for definition see Table III) which appear to contract to small geographic areas at the end of the dry season. Table IV lists the number of virus isolates from five species of mosquitoes. Pools of 50 mosquitoes were tested and very high isolation rates were obtained of >20%. *Culex annulirostris*, the vector of MVE, is by far the most widespread mosquito and has yielded the greatest number of viruses. Of the 251 isolates, 209 came from *C. annulirostris*, 56 were MVE and 22 were Kunjin (see Table V). During this study almost 200 000 mosquitoes were captured, of which 136 795 have been identified (see Table VI). These mosquito captures were made with bait traps and with EVS/CO_2/light traps. Pesticide spraying (DDT) markedly reduced mosquito captures in the irrigation areas. When spraying ceased, due to the developing resistance of the insect pests of cotton (Stanley, 1975), *C. annulirostris* rapidly

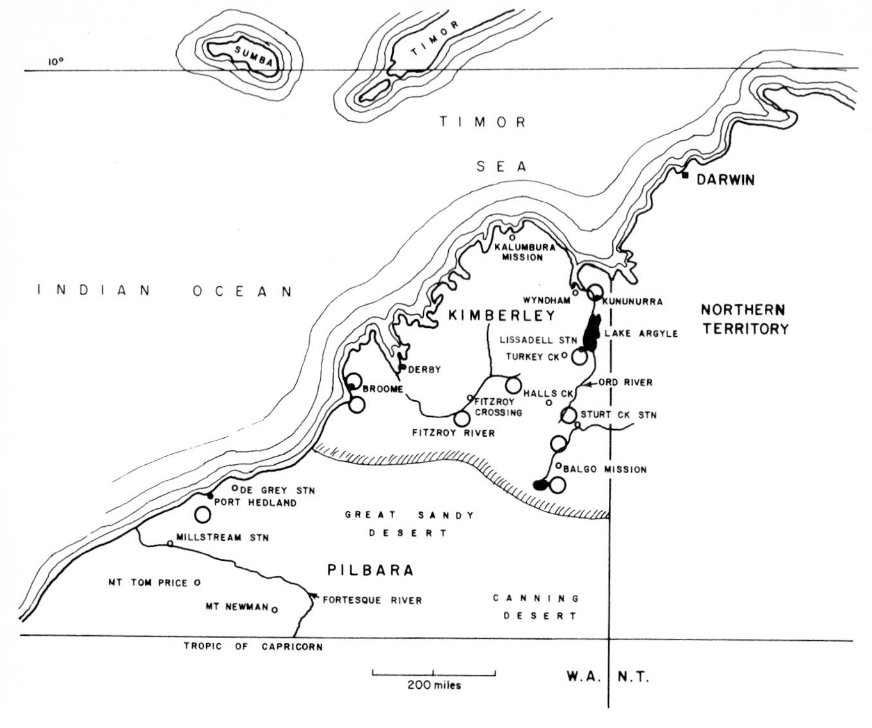

Fig. 7. Australian arbovirus encephalitis in north-west Australia. The circles indicate sites of infection.

TABLE VII. *Mosquitoes which Appear to have Increased in Density Following Creation of Man-made Lakes of the Ord River*

Coquillettidia xanthogaster	*Mansonia uniformis*
Culex annulirostris	*Aedeomyia catasticta*
C. starkiae	*Anopheles bancroftii*
C. vicinus	*A. annulipes*
C. pullus	*A. amictus*

All are species associated with permanent and semi-permanent water breeding sites

The diversity of the Ord fauna indicates the importance of the lakes to the local fauna became re-established and MVE isolations were made in this area. Following the creation of lakes in the vicinity of Kununurra (see Fig. 7), the township near the Diversion Dam and irrigation areas, the numbers of mosquitoes have increased in density (see Table VII). A similar situation is developing as the eastern and southern perimeter of Lake Argyle begins to stabilize and birds and mosquitoes adapt to the new habitat. 1978 and 1979 have seen a vast increase in water bird numbers on the lake and a high percetnage of these birds develop antibody to MVE, indicating a possible role in viral maintenance (Stanley, 1980).

Belief that MVE is enzootic over a wide area of the Kimberley is reinforced by the occurrence in 1974, 1978 and 1979 of human cases over the entire region and the transient presence of the virus in Port Hedland in the arid coastal area of the Pilbara, where intensive and large-scale mining of iron ore now demands the increased use of water and a significant increase in human population (see Fig. 7). Our observations suggest that the virus probably came down a narrow coastal strip from Broome to Port Hedland and then ceased its activity. This movement was associated with unusually heavy rainfall and the movement of birds. Continued surveillance is clearly justified if effective control measures are to be entertained in this changing scene where man's use and development of water both create and change favourable feeding and breeding habitats for birds and mosquitoes.

D. Ross River

Ross River virus (RRV) is an Alphavirus (see Table I) which causes epidemic polyarthritis in Australasia (Clarke *et al.*, 1973; Doherty *et al.*, 1977). Unlike MVE, this virus and antibody to it is widely distributed through all Australia, Papua New Guinea, the Bismarck Archipelago, Rossel Island and the Solomon Islands (Tesh *et al.*, 1975). A closely related Alphavirus, Chikungunya, has a significantly different geographic pattern as determined by antibody studies with human sera. Chikungunya is not found in Australia, but occurs in Papua New Guinea, South Vietnam, northern Malaysia, Indonesia and various islands of the Philippines group. This could be an example of mutual exclusion.

The main purpose of including RRV in this section is to draw attention to a phenomenon similar to that occurring with the recent introduction of dengue fever virus to the Pacific Islands by aircraft. In the first few months of 1979, Fiji experienced its first known outbreak of RRV infection, as a result of which >90% of the population developed antibody to RRV but not to Chikungunya virus. The only acceptable explanation of this outbreak is the introduction of RRV by aircraft carrying viraemic humans from Australia. Subsequently the virus was introduced to New Zealand by airline passengers, and it was brought back to Australia by susceptible Australians who became infected in Fiji and returned home by air while incubating the virus. The rapid movement of humans by air is thus playing a significant role in the distribution of viruses in the Southwest Pacific.

III. Discussion and Conclusions

The arthropod-borne viruses that have been selected for this essay have all been shown to have their natural ecology and transmission changed by human intervention in the naturally evolving mosquito–virus–vertebrate cycle. This has resulted in human disease and wide dissemination of these viruses throughout the planet, although all of them still remain in the original environment where they have been maintained relatively undisturbed for probably thousands of years. Movement between continents was originally by sailing ships; but jet aircraft are the present day agents of the rapid dispersal of microbial pathogens throughout the world. This movement of microbes is increasing and has resulted not only in the outbreaks of dengue fever and RRV infection described, but also in significant increases in imported malaria from endemic areas to non-endemic areas (see also Zulueta, this volume). The initial human interference has usually been (with yellow fever, dengue, Russian spring–summer encephalitis, Kyasnur Forest disease) by humans going into forests or jungles and becoming infected from the bites of virus-carrying mosquitoes or ticks. From this initial intrusion, the viruses are carried by man to his towns and from his towns to his cities (see Fig 4). This produced large urban outbreaks of disease which demanded the introduction of control measures. These took two forms—the production of a vaccine and/or vector vontrol. The only really successful vaccine has been that for yellow fever. This leaves vector control for the others, and this has only been partially successful in some urban areas. So the problems remain because there is no practical way, at the moment, of controlling these viruses in their naturally evolving ecosystems and because the prediction of epidemics and the protection of humans by vaccines have not yet been realized with the one exception cited above. Research is therefore required into vaccine production, effective mosquito control, basic ecology and evolving host–parasite relationships.

Acknowledgement

The author thanks Harry Upenieks, ARPS, RBP, for the production of Figs 1, 2, 4, 5, 6 and 7.

References

Clarke, J. A., Marshall, I. D. and Gard, G. (1973). *Am. J. trop. Med. Hyg.* **22**, 543–550.

Doherty, R. L., Filippich, C., Carley, J. G. and Hancock, J. Y. (1977). *Aust. J. exp. Biol. med. Sci.* **55**, 131–139.

Gubler, D. J. (1977). "Dengue Newsletter", Vol, 5, 10–11. South Pacific Commission.

Liehne, C. G., Leivers, S., Stanley, N. F., Alpers, M. P., Paul, S., Liehne, P. F. S. and Chan, K. H. (1976a). *Aust. J. exp. Biol. med. Sci.* **54**, 499–504.

Liehne, C. G., Stanley, N. F., Alpers, M. P., Paul, S., Liehne, P. F. S. and Chan, K. H. (1976b). *Aust. J. exp. Biol. med. Sci.* **54**, 505–512.

Liehne, P. F. S., Stanley, N. F., Alpers, M. P. and Liehne, C. G. (1976c). *Aust. J. exp. Biol. med. Sci.* **54**, 487–497.

Marshall, I. D. and Woodroofe, G. M. (1978). "Annual Report", 103–105. John Curtin School of Medical Research, Australian National University.

Port, G. R. and Wilkes, T. J. (1979). *Trans. R. Soc. trop. Med. Hyg.* **73**, 341–344.

Rosen, L. (1978). "Dengue Newsletter", No. 6, 8–9. South Pacific Commission.

Rudnick, A. L. (1977). "Annual Progress Report", 1–40. Univ. of California International Center for Medical Research.

Scott, H. H. (1939). *In* "A History of Tropical Medicine", 808–819. Arnold, London.

Stanley, N. F. (1972). *Search* **3**, 7–12.

Stanley, N. F. (1975). *In* "Man-made Lakes and Human Health" (N. F. Stanley and M. P. Alpers, Eds), 103–112. Academic Press, London and New York.

Stanley, N. F. (1979). *In* "Comparative Diagnosis of Viral Diseases" (E. Kurstak, Ed.), Vol. 3, in press. Academic Press, New York and London.

Stanley, N. F. (1980). Second Arbovirus Symposium, Brisbane. Sponsored by CSIRO Division of Animal Health and Queensland Institute of Medical Research.

Tesh, R. B., Gajdusek, D. C., Garruto, R. M., Cross, T. H. and Rosen, L. (1975). *Am. J. trop. Med. Hyg.* **24**, 664–675.

Theiler, M. and Downs, W. G. (1973). "The Arthropod-Borne Viruses of Vertebrates", 423–443. Yale Univ. Press, New Haven, Conn.

Work, T. H. and Jozan, M. (1977). *In* "Comparative Diagnosis of Viral Diseases" (E. Kurstak and C. Kurstak, Eds), Vol. 1, 621–685. Academic Press, New York and London.

10
Man and Malaria

Julian de Zulueta*
Ronda (Málaga), Spain

Malaria is . . . one of the oldest diseases of man . . . [but] the distribution of the disease over such a large area is only recent.

---

* Former Staff Member, World Health Organization.

I. Evolution of Plasmodia

Malaria is probably one of the oldest diseases of man. Other communicable diseases have been acquired by him during his long process of evolution. Taeniasis, hydatid cyst, brucellosis, possibly tuberculosis, are a result of the domestication of animals and cannot have been acquired before Neolithic times. Other diseases such as measles, mumps, smallpox, chickenpox, rubella and cholera are undoubtedly more recent acquisitions. Only the population size and living conditions of the urban age would allow for the maintenance of these diseases, which Cockburn (1967) termed "acute crowd infections".

The situation concerning malaria is different. The disease has been found among contemporary hunters and food-gatherers and it almost certainly afflicted Palaeolithic man if it did not already afflict his hominid ancestors. Monkeys and apes suffer from malaria and in the blood of the chimpanzees and gorillas of Africa are found parasites identical to *Plasmodium malariae* and *Plasmodia vivax*, the quartan and benign tertian malaria parasites of man. This indicates a common origin of these plasmodia and places the origin of the disease at the very early stages of human evolution. *Plasmodium falciparum*, the third common human malaria parasite, the causative agent of malignant tertian, is generally considered to be a more recent parasite on evolutionary grounds (Garnham, 1966; Coatney *et al.*, 1971) but there can be no doubt of its long association with man as shown by the development of sickle cell anaemia, conferring protection against malaria in the heterozygous state although lethal itself in the homozygote (Allison, 1954; Raper, 1955). The selection of this abnormal haemoglobin mutation could only have taken place in highly endemic malarious areas and over a considerable period of time.

A fourth species of malaria parasite, *Plasmodium ovale*, closely resembling *P. vivax*, is found in Africa but in our enquriy about man's role in changing patterns of the disease we will only consider the three common species of malaria parasites, which have been mentioned already. The three were found until recently in temperate and tropical areas with adequate rainfall and at altitudes of up to 2000 m above sea level. Of the malaria parasites, *P. vivax* and *P. malariae* require temperatures of at least 15°C for their development in the anopheline vector whereas *P. falciparum* requires temperatures in excess of 17 or 18°C for its development in the mosquito (Boyd, 1949; Macdonald, 1957). As a result, the July and January isotherms of 15°C in the Northern and

Southern Hemispheres have been found to be the approximate limits of diffusion of vivax and quartan malaria and the isotherms of 17 or 18°C those of falciparum malaria (Hackett, 1949).

II. Distribution of Malaria

A. Climatic Changes and Malarial Vectors

The distribution of the disease over such a large area is only recent. There are many indications that it must have spread in prehistoric times due to climatic changes and there is evidence of further spread in historic times through the agency of man. Zulueta (1973) and Bruce-Chwatt and Zulueta (1980) have called attention to the effect that the Pleistocene glaciations must have had upon the distribution of malaria in Europe and western Asia. With temperatures 8 or 9·5°C lower than those of today (Messerli, 1967; Butzer, 1972) transmission of *Plasmodium vivax* and *P. malariae* could only take place in the southernmost parts of Europe. But *P. falciparum*, requiring higher temperatures for its development in the mosquito, was almost certainly excluded from the Europe of the last glaciation.

As regards the vectors, it is also practically certain that the two most important vectors of the Mediterranean area, namely *Anopheles labranchiae* and *A. sacharovi*, were absent from the Europe of the last glaciation. The limit of distribution of the two species in the south of Europe today, corresponds to the July isotherms of 23 or 24°C. The available paleoclimatological evidence (Messerli, 1967; Butzer, 1972) indicates that nowhere in Europe were such high mean July temperatures reached during the last ice age.

The spread of malaria and its vectors towards higher latitudes must have been a slow process, for 15 000 years elapsed between the maximum extent of the ice and its reduction to its present size (Butzer, 1972). By 8300 B.C. present-day temperatures prevailed. By then the cultivation of plants and the domestication of animals had already taken place in the Levant and Near East highlands. The "Neolithic revolution" reached Greece after 7000 B.C. and other parts of Europe a millenium later (Butzer, 1972). It ensured a food supply which could sustain much larger populations than in Palaeolithic times—1000 persons per 100 km^2, according to Braidwood and Reed (1957). Such a population density could provide the necessary number of non-inmunes to maintain diseases which could not have existed in Palaeolithic or Mesolithic societies.

B. Agricultural Changes and Malaria

In the case of malaria, the increase of population and the less mobile habits of the Neolithic farmers must have resulted in an increase of the disease. This was observed in Sarawak (Borneo), where nomadic hunters and food-gatherers had lower parasite and spleen rates than slash-and-burn agriculturists living in the same forest areas (Zulueta, 1956).

Agricultural activities may also have increased the transmission of malaria in another way. The destruction of forests created conditions favourable for the breeding of anopheline mosquitoes from drier and sunnier lands, and this is probably one of the main reasons which made possible the introduction to Europe in comparatively recent times of *Anopheles labranchiae*, which during the Pleistocene must have been a North African species, and of *A. sacharovi* which must until then have been confined to western Asia.

Another consequence of the agricultural activities of man was the increase of soil erosion, resulting in turn in increased sedimentation, which had also an effect on the spread of malaria and its vectors. Some of the most malarious areas of Asia Minor and southern Europe are alluvial plains of recent formation such as the plains of Tarsus and the Meander in Turkey and those of Thermopylae in Greece and the Gargano in Italy. Exceptionally high densities of either *A. sacharovi* or *A. labranchiae* are still found in these coastal plains which until very recently remained thinly populated due to the danger of malaria.

The historical record provides us with information concerning the presence of malaria in ancient historical times. There is frequent mention of diseases in Mesopotamian records (Kinnier Wilson, 1967) but it is difficult to venture a retrospective diagnosis of malaria except in the case of a disabling ague mentioned in the Code of Hamburabi. Mention of diseases is also frequent in the Old Testament but none of them can be identified with certainty as malaria.

In the case of Egypt, according to Halawani and Shawarby (1957), there is mention of malaria in early dynastic records and the word *AAT*, found among the inscriptions of the temple of Denderah probably meant malaria (Russell, 1955). Although none of these records can be considered by itself as a conclusive proof of the existence of the disease, their cumulative effect strongly suggests its presence in the ancient Near East. On evolutionary grounds it can also be assumed that a disease which had afflicted man since his earliest days, must also have been present among the settlers of Mesopotamia and the Nile Valley.

On the same grounds it can be assumed that the Indus Civilization also suffered from malaria, although it remains completely silent on the subject of diseases as it does on many others.

The existence in the Indus Valley of a vector species, *A. stephensi*, well adapted to urban life, indicates an association of the species with man, probably dating from the time of the first urban settlements in the valley. Nowhere else in the world is found a malaria vector so well adapted to urban life as *A. stephensi*, and this strongly suggests an early association with urban development. In our view, this association, making malaria a common disease of the town-dwellers, may be one of the reasons—perhaps the principal one—for the sudden end of the Indus Civilization during the second millenium B.C.

The domestic *A. stephensi* is also likely to have enlarged its area of distribution through the agency of man. The species is found at present not only in the Indian Subcontinent, which was probably its original home, but also in oases and tracts of irrigated land of riverine countries of the Persian Gulf. When the first malaria survey of Mesopotamia was made during the First World War, *A. stephensi* was found as far north as Karbala and Amarah (Christophers and Short, 1921). A survey made during the Second World War showed that the species had by then reached Baghdad (Macan, 1950). Work carried out two decades later revealed the presence of *A. sephensi* as far north as Mosul (Muir, 1971).

Genetical evidence indicates that in this large area of distribution there is only a single species and that *A. stephensi* is in fact the same in India as in Iraq (Zulueta *et al.*, 1968). This can be safely taken as an indication of a comparatively recent dispersal. It indicates furthermore that the displacements involved are likely to have taken place through the agency of man. With the prevailing conditions of extreme dryness in the Persian Gulf area, it would have been difficult for *A. stephensi* to reach its few oases and tracts of irrigated land unless it were carried in the hold of ships, plying between its various ports since early historical times. The rapid northward displacement of *A. stephensi* in modern Iraq can also safely be attributed to the activities of man. The increased urbanization of the area and the multiplication of communications of all kinds must have facilitated the dispersal in recent times of this highly domestic species.

Returning to the world of antiquity and focusing our attention on the Mediterranean area, we find that at the dawn of Greek Civilization climatic conditions would allow for the development of the three main species of malaria parasites and some of its most effective vectors (*A. labranchiae* and *A. sacharovi*) in areas from which they had been barred during the last glaciation and its aftermath. The accounts of Herodotus and Xenophon, however, do not suggest to us that this had happened by the fifth century B.C. Although they frequently mention fevers, which almost certainly were malarious fevers, the impression gained is that classical Greece suffered much less from malaria than modern Greece, as Sir Ronald Ross (1906) and W. H. S. Jones (1909) remarked.

But perhaps the most significant information concerning the malaria situation in classical Greece is that provided by the Hippocratic texts. The clinical and epidemiological observations that they contain make abundantly clear that malaria was a well known disease in the Greece of that period but, despite assertions to the contrary, leave us in doubt as to the presence of malignant tertian (Zulueta, 1973; Bruce-Chwatt and Zulueta, 1980). What can be safely said is that, if *Plasmodium falciparum* did then exist in Greece, it must have been a rare parasite.

The situation concerning *A. sacharovi* is a similar one. The lack of anything resembling the devastating epidemics of malaria seen in Macedonia during the First World War makes it likely that the armies operating in the Balkan Peninsula in classical Greek and early Roman times were not exposed to the bites of an efficient vector like *A. sacharovi* (Zulueta, 1973). What seems probable is that the increased population movements of Hellenistic and Roman times, resulting from expanded commerce and slave trade, invading armies and returning soldiers, brought *P. falciparum* frequently to Greece and Italy until it became adapted to transmission by the local vectors. The refractoriness of *A. atroparvus*, the most widespread European vector, to tropical strains of *P. falciparum* (Shute, 1940; Zulueta *et al.*, 1975) indicates that the selection of strains adapted to transmission by this and possibly other European vectors must have taken a considerable period of time.

The introduction of *A. sacharovi* and *A. labranchiae* in Greece and Italy is also likely to have been helped by the activities of man. The coastal distribution of the two species in the two countries strongly suggests a nautical dispersal (Zulueta, 1973). This is likely to have occurred during the increase of navigation of Hellenistic and Roman times when the chances of accidental transport by ship of larvae and adults must have multiplied. The deforestation resulting from increased agriculture activities must have also favoured the introduction of species which, like *A. sacharovi* and *A. labranchiae*, originated in drier lands.

By the end of the Roman Empire, Europe seems to have suffered from malaria as much as in modern times. During the Middle Ages the disease and its vectors probably reached the prevalence and distribution that they had in modern times but in the absence of any effective treatment or prophylactic measure, mediaeval Europe must have suffered more heavily from malaria than it did recently. Italy certainly did. Failing to maintain the efficient drainage works of Roman times, rich agricultural lands like the Agro Pontino reverted to swamps, breeding Anophelines which decimated a by now scanty human population.

In the south of Europe, Italy and Greece seem to have suffered more from malaria than Spain. Celli (1901) and later Cambournac (1942) noted that the south of Spain under Arab domination seems to have suffered comparatively little from malaria. This may have been due to the almost complete absence of *A. labranchiae* and *A. sacharovi*. Only in a small zone in south-east Spain was the former species found until recently and seems now to have disappeared under the impact of residual insecticides (J. Blazquez, personal communication 1973). Elsewhere in Spain, only the much less effective *A. atroparvus* was found. The labranchiae bridgehead, if not established directly through man's accidentally bringing specimens in his ships, had only been made possibly by his agricultural activities. The Arab system of irrigation transformed the driest part of Spain into a well-watered fertile land where the newcomers could breed and live.

The absence of a potent vector in most of the Iberian Peninsula probably contributed to the successful agricultural development of Arab-ruled Spain. But it was precisely this development, based on the introduction of new methods and new cultures, which was later to produce a deterioration of the malaria situation. The Arabs are known to have introduced into Spain the cultivation of rice, although the exact date of the introduction has not been established. By the twelfth century, however, its cultivation was well known in Andalusia, as we learn from the account of Ibn Al Awan (quoted by Dubler, 1943). Its harmful effect on health was soon noted and we learn that the cultivation of rice was forbidden in Valencia in the fourteenth century, by then under Christian rule. This and other prohibitions later did not deter farmers from cultivating rice, despite its association with fevers (Rico-Avello, 1947).

In its original home in South-East Asia the cultivation of wet rice did not result in an increase of malaria, the rice fields having little attraction for the vector species. But in the case of the Iberian Peninsula the rice fields became a breeding place of choice for *A. atroparvus*. Cambournac (1939) found this species breeding in prodigious numbers in the Portuguese rice fields, counting as many as 400 larvae per m^2 of surface. Such high densities, combined with the presence of seasonal workers, sleeping in flimsy shelters or in the open, resulted in a high prevalence of malaria.

The cultivation of rice was introduced in South America by the Spaniards and its association with malaria in certain areas (e.g. northern Argentina) was known since colonial times (Gabaldon, 1949). But this brings us to the much debated question of whether malaria existed in the New World or was introduced there by the European discoverers and settlers. Among those who believe that malaria was a post-Columbian importation are Sir Harold Scott (1939), an eminent medical historian, and Mark F. Boyd (1949), one of the most distinguished American malariologists. But there are many experts, particularly in South America, who have held the opposite view like Paz-Soldan (1938) and Jaramillo-Arango (1950). We will not enter into the arguments brought forward by the two schools except to point out that their apparant contradictory views can perhaps be explained by an over-simplification of the problem. They argue about the existence or the absence of malaria in pre-Columbian America without taking fully into account that there are at least three different kinds of human malaria.

The presence of *P. malariae*, *P. vivax* and *P. falciparum* in most of the world's malarious territory in contemporary times has helped to create the misleading impression that the three species did always exist together. This may have happened in the Old World at the beginning of the Age of Discovery but there are good reasons for believing that it was not the situation in the New World at that critical moment.

The existence in the forests of South America of two monkey malaria parasites, *P. brasilianum* and *P. simium*, morphologically and biologically almost identical to *P. malariae* and *P. vivax* strongly suggests an adaptation of the human parasites to the new environment (Coatney *et al.*, 1971). In our view these anthroposes must have taken a long time to develop, longer in any case than the relatively short span of time separating us from the European discovery and colonization. It thus seems likely that, as pointed out by Bruce-Chwatt (1965), quartan and vivax malaria existed in the New World in pre-Columbian days. The introduction of the short-lived *P. falciparum* in prehistoric times seems much more unlikely, particularly if this were to happen during the last glaciation, when *P. falciparum* must have been confined to lower latitudes than it was in recent times, thus making the introduction via the Behring land-bridge or northern coastal waters virtually impossible.

In the health catastrophe produced by the introduction of new diseases from the Old to the New World by the Spanish conquistadores and their African slaves, the introduction and spread of some of them, like smallpox or yellow fever, can be followed in detail. In the case of malaria the epidemiological happenings are less clear but there is no doubt that the upheaval of the conquest generated much malaria among the conquistadores and Amerindians. If an aggravation of an existing situation did then take place, this may have been the result of the introduction of falciparum malaria by the conquistadores from southern Spain and their slaves from Africa.

The introduction of malaria in the South Pacific affords a good example of the role of man in the spread of the disease. The Portuguese navigators sailing eastward from Malacca and the Spanish explorers sailing down from the Philippines were probably the first to bring malaria to the area. To these were later added British, Dutch and French voyagers, who spread the disease further. Australia was free from malaria until comparatively recently, the first report of its appearance dating from 1849 (Lambert, 1949). Malaria and its vectors may have been relatively new introductions to New Guinea and from the available evidence it can be concluded that the anopheline mosquitoes are relatively late entrants in Melanesia (Lambert, 1949). The malaria-free zone of the Pacific, now limited to the area east of 170° (east) and south 20° (south), must have thus been much larger until comparatively recent times.

With the spread of the disease in the South Pacific through the agency of man we reach the point of maximum dispersal of malaria and its vectors as well as that of its highest prevalence. We see that the disease begins to loosen its hold in northern Europe in the middle of the nineteenth century due more to ecological changes brought about by novel practices of agriculture and stock breeding than by the judicious use of quinine. As Wesenberg-Lund (1921) pointed out, the construction in Denmark of pigsties and stables where the animals were kept most of the time, created places more attractive to feed and rest for the local vector, *A. atroparvus*, a zoophilic species, than human dwellings. Another change brought about by the increase of stock breeding was the replacement of cereals for human consumption by root crops for animal fodder. Senior-White (quoted by Hackett, 1952) believed that the introduction of turnip cultivation in England in the middle of the nineteenth century, to provide winter fodder for cattle, increased their number and made man less prone to the attacks of *A. atroparvus*, thus initiating the decline of malaria.

III. Control of Malaria

To the ecological changes brought about by improved agriculture and stock breeding and general improvement of housing and living conditions, were added, since the beginning of the twentieth century, specific measures against malaria and its vectors. Although Gorgas (1915) showed in Panama that malaria could be controlled under tropical conditions, the colossal effort made was not repeated in other tropical areas. The great gains over malaria before the advent of DDT were made in the temperate zone, in economically advanced countries, thus underlining the importance of the social factor in the prevalence of the disease. In perspective the gains made seem to have been due more to the general improvement of medical and health facilities and to improved educational, cultural and economic standards than to specific anti-malaria measures.

The advent of DDT and other resudual insecticides brought the end of malaria in Australia, Europe, the Soviet Union and USA. The worldwide effort to eradicate malaria, however, has not succeeded and we have seen in recent years an ominous increase of the disease (WHO, 1978). Eradication methods have never had more than a limited success in tropical Africa, which was and still remains the most malarious part of the world. In America and Asia the initial gains of eradication have been lost in many places by a resurgence of the disease in recent years. This, combined with the expansion of travel, has resulted in an increase of the number of imported cases in countries where malaria had disappeared for all practical purposes. Such is the situation of Australia, the USA and the European countries where transmission had ceased long ago but where imported cases of malaria are now a common feature.

One of the causes of the resurgence of the disease has been the development of chloroquine resistance in *Plasmodium falciparum* from South-East Asia and Tropical America. But perhaps more important has been the development of insecticide resistance among some of the major vectors of malaria. Such developments, however, can only partially explain the resurgence of the disease. As the experience of the Near East has shown (Zulueta and Muir, 1972), a technical problem like insecticide resistance is a less serious obstacle to eradication than those arising from defective organization and administration. Without an improvement of cultural, social and economic conditions in the large areas of the world still suffering from malaria, it is difficult to see how man, the great spreader of the disease, will finally master and eliminate it.

References

Allison, A. C. (1954). Protection afforded by sickle-cell trait against subtertian malarial infection. *Br. med. J.* i, 290–294.

Boyd, M. F. (1949). "Malariology", Chaps 1 and 26. Saunders, Philadelphia.

Braidwood, R. J. and Reed, C. A. (1957). The achievement and early consequences of food-production. *Cold Spring Harb. Symp. quant. Biol.* **22**, 19–31.

Bruce-Chwatt, L. J. (1965). Paleogenesis and paleo-epidemiology of primate malaria. *Bull. Wld Hlth Org.* **32**, 363–387.

Bruce-Chwatt, L. J. and Zulueta, J. de (1980). "The Rise and Fall of Malaria in Europe". Oxford Univ. Press.

Butzer, K. W. (1972). "Environment and Archaeology", 2nd edn. Methuen, London.

Cambournac, F. J. C. (1939). A method for determining the larval *Anopheles* population and its distribution in rice fields. *Riv. Malariol.* **1**, 17–22.

Cambournac, F. J. C. (1942). "Sobre a epidemiologia do sezonismo em Portugal". Sociedade Industrial de Tipografia, Lisbon.

Celli, A. (1901). "Malaria According to the New Researches". Longmans Green, London.

Christophers, S. R. and Short, H. E. (1921). Malaria in Mesopotamia. *Indian J. med. Res.* **8**, 508–552.

Coatney, G. R., Collins, W. E., Warren, McW. and Contacos, P. G. (1971). "The Primate Malarias". US Government Printing Office, Washington.

Cockburn, A. (1967). "Infectious Diseases: Their Evolution and Eradication". C. C. Thomas, Springfield, Ill.

Dubler, C. E. (1943). Über das Wirtschaftslebau auf der Iberischen Halbinsäl von XI-XIII Jh. *Romanica helvetica* **22**, 1–186.

Gabaldon, A. (1949). Malaria incidence in the West Indies and South America. *In* "Boyd's Malariology". Saunders, Philadelphia.

Garnham, P. C. C. (1966). "Malaria Parasites and Other Haemosporidia". Blackwell, Oxford.

Gorgas, W. C. (1915). "Sanitation in Panama". Appleton, London.

Hackett, L. W. (1949). Distribution of malaria. *In* "Boyd's Malariology". Saunders, Philadelphia.

Hackett, L. W. (1952). The disappearance of malaria in Europe and the United States. *Riv. Parassit.* **13**, 43–56.

Halawani, A. and Shawarby, A. A. (1957). Malaria in Egypt. *J. Egypt. med. Ass.* **40**, 753–792.

Jaramillo-Arango, J. (1950). The Conquest of Malaria. Heinemann, London.

Jones, W. H. S. (1909). Malaria and Greek History. Oxford Univ. Press.

Kinnier Wilson, J. V. (1967). Organic diseases of Ancient Mesopotamia. *In* "Diseases in Antiquity" (D. Brothwell and A. T. Sandison, Eds). C. C. Thomas, Springfield, Ill.

Lambert, S. M. (1949). Malaria incidence in Australia and the South Pacific. *In* "Boyd's Malariology". Saunders, Philadelphia.

Macan, T. T. (1950) The anopheline mosquitoes of Iraq and Northern Persia. *In* "*Anopheles* and Malaria in the Near East". London School of Hygiene and Tropical Medicine, Memoire No. 7. H. K. Lewis, London.
Macdonald G. (1957). "The Epidemiology and Control of Malaria". Oxford Univ. Press.
Messerli, B. (1967). Die eiszeitliche und die gegenwärtige Vergletscherung im Mittelmeerraum. *Geographica helvetica* 1967, 105–228.
Muir, D. A. (1971). Entomological evaluation of the malaria programmes of Lebanon, Syria, Jordan and Iraq. Unpublished report to WHO.
Paz-Soldan, C. E. (1938). "Las tercianas del Conde de Chinchon". Reforma Medica, Lima.
Raper, A. B. (1955). Sickling in relation to morbidity from malaria and other diseases. *Br. med. J.* i, 965–966.
Rico Avello y Rico, C. (1947). Aportacion española a la historia del paludismo. *Revista de Sanidad e Higiene Publica* **21**, 483–525.
Ross, R. (1906). Malaria in Greece. *J. trop. Med.* **9**, 341–347.
Russell, P. F. (1955). "Man's Mastery of Malaria". Oxford Univ. Press.
Scott, H. H. (1939). "History of Tropical Medicine". Arnold, London.
Shute, P. G. (1940). Failure to infect English specimens of *Anopheles maculipennis* var. *atroparvus* with certain strains of *Plasmodium falciparum* of tropical origin. *J. trop. Med. Hyg.* **43**, 175–178.
Wesenberg-Lund, C. (1921). Contributions to the biology of the Danish Culicidae. *D. Kgl. Danske, Vidensk. Selsk. Skrifter, Naturv. og Matematik.* Serv. 8, VII, No. 1.
WHO (1978). Malaria control—a reoriented strategy. *WHO Chron.* **32**, 226–230.
Zulueta, J. de (1956). Malaria in Sarawak and Brunei. *Bull. Wld Hlth Org.* **15**, 651–671.
Zulueta, J. de (1973). Malaria and Mediterranean history. *Parassitologia* **15**, 1–15.
Zulueta, J. de, Chang, T. L., Cullen, J. R. and Davidson, G. (1968). Recent observations on insecticide resistance in *Anopheles stephensi* in Iraq. *Mosquito News* **28**, 499–503.
Zulueta, J. de and Muir, D. A. (1972). Malaria eradication in the Near East. *Trans. R. Soc. trop. Med Hyg.* **66**, 679–696.
Zulueta, J. de, Ramsdale, C. D. and Coluzzi, M. (1975). Receptivity to malaria in Europe. *Bull. Wld Hlth Org.* **52**, 109–111.

11

Schistosomes, Snails and Man

David I. Grove

Department of Medicine, University of Western Australia, Perth, Australia

---

The association between man and schistosomes has been documented for at least 3000 years. . . . Migration has been one of the major human activities influencing the demography of schistosomiasis. . . .

Metazoan organisms rarely cause death, but may produce considerable morbidity . . . as . . . social and religious customs evolve, so the transmission . . . and severity of schistosomiasis . . . will continue to change. . . . [The Aswam High Dam] has led to an undisturbed stable snail population which facilitates the transmission of schistosomiasis. . . . Environmental sanitation . . . is . . . the best way of controlling schistosomiasis.

I. Introduction

Man and his helminth parasites have evolved together over countless millenia. These metazoan organisms rarely cause death, but may produce considerable morbidity, particularly in developing countries which are plagued with concurrent malnutrition and multiple infections. In contrast to other human pathogens, most worms are unable to replicate within the human host. Furthermore, the development of immunity and the acquisition of resistance to reinfection is incomplete at best. Consequently, worm burdens and severity of disease are usually related to both the intensity and duration of exposure. Some worms are transmitted directly from one person to another, some have a free-living cycle in the environment, and yet others require the participation of intermediate hosts such as insects, crustaceans and molluscs. Schistosomiasis is one of the more significant helminthiases and will be used as an illustration of this important group of human infections.

The association between man and schistosomes has been documented for at least 3000 years. Calcified eggs have been found in kidneys of two mummies of the XXth dynasty (*c.* 1184–1087 B.C.), and endemic haematuria in young Egyptian adults was mentioned frequently in a number of papyri (see Abdel-Salem and Ehsan, 1978). It is only in recent times, however, that we have begun to understand the complex interrelationships between man, schistosomes and the environment. These advances were dependent upon two fundamental observations. In 1851, Theodor Bilharz discovered that a worm was the causative agent of schistosomiasis, then in the early part of this century, Japanese workers demonstrated that the infection could only be acquired after development of the worm in certain species of freshwater molluscs (Miyairi and Suzuki, 1913).

The schistosomiases are infections of man which are usually caused by one of three species of trematodes, *Schistosoma mansoni*, *S. haematobium* or *S. japonicum*. The first organism is found in parts of Africa, South America and the Caribbean, the second in Africa and the Middle East, while the third species is found only in East and South-East Asia. It is estimated that approximately 250 million people are infected with these helminths, although only a small and unknown proportion of them have symptoms and signs of disease resulting from the infection. Since transmission of the worms is complex, and is dependent upon water and certain species of molluscs, a large number of social and environmental factors may modify the prevalence and intensity of infection in a given area. This chapter will attempt to delineate the more important ecological influences on the spread, severity and significance of human schistosomiasis. These effects can only be understood, however, in the context of the schistosome life cycle.

II. The Schistosome Life Cycle

The three major species of schistosomes infecting man have similar life cycles with a sexual generation in the definitive vertebrate host and an asexual phase in the snail intermediate hosts. The adult worms, approximately 1 cm in length, are blood-dwelling flukes; *Schistosoma mansoni* and *S. japonicum* are found predominantly in the mesenteric veins while *S. haematobium* is usually located in vesical venous plexus. These trematodes are unisexual and the longer, filiform female is held during copulation in the gynaecophoric canal formed by infolding of the sides of the male body. The female worms lay eggs in the periphery of the venules; the number produced per worm per day varies from 300 for *S. mansoni* to 3000 for *S. japonicum*. Approximately half of these eggs pass through the vessel walls to the lumen of the bowel (*S. mansoni* and *S. japonicum*) or bladder (*S. haematobium*) and thence to the exterior in the faeces or urine repectively. The remaining eggs are trapped in the tissues of the gut or urinary tract or embolise to the liver.

If viable ova reach fresh water, the egg ruptures and a larva (miracidium), which may live for up to 24 hours, emerges. If miracidia penetrate the soft tissues of a snail that is suitable for further maturation, they develop over four to seven weeks into sporocysts, then into fork-tailed forms about 1 mm long known as cercariae. Asexual multiplication occurs during this phase and one miracidium may result in thousands of cercariae which emerge from the snail under appropriate conditions over the ensuing weeks. This free-swimming stage has a life span of up to 48 hours. The cercariae penetrate the unbroken skin of man within several minutes; in the process they lose their tails and the resulting schistosomula migrate through the lymphatics and venules to the lungs, then to the portal circulation where they mature into adult worms. Within six to eight weeks of infection, mating has occurred and the females have begun to produce eggs. The adult worms probably live for about five to ten years and continue to produce eggs during that period (Warren *et al.*, 1974).

III. Mathematical Models of Transmission

Many factors relating to the worm itself, the snail intermediate hosts and the human population interact to determine the prevalence and intensity of infection and severity of disease in diverse environments. A number of mathematical models have been devised to describe the transmission of schistosomiasis (Fine and Lehmann, 1977). Some models have been constructed using sets of assumptions; they are designed to explore the relationships between different host and environment factors and to investigate their relative effects on schistosome transmission. An alternative approach has been to use models based on known age-specific prevalence rates and intensities of schistosome infections in both humans and snails. It is hoped that by delineating the more crucial and susceptible links in the chain of transmission, these mathematical approaches may assist in the formulation and organization of public health programmes designed to control schistosomiasis. Furthermore, they may give an estimate of the monetary costs involved and the benefits likely to be achieved. The following sections will discuss worms, snails and man in relation to the changing ecology of schistosomiasis.

IV. Environmental Influences on the Worms

Schistosomes are exposed to the external environment during two phases of their life cycle. Once the eggs are excreted, they need to be deposited in fresh water with suitable conditions of warmth and light for the miracidia to be released. The miracidia are attracted by light and tend to be found in the upper strata of water bodies where most of the molluscs congregate. A large number of factors determine whether they successfully penetrate snails; these include the number of miracidia and snails, the length of contact, the velocity, turbulence and turbidity of the water and the intensity of light. Furthermore, miracidia are probably attracted by chemotactic substances released from the snails (Chernin, 1970). Nevertheless, the majority of eggs which are excreted fail to produce miracidia which develop successfully in the snail intermediate host.

Similarly, cercariae are free-living forms susceptible to environmental factors. Cercariae of *Schistosoma mansoni* and *S. haematobium* usually leave the snail under the influence of heat and light, thus peak shedding occurs about midday (Webbe and Jordan, 1966), while those of *S. japonicum* are shed in the evening and in smaller numbers (Pesigan *et al.*, 1958). Since cercariae are not feeding forms but subsist on their glycogen reserves, anything which stimulates their activity such as increasing temperature will reduce their life span. They are usually found just below the surface of the water. The stimulus to finding the vertebrate host is unknown, but is probably not chemotactic. As with miracidia, the ability of cercariae to infect the host is determined by length of contact and the water velocity, turbulence and temperature. They are not resistant to dessication and are destroyed if the skin should dry before penetration is complete.

V. Snails and their Habitats

Human schistosomes are transmitted only by a limited number of species of snails. Furthermore, the various schistosome species require different mollusc intermediate hosts. Even within a susceptible snail species, some individuals are resistant to infection. The mechanisms affecting snail susceptibility are not well understood; the genetic predispositions of the snails themselves are probably important (Richards, 1970), as are strain characteristics of the schistosomes (Webbe and James, 1971). Under field conditions, snails are rarely infected by more than a single miracidium. The infection rate varies considerably; in individual foci, more than 50% of snails may be infected, but over large areas, the numbers are often less than 1%. The effect on the snail of this parasitism is variable but mortality is often increased.

Schistosoma mansoni is usually transmitted by snails of the genus *Biomphalaria*, particularly *B. pfeifferi*, *B. alexandrina* and *B. sudanica* in Africa and *B. glabrata*, *B. straminea* and *B. tenagophila* in the Americas. *Schistosoma haematobium* is transmitted by snails of the genus *Bulinus*, particularly *B. truncatus*, *B. africanus*, *B. globosus* and *B. nasutus*. Since these molluscs are obligatory inhabitants of fresh water, the distribution of this medium limits the occurrence of both snails and the human infection. Within this ecological restriction, however, the snails have adapted to a variety of environmental conditions ranging from large stagnant lakes, through flowing rivers to aqueducts, temporary roadside ditches and seepage areas (Burch, 1975). They are usually found in shallow water or near the surface of large bodies of water. They prefer water which is not turbid, allows moderate light penetration, is rich in dissolved solids, has an adequate amount of dissolved oxygen, a substratum rich in organic matter for food and the presence of water weeds for shelter and egg-laying. *Bulinus* and *Biomphalaria* are hermaphroditic, and while cross-fertilization is usual, are capable of self-fertilization. Their life span is usually less than a year and the rate of population increase is dependent upon a number of variables including the size of the habitat, degree of crowding, food supply, temperature and pH. They can survive over a wide range of water pH and prefer warm water, especially between 20 and 30°C. They may survive seasonal drying in temporary waters by burrowing into the mud and secreting mucus over their aperture. Moreover, the schistosome parasite may survive within them (Webbe, 1962).

Although the snail intermediate hosts of *S. japonicum* are morphologically and functionally quite different and are placed in a separate subclass of molluscs, they too share water or moist areas with humans and thus disease transmission occurs in the same manner as with the African and American snails. A number of subspecies of *Oncomelania hupensis* are vectors of this parasite. This snail is amphibious in its habits and is found not only in water, but also in moist, shaded places. They are especially prevalent in man-made habitats such as paddy fields, irrigation canals and drainage ditches. Oncomelanid snails, which live for several months to a year, are unisexual and copulation occurs repeatedly. The presence of an operculum facilitates their survival during dry seasons and they do not need to burrow into mud or find refuge in cracks and crevices.

VI. Animal Reservoirs

The presence or absence of an animal reservoir of human parasites may greatly alter the epidemiology of infection and modify the likelihood of success of various control measures. The importance of such a reservoir is in large measure determined by the degree of contact between man and animal. This in turn, is influenced by economic, social and behavioural factors. *Schistosoma haematobium* is primarily a parasite of man only. *Schistosoma mansoni* predominantly infects humans, but some animals, particularly primates and rodents may be infected (Amorim *et al.*, 1954; Nelson, 1960); this probably represents reverse zoonotic transmission from man to animals and is of little epidemiological significance. *Schistosoma japonicum* infection, however, is a true zoonosis and animals ranging from small rodents to water buffalo may be infected. This reservoir is of major epidemiological importance in areas such as paddy fields in which man and animals share a common environment. Consequently, the extension of rice cultivation in parts of Asia has undoubtedly led to an increase in schistosomiasis (McMullen *et al.*, 1951).

VII. Human Infection and Disease

The clinical manifestations of chronic schistosomiasis are not due to the adult worms themselves, but result from the eggs which the female worms lay. A proportion of ova are trapped in the tissues and it is the immunologically mediated inflammatory reaction and succeeding fibrosis which develops around them that produces disorder (Warren, 1972; Warren, 1978). A distinction must be drawn, however, between infection and disease; the former refers to the presence of schistosomes in the body whereas the latter indicates ill-health as a result of the parasite. The severity of the tissue disturbance is proportional to the number of eggs present; minimal infections are asymptomatic while heavy infections produce symptoms and signs of disease (Cheever, 1968; Cook *et al.*, 1974; Arap Siongok *et al.*, 1976; Abdel-Salam and Abdel-Fattah, 1977; Cheever *et al.*, 1978; Abdel-Salam and Ehsan, 1978). The number of eggs in the tissues is in turn dependent upon the number of adult worms in the veins (Cheever, 1968; Cheever *et al.*, 1977). A fundamental feature distinguishing most helminths from other infectious agents is the inability of adult worms to replicate within the human host. Consequently, the schistosome adult worm burden is limited by the number of cercariae to which the person has been exposed. It follows, therefore, that high egg counts, heavy adult worm burdens and severe disease are only likely in those who have suffered a prolonged and heavy exposure to infective schistosomes.

Schistosomiasis mansoni produces symptoms and signs referable to the gastrointestinal tract and liver (Warren and Mahmoud, 1975). Although a number of symptoms including fatigue, abdominal pain and diarrhoea have been ascribed to the infection, they are nonspecific in nature (Cook *et al.*, 1974; Warren *et al.*, 1974; Arap Siongok *et al.*, 1976). The earliest physical sign is frequently hepatomegaly. Portal hypertension and oesophageal varices may result from an intrahepatic presinusoidal block. There are few stigmata of chronic hepatic disease and liver function is usually normal. The major complication is rupture of the varices with haematemesis and melaena. Patients with severe hepatosplenic schistosomiasis may develop a portosystemic collateral circulation with trapping of eggs in the lungs and consequent pulmonary hypertension and cor pulmonale. The clinical features of schistosomiasis japonica are similar to those described above. In some instances, however, ectopic worms may lay masses of eggs in the central nervous system, thus causing focal epilepsy. In schistosomiasis haematobia, most of the clinical manifestations flow from involvement of the urinary tract. Haematuria is usually the first symptom. Frequency and dysuria are variable. Obstructive uropathy and secondary bacterial infection may culminate in uraemia and death.

A number of studies have been undertaken to define the proportion of populations in endemic areas who have significant disease. In St Lucia, West Indies, an area of lightly endemic schistomiasis mansoni, less than 5% of subjects had splenic enlargement (Cook *et al.*, 1974). Similarly, in areas of moderate prevalence but low individual intensity of infection in Ethiopia (Hiatt, 1976) and Puerto Pico (Cline *et al.*, 1977), morbidity was minimal. Even in an area of extremely high prevalence of schistosomiasis mansoni as in Machakos, Kenya, where 82% of the total population were infected, only 3% had hepatosplenomegaly, and of these, only a very small number had oesophageal varices (Arap Siongok *et al.*, 1976). In another area of high prevalence of infection in Brazil, however, 67% of the population had hepatomegaly and 20% had splenomegaly (Lehmann *et al.*, 1976). Nevertheless, no patients were found with evidence of portal hypertension. The general consensus of most authors is that only a small proportion of the population in an endemic area has significant morbidity, and even less die from the infection.

VIII. Immunity versus Ecology

Despite constant re-exposure to infection, there is relatively little severe morbidity and mortality among those who live in areas of the world that are endemic for schistosomiasis (Warren 1973). Furthermore, the peak prevalence and intensity of infection is not seen in the middle-aged and elderly, but is found in those in their teenage years. When the pattern of schistosomiasis is further analysed, it is apparent that there is a negative binomial distribution, i.e. most of the population has the lightest infection while a few people have the heaviest infections. These epidemiological observations have led to the belief that immunity to reinfection must be a factor controlling the prevalence and intensity of schistosomiasis in man. Nevertheless, the existence of such immunity is doubtful, for there is no sudden immunological crisis resulting in elimination of the parasites in animals (Smithers, 1972), nor has there been any convincing experimental demonstration of the acquisition of immunity to schistosomiasis in man (Warren, 1973; Phillips and Colley, 1978).

It has been suggested, therefore, that immunity is relatively unimportant and that biological, ecological and sociological factors are of much greater importance (Warren, 1973). The degree of infectivity of any particular environment is inconstant, for cercarial levels show marked diurnal variations as well as seasonal and yearly fluctuations. A number of economic, social and behavioural factors, which will be discussed subsequently, modify water contact thus determining the exposure to reinfection and the prevalence and intensity of schistosomiasis in each community.

IX. The Roles of Economic Status and Social and Behavioural Habits

Schistosomiasis is found predominantly in areas of low socioeconomic status where poor housing, deficient waste disposal systems, inadequate water supplies and generally substandard hygienic conditions abound. Contact with water takes place not only in relation to agricultural practices, but also during the domestic and recreational activities that are inevitable under conditions of a low standard of living. Although the pattern of these activities may vary in detail from one place to another, the same principles apply. They may result in contamination, i.e. infection of snails, exposure, i.e. infection of man, or both. Furthermore, the significance of water contact depends upon its frequency and duration and the degree of bodily exposure (Warren, 1973).

Most transmission of schistosomiasis occurs during childhood when poor hygiene and recreational factors are of major importance. Children spend long hours playing in streams and canals and frequently defaecate or urinate in or close to water sources (Farooq and Mallah, 1966; Warren, 1973). Educational achievement is a major factor, as children who spend more time in the classroom have less time for exposure and are more likely to obtain employment which involves less water contact (Farooq *et al.*, 1966). As age increases, play exposure diminishes and sex and occupational factors assume more importance. Household washing constitutes a major domestic water-contact activity among women who gather at water sources and spend long hours washing and gossiping (Farooq *et al.*, 1966). Men and women working in the rice fields, farmers washing their cattle, and fishermen all have significant contact with water. Bathing habits are important, as those who wash themselves frequently and assiduously are more exposed to infection and the risk is even greater among those who swim regularly (Farooq *et al.*, 1966). Religious influences may even come to bear, for schistosomiasis is much more prevalent in Moslems who engage in the ritual of washing before the prayers said five times each day (Farooq *et al.*, 1966). The net result of all these factors is shown in a study from Egypt which found that females, especially those less than 25 years of age, have more water contact than do males, but that the latter are more active contaminators (Farooq and Mallah, 1966). It can be seen that as economic conditions alter, and social and religious customs evolve, so the transmission of infection and pattern and severity of schistosomiasis in each community will continue to change.

X. Human Migration and the Spread of Schistosomiasis

Movement of peoples has produced widespread dissemination of many infectious agents and schistosomes are no exception. Migration has been one of the major human activities influencing the demography of schistosomiasis. In contrast to organisms which are spread directly from man to man, however, the establishment, or otherwise, of schistosomiasis in a community depends upon the presence or absence of susceptible intermediate hosts. A classical example of this is the introduction of schistosomiasis to the Americas. Schistosomiasis was presumably absent from the New World before the age of exploration. Transportation of slaves from Africa to South America resulted in the establishment of schistosomiasis mansoni on that continent. Although the introduced human reservoir was infected with both *Schistosoma mansoni* and *S. haematobium*, schistosomiasis haematobia failed to gain a foothold as susceptible snails were absent. In North America, the lack of susceptible snail intermediate hosts for both species of schistosomes has precluded the transmission of schistosomiasis, despite the immigration each year of 100 000 people from countries where schistosomiasis is endemic (Warren *et al.*, 1974). Similarly, local migration within a continent may also spread schistosomiasis, for example, an epidemic of schistosomiasis occurred in Lobay, West Africa, following the importation of manpower from an infected area (Gaud, 1958). Conversely, social and political barriers to migration may limit the spread of schistosomiasis, for example, tribal borders delimit the distribution of urinary schistosomiasis in the north and intestinal schistosomiasis in the south of Oubangui-Chari, West Africa (Gaud, 1958).

XI. The Effects of Changing Water Resources

Man and snails are both dependent upon water. As populations have increased and men's needs have changed, new water resources have been and are being developed. They range from minor works to major constructions and are found in both rural and urban areas. Small-scale agricultural processes such as the development of new ponds, channels, furrows and rice fields provide new habitats which snails may colonize with a resultant increase in transmission of schistosomiasis (McCullough *et al.*, 1968). Similarly, urbanization is associated with new water requirements and usage. For example, Belo Horizonte in Brazil has developed extremely rapidly; since neither water nor sewage disposal facilities are present in many poorer areas, streams are used for both purposes. Snails have appeared in large numbers and *Schistosoma mansoni* has been introduced by immigrants. Consequently, widespread transmission of schistosomiasis has occurred with over 60% of children being infected (Bradley, 1968).

At the other end of the scale are the large dams which are being built in tropical areas in order to provide water for irrigation schemes designed to increase crop production and to generate hydroelectric power for industrial development. Examples are dams built on the Rivers Nile (Lake Nasser), Volta (Lake Volta), Niger (Lake Kainji), Zambezi (Lake Kariba) in Africa, the Nam Pong River in Thailand and the Ord River in Australia. Such obstruction to water flow may have profound effects on water persistence and distribution for many kilometres upstream, downstream and in the newly built irrigation channels. Because of the intimate interrelationships between water, snails and schistosomes, the possible effects of these ecological disturbances on the prevalence and intensity of schistosomiasis in tropical areas is becoming increasingly recognized. Besides spreading directly along water channels, snails may also be carried by many types of animals particularly aquatic birds. Such aerial transport may accelerate the appearance of snails in newly developed impoundments. Furthermore, it allows the possibility of introducing susceptible snails to newly created bodies of water in regions in which they were previously absent. These changes are further complicated by forced mass migration of humans who may be either a reservour of schistosomiasis already, or a potential new population for infection.

The Aswan High Dam on the Nile provides an example of the effects of such environmental manipulation on schistosomiasis. *Bulinus truncatus* and *Biomphalaria* species are becoming established in Lake Nasser and in the surrounding irrigation channels (Farid, 1975). The replacement of annual flooding by perennial irrigation in the lower reaches of the Nile was associated with a rise in the prevalence of schistosomiasis from less than 5% to more than 60% (Dawood, 1951) and there is the potential for a similar massive spread of urinary and intestinal schistosomiasis in this new area around Lake Nasser. Perhaps even more important, however, will be the consequences below the dam in an area much greater than that around the newly formed lake. The dam has blocked the flow of silt with the result that planorbid snails are now found in the Nile itself. Furthermore, as the irrigation channels in the delta no longer become silted up, the annual closure with drying and dredging of silt, snails and water weeds in the canals is no longer undertaken. This has led to an undisturbed, stable snail population which facilititates the transmission of schistosomiasis (Malek, 1975). Similar changes have occurred in other areas; an explosive growth of water weeds and *Bulinus rohlfsi* led to an epidemic of urinary schistosomiasis in Lake Volta (Paperna, 1970), focal transmission of schistosomiasis occurs in Lake Kainji (Waddy, 1975), *S. haematobium* and *S. mansoni* infections rose from very low levels to 69% and 16%, respectively, of 5–14 year-olds in one settlement in Lake Kariba (Hira, 1969) and an increase in infections with *S. japonicum* has been predicted in Thailand (Harinasuta *et al*., 1970).

XII. The Economic Burden

The effects of schistosomiasis on the economy are difficult to assess. Not only do the direct costs of treatment and control programmes have to be considered, but the impairment of agricultural productivity and industrial efficiency have to be taken into account. Unfortunately, it is difficult to measure debility due to schistosomiasis alone, let alone separate the influence of that infection from the concurrent malnutrition and other endemic infections which so frequently abound in such areas. Consequently, the estimates of economic loss which have appeared must be interpreted with caution. Even in the same situations, different workers have reached disparate conclusions. For example, Farooq (1967) calculated that the annual economic loss due to schistosomiasis in Egypt was $560 million annually, while Wright (1968) "estimated" that the annual loss for the same country was $76 059 062. Similarly, in terms of the US dollar in the mid-1960s, the average annual loss per infected person was believed to vary from $3·50 in Egypt through $26 in the Philippines to $105 in Japan (Wright, 1968). There is little doubt that McMullen (1968) was correct when he observed that these estimates were based primarily on lack of information and the enthusiasm of the guesser.

A number of more detailed studies have been undertaken on smaller, well-defined groups to assess the effects of schistosomiasis on physical and intellectual capacity in order that this can in turn be related to the economic consequences. Again, conflicting opinions have been recorded. Studies of productivity loss in an East African sugar estate concluded that the difference between infected and uninfected people was small but real; there was no significant difference between the two groups while actually at work, but the former subjects had a higher rate of absenteeism (Foster, 1967). The cost of schistosomiasis to the estate was calculated at £6000 per annum, while the cost of a control scheme was estimated to require the expenditure of £3500 each year. A further study on the same estate a few years later concluded that infected persons were 3% less productive and earned 12% less income (Fenwick, 1972). Similarly, Cohen (1974) using admittedly inadequate data, has suggested that the elimination of urinary schistosomiasis in Zanzibar may give significant economic benefits by reducing mortality and extending the average working life.

In contrast, a study undertaken in the West Indies to test the hypothesis that parasitic infections reduced earnings found no evidence to indicate significant effects on agricultural labour productivity (Weisbrod *et al.*, 1973). Similarly, it has not been possible to relate schistosomiasis to growth, physical activity or intellectual ability in children (Walker *et al.*, 1970; Walker *et al.*, 1972). Finally, a somewhat subjective study of workers in a foundry, demonstrated no differences in industrial efficiency (Fine, 1975).

It is not surprising, therefore, that there is a wide spectrum of opinion concerning the significance of schistosomiasis. Sandbach (1975) has expressed the view that the economic burden of schistosomiasis is insufficient to warrant the development of highly specific measures of control. Warren (1974), on the other hand, has characterized schistosomiasis as the major chronic helminth infection of mankind and Olivier (1974) has said that "there is no reason to doubt that human schistosomiasis is a public health problem of major significance". In view of the current widespread support of schistosomiasis research and control by governments, international agencies and philanthropic foundations, it would appear that this latter belief is widely held among the medical, scientific and political communities.

XIII. Control of Schistosomiasis

Despite the reservations which have been mentioned, schistosomiasis has long been viewed as a problem requiring control. While eradication of the organism may been seen as the ultimate ideal, limitations of finance, people and technology, have made it possible only to attempt to prevent spread of infection and reduce rather than eliminate morbidity and mortality. The control measures used over the last 50 to 60 years have varied with the weapons available in the technological armamentarium and our understanding of the dynamics of transmission and the significance of infection. They have included, at different times and in varying combinations, environmental sanitation, drug therapy, snail control and health education. Each technique has been aimed at different points in the schistosome life cycle but none has been uniformly successful.

For many years, the use of molluscicides was pre-eminent. One of the major advantages of this system was that it did not require the active co-operation of the local population. Against this lies the high financial cost and possible environmental damage. Most important of all, however, is the inability of molluscicides to eradicate all vectors; the capacity of snails to reproduce rapidly necessitates the continued application of these agents in an attempt to keep snail numbers at a minimum.

Mass drug therapy was abandoned in the earlier parts of this century as the available drug, tartar emetic, was too toxic. In recent years, effective but relatively non-toxic schistosomicides such as hycanthone and niridazole have been developed. This has given a new impetus to the treatment of schistosomiasis mansoni and schistosomiasis haematobia by mass treatment campaigns. The economic, logistic and toxic side-effects have dampened enthusiasm, however (Davis, 1976). It may be that a new approach called "targeted mass treatment" may avoid some of these problems; this technique stemmed from the realization that only heavily infected people are likely to become diseased and contaminate significantly the environment with eggs. Consequently, whole populations are surveyed but only the more heavily infected individuals are treated, thus reducing costs and avoiding toxic side-effects in lightly infected persons (Warren and Mahmoud, 1976). Unfortunately, these drugs are much less effective against *Schistosoma japonicum*.

Environmental sanitation with the provision of safe water supplies and efficient disposal of sewage is obviously the best way of controlling schistosomiasis. Unfortunately, the cost is enormous and is manifestly beyond the capacity of the vast majority of people living in endemic areas. It is hoped that as the general standard of living rises, these services may become more generally available, with a resultant diminution in schistosomiasis, as has indeed happened in Japan. Given the economic and other forces militating against control, it has been suggested that health education is of paramount importance (McMahon, 1976). Theoretically, if human-water contact can be reduced and people could be persuaded to use whatever latrines are available, the prevalence and intensity of schistosomiasis would be much reduced. Nevertheless, in view of the fact that children are major contaminators, and the known propensity of men and women to do whatever is easiest at the time, it would seem that the effects of health education will probably be meagre, particularly in rural agricultural communities where most infected people live. Moreover, education in waste disposal is likely to be of less benefit in containing schistosomiasis japonica as there is a large animal reservoir of infection.

Nevertheless, the Peoples' Republic of China may be an exception to these generalizations. Schistosomiasis has been a considerable problem in that country. Claims have been made that major progress has been made in controlling infection, although a visiting American delegation was unable to evaluate with confidence the degree to which transmission has been reduced (Report, 1977). Snail control, environmental sanitation and health education have been the bulwarks of China's policy. Huge columns of earth have been used to bury snails, river and lake banks have been covered with stones or lined with concrete, and swampy land has been reclaimed. Improved water supplies and waste disposal systems have been provided and health education programmes carried out. All this has been made possible by a politically inspired utilization of a massive labour force. These efforts at schistosomiasis control devolved ultimately from the highest in the land in the form of the manifesto, "Farewell to the God of Plague" by Chairman Mao. It is unlikely that these techniques are applicable to most countries afflicted with schistosomiasis as the available labour force is much smaller and there is nothing like the degree of social control.

Jordan (1977) has recently recounted an elegant series of studies undertaken by the Rockefeller Foundation on the island of St Lucia in the West Indies in which a comparative evaluation of snail control, chemotherapy and environmental sanitation plus health education was made in three isolated valleys. Although each method achieved a measure of success, analysis of costs and benefits suggested that chemotherapy was the cheapest and most rapidly effective method but had the disadvantage of requiring patient co-operation and a stable community. It remains to be seen, of course, whether these control measures undertaken on a small island with a limited population by enthusiastic experts and considerable financial backing are applicable to the global control of schistosomiasis.

XIV. Prospects

It is difficult to predict the relationship between man and schistosomes in 50 or 100 years or so. The infection is spreading in many parts of the world and it is likely that the various control procedures just described will be ill-placed to keep up with, let alone eliminate, schistosomiasis in the short term. The answer probably lies in research leading to better methods of control. There has, in fact, been a considerable expansion in financial support for schistosomiasis research in the past few years. Two major reasons appear to account for this. Firstly, there has been a recent recognition that schistosomiasis is a major global impediment to social development. Secondly, a small cadre of dedicated researchers has greatly improved our understanding of the pathogenesis of schistosomiasis and has established it as a useful model for the study of many biomedical systems ranging from molecular biology to health education. Major efforts are now being made by the United States National Institutes of Health, The Rockefeller Foundation, the Edna McConnell Clark Foundation and the UNDP/World Bank/WHO Special Programme for Research and Training in Tropical Diseases.

There are, of course, still major differences of opinion among experts. The beacon of smallpox eradication looms high in the eyes of many, and indeed it would seem that short of the discovery of a cheap, therapeutic "magic bullet", the development of a satisfactory vaccine against schistosomiasis is likely to be the only possible short-term solution. Against this, are conservative views such as those espoused by Weller (1976), who believes that "the concept of eventual control of schistosomiasis by immunological means is a scientific star of less than the sixth magnitude on the distant horizon". For him, "the control of schistosomiasis and social development will be mutually supportive—both may require many decades". It is to be hoped that he is wrong. The future will tell.

References

Abdel-Salam, E. and Abdel-Fattah, M. (1977). *Am. J. trop. Med. Hyg.* **26**, 463–469.

Abdel-Salam, E. and Ehsan, A. (1978). *Am. J. trop. Med. Hyg.* **27**, 774–778.

Amorim, J. P. de, Rosa, D. de, Lucena, D. T. de (1954). *Rev. bras. Malar.* **6**, 13–33.

Arap Siongok, T. K., Mahmoud, A. A. F., Ouma, J. H., Warren, K. S., Muller, A. S., Handa, A. K. and Houser, H. B. (1976). *Am. J. trop. Med. Hyg.* **25**, 273–284.

Bradley, D. J. (1968). *E. Afr. med. J.* **45**, 333–340.

Burch, J. B. (1975). *In* "Man-made Lakes and Human Health" (N. F. Stanley and M. P. Alpers, Eds), 311–321. Academic Press, London and New York.

Cheever, A. W. (1968). *Am. J. trop. Med. Hyg.* **17**, 38–60.
Cheever, A. W., Kamel, I. A., Elwi, A. M., Mosimann, J. E. and Danner, R. (1977). *Am. J. trop. Med. Hyg.* **26**, 702–716.
Cheever, A. W., Ismail, Kamel, A., Elwi, A. M., Mosiman, J. E., Danner, R., and Sippel, J. E. (1978). *Am. J. trop. Med. Hyg.* **27**, 55–75.
Chernin, E. (1970). *J. Parasit.* **56**, 287–296.
Cline, B. L., Rymzo, W. T., Hiatt, R. A., Knight, W. B. and Berrios-Duran, L. A. (1977). *Am. J. trop. Med. Hyg.* **26**, 109–117.
Cohen, J. E. (1974). *Soc. Sci. Med.* **8**, 383–398.
Cook, J. A., Baker, S. T., Warren, K. S. and Jordan, P. (1974). *Am. J. trop. Med. Hyg.* **23**, 625–633.
Davis, A. (1976). *In* "Epidemiology and Community Health in Warm Climates" (R. Cruickshank, K. L. Standard and H. B. L. Russell, Eds), 223–242. Churchill Livingstone, Edinburgh.
Dawood, M. M. (1951). *J. Egypt. med Ass.* **34**, 660–669.
Farid, M. A. (1975). *In* "Man-made lakes and human health" (N. F. Stanley and M. P. Alpers, Eds), 89–102. Academic Press, London and New York.
Farooq, M. (1967). *WHO Chron.* **21**, 175–184.
Farooq, M. and Mallah, M. B. (1966). *Bull. Wld Hlth Org.* **35**, 377–387.
Farooq, M., Nielsen, J., Samaan, S. A., Mallah, M. B. and Allam, A. A. (1966). *Bull. Wld Hlth Org.* **35**, 293–318.
Fenwick, A. (1972). *Bull. Wld Hlth Org.* **47**, 567–572.
Fine, J. (1975). *Med. J. Zambia.* **9**, 96–97.
Fine, P. E. M. and Lehman, J. S. (1977). *Am. J. trop. Med. Hyg.* **26**, 500–504.
Foster, R. (1967). *J. trop. Med. Hyg.* **70**, 185–195.
Gaud, J. (1958). *Bull. Wld Hlth Org.* **18**, 1081–1087.
Harinasuta, C., Jetanasen, S., Impand, P. and Maegraith, B. G. (1970). *Southeast Asian J. trop. Med. Pub. Hlth* **1**, 530–535.
Hiatt, R. A. (1976). *Am. J. trop. Med. Hyg.* **25**, 808–817.
Hira, P. R. (1969). *Nature, Lond.* **224**, 670–672.
Jordan, P. (1977). *Am. J. trop. Med. Hyg.* **26**, 877–886.
Lehman, J. S., Mott, K. E., Morrow, R. H., Muniz, T. M. and Boyer, M. H. (1976). *Am. J. trop. Med. Hyg.* **25**, 285–294.
McCullough, F. S., Eyakuze, V. M., Msinde, J. and Nditi, H. (1968). *E. Afr. med. J.* **45**, 295–308.
McMahon, J. E. (1976). *Acta trop., Basel* **33**, 390–392.
McMullen, D. B. (1968). *Bull. N.Y. Acad. Med.* **44**, 313–316.
McMullen, D. B., Komiyama, S., Endo-Itabashi, T. (1951). *Am. J. Hyg.* **54**, 402–415.
Malek, A. E. (1975). *Trop. geogr. Med.* **27**, 359–364.
Miyairi, K. and Suzuki, M. (1913). *Tokyo Iji Shinshi (Tokyo Medical Journal)* **1836**, 1–5.
Nelson, G. S. (1960). *Trans. R. Soc. trop. Med. Hyg.* **54**, 301–324.
Olivier, L. J. (1974). *In* "Molluscicides in Schistosomiasis Control (T. C. Cheng, Ed.), 1–7. Academic Press, New York and London.
Paperna, I. (1970). *Z. Tropenmed. Parasit.* **21**, 411–425.

Pesigan, T. P., Hairston, N. G., Jauregi, J. J., Garcia, E. G., Santos, A. T., Santos, B. C., Besa, A. A. (1958). *Bull. Wld Hlth Org.* **18**, 481–578.
Phillips, S. M. and Colley, D. G. (1978). *In* "Progress in Allergy" (P. Kallos, B. H. Waksman and A. L. de Weck, Eds), 24, 49–182. S. Karger, Basel.
Report of the American Schistosomiasis Delegation to the Peoples' Republic of China. *Am. J. trop. Med. Hyg.* **26**, 427–457.
Richards, C. S. (1970). *Nature, Lond.* **277**, 806–810.
Sandbach, F. R. (1975). *Soc. Sci. Med.* **9**, 517–527.
Smithers, S. R. (1972). *Br. med. Bull.* **28**, 49–54.
Waddy, B. B. (1975). *Trans. R. Soc. trop. Med. Hyg.* **69**, 39–50.
Walker, A. R. P., Walker, B. F. and Richardson, B. D. (1970). *Am. J. trop. Med. Hyg.* **19**, 792–814.
Walker, A. R. P., Walker, B. F., Richardson, B. D. and Smit, P. J. *Trop. geogr. Med.* **24**, 347–352.
Warren, K. S. (1972). *Trans. R. Soc. trop Med. Hyg.* **66**, 417–434.
Warren, K. S. (1973). *J. infect. Dis.* **127**, 595–609.
Warren, K. S. (1974). *Nat. Hist.* **83**, 46–53.
Warren, K. S. (1978). *Nature, Lond.* **273**, 609–612.
Warren, K. S. and Mahmoud, A. A. F. (1975). *J. infect. Dis.* **131**, 614–620.
Warren, K. S. and Mahmoud, A. A. F. (1976). *Trans. Ass. Am. Phycns* **89**, 195–204.
Warren, K. S., Mahmoud, A. A. F., Cummings, P., Murphy, D. J. and Houser, H. B. (1974). *Am. J. trop. Med. Hyg.* **23**, 902–909.
Webb, G. (1962). *Bull. Wld Hlth Org.* **27**, 59–85.
Webbe, G. and James, C. (1971). *J. Helminth.* **45**, 403–413.
Webbe, G. and Jordan, P. (1966). *Trans. R. Soc. trop. Med. Hyg.* **60**, 279–312.
Weisbrod, B. A., Andreano. R. L., Baldwin, R. E., Epstein, E. H. and Kelley, A. C. (1973). "Disease and Economic Development; the Impact of Parasitic Diseases in St Lucia", p. 254. Univ. of Wisconsin Press.
Weller, T. H. (1976). *Am. J. trop. Med. Hyg.* **25**, 208–216.
Wright, W. H. (1968). *Bull. N.Y. Acad. Med.* **44**, 301–312.

12
Social Determinants in Venereal Disease

R. S. Morton*
Sheffield, England

None of the sexually transmissible diseases has been controlled.

* Formerly Director, Special Clinic, Royal Infirmary, Sheffield.

I. Basic Biology of Sexually Transmitted Diseases

Unlike so many other infections, none of the sexually transmissible diseases (STDS) has been controlled. This sad fact is one of medicine's most remarkable anachronisms. Some think the failure is compounded by a strong paradox. In spite of 35 years of availability of cheap, rapid and safe specific cures for gonorrhoea and syphilis, these diseases have actually become more prevalent throughout the world.

This chapter is an endeavour to explain both the failure and the paradox.

Table I shows that six major groups of microorganisms may be sexually transmitted and produce clinically recognizable disease in man. Not only between, but within these microbial groups, specific and different host–parasite relationships have evolved.

The basic facts are as follows. In the last 100 years syphilis has shown a tendency to decline worldwide, but throughout the period recurrent peaks of prevalence, usually associated with wars, have occurred. The Second World War was no exception. It was followed by a rapid decline in the incidence of syphilis and many believed that with the advent of penicillin the end of the disease was in sight. This assumption did not prove to be true. Between 1955 and 1958 reports from many countries to the World Health Organization showed a slow and widespread recrudescence of infectious forms of the disease. This trend has continued almost unabated in some countries and in a few has accelerated in recent years.

There have, however, been substantial gains. Mass surveys of "at risk" groups, together with the testing of sex and family contacts of those found to be syphilitic, have contributed much to control. The triumph lies not so much in the detection of the tens of thousands of infected people by dedicated health workers, but in the prevention of premature death, distress and the high cost of hospitalization of those with the chronic, crippling and killing forms of both late and congenital syphilis. The fact that morbidity rates of congenital syphilis are now low and stationary is an indication for well-sustained effort.

Gonorrhoea, variously reported as occurring between three and forty times more frequently than syphilis, currently accounts for some 200 million infections per annum. Figures are even less reliable than those for syphilis, but the trend everywhere since the mid-1950s has been unmistakable. In many areas of the world, gonorrhoea in women is increasingly recognized as the cause of a great deal of disabling pelvic infection. Sterility, ectopic pregnancy and associated surgery are prominent features. In the USA the cost of complications of gonorrhoea in

TABLE I. *Sexually Transmitted Microbial Diseases of Man*

	Microorganism	Disease
BACTERIA	*Treponema pallidum*	Syphilis
	Neisseria gonorrhoeae	Gonorrhoea
	N. gonorrhoeae	Ophthalmia neonatorum
	N. gonorrhoeae	Vulvovaginitis (children)
	Haemophilus ducreyi	Chancroid
	Corynebacterium vaginale	Vaginitis
	Calymmatobacterium granulomatis (Klebsiella)	Granuloma inguinale
YEAST	*Candida albicans*	Vulvovaginitis
PROTOZOA	*Trichomonas vaginalis*	Vulvovaginitis
	T. vaginalis	Non-gonococcal urethritis
CHLAMYDIA	LGV[a]	Lymphogranuloma venereum
	TRIC[a]	Non-gonococcal urethritis
	TRIC[a]	Inclusion conjunctivitis (newborn)
	?Chlamydia	Reiter's disease
VIRUSES	Herpes simplex type 2	Genital herpes
	Cytomegalovirus	?
	Human papilloma virus	Venereal warts
	Hepatitis B	?
	Poxvirus	Molluscum contagiosum
	Herpes simplex 2 (intra-urethral)	Non-gonococcal urethritis
	Marburg	Marburg disease
MYCOPLASMA	*Ureaplasma urealyticum*	?Non-gonococcal urethritis

[a] See Becker (1978) for characterization of these agents as *Chlamydia trachomatis*.

women is estimated to be at least $200 million per annum.

Non-gonococcal urethritis (NGU) in men, with its many associated genital and general conditions in both sexes, shows a growing prevalence in those countries where the disease is reported, e.g. in the United Kingdom, Ceylon and France. In England 11 000 cases of NGU were reported in 1951 and 70 000 in 1977. The Center for Disease Control in

Atlanta estimates that 2·5 million episodes of NGU occur annually in the USA.

Chancroid, lymphogranuloma venereum and granuloma inguinale have fortunately been reported less frequently than pre-war, but these diseases are still common in many subtropical areas of the world.

Trichomoniasis and candidiasis are widespread throughout the world. Of those countries that report the number of cases, all show increases. The same situation applies to the viral STDs, such as genital warts, cytomegalovirus disease and hepatitis B. Increases have been particularly marked in genital herpes which in some unknown way is associated with cancer of the cervix. Other less common STDs, such as scabies and infestation with pubic lice, are likewise regarded as becoming more prevalent.

II. Social Environment, Economic Prosperity and Sexually Transmitted Diseases

The man-made contributions to the nature of the present STD problem can be discussed: firstly, in terms of the changing social environment as it influences attitudes; and secondly as the result of how changing attitudes are reflected in altered behaviour patterns. In "feedback" fashion these in turn alter the social climate. The precipitate formed by these interactions is the local STD morbidity rate. Population growth and movement, like identifiable "at risk" groups, give us some of the numbers which enable us to measure the changes.

History tells us that this is not man's first era of sexual freedom; it may be seen as Western man's third. The first of these eras came with the Renaissance in the latter part of the sixteenth and the early part of the seventeenth century. It was an era noted for its heady licentiousness, great feasting, wild intoxication and widespread toleration of prostitution. The second age of sexual freedom came in the late eighteenth century—The Age of Reason, or Enlightenment. Demands for freedom from all kinds of restraints affected the New World as well as the Old. Self-indulgence took precedence and sexual expression was uninhibited at all levels of society.

The last 20 years and the former two ages of freedom have several common features. All three periods took place in times of growing economic prosperity. Furthermore, each is characterized by a questioning of authority in which religious, social, financial, legal and political concepts are challenged. Demands for sexual freedom are therefore but one facet of a call for release from all kinds of restraints. The third feature common to all three eras is that each has been in a time of rapid scientific advance and technological innovation.

The liberalism, or tolerance of these ages, has in its day been welcomed as realistic. Minority groups have tended to misinterpret liberalism as licence, and abuses have led to increasing numbers of people being embroiled in age-old medicosocial problems, such as are exemplified in rising illegitimacy rates, alcoholism and a growing incidence of sexually transmitted diseases. Such disasters have led in the past to costly disillusionment and a reversal of attitudes. Thus in England the first age of freedom was followed by Cromwell's puritanical Commonwealth, in which corporate good was favoured over personal desire. The second era of freedon was followed by uptight Victorianism with its emphasis on abstract virtues, including chastity, and with the work ethic and family life highly prized. The sexually transmitted diseases were far from absent in these post-freedom periods. Although no accurate figures are available the writings of the time which addressed themselves to the problem of contemporary attitudes and behaviour lead us to believe that casual sex and the frequency of partner change diminished slightly, resulting in a fall in sexually transmitted disease rates or at least a levelling off of their prevalence.

The present era of sexual freedom with its greater STD prevalence began with post-Second World War recovery and the economic prosperity which started to manifest itself in the mid and late 1950s. Social improvement led to greater financial independence, which in turn led to overt expressions of and demands for freedom—particularly among young people. As a corollary, the widespread fall-off in the rate of economic growth in the early 1970s was accompanied by a deceleration, a levelling off or a fall in gonorrhoea morbidity rates in several Western countries. It is of interest that trends in other manifestations of medicosocial pathology, such as high pre-marital conception rates, evidence of alcohol and drug abuse and attempted suicide rates, follow those in sexually transmitted disease when gonorrhoea is used as an index. Whereas in the earlier part of the century the physical environment, as exemplified by poverty, overcrowding, malnutrition and death from infection, produced a preponderance of medicosocial problems affecting infants and children, today it is the social environment which is hazardous and is the determinant of medicosocial problems in adolescents.

III. Political Ideologies and Sexually Transmitted Diseases

Political ideologies, with their availability or absence of choices and freedoms, influence trends in sexually transmitted diseases. Strict comparisons are not possible, for even in countries with a nationwide network of clinics there are obvious disparities, e.g. between Russia and England. In Russia, the incidence of VD in the late 1950s and in the 1960s was at an apparently irreducible minimum, whereas in England the incidence moved relentlessly up from the mid-1950s to 1970. In general, strong governments, whether Right or Left, tend to reduce choice and self-expression, both social and sexual. The democratic governments of the Western countries have relaxed the harshness of many of their laws, e.g. suicide is widely regarded as no longer a crime. There has also been a less punitive element in sentencing policies; and laws regarding censorship have been relaxed. In sexual matters, legal changes of a comparable nature have taken place regarding homosexuality, abortion, prostitution, provision of free contraceptives, etc. Moves towards greater egalitarianism have also spread into social, political, financial and religious aspects of life. The sexual freedom movement started by Freud, augmented by the work of Kinsey and his colleagues and more recently by Masters and Johnson, has led to more homogeneous attitudes and behaviour patterns which begin to break through barriers of creed, colour and custom. In the present era, the influence of scientific advance and technological innovation has been specifically applicable to sexual expression, in the form of the contraceptive pill and the intrauterine device. Removal of the fear of pregnancy means that women are now more free to enjoy their sexual involvement. Social constraints and restraints exacted by neighbours, religions or marriage ties have all declined. The need for such restraints was determined by the recognition of the many problems engendered by illegitimacy, such as the entailment of property. Today in Western countries, pre-marital sexual activity for females as well as males is widely regarded as the norm.

The potency of these legal and social changes can be measured only roughly. The first index of change is the STD morbidity rates, the second is the pre-marital conception rates. The latter rates have risen in many countries in spite of the availability of modern contraceptives. In England, a third measure of change has been sought by Schofield (1976). In 1965 he found that 45% of teenagers in the UK were in favour of pre-marital sex. Some 7 years later the figure was 87%. Schofield goes further: after much discussion, he defines a promiscuous person as anyone who has had more than one sexual partner in a year. He recognizes that the definition is imprecise and distorts the real meaning of the word. Using the definition, 12% of boys and 2% of girls aged 15 to 19 years were promiscuous in 1965. In the early 1970s,

Schofield studied 376 25 year olds and found that 17% were promiscuous. He estimated that there are now 4 million promiscuous people in the UK. He concludes that there are going to be more promiscuous young people in the future.

IV. Urbanization, Population Movement and Sexually Transmitted Diseases, "At Risk" Groups

Just as man influences the views of his society, so his society influences him. New ideas and discoveries alter the social environment, which in turn leads to changes in attitudes and so to alterations in behaviour patterns (Guthe, 1974). This applies as much to fashions in sex as to those in dress or architecture. There is some evidence that the rate of reciprocal interaction between man and his society is more rapid today than in earlier centuries.

Today's attitudinal and behavioural changes can to some extent be measured by a study of groups of people recognized as more "at risk" to sexually transmitted disease than the average. Such studies are now considered as prerequisites for a rational approach to the containment of sexually transmitted diseases within manageable proportions.

"At risk" groups are products of the general trends we have been discussing. They emerge from a background of ever-growing populations with a rising proportion of sexually active young people. More and more of these young people are crowding into new and renewed urban areas with their concentration of industrial opportunities and educational facilities. Worldwide, tribal or family ties are broken as young people move into cities in search of work or learning. Such areas attract the prostitute and the homosexual in search of anonymity and sex partners. The bigger the city the higher the STD morbidity rate tends to be. The geography of gonorrhoea like its seasonality needs further study. Regarding the latter, we only know that in temperate zones peak morbidity rates occur in the third quarter of the year.

Population movement has been a worldwide phenomenon in all continents over the last 20 years. The migrant population of Europe is now approaching six million. Multiracialism is becoming an established fact, particularly in France, Holland and the UK. Immigrants rarely bring infection to the land of their adoption. The infection is more commonly acquired after their arrival. This applies particularly to the young unattached male. The attitudes and behaviour of immigrants vary according to their ethnic origins, but all are more at risk than matching endogenous groups. For example, in the UK West Indian men are nearly nineteen times more likely to get gonorrhoea than their British-born counterparts.

Other itinerants are also noted as being "at risk", e.g. long-distance lorry drivers, seasonal workers in agriculture, and tourists. The numbers of the last group have increased fourfold in a decade, with over 200 million stopovers being made annually by those travelling by air. In some European countries between 20 and 25% of infectious syphilis is imported by returning tourists. In the UK between 3 and 4% of gonorrhoea is similarly imported. Merchant seamen form an "at risk" group which has received special study. Seafarers are 15–20 times more liable to acquire infection than land-lubbers.

The role of the prostitute as a vector of the STDs varies greatly from one part of the world to another. In the Western Pacific region and South-East Asia, they are said to account for 80–90% of the gonococcal infections occurring in men. Similar figures pertain in some South American countries and in some African countries. In North America, Europe and Commonwealth countries, the reported figures vary from between 5 and 20%. It has been generally believed in these latter countries that the prostitute is losing out to the "good time" girl. Recent studies in the UK suggest, however, that although the percentage of infections attributed to prostitutes is declining the actual numbers of infections so acquired is increasing.

V. Homosexuality, Age and Sex Ratios of Sexually Transmitted Diseases

Homosexuals play a prominent part in the epidemiology of the STDs. This is particularly noticeable in Europe and the USA. Their rates of partner change, whether they are active or passive or facultative, is currently greater than that of heterosexuals. A measure of this is their reinfection rate, which is five times that of heterosexuals. In the provincial cities of the UK, where homosexuality between consenting adult males is no longer illegal, 5% of gonorrhoea occurring in males is in homosexuals. As already noted, homosexuals tend to congregate in large cities. In five clinics in the centre of London, 27·6% of gonorrhoea in males is homosexually acquired. In fifteen other London clinics the figure is 7·7% (British Co-operative Clinical Group, 1973). In one central clinic 14% of the homosexuals seen were other than British born (Thin and Smith, 1976).

Sexually transmitted diseases are diseases of young people. In most countries at least 60% of all infections occur in people under the age of

24 years. Each town or city produces special "at risk" groups, e.g. seafarers, students, nurses, itinerant workers, etc. In a growing number of countries collection of statistical data is now by age groups (based on the frame defined in the International Classification of Diseases) so that specific rates of attack may be more accurately calculated and yearly differences reported more precisely. Such data will be particularly useful for forecasting morbidity rates in countries where birth rates have been falling.

In the present era of sexual freedom, the most dramatic demographic change reported from clinics in Westernized countries has been the relentless, year by year progression of the male : female ratio from 3 or 4 : 1 of 15–20 years ago to the near 1 : 1 of today. The trend is not only confined to the infected, it applies also to those found free from infection, and it has been found to be independent of the quality of contact tracing (Morton, 1970). The conclusion is that more and more women are seeking tests because more and more of them are placing themselves at risk. Changes in behaviour and attitudes are more obvious in women than in men. In an age of sexual freedom, this should surprise no one. Another factor is also operational; studies in Scandinavia and the UK have shown how modern contraceptive methods augment the general sexual freedom trends. Women on the Pill are likely to have sex more often and with more partners than their non-Pill-taking sisters (Juhlin, 1968). For many women sex equality means equality in sex, and that is now a reality.

In conclusion, we may say from this brief review, that eras of sexual freedom are inseparably associated with high and rising STD rates. Demands for sexual freedom are only part of a more widespread clamour for freedom from legal and social restraints and constraints. Changing sexual attitudes are expressed in altered behaviour which is hazardous to health, particularly in some groups of young people.

History suggests that the liberalism of past eras of sexual freedom has been misinterpreted by some as licence, that this has proved costly and eventually socially unacceptable. The result has been a reversal of trends. Such data as we have concerning the present era of sexual freedom suggests that the advent of modern contraceptives is capable of minimizing the problem of pre-marital conception. However, by making sexual intercourse much more a recreational than a procreational activity, modern contraceptives make no contribution to the control of sexually acquired infections. There is some evidence that these contraceptives may promote the prevalence of the STDs. The indications are that these infections will continue to present themselves in large albeit fluctuating numbers for some years to come.

References

British Co-operative Clinical Group (1973). *Br. J. ven. Dis.* **49**, 329–334.
Guthe, T. (1974). "Sexually Transmitted Diseases (STD): Scope and Control Measures". European Public Health Committee, Council of Europe, Strasbourg.
Juhlin, L. (1968). *Acta derm. ven.* **48**, 75–81.
Morton, R. S. (1970). *Br. J. ven. Dis.* **46**, 103–105.
Schofield, M. (1976). "Promiscuity". Gollancz, London.
Thin, R. N. T. and Smith, D. M. (1976). *Br. J. ven. Dis.* **52**, 161–164.

13

Smallpox and Its Eradication

Frank Fenner

Centre for Resource and Environmental Studies, Australian National University, Canberra, ACT, Australia

---

Smallpox was one of the great scourges of mankind. . . . It has now been eradicated . . . with an estimated annual savings of over $1000 million.

I. Introduction

No disease has had a longer history of human intervention, nor one where more sharply contrasting motives have held sway at different times and places, than smallpox. Long before the germ theory of infectious diseases had been elaborated, deliberate inoculation with material from scabs and pustules (called variolation) was practised as a preventive measure, first in China and India, then in the Middle East, and from the early eighteenth century in Europe and North America. Late that century Edward Jenner scientifically tested and publicized the country tale that had been confirmed some 20 years earlier by Jesty, namely that dairymaids were spared smallpox because they had earlier suffered from cowpox. He introduced vaccination as a much safer preventive measure than variolation, and forecast the eradication of endemic smallpox by this measure. During the first half of the twentieth century this was achieved in many countries, mostly in Oceania, North America and Europe, but the disease remained endemic and common in many parts of Asia, Africa, and South America. Then in 1967 an intensive campaign was mounted by the World Health Organization to achieve global eradication of smallpox; an epoch-making event which was accomplished by late 1977 and officially certified in December 1979.

Human activity in relation to smallpox has not always been benign. The English settlers of North America, themselves immune from prior infection, deliberately used smallpox as a weapon in their fight against the Indians; the Spanish conquests of Mexico and Peru owed more to smallpox than to any other single factor, and resentful convicts in Australia appear to have deliberately infected the local Aborigines with smallpox within a year of landing in Sydney Cove.

Smallpox is caused by an orthopoxvirus, and is usually a severe febrile disease with a widespread rash that goes through macular, vesicular and pustular stages, affects the mouth and nasopharynx and skin, usually with a preponderance of lesions on the extremities, including the soles and palms. The syndrome can be caused by two species of *Orthopoxvirus*: variola virus, of which many strains of differing virulence have been recognized from different geographic areas (Table I); and monkeypox virus, recognized since 1970 as a very rare cause of sporadic self-limited outbreaks of clinical smallpox, but only in West and Central Africa.

Epidemiologically important features of smallpox that permitted its

TABLE I. *Smallpox: Case Mortality Rates*[a,b]

Place	Year	Cases	Deaths	Percentages
India	1974–75	2 826	575	20·3
Pakistan	1971	1 674	249	14·9
West Africa	1967–69	5 628	540	9·6
Indonesia	1969	11 966	950	7·9
Uganda	1966–70	1 045	54	5·2
Ethiopia	1972–74	21 250	243	1·1
Brazil	1969	6 795	37	0·5

[a] Includes both vaccinated and unvaccinated cases.
[b] From the Final Report of the Global Commission for the Certification of Smallpox Eradication, December 1979 (*Wld Hlth Org./SE/*79.152).

eradication in the first half of the twentieth century in several countries of Europe, North America, Australia and New Zealand, are set out in Table II (items 2, 3, 4, 5 and 6). The incubation period is 12–14 days and cases are rarely infectious before they can be diagnosed, so that when combined with vaccination, surveillance and containment is an effective method of control if the majority of the population has been successfully vaccinated or where the public health measures are highly efficient.

Global eradication was possible only because other features of smallpox, mainly sociopolitical (items 1, 7, 8 and 9 of Table II) were supportive of the epidemiology of the disease.

TABLE II. *Why Global Eradication of Smallpox Succeeded*

Biological Reasons
1. Severe human disease (high mortality; blindness in many survivors)
2. No subclinical cases
3. No recurrent excretion of virus
4. Can usually be diagnosed before it becomes infectious
5. No known animal reservoir host
6. An effective, stable vaccine is available

Sociopolitical Reasons
7. No social barriers to prevention, as there are in sexually transmitted diseases
8. Global eradication offered considerable financial advantages for rich as well as poor countries
9. Inspired leadership of the intensified programme of WHO

II. The Smallpox Eradication Campaign of WHO

Within a few years of the establishment of the World Health Organization in 1948, the Pan-American Sanitary Bureau (now the WHO Regional Office for the Americas) initiated a campaign to eradicate smallpox from the Americas. By 1959 this had produced encouraging results; smallpox remained endemic only in Argentina, Brazil, Bolivia, Colombia and Ecuador. In that year the Soviet Union sponsored a WHO resolution calling for global eradication of smallpox, to be supported by voluntary contributions of vaccine and funds. Almost nothing was achieved over the next decade, because financial support was totally inadequate.

In 1966 the World Health Assembly recognized the failure of its efforts and after much argument launched an intensified Smallpox Eradication Programme to operate for a decade from 1 January 1967, for which proper financial support was provided. A small Smallpox Eradication Unit was established in WHO Headquarters in Geneva, led from 1967 to 1976 by Dr D. A. Henderson, of the USA, and since 1977 by Dr I. Arita of Japan. Smallpox was endemic (in 1967) in thirty-three countries and imported cases had occurred in another eleven countries (Fig. 1). The scale of the problem can be recognized when it is realized that cases were grossly underreported—there were probably 13 million cases in 1967, mostly in the poor countries, although only 130 000 were reported.

The Smallpox Eradication Unit set about systematically dealing with the matter of eradication, drawing upon the international community for expert help, and as the programme appeared to be succeeding, calling successfully for additional "voluntary" funds that could be used in a flexible way. Attention was devoted initially to four problems—the provision of a good vaccine, the systematic study of the possibility of an animal reservoir (the "rock" upon which yellow fever eradication had foundered), the development of adequate national programmes and infrastructure in the then-endemic countries, and the availability of a good laboratory diagnostic service to all countries.

A. Vaccine

Liquid vaccine was quite satisfactory for vaccination in countries where the climate was temperate, and where smallpox had long since disappeared as an endemic disease. But it was useless where smallpox still persisted, in the poor countries of the tropical world. Collier had shown in 1955 that the vaccine could be freeze-dried and

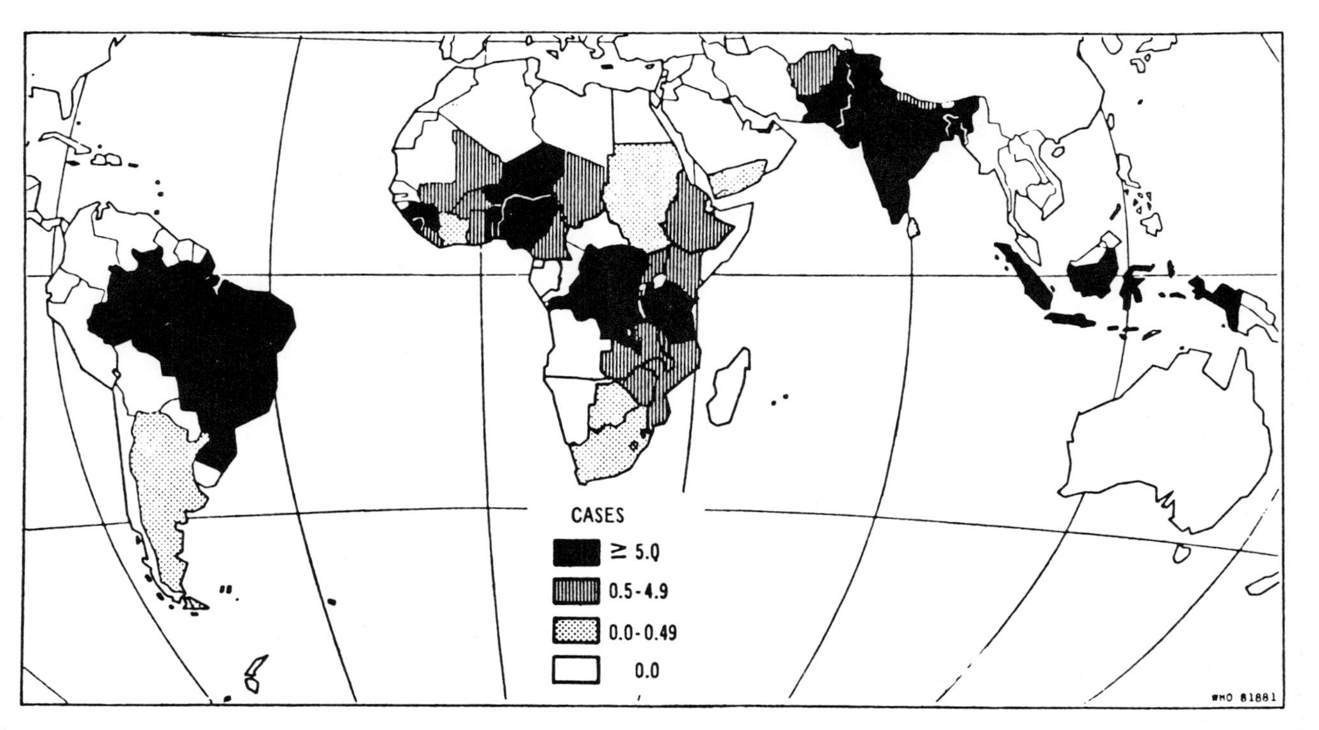

Fig. 1. Map of the world, showing the incidence of reported cases of smallpox (per 100 000 population) in the 33 countries in which it was endemic in 1967. The actual incidence was probably about 100 times greater. (From Breman, J. G. and Arita, I. (1978) Poxvirus infections in humans following abandonment of smallpox vaccination. *In* "Proceedings of the 3rd Munich Symposium on Microbiology on 'Natural History of Newly Emerging and Re-Emerging Viral Zoonoses'", 137–159).

then kept indefinitely, yet in 1967 only 12% of the batches of vaccine used in the field in endemic countries were potent. WHO established vaccine standards and persuaded laboratories in Holland and Canada to serve as international vaccine reference centres. Endemic countries with large populations were encouraged to produce their own freeze-dried vaccine. By 1970, all the vaccine in use met the accepted standards and soon after that a good quality vaccine was being produced in endemic countries like India, Indonesia, Burma, Kenya and Brazil.

Another early objective was to improve the vaccination technique. Two methods were introduced: a jet injector, originally designed by the US Army, and a bifurcated needle, developed by Wyeth Laboratories in the 1960s. Jet guns were effective and useful for mass campaigns in places where large groups of the population could be assembled, and where good service facilities were available, but they were of limited value in Asia, where vaccination was traditionally carried out on a house-to-house basis. The bifurcated needle, eventually made of special steel so that it could be repeatedly boiled or flamed, became the ultimate solution, and was effective, cheap, economical of vaccine, and could be used safely without prior sterilization of the skin site.

B. Animal Reservoir

The experience of yellow fever made the Smallpox Eradication Programme very much aware of the threat to the campaign that an animal reservoir of variola virus would pose. There was a candidate disease, known as monkeypox because of outbreaks in wild monkeys that were held in laboratories in Europe and USA for the production and testing of poliovirus vaccines. An advisory committee of virologists met first in 1969 and kept this problem under regular review, with considerable anxiety when, following the eradication of smallpox and variola virus from West and Central Africa, human monkeypox, clinically resembling smallpox, was recognized there in 1970. A few cases have occurred annually in those parts of Africa each year since then (Fig. 2), and such incidences can be expected to continue. Although clinically identical with smallpox caused by variola virus, human monkeypox is very poorly transmitted between humans; it does not pose a public health threat although continuing surveillance is clearly warranted.

In the course of work with monkeypox, another virological problem has emerged which is so far unresolved, a virus designated "whitepox virus". By all laboratory criteria it is variola virus that has been recovered from several unusual sources; on two occasions from healthy cynomolgous monkeys, in 1964 in a clinical diagnostic laboratory in the

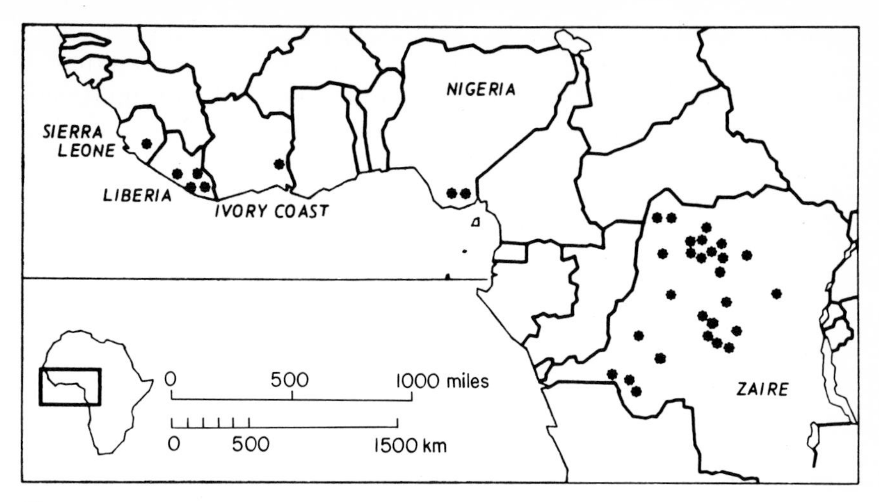

Fig. 2. Location of the thirty-five human monkeypox cases diagnosed in West and Central Africa between 1970 and 1978. Secondary infection observed in only two cases. Most cases occurred in unvaccinated children living in small villages in dense tropical forest. (From Breman J. G. (1978) Human monkeypox: updated 1978. *Wld Hlth Org. SME*/78.15.)

Netherlands, on four occasions from tissues for four different species of wild animals captured in Zaire between 1973 and 1975 and tested in Moscow, and recently as a so-called "white pock variant" of monkeypox virus, again in the Moscow laboratory. The significance of whitepox virus is unknown and may never be resolved with certainty; it is important to realize that no human infection with this virus has ever been reported. It is not impossible that all isolates of whitepox virus represent laboratory contaminants of cultures with variola virus, although this is clearly impossible to prove. But the existence of whitepox virus and of clinical smallpox caused by monkeypox virus makes it essential that "authentic" strains of variola virus (or their genetic material) should be preserved indefinitely so that comparative tests of viruses suspected of being variola virus can always be performed.

C. Laboratory Research and International Diagnostic Laboratories

Research on variola and monkeypox viruses was clearly necessary after the recognition of human monkeypox in 1970, and was promoted by WHO and coordinated at meetings of the specialist virologist group. It was also essential to have a few laboratories able and willing to carry out laboratory diagnostic tests, by electron microscopy and culture, of scab material from all parts of the world. The USA and the USSR provided such facilities, at Atlanta and in Moscow; they were called WHO Collaborating Centres, and they have processed a great number of specimens, especially during the last five years of the campaign, in relation to the international certification progamme (see Table V).

D. National Infrastructure

Smallpox eradication had been achieved before 1950 in countries that had a well-developed public health service, or isolated countries that were protected by their isolation, helped by quarantine. WHO put an intensive and successful effort, supported by international consultants from many countries, to developing national smallpox eradication programmes in all endemic countries, and a national infrastructure to carry out the planned procedures and subsequently to search for residual cases.

III. The Progress of Eradication

WHO is an intergovernmental agency, and it therefore looked upon its eradication programme in terms of countries in which eradication of endemic smallpox was progressively achieved. The steady fall in the number of endemic countries is illustrated in Fig. 3. This was achieved by two strategies; mass vaccination and surveillance and containment. Mass vaccination and "normal public health surveillance" had long before eradicated smallpox from many countries. The problem was how to achieve eradication in countries that lacked an effective public health service. Initially stress was laid on the provision of a good vaccine and the achievement of widespread mass vaccination and revaccination. In some countries this was enough to achieve eradication. But it looked hopeless in Indonesia, India and Bangladesh, and in the poor countries of Africa. For example, in a population of 23 million people in central Java, in spite of 95% vaccination coverage, over 1000 cases of smallpox were found in 1969, 85% of them in persons who had not been successfully vaccinated. Vaccination of the "last 5%" was logistically impossible.

The strategy was changed. Having greatly lowered the size of the susceptible "herd" by mass vaccination, eradication was achieved by a highly organized campaign of surveillance and containment. As soon

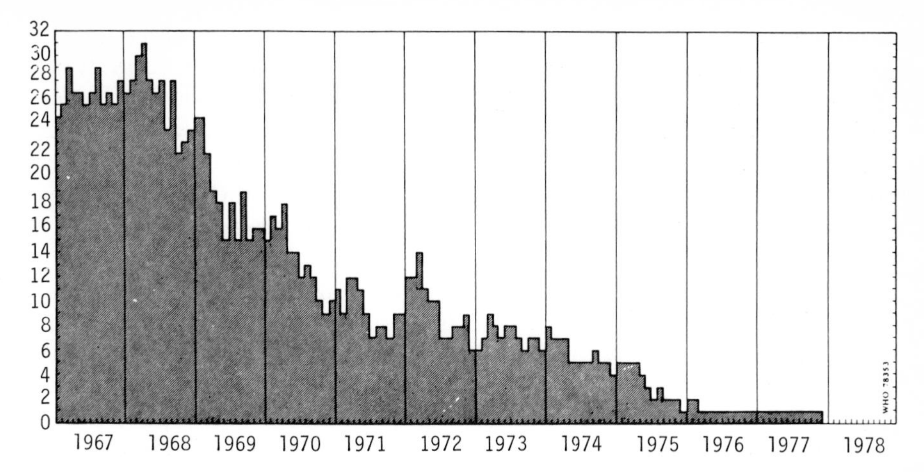

Fig. 3. Numbers of countries reporting endemic smallpox each month, between 1967 (33 endemic countries; 11 countries with imported cases) and 1977 (last endemic case in Somalia in October 1977). (From Breman, J. G. and Arita, I. (1978) Poxvirus infections in humans following abandonment of smallpox vaccination. *In* "Proceedings of the 3rd Munich Symposium of Microbiology on 'Natural History of Newly Emerging and Re-Emerging Viral Zoonoses' ", 137–159).

as a case was recognized it was isolated in the family hut, all persons in the village were vaccinated, the house was placed under 24-hour guard, and surrounding households for a distance of about 5 km were vaccinated. Initiated in West Africa by Dr W. Foege, this programme has proved successful everywhere, as was exemplified dramatically in India, where there were 11 000 notified cases in one week in May 1954 and the last case in the country occurred in May 1975.

IV. The Certification of Eradication

By the early 1970s it became clear that endemic smallpox was likely to be eradicated in several countries, and groups of neighbouring countries, where it had been endemic in 1967 and for hundreds of years before that. Global eradication could be assured, and achieved, only by eradicating smallpox from each of the thirty-three countries where it had been endemic in 1967. The problem the Smallpox Eradication Unit now faced was to devise a way of establishing with a high degree of probability, and demonstrating to the world community, that endemic smallpox had indeed been eradicated in these countries.

Given the international importance of eradication for each country, some method of international examination and certification was needed. The first task was to decide what period of time should elapse before an international team should be called to examine the situation. Reviewing the intervals that had elapsed between an apparent "last reported case" and recognition again of the endemic disease (Table III) the WHO Expert Committee on Smallpox Eradication in 1971 decided on two years; that is, three times as long as the longest recognized interval. A series of International Commissions for the Certification of Smallpox Eradication were established, and procedures were developed that were suitable for highly endemic countries like India and Somalia. Other procedures were used in countries where the last reported case had occurred many years before. Both kinds of procedure needed to be flexible, because some countries had experienced only severe smallpox, others only mild smallpox, and some both kinds of disease. Furthermore, the health infrastructure and epidemiological circumstances in different countries differed enormously.

TABLE III. *Summary of Episodes in which Smallpox Foci Remained Undiscovered for Long Periods*

Country	Duration of missed focus	No. of cases	Date of[a]	
			Discovery	Last case
Brazil	15 weeks	18	2.3.71	5.3.71
Botswana				
No. 1	13 weeks	19	7.3.73	15.4.73
No. 2	27 weeks	15	20.9.73	14.9.73
No. 3	10 weeks	6	21.11.73	15.11.73
Indonesia	34 weeks	163	14.12.71	23.1.72
Nigeria	22 weeks	84	21.3.70	10.5.70

[a] Hidden foci were usually quickly contained once they were discovered; sometimes (Botswana Nos 2 and 3) discovery occurred after the onset of the last known case.

A substantial part of the funds provided to the Smallpox Eradication Programme had been devoted to providing international expert consultants to back up the national campaigns, and ensuring that good vaccines and needles could be got to even the most remote places. Devoted field workers, four-wheel drive vehicles and helicopters all played their parts, both in the eradication campaign itself and in the extensive and intensive "searches" that were mounted in the previously highly endemic countries to ensure that smallpox had indeed been eradicated. Most important, from this point of view of certification, was that the paperwork (notification of suspected cases, follow-up visits, collection of material for laboratory study, containment and vaccination where suspected cases were found) was well done and was well checked and supervised. The impending visit of an International Commission served as a very effective stimulus for this work, and in countries like India, where smallpox had long been a scourge, the International Commission was received with great ceremony, at the Centre (New Delhi), in the individual state capitals, and in the villages. International Commissions, and other forms of visits adapted to the epidemiological and political circumstances of particular countries, had by June 1979 visited fifty-five countries, sometimes a Commission to a country (e.g. India, Bangladesh, Somalia, Ethiopia), sometimes to a group of countries (South America, West Africa, Central Africa, etc.) (Fig. 4).

A. The Global Commission for the Certification of Smallpox Eradication

As worldwide eradication became a near-reality, symbolized dramatically by the certification of eradication of smallpox from India in April 1977, WHO set up the World-Wide Consultation of Experts to advise it on how WHO should certify, and assure all countries of the world, of global eradication. The Consultation met in October 1977 and recommended that it should be constituted as the Global Commission for the Certification of Smallpox Eradication, to which the World Health Assembly agreed. The Global Commission's task was to work towards its own demise, hopefully in May 1980, with the acceptance of worldwide eradication by the World Health Assembly.

B. Surveys Prior to Certification

Following intensive "country reports", prepared in consultation with WHO expert advisers, the International Commission visits were designed, not to find cases of smallpox, but to see whether the system of surveillance and reporting, from the capital cities out to the most distant villages, would have been adequate to detect smallpox had it occurred. Two kinds of surveys were developed to supplement the information available from active searches for smallpox cases and from the paperwork. Severe smallpox almost always leaves those who survive with pockmarks, easily visible on the face (Table IV). Pockmark

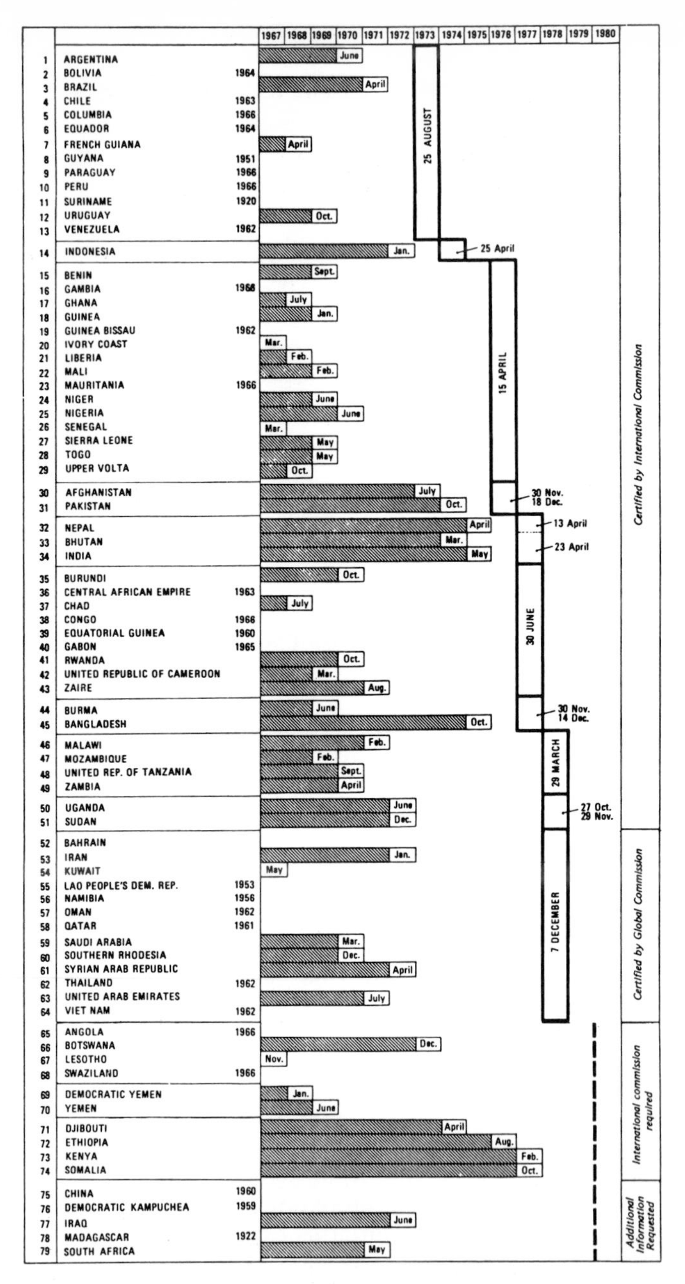

Fig. 4. Diagram illustrating 79 countries and areas designated by the Global Commission in December 1978 as requiring special procedures for the certification of smallpox eradication. The date shown opposite each entry is the year of the last reported case; the date of certification is also shown. At the end of 1978 only 15 countries remained to be certified; 7 of these had been certified by June 1979 (From *WHO Wkly Epidem. Rec.* No. 1, 5 Jan. 1979).

surveys, including adults and adolescents (so that the observers knew what they were looking for) but extending down to pre-school children, were an excellent way of determining when smallpox had last occurred in a village or town, in Asia and most parts of Africa. But mild smallpox (variola minor) has been the only form of the disease seen in recent years in South America, Ethiopia, Somalia, Botswana and Sudan. This rarely leaves facial pockmarks, at least of the number (five or more) accepted by the Commission as positive (Table IV).

TABLE IV. *Facial Pockmarks After Severe Smallpox (Variola Major) and Mild Smallpox (Variola Minor)*

Group	Total number	Facial pockmarks		
		0	1–4	5 or more
Severe smallpox, unvaccinated	224	23 (10%)	10 (5%)	191 (85%)
Severe smallpox, vaccinated	240	53 (22%)	32 (13%)	155 (65%)
Mild smallpox, unvaccinated	175	134 (76%)	29 (17%)	12 (7%)

For such countries another kind of check was needed. Since the disease most likely to be confused with smallpox was chickenpox, "chickenpox surveys" were developed for these and some other countries. Scab or vesicle material was collected from suspected chickenpox cases, especially the rare severe or fatal cases, and from cases in unvaccinated children. Usually, one specimen only was obtained from each outbreak, and attention was concentrated on "vulnerable areas", where epidemiologists thought smallpox most likely to have occurred in the recent past. The collected material was sent through WHO to the WHO Collaborating Centres in USA and USSR, and there examined electron microscopically for pox- or herpesviruses and by culture for poxviruses. The scale of recent surveys is indicated in Table V.

So far, no country that had received an International Commission has failed to provide evidence of eradication, and no cases have occurred subsequently in countries that have been certified. At the time of writing (May 1979) it seems certain that global eradication will be announced by the World Health Assembly in May 1980.

TABLE V. *Chickenpox Surveys: Specimens Collected in the Horn of Africa and Tested for Variola Virus, 1977–79*[a]

Country	Population in millions	Number of specimens collected		
		1977	1978	1979 (15 April)
Djibouti	0·5	17	69	37
Ethiopia	30	565	1004	941
Kenya	16	147(4)[b]	113	475
Somalia	4	864(265)	1691	803
Total	50·5	1593(269)	2877	2256

[a] From *WHO Wkly Epidem. Rec.* No. 18, 4 May 1979, 137–142.
[b] Number of specimens positive for variola virus.

V. Post-eradication Strategy

In spite of the dramatic success of the Intensified Smallpox Eradication Programme, it would be foolish not to provide some insurance against future unexpected happenings. Various steps have been taken or are in train.

A. Vaccine

Freeze-dried vaccine stored at −20° maintains its potency for at least 15 years, and probably much longer. Many individual countries have set aside stocks, and WHO has a reserve of 200 million doses, plus needles and accessory equipment, stored in Geneva and New Delhi.

B. Animal Reservoir

The whitepox viruses remain an enigma, and monkeypox virus is a reality that could conceivably initiate human smallpox again. Continued surveillance in West and Central Africa, especially in Zaire, is required. Furthermore, it is necessary to have some way of comparing a suspected "variola virus", 5 or 10 years hence, with "authentic" variola virus. There is clearly a need to maintain high security diagnostic laboratories, probably at the WHO Collaborating Centres in Moscow and Atlanta. The need for comparison seemed at first to require the continued storage of variola virus stocks in such laboratories, but the development of genome maps of the orthopoxviruses and the possibility of cloning and storing restriction enzyme fragments of the variola DNA molecule in plasmids of *Escherichia coli*, may provide another way of keeping the necessary information (DNA) readily available. The escape of virus from a laboratory in the University of Birmingham (England) in August 1978 made it clear that the number of laboratories holding and using variola virus should be reduced to the essential minimum.

VI. Conclusions

Smallpox was one of the great scourges of mankind. It exerted obvious effects on geopolitics in middle and south America, and more subtle effects in other places. Besides the wasted lives, it left a legacy of pockmarks and blindness in many of those who survived. Its exclusion from countries where it was non-endemic, in times of world wide air travel, necessitated an elaborate health inspection system at sea- and airports, and vaccination itself carried some morbidity and a low mortality. It has now been eradicated, and at an annual cost (additional to national costs of about $20 million a year) of about $10 million since 1967 (plus the uncosted devotion of an army of national and international health workers, advisers and consultants) with an estimated annual saving of over $1000 million. The World Health Organization as the instrument, and the international community as the operators, can be proud of the achievement, foreshadowed in 1801 by Edward Jenner: "It now becomes too manifest to admit of controversy that the annihilation of the smallpox, the most dreadful scourge of the human species, must be the result of this practice [vaccination]."

14

The Emergence of New Infectious Diseases

Cedric Mims

Department of Microbiology, Guy's Hospital, London, UK

The best safeguard against the fourth rider of the apocalypse in the form of a devastating new infectious disease is increased understanding and constant vigilance on the part of microbiologists, physicians and veterinarians. Since the world is now one place for infectious diseases, international co-operation under the benevolent auspices of the WHO will be essential.

I. Introduction

Microorganisms are constantly undergoing evolutionary change. As with higher forms of life, many varieties become extinct while others are better adapted to survive and are successfully perpetuated. This evolutionary process takes place with all parasitic microorganisms whether the host is a mouse, apple tree or man, and the rate of evolution is generally rapid compared with the rate in the host. Because of this, parasitic microorganisms are most of the time one step ahead of the host, and have many methods for evading host defences. But microorganisms, like all parasites, are dependent on the host, and are greatly affected by changes in host biology and activity. In man, when these changes are cultural rather than genetic in origin they can be rapid and dramatic on an evolutionary time scale. Thus in the course of a mere 100 000 years paleolithic men living in small hunter-gatherer groups have been replaced by more than 1000 million modern men with their cities and civilization. During this period genetic changes can only have been small, but advances in culture have formed the basis for a novel and much more rapid type of change which has amounted to the transformation of a species. As a result, some of the infectious disease agents parasitic in man have been presented with new difficulties, but at the same time those parasitic in animals or free-living in the environment have had opportunities to establish themselves in the human species. This chapter deals with the emergence of infectious diseases in relation to human evolution.

The alterations in human life-style have been greater in the past 100 years than in the preceding 100 000, but those with the biggest impact on host–parasite relationships have been taking place for several thousand years. They can be classified (Table I), and will form the basis for my account of the emergence of infectious diseases of man. This approach gives good indications as to possible sources of new infectious diseases of man. Prehistory and archaeology provide poor evidence, and speculation is therefore inevitable.

II. Crowding

Together with an overall increase in human numbers there has been a concentration of individuals in towns and cities.

Most microorganisms are transmitted more readily when the host species is present in greater numbers; increased density of the host especially affects transmission by the respiratory and enteric (gastro-intestinal) routes. Respiratory viruses, for instance, spread rapidly and become more common when man is crowded in cities, particularly in enclosed spaces during cold weather. The same thing happens when chickens are maintained in close proximity in batteries or when horses are brought together in race meetings. New strains of influenza virus are constantly appearing and although most of these cause mild illness, a strain with high transmissibility and pathogenicity could emerge (see Mackenzie, this vol).

The rhino(nose) viruses are also evolving rapidly in association with crowding. They cause "hit and run" upper respiratory infections. The incubation period is rapid (a few days) and after growing in nasal epithelial cells these viruses are shed in vastly increased numbers to infect fresh individuals before host immune defences have much of an opportunity to control the infection. The same condition (the common cold) can be caused by various other viruses but the rhinoviruses are an important group.

Crowding also provides opportunities for the increased spread of gastrointestinal infections and infestations. It not only encourages parasites that are shed from the infected host as highly resistant eggs or spores, but also favours parasites that are shed in less stable form. The first example is cholera. This must be a relatively recent parasite of man, because in its classical form cholera could not have maintained itself before men lived in towns and cities. In the past it has spread mainly by the contamination of water supplies with infected faeces. As the devout gather in their tens of thousands on the pilgrimage to Mecca, or Hindus enjoy the Holy Water of the Ganges, the cholera vibrio takes its opportunities. There are signs that cholera is continuing to evolve, as public health measures provide fewer opportunities for water transmission, by adapting itself to transmission via fingers and food rather than water. Thus, the El Tor strain is less pathogenic than classical severe cholera. It is shed from the intestines for a longer period, enabling the sufferer to carry the infection in the community and distribute the bacteria more effectively to other individuals. It is also less readily inactivated on drying and is more easily spread via fingers or dates.

The second example is the large number of gastrointestinal viruses that infect modern man, in many ways comparable to the respiratory viruses mentioned earlier. These, too, are of the "hit and run" variety, and, like the rhinoviruses, cause little or no serious illness. There are three strains of human poliovirus, 26 strains of Coxsackie virus and 32 strains of echovirus. The person who develops a neurological illness

TABLE I. *Factors behind the Emergence of New Infectious Diseases of Man*

Changes in human life-style or activity	Examples of new infections that have emerged or are still emerging	Mechanism
1. Crowding	Respiratory virus infections	
	Rhinovirus	Increased density of susceptible hosts
	Legionnaire's disease	Air-conditioning?
	Gastrointestinal infections	
	Cholera	Increased density of susceptible hosts and use of water
	Enteroviruses	
2. Domestication of animals	Probably most human infections including:	
	Psittacosis	Close association between man and domestic animal
	Distemper	
	Influenza	
	Q fever	
	Salmonellosis	
3. Moving into new habitats: new encounters with infectious cycles	Scrub typhus	Close contact with wild animal infectious cycle
	Plague	
	Lassa fever	
	Bolivian haemorrhagic fever	
4. Increased rate of movement	Influenza as a global infection	
	Lassa fever or yellow fever in Europe	

5. New patterns of sociosexual activity	Sexually transmitted infections Herpes simplex 2 TRIC agents Syphilis Glandular fever	Multiple sexual partners
6. Increased survival of susceptible individuals	Immunosuppressed kidney transplant recipients *Pneumocystis carini* Cytomegalovirus Aspergillosis	Harmless commensal micro-organisms cause disease in host with depressed resistance
	Children with leukaemia Fatal chickenpox	Common, harmless infection becomes lethal
	Severe mumps, polio, varicella and EB virus infections in adolescents or adults	Infection harmless in child is more serious when infection is put off until later in life
7. Manufacture of new infectious agents by man	Indirect—production of antibiotic-resistant bacteria Antibiotic-resistant staphylococci in hospitals Tetracycline-resistant typhoid bacilli Penicillin-resistant gonococci Direct—genetic manipulation Not yet accomplished	

(meningitis, paralysis) with poliovirus, or whose heart is affected by a Coxsackie B virus, is the exception. In most of us these infections are restricted to the intestine and are mild or unnoticed. It is impossible to delve into the evolutionary history of these viruses in man, but they could not have maintained themselves in their present form before the development of cities, and still cannot do so in small isolated groups of human beings (see Chapter 3). Presumably they have appeared since the big changes in human numbers and densities, and their abundance and variety suggest that they are continuing to diversify and evolve. One recently discovered group of human gastrointestinal viruses, the rotaviruses, are an important cause of diarrhoea in infants and children. Remarkably similar viruses affect mice, foals, piglets and calves, and an origin from one of these associates of humans seems likely (see Section II).

Although crowding itself generally favours the spread of infection, the concentration of people into modern buildings has made it easier to control certain types of infection. For instance, enteric infections are reduced when faeces are disposed of through sewage systems and when there is uncontaminated water for washing and drinking. Cholera fails to spread through the community under these circumstances, but enteroviruses and rotaviruses still do so, although on a greatly reduced scale, so that infection tends to occur later in life than under less hygienic conditions. Nevertheless measures to control the environment in buildings can lead to new problems. In the original outbreak of Legionnaire's disease, 182 legionnaires attending a convention in Philadelphia developed severe pneumonia, and 17% of them died. The cause was a newly discovered bacterium which appears to have contaminated the air-conditioning system of the hotel in which they were staying, and was thereby delivered to their lungs.

In modern towns and cities the microbiological quality of food and water is carefully controlled and our freedom from many infections depends on the efficiency of this surveillance. But this means that the entire population is now vulnerable to contamination from centralized supplies. The distribution of pathogenic microorganisms or their toxins in food and water occurs occasionally and reminds us of our vulnerability, but is largely a subject for science fiction or biological warfare.

III. Domestication of Animals

Domestication led to an exceedingly close association between man and certain animals, and there was an inevitable transfer of parasites, including microorganisms. Examples include measles, quite probably originating from distemper virus in man's canine associate (see Chapter 7) and influenza A, new strains of which continue to arise from closely related viruses in birds (see Chapter 9). I shall mention two other interesting examples.

First psittacosis, an infection acquired by man from cage birds. The parasite is one of the chlamydia, more like a bacterium than a virus, but quite distinct from either of these. It causes an initially harmless infection in birds such as parrots and budgerigars, and the infectious agent then persists in the spleen of the bird. As a result of certain stresses, such as transport in cages, changes in diet and so on, the infection is reactivated, and the chlamydia are shed from the respiratory tract and in the faeces. The bird often looks unwell, and people in close contact with it now inhale the chlamydia and develop an unpleasant type of pneumonia. Fortunately the infected individual rarely transfers the infection to others, human cases being nearly always acquired from birds. A man as isolated as Robinson Crusoe would have been free from the common cold and from enteroviruses, but he might have caught psittacosis from his parrot. There are many other infectious diseases that come from man's animal associates but are not transmitted directly from man to man. For this reason infections such as psittacosis, Q fever (caused by a rickettsial parasite) or Lassa fever (see below) can never in their present form be major causes of human disease. On the other hand, if a new variant arose that was transmitted directly from man to man this would be the starting point of a new and more serious human infection. By staying exclusively in the human host, the infectious agent would be able to evolve and develop new features that distinguish it from the ancestral form in animals.

The second example of an infection acquired from man's animal associates is salmonellosis. There are more than 1000 distinct species of bacteria in the Salmonella group, but only typhoid and paratyphoid are primarily infections of man. The rest parasitize a great variety of animals, including birds and reptiles, and some infect domestic animals which then act as a source of human infection. But they are much less infectious for man than typhoid or paratyphoid, and at least a million bacteria must be ingested to produce disease, which is generally some form of gastroenteritis. *Salmonella agona*, for instance, probably originated as a bacterium associated with fish and birds off the Peruvian Coast of South America. Intensive fishing by man yielded a surplus of fish which were converted to fish-meal and exported to Europe for incorporation into food pellets fed to poultry. In the 1960s *S. agona* established itself in the intestines of domestic chickens in

Europe, and chicken carcasses prepared for human consumption were often contaminated. Inadequate cooking of frozen birds allowed some of the bacteria to survive, and multiplication took place, especially when carcasses were then left for some time at room temperature. People eating such chickens developed Salmonella gastroenteritis. Salmonellosis, which sometimes causes a more serious disease, is an infection acquired from man's domestic animals as a result of modern methods of keeping, feeding and preparing their carcasses for consumption.

IV. Moving into New Habitats: New Encounters with Infectious Cycles

Man constantly explores and colonizes new areas of the earth. In doing so he makes new encounters with animals and their parasites, and, if he is susceptible to any of these parasites a new human disease may be produced. Scrub typhus is an example. Many rodents have their own rickettsial infections, transmitted from individual to individual by fleas, mites or other bloodsucking arthropods. There is generally little damage caused in the rodent host because the association is an ancient one and has had time to settle down to a state of "balanced pathogenicity"*. In the Second World War, when Australian, American and Japanese soldiers were struggling for the possession of certain islands in the Pacific, and when men were lying, sleeping or hiding on the ground, there was an unprecedented amount of interation between man and one of these rodent-rickettsial parasite cycles. Men bitten by ticks from rodents became infected with the rickettsia and developed a serious disease called scrub typhus.

Plague provides another example. *Yersinia pestis* is a bacterial parasite of rodents spread from rat to rat, gerbil to gerbil, or from marmot to marmot by bloodsucking arthropods. The great human experiences with this bacterium have at all times followed his interaction with the naturally occurring rodent–flea cycle. This has occurred for thousands of

* The first encounter of a parasite with a new host may lead to a devastating illness or death, as a result of which the parasite has difficulty maintaining itself in the host species. There are strong evolutionary forces favouring the emergence of a less virulent variety of parasite or a more resistant variety of host, and eventually the parasite and the host tend to reach a state of balance. Myxomatosis in the Australian rabbit provides a classic example of the evolutionary transition from a highly virulent to a relatively avirulent state of parasitism (see Chapters 1 and 4). Both the virus and the host species have undergone genetic changes as a result of which the virus now multiplies, is transmitted and maintains itself in the host species in a less harmful fashion.

years in Asia (see Chapters 3 and 4), and also in Africa and other countries. The major devastations in man were in the form of the Black Death, and in Europe this resulted from the invasion of human dwellings by the black rat, a rodent brought back to Europe from the Middle East (together with leprosy, trachoma and the donkey) by the returning Crusaders. Fleas from infected rats bit a man's arm or leg and thus introduced the bacterium into his body. Following spread to the local lymph node the bacteria multiplied causing a painful swelling, or bubo, in the armpit or groin. After this they reached the bloodstream, spread through the body, liberated toxins, and usually caused death. But the infection was not passed on directly from man to man (see also psittacosis above). On occasions, however, the bacteria reaching the lungs multiplied extensively in this organ and were then able to exit from the body in large numbers by the respiratory route. When this happened the exclusively rat-borne bubonic plague changed to a pneumonic form in which the disease spread with great rapidity directly from person to person. Pneumonic plague has been a major influence in human history (see Chapter 3). I mention plague, an infection which still emerges when man encounters the rodent–flea cycle (it was a significant cause of death in US soldiers in Vietnam) in order to compare it with Lassa fever.

Lassa fever is a recently described and striking infection of man. The virus of Lassa fever exists in Africa as a harmless infection of a small rat called *Mastomys natalensis*. It is well adapted to this particular rodent, causing no harm and remaining in the body throughout life. It is excreted in the urine, saliva and faeces. As a result of close contact with infected rats, either in rat-infested dwellings or in the course of hunting these animals, man acquires the infection. The disease is often mild, but medical attendants who are unwittingly and intimately exposed to blood or secretions from an infected patient often suffer a severe and fatal infection. Person to person spread via natural routes has not so far occurred in spite of numerous opportunities. The virus is present in the throat, but presumably there is insufficient multiplication in throat and lungs for there to be effective transmission via the respiratory route. By analogy with plague (see Fig. 1) a change in respiratory pathogenicity could transform Lassa fever into a major infectious disease of man.

A very similar virus exists in the same fashion in Bolivia in association with another small rodent called *Callomys callosus*. Close contact of the infected rodent with man leads to a severe, sometimes fatal, illness (Bolivian haemorrhagic fever) but once again man to man spread is rare. *Callomys callosus* is a "bush" mouse, and during the original outbreak in San Joaquin, Bolivia, the association with man occurred in

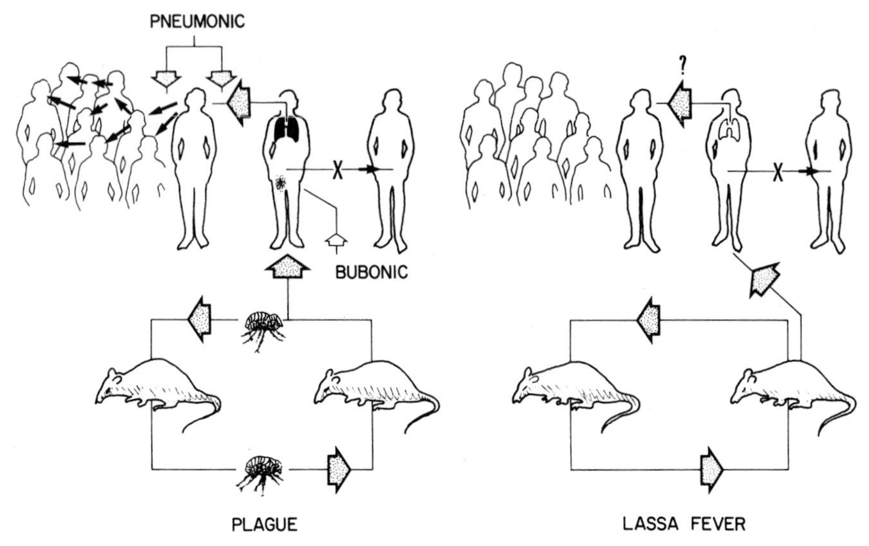

Fig. 1. *Comparison between plague and Lassa fever.*

an interesting way. An intensive mosquito spraying programme had been undertaken with DDT, and in the houses the geckos eating the DDT-containing insects were themselves eaten by the resident cats. As DDT accumulated in the cats and exceeded the lethal dose, the cats, who normally prevented wild rodents from invading the houses, died. The subsequent infestation of houses with virus-carrying *Callomys callosus* and the death of 126 infected inhabitants thus had an interesting ecological association with the anti-mosquito campaign.

Another recently described and severe infectious disease, which presumably originates from an infectious cycle in animals, is caused by Marburg and Ebola viruses. Marburg virus disease first appeared in 1967, when there were 31 cases with seven deaths in West Germany and Yugoslavia. The infection was acquired by contact in research laboratories with tissues from African Green Monkeys. But in Uganda, their country of origin, these monkeys are not infected, and the source of the virus is unknown. Three more cases of the disease were seen in South Africa in 1975, but there is no information as to how the first patient, an Australian hitch-hiker, was infected. Further outbreaks of a severe haemorrhagic fever due to a related virus (Ebola) occurred in 1976 in the Sudan (299 cases, 150 of which were fatal) and in Zaire (237 cases, 211 of which were fatal). In spite of extensive investigations, the source of Marburg and Ebola viruses is still unknown. Neither of them are transmitted very effectively from man to man by natural routes. As with Lassa fever and other infections, a change in transmissibility could enable them to have a major impact on mankind.

V. Increased Rate of Movement

In the beginning men walked; then there were horses with or without the wheel, which in turn gave way to trains and motor cars. Steamships replaced sail, and now we have jet aircraft. Thus a new strain of influenza A virus, if it had arisen in Central America or Indonesia in the year 1000, would have had little or no opportunity to reach Europe, Africa or the Far East. The 1919 strain of virus travelled across the world over the course of months at the speed of steamship and train, and a new strain now crosses the continents by jet in a matter of hours. This example is dealt with in Chapter 9, but the principle has been of major importance in the emergence of infectious diseases in new areas of the world. A new disease like Lassa fever from Africa, which 50 years ago would have killed the bearer before he arrived in Europe, can now suddenly appear in London or New York, a matter which is a source of great anxiety for public health authorities.

Nowadays any human pathogen, unless it rapidly causes unmistakable illness so that it can be identified and the patient quarantined, has rapid access to Europe or North America. Cholera, an ancient infection in the Far East, did not reach Europe until the nineteenth century. For some reason it had been unable to make this journey by land, and was brought by ship to Arabia in 1817, spreading to Persia and Europe, reaching England in 1831. Rabies originated in Africa, where four similar viruses exist today. It reached the Americas by sea and the first infected dogs are recorded from Virginia in 1753, and in South America (Peru) in 1803. Outbreaks of yellow fever in Marseilles or Philadelphia were possible when ships sailed to these ports from Africa and South America. In 1979 a woman residing within a mile of Amsterdam airport suddenly developed malaria. She had almost certainly been bitten by an infected mosquito carried by jet from Africa or the Far East.

VI. New Patterns of Sociosexual Activity

The first movement of men into towns and cities led to alterations in social and sexual life, but more fundamental changes have resulted from increased mobility and from shifts in moral attitudes. The present flowering of sexually transmitted infections is referred to in Chapter 12 and I only wish to suggest that these infectious agents are continuing to evolve, making the most of the opportunities for transmission during sexual activity. Chlamydia in particular, represented by the TRIC agents, now have great opportunities for evolution and diversification, and new types are probably emerging.

Syphilis provides a good example of the evolution of a sexually transmitted disease. It has been suggested (Hackett, 1963) that syphilis originated in warm countries as a non-venereal infection causing skin lesions and was transmitted from person to person by contact, in much the same way that the closely related bacterium causing yaws is transmitted nowadays. As man moved into cooler climates and covered most of his skin with clothes, the bacterium evolved and developed the capacity to spread during sexual intercourse.

Herpes simplex type 2 is a sexually transmitted virus infection which may have originated more recently. The original herpes simplex virus of man causes lesions (cold sores) in the region of the mouth, and spreads from person to person via contact and saliva. If the genital regions become infected the virus can now be transmitted directly to the genitals of another individual during sexual activity. In the distant past this was a sporadic occurrence, but in more recent times sexual transmission began to take place more commonly. This was independent of oral transmission, and at a different age, enabling the sexually transmitted virus to evolve independently. It developed antigenic and other characteristics that now distinguish it (herpes simplex type 2) from the original (herpes simplex type 1) strain. Infection with the latter does not prevent infection with the former, which has become one of the commonest sexually transmitted diseases. Cytomegalovirus is another human herpes virus, normally spread via saliva, that seems to be in the process of giving rise to a sexually transmitted variant. There are scores of distinct herpes viruses infecting most species of animals, and one can trace their evolutionary history according to biological properties and DNA analysis (Nahmias, 1974; Nahmias and Reanney, 1977; Honess and Watson, 1977). A particularly powerful technique (restriction enzyme analysis) has recently been developed, which fingerprints viral DNA and detects quite small differences. This may provide further information about the evolution of herpes viruses. Nucleic acid homologies and the host range pattern can also be used to study the evolution of leukaemia viruses in relation to the evolution of the host species (Benveniste and Todaro, 1976). The papovaviruses also lend themselves to studies of this sort. The DNA of mouse (polyoma) monkey (SV40) and human (BK) viruses have been sequenced, and their relative evolutionary distance calculated by computer analysis (Soeda *et al*, 1980). These distances agree with what is known of rodent and primate evolution and it is clear that these are exceedingly ancient parasites and have evolved with the host species, diverging from each other as the host species diverged. The calculations indicated that the rate of evolution of the virus genes was $4{\cdot}5 - 6{\cdot}5 \times 10^{-9}$ per year per nucleotide site, which is slightly faster than that estimated for haemoglobin genes.

Glandular fever is another virus disease that has appeared quite recently, in this case because of changes in hygiene as well as in sociosexual activity. The causative agent, EB virus, is shed from the infected individual in the saliva. Originally it was a universal and unnoticed infection of small children whose behaviour and life style had always favoured the salivary spread of infectious agents. In developed countries, however, intimate contacts between small children have become less common. There is more washing and "hygiene" and this has meant that saliva is less freely exchanged. In these countries, therefore, most individuals fail to become infected with EB virus during childhood, and the next opportunity for extensive salivary exchanges is in kissing during sexual activity. The infected adolescent or adult now develops the troublesome disease glandular fever, instead of the very mild or inapparent infection seen in infants and young children. The disease glandular fever has therefore emerged because of changes in human activity, and it is an example of an infection that is much more severe in adults than in young children (see below).

VII. Increased Survival of Susceptible Individuals

Throughout evolutionary history, those susceptible to lethal infectious diseases have been ruthlessly eliminated. All species, including man, have genetic characteristics reflecting this relentless weeding out process. As new infections emerge the process of selection affects both parasite and host so that initially virulent infections tend to become less harmful, as pathogenicity settles down to a more balanced state (see footnote on page 238. Syphilis, for example, appears to have been a much more severe infection immediately after its invasion of Europe in the sixteenth century. It was referred to as the "great pox", in contrast to the relatively less virulent smallpox, and the milder disease we see today is perhaps a result of changes in the bacterium and possibly the host. The sweating sickness was a dramatic infectious disease that caused five epidemics in England between 1485 and 1551 (Sloan, 1971). Those affected developed headache, chest pain, severe sweating and often died within 24 hours. The first epidemic began three weeks after the entry of the Earl of Richmond's army (which included mercenaries from France) into London. The Lord Mayor of London, his successor, and six Aldermen, died within a week. It does not sound like any known infectious disease and disappeared after the last epidemic. Either the infectious agent changed suddenly to give a less virulent and less recognizable disease, or it failed to settle down to a state of balanced pathogenicity and "burnt itself out" after infecting most people.

Recently, however, the ancient process of weeding out has been dramatically interfered with as a result of medical advances. Individuals with genetic susceptibility to diseases such as tuberculosis, measles, syphilis or diphtheria are now in many parts of the world protected by vaccination, and genes conferring susceptibility can be handed down to offspring and thus accumulate in the gene pool of the species. If at some future date vaccination ceased and these infections or closely allied ones reappeared, then new diseases could emerge, highly virulent in susceptible human communities. So far this has not happened.

Medical intervention, as well as promoting the survival of susceptibility genes in the human species, also allows the survival of susceptible individuals. Immunosuppressed kidney transplant recipients have low resistance to many infections that are harmless in normal individuals. Virtually new infectious diseases therefore emerge, such as pneumonia caused by cytomegalovirus or the protozoan parasite *Pneumocystis carinii*, and infection is a common cause of death in these patients. In the same way, children with leukaemia often suffer fatal infections with the normally harmless chickenpox or common cold viruses. A large number of commensal or non-pathogenic microorganisms cause novel infections in patients who are kept alive with impaired antimicrobial defences. They are appropriately called opportunistic infections.

There is another interesting source of hypersusceptible individuals. In the past, many infections occurred almost exclusively in childhood, but as a result of changes in hygiene and way of life there has been a tendency for them to be postponed until adolescence or adult life. The resulting disease is then often more severe and at times what can be regarded as a new disease has emerged. Poliomyelitis, for instance, is a universal and mostly unnoticed infection of infants and small children in developing countries. When primary infection is delayed until later in life as a result of improved public health and hygiene, paralytic disease becomes more common. Similarly chickenpox, mumps, hepatitis B and EB virus (see above) cause more severe infections or new clinical features in adolescents and adults, and new diseases can be said to have emerged. As the same thing happens with other infections, new diseases are likely to be seen in adults. Infection in childhood is also prevented by vaccination programmes and in developed countries certain infections are becoming uncommon enough for children who missed being vaccinated also to miss natural infection. These individuals are fully susceptible to infection in later life, and adult measles for instance, is already becoming a less rare clinical condition. Adults might also become susceptible to childhood infections if there was a serious waning of the immunity conferred by vaccines.

VIII. Manufacture of New Infectious Agents by Man

A. Indirect (Antimicrobial Drugs)

Since antimicrobial drugs were first used, selection pressures have favoured the survival of microorganisms resistant to these drugs. Bacteria such as staphylococci have shown great versatility and adaptability, developing resistance to almost every antimicrobial agent soon after it was discovered. Other bacteria, such as the gonococcus, took a long time to become resistant to drugs (penicillin), but increased resistance is probably inevitable, especially in hospitals where the drugs are so commonly used (Finland, 1979). Resistance is not necessarily stable, and resistant forms often die out when the drug ceases to be used. Medical use of antimicrobial drugs can be said to have created new strains of resistant bacteria. Fortunately they are no more pathogenic than the original strains but drug resistance makes treatment more difficult. A classical example was the appearance of tetracycline-resistant strains of typhoid bacilli in Mexico in the 1960s as a result of the widespread availability and use of tetracyclines for diarrhoea.

B. Direct (Genetic Engineering)

Scientists are now capable of manufacturing new infectious agents. Pieces of DNA can be synthesized or broken off and joined up again at will, and novel combinations of genetic characters are thus obtained. Theoretically, as has been pointed out by the opponents of genetic engineering, one could make a breed of *Escherichia coli* (the common human bowel bacterium) that colonized man and produced a deadly product such as botulinus toxin.

TABLE II. *Possible Origin[a] of some Human Infectious Disease Agents*

	Vertical evolution from ancestral primates[b]	Origin from animals associated with man[b,c]	Man infected "accidentially". Primary infectious cycle (zoonosis) in animals ± vectors	Origin obscure
Viruses	Varicella-zoster	Influenza A (birds)	Marburg, Ebola viruses	Rubella
	Herpes simplex	Respiratory syncytial virus (cattle)	Arenaviruses (LCM, Lassa fever, etc.)	
	Cytomegalovirus	Measles (dog distemper, cattle, rindepest)	Arboviruses (yellow fever, etc.)	Hepatitis A and B
	EB virus	Rotavirus (cattle, cats, mice, horses)	Rabies	
	Parainfluenza virus 2	Coxsackie B (dogs)		
	Polyoma-like virus (BK, JC)	Parainfluenza virus A (mice, pigs)		
	Wart viruses	Parainfluenza virus B (cattle)		
	Adenoviruses ⟷	Adenoviruses (cattle, pigs, dogs)		
	Mumps ⟷	Mumps (NDV in poultry)		
	Variola (smallpox) ⟷	Variola (cattle, sheep, etc.)		
	Reoviruses ⟷	Reoviruses (dogs, mice, sheep, pigs)		
	Leukaemia virus ⟷	Leukaemia virus (cats, mice, cattle)		
	Coronaviruses ⟷	Coronaviruses (mice)		
	Rhinoviruses ⟷	Rhinoviruses (horses, cattle)		

Mycoplasma	Mycoplasma pneumoniae		Mycoplasma pneumoniae (cattle)			
Chlamydia				Ornithosis		Trachoma, TRIC agents
Rickettsia				Most rickettsiae		
Bacteria	Staphylococci, streptococci	⟷	Staphylococci, streptococci	Brucella		Neisseria
	Escherichia coli	⟷	*E. coli*	*Yersinia pestis* (plague)		*Salmonella typhi*
	Mycobacterium tuberculosis	⟷	*Mycobacterium tuberculosis* (cattle, mice)	Actinomycosis	Origin from free-living bacteria ?	Corynebacteria (diphtheria)
	Bordetella pertussis	⟷	*Bordetella pertussis* (dogs)	Leprospirosis		Cholera
	Haemophilus influenzae	⟷	*Haemophilus influenzae* (dogs, pigs)	Anthrax		Clostridia (tetanus, botulism)
	Treponemal infections (syphilis, pinta)	⟷	Treponemal infections	Salmonellosis		Pseudomonas
	Shigella?		Campylobacter (cattle)	Tularemia		Proteus
				Listeria monocytogenes		
Protozoa	Malaria	⟷	Malaria	Toxoplasmosis		Trichomonas?
	Entamoeba histolytica		Leishmaniasis ⟷	Leishmaniasis (dogs, etc.)		
			Trypanosomiasis ⟷	Trypanosomiasis		

[a] Origin of pathogenic agents from harmless commensals, and vice versa, is also possible.
[b] Who have related or similar infectious agents.
[c] Note: Origin of animal strains from man is also possible.
⟷ = an origin from either of these sources is possible.

But genetic engineering also means that it is now possible to manufacture exceedingly useful new bacteria, capable for instance, of providing us with cheap and pure insulin. It seems unlikely that these laboratory manoeuvres, undertaken with appropriate care, carry a risk worth worrying about. In any case, the deliberate production of a devastating new infectious agent, a possible aim of biological warfare, would be far from easy, nature having accomplished much that it is possible to accomplish. But this is now more than a subject for science fiction and, because men do evil things, it is not inconceivable that the most catastrophic infectious agents will one day be synthesized by man himself.

IX. Conclusions

The factors behind the emergence of new infectious diseases are summarized in Table I and the possible origins of human infections are tabulated in Table II. The latter, especially, is designed to stimulate interest rather than reveal the truth.

Generally speaking, infectious agents that emerged and evolved with man during his descent from ancestral primates are less pathogenic. Like all good parasites they have had time to settle down to a state of balanced pathogenicity (see page 238) with only the type of change listed under category 6 (Table I) to make them more harmful for man. Theoretically a new virulent strain could at any time emerge from one of them, but this can be said of any infectious agent.

Taking a look at the future, it can be predicted that high population density will continue to favour the emergence of new respiratory infections, and those able to infect healthy people with intact defence mechanisms will be for the most part viruses. Such rapidly evolving and resourceful microorganisms will often be a step ahead of vaccines and chemotherapeutic agents. A future Andromeda strain would be the sort that spread rapidly by the respiratory route and caused serious illness. Respiratory viruses therefore present a notable threat to the health and survival of man. Gastrointestinal infectious agents, on the other hand, will have a harder time of it as the route from faeces to mouth is made more difficult for them to negotiate.

If human beings are to remain as they are, with close skin and mucosal contacts forming the basis for affection, love and social bonding (Montague, 1972), then the infections spread via skin and mucosae will continue to emerge, as illustrated by the TRIC agents and herpes simplex type 2 (see above). But infections spread by sexual activity are unlikely to cause such sudden devastating outbreaks of disease as those transmitted by the respiratory route. By the latter route an individual can infect a dozen others in a few minutes, a feat far beyond the capacity of the most energetic lover. The skin itself is a source of infection in the case of the human wart viruses for instance, but more commonly the skin merely transfers (via fingers) infectious agents present in urine, saliva, tears or faeces. There might be a great future for a stable infectious agent that was transferred effectively by coins and bank-notes.

The increasing survival of susceptible individuals and the emergence of antibiotic resistant bacteria will, no doubt, still give serious problems in hospitals, but this is unlikely to breed new infectious agents with a significant impact on mankind.

Whatever else happens, infectious microorganisms will continue to evolve, exploiting weaknesses in defence both in the individual and in the community. New infectious agents can always arise from those already infecting man. Apart from this there have been two major origins for infectious diseases (Table II). First the infectious cycles in wild animals (zoonoses). Many of these infections have been particularly severe in the human host. It seems likely that this source will slowly dry up as man more thoroughly colonizes and develops the surface of the earth. The habitats supporting these infectious cycles will be eroded and ultimately destroyed so that the zoonoses disappear. But before this happens there is ample time for the emergence of new and virulent infectious agents. The example of Lassa fever shows how they could arise, because a relatively small change in pathogenesis could have made this infection into a major human pandemic (see Fig. 1). Psittacosis could cause explosive outbreaks of respiratory disease if it spread readily from person to person like measles. Rabies virus might do a good deal of damage if it caused a persistent subclinical infection in certain individuals and spread with efficiency via saliva.

The second major source of new infectious diseases has been from the animals domesticated or otherwise associated with man. Will they continue to pose a threat to human health? Man's tenacious murine companions (rats and mice) are not going to be easy to eliminate, and meanwhile they remain potential sources of new human diseases. London for instance, still has millions of rats, now banished from ordinary dwelling places to the warehouses, docks and sewers. Important changes can be foreseen in the case of the other human associates. Pets and domestic animals still present a microbiological threat to human health in so far as novel human pathogens could arise from the great variety of infectious agents carried and still evolving in these animals. On the other hand the infectious diseases of domestic animals will be better controlled, and intensive husbandry will remove them more and more from intimate contact with man. And although people will probably always have pets, vaccines and other practices will improve their cleanliness, at least from a microbiological point of view.

The best safeguard against the fourth rider of the apocalypse in the form of a devastating new infectious disease is increased understanding and constant vigilance on the part of microbiologists, physicians and veterinarians. Since the world is now one place for infectious diseases, international co-operation under the benevolent auspices of the WHO will be essential.

References

Benveniste, R. E. and Todaro, G. J. (1976). Evolution of type C viral genes: evidence for an Asian origin of man. *Nature, Lond.* **261**, 101–108.

Finland, M. (1979). Emergence of antibiotic resistance in hospitals 1935–1975. *Rev. infect. Dis.* **1**, 4–21.

Hackett, C. J. (1963). On the origin of the human treponematoses. *Bull. Wld Hlth Org.* **29**, 7–41.

Honess, R. W. and Watson, D. H. (1977). Unity and diversity in the herpesviruses. *J. gen. Virol.* **37**, 15–37.

Montague, A. (1972). "Touching". Harper and Row, New York.

Nahmias, A. J. (1974). The evolution (evovirology) of herpesviruses. *In* "Viruses, Evolution and Cancer" (I. Kurstak and K. Marararosch, Eds), 605–624. Academic Press, New York and London.

Nahmias, A. J. and Reanney, D. C. (1977). The evolution of viruses. *A. Rev. ecol. Systematics*, **8**, 29–49.

Sloan, A. W. (1971). The sweating sickness in England. *S. Afr. med. J.* **45**, 473–475.

Soeda, E. *et al.* (1980) Host-dependent evolution of three papovaviruses. *Nature* **285**, 165.

Part III

Some Patterns of Health Care

Introduction

The emphasis in this section changes. It is concerned with man's response to disease and methods of dealing with disease, rather than with disease itself. The various chapters consider societies and types of society and their methods of meeting changing health problems.

In the first chapter of this section Professor Kamien describes the impact of advancing Western technosociety upon the Australian Aboriginals' hunter-gathering society. It is a recent enactment of the inevitable tragedy described by Dr McNeill in Chapter 2. Neither of these authors, however, considers the possible role of genetic factors in these circumstances. The small physical differences between Aborigines of different localities are surprising since one would expect more diversity to have resulted from the genetic changes which occur in small populations with their correspondingly small gene pools.

Chapters 16 and 18, by Dr and Mrs Underwood and Dr Radford respectively, continue this theme, and again emphasize the roles of understanding and cultural differences in taking health care from one place to another. The diversity of indigenous African culture makes the contribution of Dr Ofosu-Amaah (Chapter 17) more difficult to summarize, but the same problems are apparent: the relations between disease, migration, technology and cultural interaction and conflict.

The last two chapters in Part III, by Dr Ladnyi and Dr Hordern move the discussion from the developing to the more developed societies, describing patterns for the provision of health care which vary from the completely bureaucratic system of the USSR to the mixed systems of Australia and the USA.

The conclusions which emerge from this section are surprising. There is among professionals a general dissatisfaction with health care. Sometimes this derives from unfortunate but well-meaning attempts to impose methods and goals of health care developed in one country upon the people of a different culture and country, or to provide "curative" medicine where the needs are for preventive medicine, health education and population control. In some cases the results of such attempts have ultimately been "counter-productive". Examples of this were cited in the previous section.

Problems have also arisen from political and bureaucratic failure to realize that provision of health care is open-ended, and not subject to traditional supply-and-demand economics. This is most clearly seen in the National Health Service of the United Kingdom. Cost is becoming progressively more important in systems of health care, and may ultimately become the limiting factor.

The lesson is that provision of health care is never easy and may even be dangerous: each advance or change brings new problems, often harder to solve than the ones they replace.

15

The Aboriginal Australian Experience

Max Kamien

Department of Community Practice, University of Western Australia, Perth, Australia

---

"When the white man came he sort of mucked things up." (The words of Mr George McDermott, a full-blood Aboriginal of the Wanggumara tribe, shortly before he died in 1972 at the age of 88 years.)

I. Historical Factors

A. Origins

Although Aborigines have lived in Australia for at least 40 000 years little is known about their history before their relatively recent contact with whites just over 200 years ago. It is thought that the Aborigines originated in Java and reached Australia by raft or canoes made from hollowed logs. This was then possible because the sea level was low and the greatest distance between land masses was only about 100 km (Calaby, 1976).

Although some early Aboriginal skulls exhibit a high frequency of the traits of primitive man (*Homo erectus*), anatomists and paleontologists who have studied them currently conclude that the Australian Aborigine is a genuine branch of modern man (*Homo sapiens*). He is generally classified as an Australoid. Other such groups are found in Malaysia, Ceylon and southern India (Elkin, 1964; MacIntosh and Larnach, 1976).

B. State of Health

The health of Aborigines before contact with whites is a matter of conjecture. It is pieced together from the descriptions of the early white explorers and more recently by photographs taken of Aborigines who had experienced little white contact (Basedow, 1915). Nearly all these explorers regarded the Aborigines as fine athletic specimens. This description holds true for Aborigines in the coastal areas as well as for those in the Australian hinterland. Even the ex-buccaneer William Dampier, who wrote that the Aborigines were "the miserablest people in the world", quickly recovered from his undoubted culture shock and observed that those same Aborigines were "tall, strait-bodied and thin. . . ." (Dampier, 1729).

This apparent good health could well have arisen by a process of natural selection which weeded out the weak and deformed. There is little doubt that the nomadic life was physically difficult, especially in inland areas which were subject to extremes of climate. There would have been no place for those who could not keep up or play their part in the daily quest for sustenance. At the same time the nomadic life carried out in small groups of people would have contributed to their good health by discouraging the evolution of communicable disease.

There is still speculation about which diseases, if any, were endemic in Australia before Asian or European contact. In 1837 George Grey observed that the Aborigines on the MacDonald range in the north of Western Australia, kept their eyes half closed and he assumed that this was to protect them against flies which by his description were as numerous then as they are now (Grey, 1841). It is probable that these Aborigines were suffering from trachoma. This eye disease could have been introduced by contact with Macassan trepang fisherman, as suggested by Dame Ida Mann (1957), or it could equally have been endemic in Aborigines for many thousands of years (Abbie, 1969). The anthropologist Dr Isabel White (1977) points out that in the western desert the Pitjantjatjara words for old and for blind are used interchangeably. Because of this she tends to favour the view that trachoma has been endemic in Aborigines for a very long time.

A similar dilemma exists about the treponemal disease of yaws, which was a major public health hazard in Aborigines until about 30 years ago. This has been vividly described by Hackett (1936), who also found yaws-like lesions ("irkinjta") in old Aboriginal bones in both southern and eastern Australia. It is hoped that further evidence about the antiquity of yaws will come from current paleopathological studies. Malaria and leprosy were undoubtedly introduced into Australia in the last 400 years through Macassan fishermen and at the turn of this century by infected Chinese and Pacific islanders who were brought to Australia to work on railway construction in the Northern Territory and in the sugar cane fields of Queensland (Cook, 1927).

Whatever the true prevalence of these diseases, it still appears likely that the Aborigines had reached a state of ecological equilibrium with their environment which not only provided them with a framework for a satisfying human existence but also kept them in a state of good health. In this regard their collective health in the late eighteenth century was almost certainly better than that of the English, whose occupation of Australia led to the Aborigines' rapid decline.

C. Contact

The early demise of the Aborigines resulted from disease, dispossession of land with resulting famine and to a lesser extent from massacre and the breakdown of their cultural support systems. The Aboriginal population fell from an estimated 300 000 in 1788 to 67 000 in 1933. This latter figure also includes part-Aborigines (Radcliffe-Brown, 1930; Population and Australia, 1975). Since this chapter must be necessarily short, I shall illustrate my theme by reference to the area of western New South Wales (Fig. 1) in which I have done most of my field work.

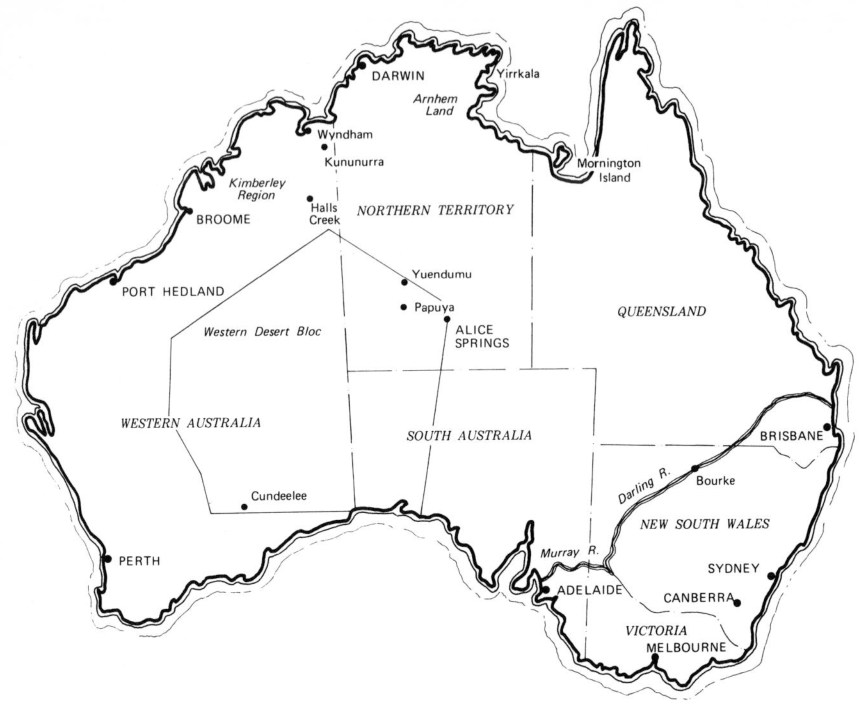

Fig. 1. Map of Australia.

1 Smallpox

In 1829 Captain Charles Sturt was the first recorded white man to have come into contact with the Ngjamba tribe who lived around what is now the town of Bourke. He noted that many of the Aborigines were pock-marked, and he was able to elicit that a "violent cutaneous disease had raged through the tribe and killed great numbers of them" (Sturt, 1833a). Six years later this observation was confirmed by Thomas Mitchell the then Surveyor-General of New South Wales who was of the opinion that he was seeing the remnants of a depopulated tribe (Mitchell, 1839). An epidemic of smallpox in both whites and Aborigines did occur in the first year of the Port Jackson settlement in 1789 and by 1790 Governor Phillip noted that about half of the Aboriginal population around Port Jackson had died from smallpox (Cumpston 1914; Bridges, 1970; Gandevia, 1974). It is possible that smallpox was carried by Aborigines fleeing from the disease and by intertribal contact such as at the large clan gatherings which occurred on ceremonial occasions. The real point at issue is that the white man's influence preceded his physical advance along the frontier of settlement. In some areas the major devastation to Aboriginal society had occurred years before they first came into contact with what they probably regarded as some malevolent ghostly white ancestral figures.

2 Other Contagions

Other infectious diseases also played their part in the decline of the Aborigines. On his second trip up the Darling River, Sturt recorded that "syphilis raged amongst them with fearful violence; many had lost their noses and all the glandular parts were considerably affected" (Sturt 1833b). This description is closer to that of yaws than of syphilis but again there can be no certainty of how a totally non-immune population would have responded to a newly introduced disease.

Settlements and missions had the effect of bringing Aborigines into close proximity with each other and with whites. This favoured the spread of those diseases which are contracted by inhaling infected droplets, breathed, coughed or sneezed by those with an active infection. By the late nineteenth century, tuberculosis had become a major cause of disease and death and in some settlements it accounted for up to 28% of all deaths (Moodie, 1973). Influenza epidemics are recorded in whites as early as 1837 and it is a reasonable assumption that Aborigines were also afflicted. The pandemic of Spanish influenza in 1919 raged through settlements in central and northern Australia and caused many deaths (Urry, 1979).

The lessons which could have been learned by an examination of the public health aspects of settlement were lost on or ignored by the administrators of Aborigines. The immediate effect of forming a new settlement was the spread of respiratory infections with a resulting high death rate. This was as true for part-Aborigines from the far west of New South Wales who were settled in a "mission" in 1936 as it was for the nomadic Pintubi tribe who were moved to the central Australian government station of Papunya in 1965 (Kamien, 1978; MacFarlane 1978).

3 Massacre

Although Aborigines were skilful hunters, up to 70% of their diet was obtained by gathering seeds and trapping small marsupials. The cattle and sheep of the white settlers ate and trampled the vegetation and the introduced rabbit competed more than successfully for food with the smaller marsupials (Latz and Griffin, 1978; Frith, 1978). Kangaroos and emus were regarded by the white settlers as vermin and many were destroyed. The traditional food sources of the Aborigines rapidly diminished. Aborigines sampled the new food sources and found them satisfying. This competition for land and the subsistence it offered resulted in bloody conflict. The Aborigines killed a few whites and the whites retaliated. Sometimes this was by sporadic killing but often it was by mass murder. Poisoned flour, punitive expeditions and wholesale shootings occurred (Rowley, 1970). In 1870 in the Darling River area alone, some 400 Aborigines young and old were rounded up and systematically shot in retaliation for killing cattle (Kamien, 1978).

The end result of this disease, dispossession and massacre was the almost total decimation of the Aboriginal population in the Bourke area. In 1845 there were about 3000, by 1863 this had fallen to 1000 and by 1884 there were only 25 men, 35 women, 10 boys and 10 girls left. "There had been a decrease to an extent scarcely short of annihilation (the majority of the remnant being decrepit in the extreme), owing in part to the diseases that accompanied the white man; in part to whatever must be the result of putting a piece of new garment upon an old" (Teulon, 1886).

It is little wonder that the new occupiers of the Australian continent thought it inevitable that the Australian Aborigine would soon cease to exist. In the case of Tasmania they were right. Truganinni, the last Tasmanian Aborigine, died in 1876, thus giving to white Australia the dubious distinction of having completed the first and only utter genocide of a racial group.

4 Settlements

The first half of the twentieth century saw the Aborigines living in an uneasy equilibrium with a dominant white society. Those who were tribal or semitribal were gradually being settled in Church-run missions or State government settlements. This was sometimes for humanitarian reasons such as protection from the white man or because of failing food supplies resulting from drought. More often it was for administrative expediency and because it was assumed that assimilation would occur more easily in Aboriginal towns.

A natural development of living on settlements with poor, overcrowded accommodation and a lack of facilities for adequate hygiene was the continuation of infectious disease. Although Aborigines had by now developed some immunity to the more common exanthems such as chickenpox, other infectious diseases still played a part in their high rates of mortality and morbidity. Tuberculosis was common and epidemics of measles predisposed young Aboriginal children to pneumonia and gastroenteritis which were and still are the main reasons for the high rate of infant mortality (Moodie, 1973).

II. Social Disintegration

The occupation of the Australian continent by the white man did more to the Aborigines than bringing new diseases and reducing their food supply. The whites dominated the Aborigines, and not understanding their beliefs and their culture, disparaged their way of life. Many missions and government settlements developed a dormitory system in which children were removed from their parents and held virtually as prisoners in a boarding school situation. The rationale behind this was to separate the children from their parents' "noxious" culture and inculcate into them some white skills and apparent virtues. Another common purpose was to postpone sexual activity and so limit the number of early pregnancies in Aboriginal teenage girls. Government settlements were generally decrepit and were ruled over by managers the majority of whom were nothing less than scoundrels and tyrants (Hiatt, 1965). In many cases the manager or his wife were also responsible for the children's education. Their lack of ability and conscientiousness in this field was a major contributing factor to the high rate of illiteracy exhibited by their former pupils. The reader who wishes to obtain an Aboriginal view of life on a government settlement need go no further than to read the book "The Two Worlds of Jimmy Barker" (Mathews, 1977). However, the settlement and mission system was not wholly bad and in many areas it contributed to the survival of the Aborigines by providing food, water and more recently medical attention. At the same time it was a major factor in institutionalizing the Aborigine.

A. Institutionalization

The general effect of institutionalizing people is that they lose their desire and ability to be self-sufficient. They withdraw into a state of apathy expressed through dependent behaviour with an accompanying loss of initiative. The only form of protest that is safe for them is passive resistance, often disguised to appear as incompetence or stupidity.

Many of these settlements were and are overcrowded. Aborigines were never asked where and with whom they should settle, with the consequence that some settlements comprise the remnants of tribes who were traditional enemies. These two conditions lead to disputes, fighting and occasionally to riots.

In addition to this institutionalization and the insecurity and suspiciousness engendered by living alongside a different tribal group, the

Aborigines were excluded from any real contact with whites. They were actively discouraged from travelling into a city and in many areas had to get a police permit to do so. The end result of this institutionalization, social disparagement and sociocultural exclusion was to help complete the disintegration of their society with its accompanying confusion in their normal patterns of behaviour. Such a society does not perceive of itself as having mental comfort.

Three surveys of Aborigines have been conducted using a modified Cornell Medical Inventory Health Questionnaire. One was performed in the vernacular in a tribal community on Mornington island, the other in a fringe-dwelling part-Aboriginal population and the third in urban Aborigines in Sydney. All showed high levels of complaints with regard to chest pains, headaches, fatigue and the symptoms of anxiety and depression. Anger, resentment and irritability rated very highly, being found in just over half of each of these communities (Lickiss, 1971; Cawte, 1972; Kamien, 1978).

There are similar studies of disintegrated communities in the world such as the Eskimo and the American Indians. Like the Australian Aborigine, their members too exhibit high levels of stress which they try to relieve by such maladaptive responses as getting drunk and fighting.

B. Alcohol

Pre-contact Aboriginal society was one of the few which did not brew an alcoholic beverage. Aborigines were first introduced to alcohol by some of the more rowdy elements of Port Jackson, who made an entertainment out of getting Aborigines drunk and watching them demean themselves. This "pastime" was also carried on in other areas of settlement where Aborigines learned to copy the excessive white drinking patterns which were common in the nineteenth century and which are still common in many parts of rural Australia.

The end result is that alcohol is one of the major social and health problems facing the Aborigines and in many areas of Australia it is the main and most immediate threat to their survival. It disrupts their family life and interferes with the care of their children. It is a principal factor in precipitating minor crime and it is a leading cause of early death through physical disease and accidents. The degree to which this occurs is illustrated by my own medical experience in September 1971, when I stitched lacerations or set the broken bones of 25% of the adult male Aboriginal population of Bourke. The Bourke Aborigines spent about a quarter of their total weekly income on alcohol. They were also obliged to pay a sizeable amount in fines incurred as the result of disturbing the peace or some other petty misdemeanor committed while drunk. This deficit in their already meagre income made the poor that much poorer and interfered with their ability to purchase necessary food and medicine.

C. Diet

I have already mentioned that many of the missions and settlements provided food and water which helped the Aborigines to survive. Transport to these outlying settlements was difficult and the most practical compact and non-perishable foodstuffs were those which usually comprised flour, sugar, jam, tea and canned meat. Aborigines were attracted to such a diet because it was sweet and more easily and regularly obtainable than foraging for grain and small animals or hunting for meat. The end result is that Australian Aborigines now have one of the most unhealthy diets currently known to man. Nutritional surveys show that after excluding alcohol, flour and bread provide up to 56% of their calories and 60% of their protein (Kamien *et al.*, 1974; Hitchcock and Gracey, 1975). Other empty calories come from the several spoonfuls of sugar that are added to the tea which is drunk frequently throughout the day with the average sugar consumption for an adult lying between 0·5 and 1 kg per week (White, 1977). Some Aboriginal groups exceed this and dentist Tasman Brown (1976) recorded that in 1972 the sugar consumption for the 950 men, women and children in the central Australian settlement of Yuendumu was 6400 lb (2909 kg) per month.

The recent outstation movement of some Aborigines leaving settlements and going back to their tribal areas has not had that much effect on their high carbohydrate intake. Geneticist Mr Neville White noted that during a 12-day period in 1977 one outstation in eastern Arnhem Land consumed 72 kg white flour, 40 kg self-raising flour, 96 kg white sugar and 4·5 kg tea. The "maximum number of people at the camp at any one time was 31 but most often it was about half that number" (White 1978).

It became obvious to welfare officials that the diet of settlement Aborigines was poor, especially for children, pregnant women and lactating mothers. Their answer to this was to set up a system of communal feeding in which hygienically prepared and served meals were made available to Aborigines at little or no cost. Although this communal feeding was unpopular with many Aborigines, it was often the only food available especially since prior to 1969 Aborigines did not receive all their wages in cash. One adverse effect of communal feeding was to lessen a mother's responsibility for the economic management of food and for the feeding of her children. More subtle, but equally damaging, was the disparaging way in which some white nursing sisters regarded the methods used by Aboriginal mothers to feed their children. These nursing sisters discouraged Aboriginal mothers from supplementing their breast milk with high protein and fat-containing native food such as witchetty grubs (grubs of moths of the family Cossidae) and encouraged them to wean their children onto the less nutritious bottled and tinned commercial baby food.

The loss of land to graziers or the geographical relocation in settlements led to a marked reduction in hunting and in gathering food. This new sedentary existence coupled with a highly refined flour and sugar diet has also changed the pattern of disease in present-day Aboriginal adults.

Various surveys have shown the prevalence of diabetes to lie between 10 and 20% in those over 20 years of age (Wise *et al.*, 1970; Finlay-Jones and McComish, 1972; Bastian, 1979). The reason postulated for this high rate of diabetes is that possession of the diabetic gene would have been an advantage to a hunting people whose dietary pattern was that of feast and famine. When food was plentiful there would be an increased tendency to deposit fat and when food was scarce the diabetic tendency would have a protective effect in warding off hunger. The process of acculturation with its resultant change in eating habits, reduced physical exercise and an accompanying high birth rate, would tend to produce symptomatic diabetes in those people who possessed this genetic make up (Neel *et al.*, 1965).

This tendency to diabetes is also reflected in the high serum levels of cholesterol and triglycerides found in Aborigines. Another coronary risk factor becoming more common in Aborigines is hypertension. In 1958, Casley-Smith found normal blood pressures and low cholesterol levels in Aborigines still living a tribal life in the central desert (Casley-Smith, 1959). The ready availability of salt, the increasing obesity associated with a high carbohydrate diet and a sedentary life have resulted in high rates of hypertension (Wise *et al.*, 1970; Kamien 1976; Bastian, 1979).

As yet there is little documented evidence about the incidence of ischaemic heart disease in Aborigines. However, a recent study of full-blood tribal Aborigines in the west Kimberley region of Western Australia, found frank ischaemic changes in the electrocardiographs of 7% of the population and probable coronary heart disease in 7% of the men and 11% of the women (Bastian, 1979). My impression from discussions with doctors who work with Aborigines is that coronary heart disease is a leading cause of premature death in Aborigines. My own experience was that between 1967 and 1971 myocardial infarction accounted for 14 out of the 23 adult deaths in Bourke Aborigines. This had a marked effect on that community especially since nearly all those who died were under the age of 50 years.

Another possible effect of the change to a refined diet is an earlier age of menarche in Aboriginal women. In the hunter-gatherer state, Aboriginal women were reported as having their first babies about the age of 18 years and the Kung and Kalahari bushmen of Botswana, who are still hunter-gatherers, have a late age of menarche of about 15 years (Meggitt, 1965; Truswell, 1977) (see also Black, this volume). This is alleged to be a result of their low body fat. There is some evidence that a change to a high carbohydrate diet results in high insulin levels with a corresponding hypoglycaemia which in turn stimulates the release of growth hormone from the anterior pituitary (Brown, 1976). Aboriginal women currently have a high birth rate, and an early menarche contributes to early, closely spaced and often unwanted pregnancies which in their turn play a part in the despondency and chronic weariness of so many Aboriginal women.

III. Health Care

A. Cultural Chasm

Providing medical and nursing care to Aborigines has been a planned attempt at improving their health. There can be little doubt that in most settlement areas immunization and public health measures have reduced or controlled such diseases as tuberculosis, poliomyelitis and measles. An even greater effort has gone into providing curative services for all Aborigines. Even the most remote communities have access to Flying Doctor Services which can give advice and treatment or, if necessary, arrange emergency evacuation to a larger medical centre. However, medical services in themselves are unlikely to affect the incidence of those diseases due to respiratory and gastrointestinal infections which are relatively resistant to medical technology. Nevertheless the early application of modern medicine can usually save lives and reduce the severity of an individual episode of illness. It is unfortunate and sometimes tragic that this type of medicine is often applied so late. Too many Australian doctors and nurses regard this late presentation of illness as a manifestation of Aboriginal fecklessness. Few consider that their judgemental attitudes and actions could have contributed to an Aborigine postponing for as long as possible, a medical consultation.

Australian medical students stem overwhelmingly from middle and upper middle-class backgrounds. They receive a medical education which quite correctly concentrates on the physical pathology of illness. Unfortunately this is usually at the expense of any great degree of understanding about the social and psychopathology of people whose life-style differs from that of the middle-class white Australian.

It is my view that more Aborigines die as the result of this ethnocentric sociomedical blindness than do so because of a failure to diagnose an illness or to apply to it the correct medical treatment. This assertion is of course a simplification of a very complex issue. There are many other reasons why an Aborigine may postpone seeking Western medical attention. One such reason is that he may choose to be treated by an Aboriginal healer. These charismatic figures have been extensively studied by anthropologists and some doctors. Their abilities, especially in the fields of social and psychological illness are considerable, and their status in Aboriginal communities is high (Cawte, 1974; Elkin, 1977). Until recently their role was largely ignored by Western medical practitioners and administrators. In the few instances where they were employed by a health authority or a hospital they have been used as ward orderlies or as general roustabouts. This is analogous to employing an eminent psychoanalyst from a European country to clean the toilets of an Australian country hospital.

The ethnocentricity of the bulk of Australian medical graduates does not seem to be changing from that which I have described. New doctors and nurses go unprepared to country areas where, whether they like it or not, much of their work will be with Aborigines. Most of them know nothing of the local history of these people and nothing of their medical beliefs and practices. They make the same stupid, crosscultural mistakes and the same social blunders as the equally ignorant doctors and nurses who preceded them. The more empathic learn from their errors and gradually make up the ground lost by their earlier actions. The less sensitive are refractory to social or to cultural learning. They grow more judgemental and impatient in their dealings with Aborigines who in their turn, do everything possible to avoid contact with such a doctor or nurse. It is not medical technology that is such a misfit in the health care of Aborigines as it is that so many white health professionals by training and personality are unfitted for working with Aborigines. They talk and act as if they are programmed for failure almost before they have begun.

It is naive to assert that a suitable tertiary educational training will effectively change a student's attitudes. It is, however, an indictment of our educational system that our future doctors or nurses rarely get the opportunity to discover what their racial attitudes really are and how these are likely to influence the quality of the medical care that they will provide when they have graduated.

The inception of Aboriginal Medical Services in some eleven urban centres in all states of Australia, except Tasmania, is a reflection of the felt needs of Aborigines. They have not felt welcome or psychologically safe in the medical services of the majority white culture. Not infrequently they will travel several hundred kilometres just to have their children treated by what they recognize as a sympathetic doctor employed by an Aboriginal Medical Service. It is hoped that the confidence they gain through dealing with these services will extend to their contacts with other non-Aboriginal run medical services. Until Aborigines become demanding consumers of medical care, it is unlikely that the white providers of that medical care will learn to make it fit the real and the felt health needs of the Aborigines.

B. Bureaucratic Responsibility

At the level of the individual a cultural chasm exists between most of the white providers of health care and the Aboriginal recipients. This makes the Aborigines reticent to use white medical services. In the urbanized or fringe-dwelling situation this contributes to low immunization rates and on occasion to a more severe degree of illness than would have occurred had treatment been applied earlier in the illness episode.

At the community level the real health needs of Aborigines often get lost in white bureaucracy. The administrative structures of white society are largely vertical. The needs of an Aboriginal community (or any community for that matter) are usually horizontal. Take, for example, a community in which the water has been shown to have an unacceptably high bacterial count, one-third of the taps do not function and for the remainder the water pressure is so low that only a trickle of water can be obtained. (For a variety of such examples see the report from the House of Representatives Standing Committee on Aboriginal Affairs, 1979.) The Health Department will realize that this is a potential health hazard. However, they are not funded to intervene in water supplies. This is a matter for the Department of Supply. Several letters will be exchanged and in all likelihood nothing will happen. The community may complain and their objections may be noted in reports of the House of Representatives Standing Committee on Aboriginal

Affairs, as well as in other government reports. Still nothing may occur (e.g. compare reports of the 1974 and 1979 House of Representatives Standing Committees on Aboriginal Affairs about the Water and Sewage Supply of Yirrkala). The same type of buck-passing occurs with the division of responsibility for Aboriginal reserves which may occur between state, federal and local government. A local government authority may claim that they have no responsibility for Aborigines on reserves because they are not ratepayers and because the reserve is the responsibility of a State or Federal governmental authority. Here again Aboriginal requests may be lost in the ample grey areas between the vertical administrative structures. Unhappily, this mode of thinking can still occur when Aborigines are given control of such an organization.

I recently visited the reserve in Bourke in which Aboriginal people did not consider they were receiving an equitable piece of the housing action that was occurring in the town. The Aboriginal directors of the housing co-operative explained that this was because the reserve now belonged to the New South Wales Aboriginal Lands Trust and this organization had not given the housing co-operative funds with which to upgrade the facilities on the reserve.

These problems will only be solved when Aboriginal groups are given reasonable financial resources together with real power to decide upon and to implement their priorities. The amount of money allocated to each community may not necessarily exceed that currently spent by Government Departments such as Health, Education, Supply and Welfare. The crucial factor in putting this money to proper use will be that Aboriginal leaders will be responsible to their own people. Similarly any white people employed to help the Aborigines will be employed by that Aboriginal community and so will be responsible to them rather than to the Government Department which now employs them.

IV. Conclusions

Aborigines have lived in Australia for a long time. They had reached a stage of spiritual and ecological equilibrium with the often harsh Australian landscape and climate. This was shattered by white settlement with its accompanying infectious diseases, by dispossession from their land to which they had close spiritual and economic ties, by miscegenation and by the general social disintegration which occurred in the remnant of a dispirited and disparaged people. This disintegration has not been improved by short-sighted governmental policies and even when these policies have become more altruistic, the ponderous bureaucratic structures of white society have generally produced a less desirable result than was intended. Medical services have often been at variance to the true needs of Aborigines with the accent on curative medicine and evacuation to large hospitals, and medical and nursing personnel have equally often taken the same ethnocentrically narrow view of Aborigines so commonly found amongst less educated white Australians.

In the last eight years there has been a resurgence of pride amongst Aboriginal people. Some are learning to find their way through the maze of the Australian legal and political system and are pressing for a greater recognition of their depressed situation and for ways to alleviate it. For tribal Aborigines in the Northern Territory and South Australia this may be helped by the recent achievement of land rights. For part-Aborigines living on the fringe of country towns or large cities, the answers are less obvious. They are a self-propagating subculture who occupy the lowest rung on the social ladder of Australia. Their health has improved a lot over the last decade. Nevertheless their current vital health statistics are only on a par with that of whites who lived in New South Wales between 1900 and 1910 (Kamien, 1978).

White Australians have always been xenophobic and never more so than to the original inhabitants of this continent. It is going to take strong and concerned political leadership to set the scene for Aboriginal development and then to brave the forces of reaction that always see help to Aborigines as discrimination against whites. No amount of help from altruistic whites can make up for this lack of political will. Aborigines have a birth rate more than twice that of white Australians. The descendants of the oldest known, continuous living culture will not die out. Their future situation will act as a reflection and as a form of quality control on the moral health of the rest of Australia.

References

Abbie, A. A. (1969). "The Original Australians", 86–87. Reed, Sydney.

Basedow, H. (1915). *In* "Proceedings of the Royal Geographical Society of Australasia: South Australian Branch", Vol. 15, 57–242. Thomas, Adelaide.

Bastian, P. (1979). *Aust. N.Z. J. Med.* **9**, 284–292.

Bridges, B. (1970). *Med. J. Aust.* **2**, 879–883.

Brown, T. (1976). *In* "The Origin of the Australians" (R. L. Kirk and A. G. Thorne, Eds), 195–209. Australian Institute of Aboriginal Studies, Canberra.

Calaby, J. H. (1976). *In* "The Origin of the Australians" (R. L. Kirk and A. G. Thorne, Eds), 23–28. Australian Institute of Aboriginal Studies, Canberra.
Casley-Smith, J. R. (1959). *Med. J. Aust.* **1**, 627–633.
Cawte, J. E. (1972). "Cruel, Poor and Brutal Nations". Univ. Press of Hawaii, Honolulu.
Cawte, J. E. (1974). "Medicine is the Law". Rigby, Adelaide and Sydney.
Cook, C. (1927). "The Epidemiology of Leprosy in Australia". Commonwealth Department of Health. Service Publication No. 38, Government Printer, Canberra.
Cumpston, J. H. L. (1914). "The History of Smallpox in Australia 1788–1908". Quarantine Service Publication, No. 3. Government Printer, Melbourne.
Dampier, W. (1729). "A Collection of Voyages", Vol. 1, 463. Knapton, London.
Elkin, A. P. (1964). "The Australian Aborigines: How to Understand Them". Angus and Robertson, Sydney.
Elkin, A. P. (1977). "Aboriginal Men of High Degree". Univ. Queensland Press, Brisbane.
Finlay-Jones, R. A. and McComish, M. J. (1972). *Med. J. Aust.* **2**, 135–137.
Frith, H. J. (1978). *In* "The Nutrition of Aborigines in Relation to the Ecosystem of Central Australia" (B. S. Hetzel and H. J. Frith, Eds), 87–93. Commonwealth Scientific and Industrial Research Organization, Melbourne.
Gandevia, B. (1974). *Aust. N.Z. J. Med.* **4**, 111–125.
Grey, G. (1841). "Expeditions in Western Australia 1837–1839". Australiana Facsimile Editions (1964), No. 8. Libraries Board of South Australia, Adelaide.
Hackett, C. J. (1936). *Med. J. Aust.* **1**, 733–744.
Hiatt, L. R. (1965). *In* "Australian Society" (A. F. Davies and S. Encel, Eds), 274–295. Cheshire, Melbourne.
Hitchcock, N. E. and Gracey, M. (1975). *Med. J. Aust.* Special Supplement **2**, 12–16.
House of Representatives Standing Committee on Aboriginal Affairs (1974). "Present Conditions of Yirrkala People" 94. Australian Government Publishing Service, Canberra.
House of Representatives Standing Committee on Aboriginal Affairs (1979). "Aboriginal Health", 38–41. Australian Government Publishing Service, Canberra.
Kamien, M., Nobile, S., Cameron, P. and Rosevear, P. (1974). *Aust. N.Z. J. Med.* **4**, 126–137.
Kamien, M. (1976). *Med. J. Aust.* Special Supplement **1**, 38–44.
Kamien, M. (1978). "The Dark People of Bourke: A study of Planned Social Change". Australian Institute of Aboriginal Studies, Canberra.
Latz, P. K. and Griffin, G. F. (1978). *In* "The Nutrition of Aborigines in Relation to the Ecosystem of Central Australia" (B. S. Hetzel and H. J.

Frith, Eds), 77–85. Commonwealth Scientific and Industrial Research Organization, Melbourne.
Lickiss, N. (1971). *Oceania* **41**, 201–228.
MacFarlane, W. V. (1978). *In* "The Nutrition of Aborigines in Relation to the Ecosystem of Central Australia" (B. S. Hetzel and H. J. Frith, Eds), 49–62. Commonwealth Scientific and Industrial Research Organization, Melbourne.
MacIntosh, N. W. G. and Larnach, S. L. (1976). *In* "The Origin of the Australians" (R. L. Kirk and A. G. Thorne, Eds), 113–126. Australian Institute of Aboriginal Studies, Canberra.
Mann, I. (1957). *Bull. Wld Hlth Org.* **16**, 1165–1187.
Mathews, J. (1977). "The Two Worlds of Jimmy Barker". Australian Institute of Aboriginal Studies, Canberra.
Meggitt, M. J. (1965). "Desert People", 270–271. Univ. Chicago Press, Chicago.
Mitchell, T. L. (1839). "Three Expeditions into the Interior of Eastern Australia: with descriptions of the recently explored region of Australia felix, and of the present colony of New South Wales." Australian Facsimile Editions No. 18, 1965. Libraries Board of South Australia, Adelaide.
Moodie, P. M. (1973). "Aboriginal Health". Australian National Univ. Press, Canberra.
Neel, J. V., Fajans, S. S., Conn, J. W. and Davidson, R. T. (1965). *In* "Genetics and the Epidemiology of Chronic Diseases" (J. V. Neel, M. W. Shaw and W. J. Schull, Eds), 105–132. US Department of Health, Education and Welfare. Public Health Service Publication No. 1163, Washington, D.C.
Population and Australia: a demographic analysis and projection. First Report of the National Population Inquiry (1975). Vol. 2, 478. Government Printer, Canberra.
Radcliffe-Brown, A. R. (1930). *In* "Australia, Official Year Book No. 23, (1930)", 687–696. Australian Government Printer, Melbourne.
Rowley, C. D. (1970). "The Destruction of Aboriginal Society". Australian National Univ. Press, Canberra.
Sturt, C. (1833a). "Two Expeditions into the Interior of Southern Australia during the years 1828, 1829, 1830 and 1831", Vol. 1. Australiana Facsimile Edition No. 4. 1963. Public Library of South Australia, Adelaide.
Sturt, C. (1833b). "Two Expeditions into the Interior of Southern Australia during the years 1828, 1829, 1830 and 1831", Vol. 2. Australiana Facsimile Edition No. 4, 1963, 1–5. Public Library of South Australia, Adelaide.
Teulon, G. N. (1886). *In* "The Australian Race . . ." (E. M. Curr, Ed.), Vol. 11, 186–223. Government Printer, Melbourne.
Truswell, A. S. (1977). *In* "Health and Disease in Tribal Societies" (Ciba Foundation Symposium—new series 49), 213–221. Elsevier/Excerpta Medica/North Holland, Amsterdam.
Urry, J. (1979). *J. Aust. Studies.* **5**, 2–16.

White, I. M. (1977). *In* "Health and Disease in Tribal Societies" (Ciba Foundation Symposium—new series 49), 269–292. Elsevier/Excerpta Medica/North Holland, Amsterdam.

White, N. G. (1978). *In* "House of Representatives Standing Committee on Aboriginal Affairs (Reference: Aboriginal Health)", 2429. Official Hansard Report, Commonwealth Government Printer, Canberra.

Wise, P. H., Edwards, F. M., Thomas, D. W., Elliot, R. B., Hatcher, L. and Craig, R. (1970). *Med. J. Aust.* **2**, 1001–1006.

16

New Spells for Old: Expectations and Realities of Western Medicine in a Remote Tribal Society in Yemen, Arabia

Peter Underwood and Zdenka Underwood

Department of Community Practice, University of Western Australia, Perth Australia

---

There is a considerable difference between a good doctor and a bad doctor, but no difference between a good one and no doctor at all. Dalton

---

I. Yemen and Raymah—The Background

Between September 1975 and September 1977 the authors were part of a team which set up a Community Health Project in Raymah, a remote area within the Yemen Arab Republic (formerly North Yemen). Yemen is a small country on the south west tip of the Arabian peninsula (Fig. 1). As a consequence of its formidable geography (rugged mountains cut off on all sides by barriers of desert) and the legendary xenophobia of its rulers, Yemen's 6 million people, the inheritors of a unique culture extending back over several millenia, have lived out their lives untouched until recently by the changing passions of the outside world. Within this remote country the inhabitants of Raymah, a tangled massif rising to 3000 m and about 60 × 40 km in area, are some of Yemen's most isolated people. No roads penetrate the region, which is surrounded by desert on one side and precipitous wadi systems (valleys) on the others. The extreme ruggedness of the massif and the natural barriers of mountain, wadi and desert on all sides account for the immemorial isolation and independence of the region.

Isolation and inaccessibility, together with an exclusive dependence on agriculture, combine to provide Raymah with its special characteristics. The 150 000 inhabitants of Raymah are almost all poor peasants or landowners who live in the 1200 isolated villages and hamlets that dot the cliffs, terraces and high wadis of the massif (Fig. 2). Agriculture is the only industry in Raymah. It is an ancient system based largely on the intensive production of cereal crops, mainly sorghum, from the terraces nourished by the summer monsoons and carved from the mountains by hundreds of generations of farmers.

When we arrived in Raymah in 1975 most Raymis appeared to have had no contact with Westerners, with Western ideas, or Western technology. Their lives were governed by the rhythms of the seasons and the rules and customs of their dense and complex society.

This society has shown little change in its fundamental patterns over many centuries. In fact, there is a striking continuity between this society and the rich South Arabian civilizations which flourished before the time of Mohammed the Prophet, and even before Christ. According to Ronart and Ronart, there are direct geographical, linguistic and cultural links between at least one tribe living near Sana'a, the capital of Yemen, and the Mineans, a very early South Arabian civilization which existed from the eighteenth to the tenth century B.C. (Ronart and Ronart, 1966). In Raymah itself there is a proliferation of place names,

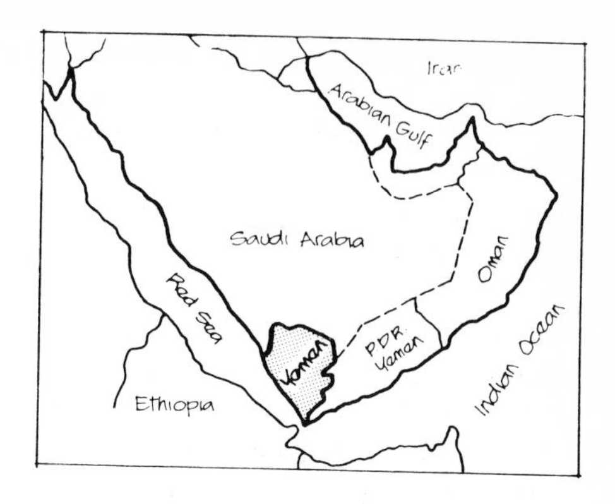

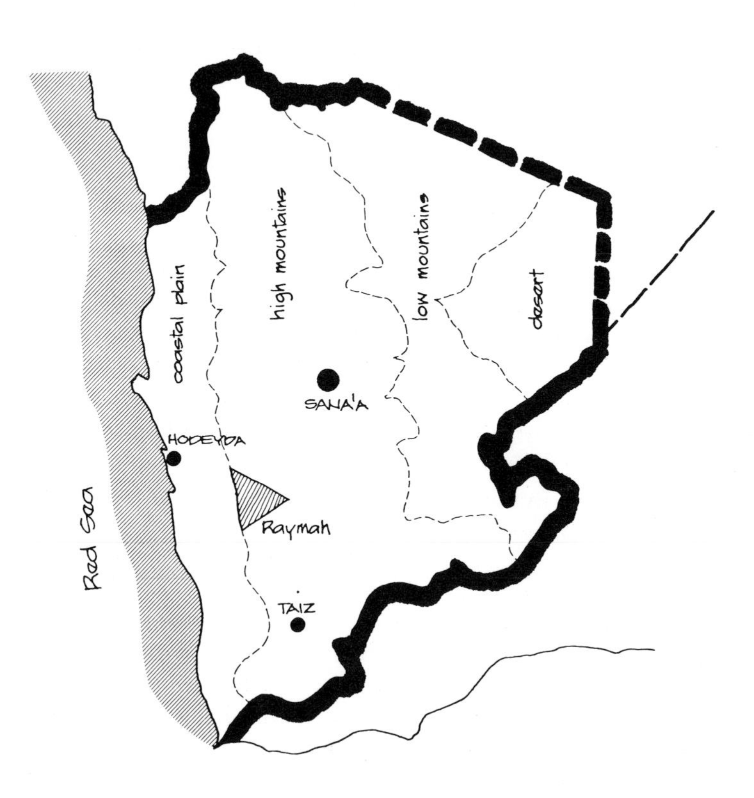

Fig. 1. Maps (Arabian Peninsula, Yemen Arab Republic).

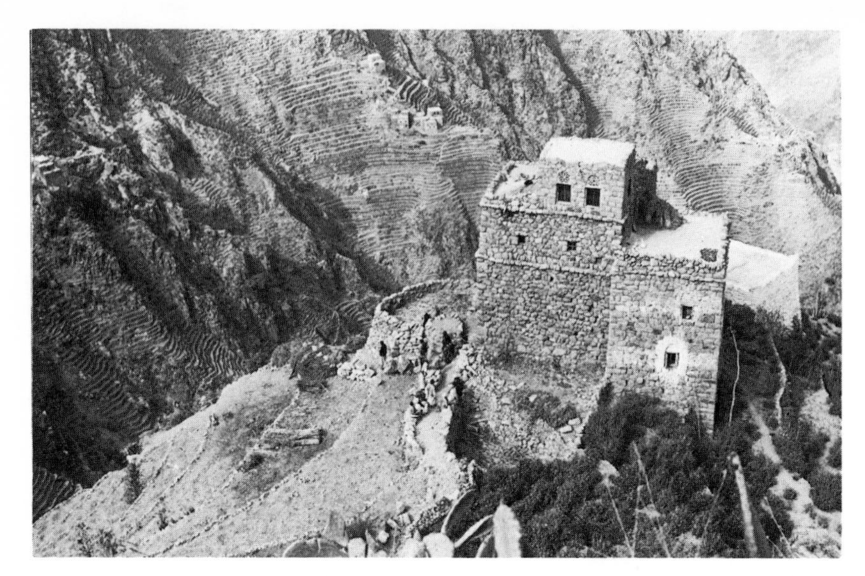

Fig. 2. An isolated hamlet in Raymah. The majority of Raymah's 150 000 people live in the 1200 villages that dot the cliffs, terraces and high wadis of the massif.

dams and cisterns dating from Himyaritic times (second to sixth century A.D.). While there have been numerous foreign invasions of Yemen, starting with the Romans in the first century B.C. and ending with the Turks in this century, none seem to have made a lasting mark on the basic rhythms of Yemeni life. For most of the twentieth century Yemen remained one of the world's most isolated and least-known countries. This lasted until 1970, when the country began to recover from the effects of its Civil War (1962–68). Then the new Republican Government declared that the isolationist policy of the Imams had formally ended and that trade and cultural relations were to be established with the outside world. Since that time Yemen has received massive aid from both the East and the West.

This brief outline of Yemen's history reveals why this country has remained so much more isolated than most Third World countries. The Yemenis are the inheritors of a remarkable culture going back at least 1000 years before the birth of Christ. During the past 2000 years dynasties have risen and fallen, but a deep continuity has been maintained. This rich and individual inheritance explains much of the character of the people, not in the least cowed or inferior as they face the modern world. It also accounts for the absence of the rudiments of an administrative or political infrastructure to handle the sudden, massive inflow of foreign aid, foreign money, foreign influence and foreign ideas.

What impact has the outside world had on Yemen in this short space of a few years, and what in particular has been its influence on illness and health? Outwardly Yemen still gives the appearance of a robust traditional society. However, the modern world has already made a more significant impact on the culture than any of the other numerous invasions of the past 2000 years, with the possible exception of the "invasion" of Islam. The influence of the modern world is clearly seen in the towns of Yemen, but is now noticeable in the tiniest hamlet in remote Raymah. In this chapter we outline some of the major effects of foreign influence, both on the country as a whole and on the village and the villager. We will concentrate particularly on the changing expectations and the changing realities within the field of health. In our opinion, Yemen and Raymah are particularly worthy of examination in this respect because of the unique combinations of ancient isolation and very recent change producing a convulsion in a society which remains fundamentally in the Middle Ages.

The "Statistical Year Book of the YAR, 1976" reveals the steady, indeed inexorable decline in Yemen's foreign trade balance over the past ten years. For most of its long history Yemen has been largely self-sufficient, but by 1974 imports outweighed exports by a factor of 15. The gap has steadily increased year by year since 1964. The trade deficit is made good by foreign aid (said to be largely from Saudi Arabia). Food makes up over half of the total imports. Thus it would seem that in this short period the immemorial independence of Yemen has already been so drastically altered by its fledgling contacts with the outside world that it is no longer minimally self-sufficient, even in such a basic requirement as food.

This change at the national level of housekeeping is mirrored in the domestic housekeeping of thousands of Yemeni families. At the level of the family, many of the men work abroad and send back their money to support the family who remain behind. Perhaps the single most profound change in Yemen's long history will turn out to be the growing efflux of men from the countryside to the towns of Yemen and to the towns and oilfields of Saudi Arabia and the Arabian Gulf.

According to Government sources, over a million of Yemen's 6 million people are estimated to live outside the country (Statistical Year Book, YAR, 1976). When we first arrived in Raymah, there was little evidence of this emigration, but by the time we left, two years later, the trickle had begun to turn into a torrent. In short, the country as a whole, and tens of thousands of families within it, balance the growing gulf between their expenditure and income with foreign money. According to legend, Imam Yayha (who ruled from 1904 to 1948) declared: "We would rather be poor and eat grass, than live under the foreign boot." His famous dictum now has a strangely prophetic ring.

The consequences of the efflux of men from the countryside on the fabric of the culture are not only economic. The terraces of Raymah, monuments to the skill and toil of a hundred generations of peasants, have a deceptively fragile grip on the near vertical slopes of the mountains. Without an abundance of labour the terrace walls crack open with the rains and soon the terraces and the soil they cosset, tear away down the wadi. Figure 3 reveals the loss of a whole mountain side of fertile soil in a space of six weeks. This occurred in a remote area of Raymah where most of the men were away working in Saudi, and so were unable to repair the terrace walls before the torrential rains split them open.

The traditional society with its basic life-style, beautifully and intricately adapted to a terrain and climate of extremes, is now faced with a different kind of threat to its survival. Against this new threat the ancient strengths of the culture seem to be of little avail. Economic independence has already been compromised, if paid for by a greater freedom of movement and a great influx of money. However, the cost may be the destruction of the traditional culture. Without abundant labour the terraces, which provide the basis of the agriculture on which the society depends cannot survive.

II. Changes in the Pattern of Family Life in Raymah

How then has the life of the individual family in Raymah changed as a result of the forces we have outlined? It is beyond the scope of this chapter to discuss the many profound changes at the level of the individual and the family which grow out of these economic and demographic changes. Beneath the obvious changes as a result of increased ready cash (usually swiftly channelled into a better house and the ubiquitous transistor radio), lie more subtle and more significant changes in the way the people live, eat and work. Before discussing the changing cultural patterns with respect to illness and health, it is necessary to analyse a few of the more general changes which are emerging within domestic life in Raymah.

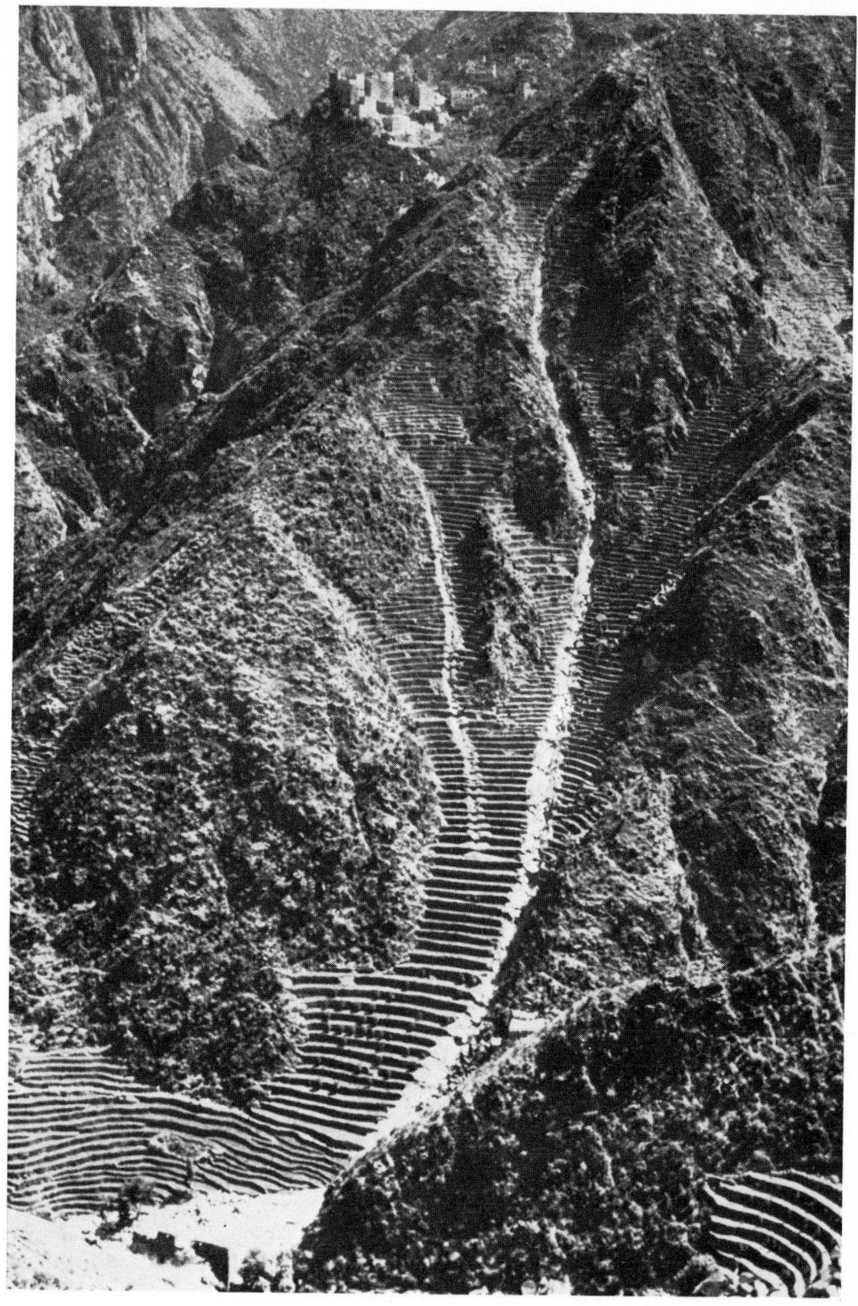

Fig. 3. Man and ecology—devastating erosion in a remote valley in Raymah. A whole slope of terraces has been destroyed due to inadequate maintenance of the terrace walls; the men had left to work abroad.

A. Some Changes in Diet and Social Habits

Our first example concerns the massive imports of foreign grain (either bought cheaply or provided "free" as "aid"). Combined with the steeply rising cost of labour, these imports have made sorghum an increasingly uneconomic crop to produce. This has meant a shift in the choice of staple grain for the family. They tend to buy more foreign grain, or even white flour, in place of their own or local sorghum. This has an economic influence on the farmer as a producer, and a direct influence on his family's diet.

Second, in contrast to the first example, is the changing prevalence of the habit of chewing qat *(Catha edulis)*, a mildly narcotic shrub. According to our observations qat chewing had been largely confined to the towns in the past and was quite uncommon in a rural area like Raymah. Generally it was either the habit of a few well-known chewers (almost invariably the better off), or used by the general populace on festive occasions. Over the past ten to fifteen years, and particularly the past five years, the habit has mushroomed, so that in the village in which we lived about 80% of the adult population, male and female, chewed at least once per week. Qat chewing, originally almost entirely confined to men in Raymah, is now also widespread amongst the women and not uncommon among children. (The source of the data on Raymah is explained in the references). The high cost of qat, as well as its pharmacological effects which include dependence and anorexia, have a direct influence on the everyday life of many thousands of Raymi peasants. The increase in the habit seems to be largely explained by the greater contact with the towns and the greater availability of cash. However, the almost orgiastic abandonment with which at times whole villages give themselves up to the fantasy world of qat seems to us to have some elements of a conscious or unconscious reaction to the growing dislocation of the traditional culture. The parallels with alcohol amongst Australian Aborigines are striking (see Kamien, Chapter 15, this volume).

Among other changes occurring in the culture two others need special mention, for they bring us closer to our essential concern of illness and health. These are the veiling of women and the changes in infant feeding practices.

Like qat chewing, veiling of women used to be uncommon in Raymah. The practice was confined to the few very wealthy families in the four or five larger towns of the Raymah district. It has become much more widespread over the past ten years. The same two major reasons seem to be operating here, namely, much greater contact with the towns of Yemen and the Arabian Peninsula (where veiling is the rule), and much more available cash. As one becomes wealthier, or more travelled, one aspires to veil one's wife, much as in the West as one moves up the social ladder, one improves one's car. In Raymah veiling is confined to the rich, the aspiring rich, or the relatively poor snobs. It is an economic handicap, because the wife is not only veiled, but unable to move outside the house. She spends the majority of her time in the "harem" and so is unable to work in the fields or to carry water. Someone must be paid to do that for her. Thus veiling is expensive.

The aspect of veiling with which we are concerned here is the influence of the veil on the health of the woman and her children, rather than its effect on woman's freedom. According to our observations, the emotional and physical health of the women of the harem suffers as a consequence of their social and physical isolation. This factor overrides their relatively greater wealth which by itself might be thought to offer advantages in health. Veiled women suffer more from tuberculosis, anaemia, and osteomalacia than their poorer cousins, who are not confined to the dark interiors of their houses but can have robust social intercourse with the outside world. Naturally the health of the children of the harem suffers too, for the health of the dependent child depends directly on the vitality of the mother, as it is the mother who provides the essential element in the child's environment. Our data on child nutrition indicates that both marasmus and rickets are more common in the wealthy homes where the women are veiled than in families of moderate (though not inadequate) means, where veiling is absent. In this case a chain of events evolves from the loosening of Raymah's age-old isolation. This chain ends up in a different pattern of child rearing and a measurable change in health. The link between the original influence and the observable result is a subtle cultural change at the very heart of the society.

The second example is the increasing practice of bottle feeding with artificial milk. Little more needs to be said on this catastrophe which has been documented in many Third World countries (see Jelliffe and Jelliffe, 1975). We can merely summarize the position by pointing out that imported powdered milks were little known in Raymah a few years ago, that they are now widely used in the larger towns and increasingly in the villages, and that the substitution of polluted, infected and diluted artificial milk for the breast frequently has fatal consequences for the child. In this particular example, the chain linking Western influence, a change of behaviour and a deterioration in health is clearer and more direct.

B. Ramifications of Change in Terms of Illness and Health

We will now move directly to the relationship between this changing society and its health. To do this there are three questions we must examine. The first concerns the beliefs and expectations of the individual Raymi in the field of health, the second, how these beliefs have changed in the changing society and the third, how the people's expectations match the changing reality.

We will begin to answer these questions by describing in a rather personal and anecdotal way how we began to develop an appreciation of the nature of the people's beliefs on illness and health. For it was as the result of these surprising, indeed disturbing, insights that we began to question seriously the putative system as seen by most foreigners, and so redefine the role that Western medicine was coming to play within the society.

1 The Local Practitioner

From the very beginning of the Health Project's existence one of the authors (P. U.) made frequent emergency medical calls to remote villages and hamlets within the massif. In these areas, where most of the people had never seen a foreigner, traditional life seemed preserved without blemish. However, to my astonishment, as I walked through the village to the home of the sick, I would often find information inserts and empty drug packages strewn on the path. The packages or inserts would describe their contents in English. For a long time there was a puzzling incongruity between the seeming pervasiveness of an entirely traditional culture, in which very few of the people could read Arabic, and this ubiquitous flotsam from Western drug houses. Eventually, however, it became apparent that the visits had usually been preceded by a Yemeni practitioner, who had already administered Western drugs to the sick patient and, characteristically, discarded the packaging in the street.

Further enquiry and experience revealed that throughout Yemen and even in Raymah every larger village possessed someone who treated sick people with Western drugs. If he lived mainly from this work he was called in Arabic *sahi*, health worker, a word derived from the Arabic *Saha*, meaning health. The phenomenon of the *sahi*, a man who practises a form of Western medicine in his local community, has grown up very quickly over the last five years. It is of central importance to a discussion of local beliefs on illness and the changing patterns of health care.

Individual sahis, of whom there are dozens in Raymah (and more like hundreds if one includes part-timers), have had a very variable training. However, the essential requirement is some association, no matter how brief, with a doctor, pharmacist, hospital or other sahi, in one of the larger towns of Yemen or Arabia. Some sahis have had an "education" of two or three years nursing in one of the hospitals in Yemen, Saudia or the Gulf. The experience of others may be much less than this; for instance a month's job as a cleaner in one of Yemen's less than salubrious hospitals during the period of the Imam, years before. The training, in fact, is really beside the point. It merely provides the budding practitioner with his sine qua non. This is the ability, or better the confidence, to administer an injection.

The sahi's practice consists largely of giving injections of various drugs. In fact, the sahi is called by the patient to administer an injection. The most common of the injections given are calcium, liver extract, chloroquin, vitamins C and B_1 and B complex, penicillin or chloromycetin. However, bizzare combinations of steroids and other hormones, erythropoietic agents, enzymes and various animal vegetable extracts are in vogue from time to time. Calcium and chloroquin can have dangerous, even fatal side effects if given intravenously; they often are. Calcium gluconate is given in most cases regardless of the symptoms. This seems to be related to the fact that intravenous calcium gives autonomic effects including flushing and faintness, clear evidence to the Raymi of the drug's power. Even the best sahis possess very limited diagnostic skills, and those that do hardly use them. Most of the time the sahi gives the patient what he requests. Otherwise he administers a drug deemed appropriate to both the patient's condition, as revealed by a few simple questions, and the drugs in his possession at the time. The sahi charges large sums for his services and the drugs he supplies. Even very poor people usually manage to raise the money and pay without demur. An average consultation in 1976 cost about $10·00 and the drugs at least another $10·00.

The sahi uses very little counselling or psychological skill; his role is to inject the elixir. He is not seen as a source of advice, guidance, knowledge or support. Consequently the sahi plays no role whatsoever in preventive medicine. To the Raymi, the sahi practises what is considered to be Western medicine; the quintessence of Western medicine is therefore the treatment of illness by injections.

The recognition of the importance of the phenomenon of the sahi througout Raymah led to our re-evaluation of the nature and degree of Western influence in this traditional culture. It seemed that here was an example of a Western model of medicine, imported, debased, then grafted to the local society with truly remarkable speed. Consequently it seemed to us that the nature of the phenomenon could not be understood unless a much greater amount of knowledge was gathered about the nature of local beliefs about health and disease, treatment and cure. This seemed a fundamental step, not only in understanding what was happening, but in attempting to lay the foundations of an appropriate and effective health service for Raymah. From this point we began a deliberate attempt to study local beliefs.

2 The Nature of Local Beliefs on Illness

Gathering information on illness was a complex and slow process. One of the major reasons for this was that the discussion of illness was thought likely to bring retribution from the powers that produced it. Discussion with a foreigner was especially fraught with danger. Nevertheless, a picture of local beliefs was painfully pieced together, though it must be considered at this stage as partial and provisional.

Most Westerners in Yemen would say that the Islamic society of Yemen is essentially practical and down to earth and that superstition and magic are not deeply important parts of the culture. Those with closer contact with Yemeni people recognize that the local people are quite markedly superstitious. However, there is usually no suspicion whatsoever of the existence of any organized system of magical belief.* As we eventually discovered, such a system exists. Beneath the worldly practicalities of Islam and the materialism of Raymi peasant society is a bubbling, complex, and often terrifying magical world. It has profound ramifications in the field of illness and medicine.

This magical world provides the Raymi with his views on illness, giving him the explanation of the causation of disease, on why it affects some people and not others, on why the manifestations of disease are variable and on why some diseases and not others are curable. Raymis to not believe that illness is caused by a germ, or by contaminated food or water or even less by their practices of ablution. Rather, they believe that they are ill as a result of a confluence of events. In each individual case there is a great variety of forces, some external to the sufferer, some internal, that work together to induce illness. In this chapter we cannot detail the various mechanisms that operate, but we can quote some examples and draw some generalizations.

* We use the word magic to mean the system whereby the course of events is influenced by compelling the agency of spiritual beings or occult forces. We stress at different times in this chapter that in the eyes of the Raymi the system is pervasive, comprehensive and internally consistent and its manifestations palpably observable.

Illness can be the result of the direct and deliberate machinations of people who wish to harm the sufferer. Sometimes this can be performed by straightforward poisoning or more commonly by sorcery. For instance, a girl told us how an old woman with special powers cast a spell on her so that her wrists were instantly broken and remained from then on weak and painful; from time to time they were capable of spontaneously refracturing. In this case the sufferer was not blameless, for the spell had been cast upon her during an exhibition of dancing to a group of women. The dance was one the girl had learnt in Saudia and was rather more erotic than the local style. The girl had offended the old women and one of them had taken her retribution.

In this case the external agency operating on the girl had no material motive. The witch gained nothing from punishing the girl, bar satisfaction. The next example, the case of the death of a friend's brother, contrasts with the first. The family believed that the brother had been mysteriously and semi-magically poisoned by other relatives, whose motive was monetary and sexual. The accused pair, a man and the victim's wife, not only subsequently inherited the dead man's terraces, but eventually married. Our informant was convinced that the poison used was menstrual fluid. Subsequently we were able to establish that the likely cause of death was typhoid fever.

We are not here implying that the man's death was not also influenced by his belief that occult powers were working against him. Although we have described the system of belief as "magical", the causation of disease as "supernatural" and the process of casting spells as "sorcery", we do not mean to belittle the power of the beliefs, or the capacity of the spells to hurt or heal.

Although there is a difference between the two cases in terms of the expectations of the accused and the culpability of the victim, they are similar in that the outside agencies were thought to operate deliberately and vengefully on the victim. The widespread belief in the Evil Eye is different. Although the Evil Eye represents a "real fear of evil influence through other people" (Spooner, 1970), the possessor of the Evil Eye as a general rule harms unintentionally. Such a person is not usually aware of his powers and has little control over them. The possessor of the Evil Eye is usually either a stranger or a local person whose social activity, appearance, attitudes, or behaviour is to some degree unorthodox or different. This makes such a person prominent in a highly traditional and conformist society. Usually the possessor of the Eye (in arabic *ʿayn*) is not a part of a faction, but someone who operates indiscriminately, almost inadvertently. We agree with Douglas that the possessor of the Evil Eye is a person "singular in appearance, apt to stare rather than speak and who shoots out danger" to any unfortunate around him (Douglas, 1970).

The belief in the Evil Eye is powerful and pervasive in Raymah. The consequences of this belief are very important for all people living and working in this culture, perhaps most of all for foreigners who are not only singular in appearance, but tend to stare rather than speak as they struggle with the language. They are easily seen as the sources of the Evil Eye. In passing, it is worth mentioning a few ways in which a foreigner can avoid this: he should make a serious and continuing attempt to follow social etiquette, especially as regards salutations, greetings and farewells; he should refrain from comments on people's appearance, or health; and above all, he should never mention illness, except in the most indirect and impersonal way.

The belief in the *ginn* is different again. The ginn are ubiquitous and capricious spirits. They are semihuman rather than supernatural, with their tiresome bumps and yells in the night and their petty thievery. However, their mischief can cause harm and even serious injury and death, as they playfully swoop into the human world, create havoc, and then retire to their own world beyond human intervention or restraint. The Raymi is frightened of the ginn but retains for them the sort of humorous, even affectionate awe which one holds for an irrepressible, if naughty child.

From these few examples a picture emerges of the rich and complex beliefs which underlie the Raymi's attitude to illness. It is extremely important to understand that these beliefs are well organized and structured into a system which is internally consistent and logical. In any one case the disease or injury can be fully explained by a spell, a semi-magical poisoning, the Evil Eye, the ginn, or a combination of these beliefs. The pattern in individual cases varies enormously.

As we have seen, there is also variation in the onus of responsibility on the sufferer. This may vary from a straightforward retribution as the result of the victim's own misdemeanours, to an utterly unmerited punishment. Essentially, however, illness arises from a confluence of events with outside forces or agencies.

3 Western Medicine as the New Magic

The next questions to ask are: How does this magical world fit in with the growing passion for Western medicine? If the cause of illness is beyond the material, why is it that Western practitioners, either the sahi or real Westerners if available, are not considered irrelevant? Indeed, the people express a deep need for their services and are prepared to pay relatively enormous amounts for them.

Part of the answers to these questions lie in the fact that there is no powerful system of traditional medicine in Raymah. It is striking and paradoxical that in such a sophisticated and ancient culture as Raymah there is a remarkable lack of any body of indigenous well-organized medical knowledge and practice. Traditional practitioners are very few; there are only two well-recognized Arab doctors in Raymah. They use herbal preparations and do some very minor surgery. They do not appear to enjoy either special prestige or great popularity. At the village level, although there is a general belief in the value of certain herbs, there is usually no one special person with expertise in their use and trusted because of his knowledge. Thus any moderately serious illness is met with a sense of fearful resignation. Usually one of the family scarifies the skin. Then, depending on the severity of the illness and the wealth of the family, a request is made to a Western practitioner.

At the same time, of course, the bad magic is tackled by the performance of a number of incantations and even spells-in-return, and the use of other rituals such as the recitation of the Koran, and the use of amulets. However, all these procedures, though believed to have power, are not systematized or embodied in one group of people, so constituting what is normally defined as a system of medicine. Thus the lack of a developed indigenous system of medical practice may explain in part the strong desire of the local people for Western medical intervention, despite their profound belief in the supernatural causation of disease.

But there is more to it than that. One of the more disconcerting, and at first inexplicable, aspects of treating very ill people in Raymah was the feeling that although it was clear the practitioner was desperately wanted by the sick man and his family, he was at the same time viewed as somehow profoundly peripheral to the central action. An understanding of the nature of local beliefs eventually made this apparent paradox explicable: the Western practitioner is peripheral in the sense that he is unable to influence the cause of the illness. He is called only when symptoms have appeared; that is, in the post-causation phase.

However, herein lies the rub. Although the Western practitioner cannot modify the cause of the disease, which has arisen from the magical confluence and so is manifestly beyond his influence, he is seen to be sometimes capable of influencing its course, its outcome. In our opinion, the fact that the practitioner is believed to be able to modify the course of illness has brought his own powers into the realm of the magical.

The powers of the doctor to heal are to an enormous extent related to the giving of the injection; the needle is of overwhelming importance in the eyes of the Raymi. The intervention by the sahi or the doctor and the administration of the injection has taken on magical properties and magical power, and the strength and status of a ritual. This New Magic, derived from an exotic culture, and possessing its own rites and mysteries, and practised by a body of initiates, is seen to have power to combat the Old.

There are some parallels here with the Cargo Cults of New Guinea (see Lawrence, 1964). We were always being asked what injections we gave our son who was so manifestly big and healthy. Most disbelieved us when we said the cause is good food, although one old lady believed us sufficiently to request some pork, forbidden to Moslems. There was clearly a feeling among many Yemenis that we possessed secrets that enabled us to be rich and healthy. These we appeared to guard closely.

For two major reasons the New Magic, as practised coarsely by the sahi in Raymah and with some relative sophistication by Western-trained doctors in other parts of Yemen, produces little benefit in terms of the people's health. In fact, the growing power of the belief in the doctor and his drugs is a major handicap to any real improvement in their standards of health.

The first reason for this arises from the origin of the major diseases prevalent in the area. Like most Third World countries, the overwhelming proportion of Raymah's illnesses can be grouped into three broad categories. They are: childhood malnutrition; infective and parasitic disease; maternal disease and accident. These three groups are widespread and serious. Although morbidity and mortality data are absent in Yemen, it would seem that these illnesses combine to produce one of the shortest life expectancies in the world. Certainly our data indicate that more than half of the children die before they reach five years, while half of the children under five and 70% of the children under two, suffer from severe protein and calorie malnutrition (PCM). This is based on Jelliffe's criteria where severe PCM is classified as body weight less than 60% of standard weight (Jelliffe, 1966). Among adults, infections and infestations with tuberculosis, bilharzia, malaria, various nematodes (especially *Ascaris*), amoebae, *Giardia* and typhoid fever, cause widespread ill-health, disease, deformity and death. Apart from the complications of childbirth, women suffer invariably from nutritional anaemia. In addition to marasmus, children have high rates of rickets and anaemia. There are also epidemics of measles, whooping cough and gastroenteritis which periodically sweep devastatingly through the young population.

The origin of these three groups of diseases lies embedded in the culture. To demonstrate this we will briefly examine the origin of each of the three groups.

Childhood malnutrition is prevalent in all social classes. It does not appear to be simply the consequence of insufficient available food. As we have indicated, it is particularly prevalent in the richer families where the women are veiled. While it is true that the prevalence is again higher among the (relatively few) very poor families, where food is scarce, there is usually no lack of available food suitable for consumption by young children. The reason for the malnutrition lies in the fundamental beliefs the society holds about food and child rearing and the role and position of mothers within the society. Children become malnourished because breast-feeding is short and often inadequate, because a feeble episode of breast feeding is commonly followed by bottle feeding, with all its dangers and inadequacies, and because weaning foods are invariably grossly inadequate. This last point is perhaps the most important of all. Children are usually not given prepared weaning food during the vital period between the age of six months and three years. During this time they exist on overdiluted milk and a few scraps of bread. By the age of three or four they are mobile and can then physically help themselves to the family's food. After this their level of growth and nutrition starts to improve. It is very important to stress once again that suitable weaning foods are available, e.g. there is abundant and relatively cheap grain. They are not used because mothers do not recognize the need for their use. In addition to these fundamental defects in nutrition, the depredations of recurrent infections and parasites make a significant contribution to the children's gross failure to thrive.

Infectious and parasitic diseases, the most serious problems of adults, have their origins in the level of personal and public hygiene in the community. In Raymah there is virtually no system of hygienic disposal of human excreta and no adequate system of water supply for domestic use, so that food and drinking water are very often contaminated. So commences an endless cycle of reinfection and recontamination.

The *women's level of health* is much below that of men, for they bear the added stresses of poorer food, frequent and hazardous childbirth and arduous physical work in the case of the poor, and social isolation in the case of the rich.

Thus the three major illnesses of Raymah arise from the very soil of the culture, from what the people believe, and how they behave and interact. A disease in an individual Raymi is the end stage of a long and complex chain which starts in the heart of the culture. Children are underweight because they are not fed, which is because the culture does not recognize their special needs for food; they have rickets because they are swaddled and kept inside. Similarly adults contact bilharzia because there is no recognition that it is harmful to urinate and defaecate in water used for washing. Women become anaemic because the culture decrees that men eat first, and the best. Thus Western curative medicine, whether practised by the largely incompetent and corrupt sahi in the village or by the somewhat more competent Westerner, or Western-trained doctor in his hospital, is powerless to modify the pattern of illness, for it can only juggle with the very end stage of the chain. The patient "cured" of bilharzia by his injections goes back to his village to wash and void in the same water, while the rickety child of the paramount Sheik, bearing a load of vitamin D in his buttocks, returns to the sunless caverns of the family mansion. If he had seen a poorly trained sahi rather than one of the better Western-trained doctors, his buttocks would more likely to have contained not the essential vitamin D, but penicillin or chloroquin! (Rickets is a disease of children characterized by weakness of the bones; it is due to lack of vitamin D, which is provided either from the diet, or synthesized in the skin in the presence of sunlight.)

Thus the New Magic of the sahi, or the orthodox model of health care based on doctors, hospitals and cure, which is now growing up in the cities of Yemen and spreading into the country, is fundamentally incapable of coming to terms with the basic causes of illness, which are rooted in the culture. In our view the New Magic is not only impotent in tackling the roots of illness, it has manifestly harmful effects in drawing attention away from these roots and so substituting a slick panacea, or alternatively a simulacrum, in place of the real changes that are required. These real changes include improvements in water supply, in nutrition, in housing, changes in the attitudes and relationships of the people, as well as a more equitable social and political system.

We began this section by saying that there are two reasons why the New Magic is counterproductive. The first reason, discussed above, is that it cannot decrease the amount of *illness* in the community. The second reason is related to its influence on *health*. As we have demonstrated, the people in their traditional culture have developed an elaborate system of explanation of the nature of illness based on a framework of magical belief. With remarkable speed they have incorporated what they understand to be Western medicine into the same framework. If the traditional beliefs on the aetiology of disease made it very difficult to attack the real roots of illness, the new relationship with Western medicine reduces the chances even further. For Raymis are coming to believe that health is the absence of disease and that disease can only be reduced or overcome by more drugs, more doctors and more hospitals. (In this, the average Raymi is at one with the average Westerner: it is not only the superstitious peasant from Yemen who reveals a touching faith in the miraculous). The injection, the New Magic, will miraculously fix everything. Moreover, it will do so without the need for the patient to do anything at all, but lie down, roll over and pay the bill. The New Magic induces a burgeoning expectancy that health is at the end of a syringe. It is available to anyone who can get to and pay for the needle. Thus begins a process of dependency and a desire for more, better, and more expensive cures. In contrast, the Raymi grew up in an intimate relationship with the Old Magic, which blossomed richly around him like a prolific tropic garden beneath the strong if austere carapace of Islam, and was as freely available and accessible as the mountain air.

III. The Impact of Western Medicine

In summary it can be seen that the Western cure-orientated intervention does nothing to reduce illness, except sometimes temporarily in individual cases, for it cannot influence the cause of the illness. But more than this, at a more profound level, we believe that its influence is counterproductive by inducing a state of increasing dislocation between a man and his environment. It cannot reduce illness, because illness derives from the fabric of the culture, and it cannot improve health, because health is essentially about a man's capacity to cope autonomously with his environment. Looking at Dalton's quotation which heads this chapter, we can say that a good doctor of the orthodox mould is better than a bad doctor because he is more likely to help the illness of the individual patient. He is also less likely negligently to harm a patient; the bad doctors of Yemen and Raymah frequently do so (in terms of the example above he is more likely to give vitamin D rather than penicillin to the rickety child), but he is worse than no doctor because of the distorted dependency and false and expensive expectations his presence induces. To us the debased form of Western medicine practised by the sahis in Raymah is a grotesque example of how a Western institution can be caricatured, then speedily grafted, with harmful results, to another culture. The sahis are an extreme example for they carry the curative role to its extreme. However, the model of health care adopted for the rest of Yemen is overwhelmingly dominated by the curative/doctor/hospital/drug/technology philosophy and though practised with relatively less incompetence and corruption, has most of the same defects, and virtually all the same effects, as the medicine of the sahis.

IV. Implications for a Health Service

In what ways can the above analysis be used in designing an appropriate health service for a place such as Raymah? Are there any rules of thumb that can be followed in attempting to devise a system which more effectively reduces illness and yet remains sympathetic to the culture? What practical lessons have been learnt from the first two years of the Raymah Health Project's existence? To answer these questions we will now discuss the implications for a health service under two headings.

A. The Need for Information

The fundamental step of pioneer health workers is to gather information about the community. This is not normally considered a major role for a health project. Such research should have two principal foci:

1. Research related to the structure of the society in its broadest sense, as well as an analysis of the health problems of the community; this includes an epidemiological assessment of the prevalence and causation of the major illnesses.
2. Research based on the evidence that has been gathered, to identify the areas that may benefit from intervention.

It may seem obvious that nothing useful can be done until one knows with what one is dealing. However, in our experience this primary step is often forgotten. It was certainly little emphasized in the early days of the Raymah Project, a project which set out with somewhat radical views as to its priorities, and an acute awareness of the shortcomings of many other medical aid projects. We will cite only two examples in which careful research identified and clarified hitherto unknown or poorly understood problems.

The analysis of malnutrition showed that it was largely confined to young children and adult females. It was not simply the result of poverty and would not respond to increasing food imports to the region.* In fact, such food inputs would have destructive effects by reducing the economic viability of farmers. The solution to improved

* We wish to make it clear that our argument is based on our experience in Yemen: in other countries, other factors, particularly poverty, seem to be more important in the aetiology of malnutrition (see George, 1976).

nutrition in Raymah depends firstly on a painstaking programme of nutrition education and secondly on improving the variety of food available. It would be hoped such education would lead to an improved knowledge of infant feeding. However, improved infant nutrition also depends on an improved status for the women of Raymah.

While in such a short period it would be impossible to expect major changes in these areas, we believe that a useful beginning was made by the development of Under Fives Clinics and a corps of primary health workers, both concentrating on nutrition, together with the Project's experimentation and extension work with vegetable growing. Also, despite the enormity of the problem of the role and status of women in Raymah and the malicious influence of the increasing prevalence of veiling, the Health Project demonstrably revealed its attitude by employing and training several women in responsible roles. This was the first time such a thing had happened in a millenium; it made a visible impact.

A second example in which active information gathering modified the whole approach of the Project was the subject of the people's beliefs about illness. The insight derived from this study should modify the practical way in which health workers live and work in Raymah by showing them that what they think they are doing and what they are seen to be doing by local people are often quite different. It also reveals in even starker form the disastrous potential of a naive Western model of health intervention.

Numerous other examples could be quoted to support our thesis that the gathering and evaluation of information is a major role of the health team. Knowledge in itself may not lead inevitably to wisdom, but it is the end of ignorance.

B. Prevention Versus Cure

For another culture Hamilton suggested Four Keys to Prevention (Hamilton, 1974). We give them as closely approaching our own budding thoughts in this field.

(a) A continued, close, humanly involved relationship between the person primarily involved in health care and the community.

(b) A concerted, sympathetically devised programme of health education in its broadest sense, staffed by workers who are not only concerned with routine medical work, directed at the existing community level and not with some Western model of efficiency as a guide. That is, health education must use the community's existing resources, human, social and technological.

(c) The most complete as possible involvement of local medical practitioners, respect for their proficiencies, and their enlistment as professional partners in the health service, not as "assistants" or menials.
(d) The fullest possible community participation and consultation in all decisions affecting its welfare, and a careful consideration of possible destructive effects resulting from externally introduced programmes of change in any sphere.

Between the acceptance of these keys and their elaboration lie a number of deep difficulties, one of the most significant being that two of the major ideas embodied in the Four Keys may appear mutually incompatible.

We have been at pains to show what health care means to a Raymi. It means curative medicine. There is thus a gulf between a health team, which becomes imbued with preventive zeal, and the populace, who not only fail to recognize the importance of prevention, but have a very clear idea as to what is important. And yet one of the Keys to Prevention says that community participation and consultation is essential to improvements in health. The community, if given the chance and the choice, would opt for more doctors and hardware and hospitals as the main way of improving health.* How is it possible to resolve this incongruity?

Although much of what we have been saying in this chapter has been an argument for prevention, it is our view that the needs of the people for medicine can never be ignored by those who live in and care for the community. It seems to us that the primary key to prevention lies in the "continued close humanly involved relationship between the person primarily involved in health care and the community". Such a relationship brings the health team member to a position where he understands to some extent what it is to be a member of a different culture. This enables him to recognize and understand the need of the sick for medicine. A health project is meant, after all, to serve the people. A model of health which excludes their beliefs and their needs is not only an arrogance, but also will not work. This means that while a major shift in emphasis must be made towards prevention, curative medicine is important, and much harm can result from making a categorical and exclusive distinction between the two. Indeed there is a great danger that preventive medicine is becoming a slogan. The old model of cure has not worked and a new model of prevention is being put in its place. At its most banal the new model is merely a different dose of medicine, again providing "the answer" in terms of a prescription, so to "deliver health more efficiently, more cheaply and more equitably". The point

* The choice has already been made by the *Western* community . . .

of this chapter is that useful change is dependent on knowledge of the culture and that prescriptive Western solutions are dangerous. It is hoped preventive medicine will not be taken over by people who know what is inevitably right for others whom they have never touched and who have never touched them.

We can summarize our views on curative medicine by saying that it should be as basic, as cheap, and as self-sustaining as is possible, but it should be organized, funded, and staffed to provide a decent service to care for sick people. Moreover the curative work must be integrated with the preventive work at all levels and especially with teaching and health education.

While it is true that preventive measures hold the key to the alleviation of most serious diseases in Raymah, the chances of success in the wider field of prevention will greatly increase if the project has been seen to respond to the felt needs of the community. Only by doing this is it possible to establish the necessary mutual trust and understanding.

Key Three, concerning the use of local practitioners, is highly relevant to the Raymah experience. The sahi provides the great majority of Raymis and Yemenis with their first contact with Western medicine. If he has been largely responsible for the elaboration of the New Magic, with all the attendant ill-effects we have charted, he also holds the key to any real improvement in health care. This is because he knows the culture and is accepted. The problem is to get him to apply what is useful, not misapply the frippery of Western medicine. Stated differently, the problem is to devise a strategy which enables the Western model of illness, based on germs and physiology, to interact constructively with the Yemeni model of illness based on supernatural belief.

To this end, a programme of training local primary health workers selected largely but not exclusively from practising sahis, was instituted in Raymah. The aims of the project were to provide the auxiliaries with an understanding of the diagnosis and treatment as well as the principles of causation and prevention of the major diseases that prevail. There was an emphasis on the importance of nutrition and immunization. The results of this project even at its early stages appeared optimistic.

V. Health Development—Integration or Fragmentation

It may be argued that if the origin of much of Raymah's illness lies in the structure of the society, there is no place for health workers in Raymah. Indeed, such is one interpretation of Dalton's quote at the head of the chapter. According to this argument, improvement in disease will follow only as the result of improved nutrition, water supply, housing and more equitable and more just systems of government. It follows that these fields are viewed as beyond the realm of influence of the health worker. For a number of reasons, we do not hold this opinion, though we recognize its weight.

The first reason why health workers have a useful role lies in the fact that they are seen by the local people as meeting a clearly recognized need. This means that they are more easily accepted by the community and so can more readily establish the "close humanly involved relationship" which we believe is basic to the development of any worthwhile and appropriate development. This ease of intimate contact, so much more difficult for the engineer, economist or agriculturist, should provide the health worker with both special insight into the workings of the society and some special power to influence it. Thus individual cures can be made a springboard for the beginnings of change in the society.

We will give several examples of this: the treatment of sick children can be broadened into an Under-Fives Clinic with nutritional assessment and education and immunization; contact with an ill child provides the chance for a discussion on family planning (see Morley, 1973); the recognition and treatment of a number of cases of guinea-worm (transmitted in this case via religious ablutions in communal Mosque pools) provides the opportunity for a meeting with the affected community at a level at which concepts of public hygiene can be introduced. In such ways medicine can move from its exclusive domain of treating the sick into the wider fields of prevention of illness and of community development. In a community like this prevention and community development are very difficult without curative medicine.

The case of the *Rinderpest epidemic* is a special example of how the Raymah Project broadened its role with unexpected benefits.

In early 1976, Rinderpest, a serious cattle disease, broke out in Yemen and the epidemic eventually reached Raymah. Mortality was very high, reaching 80% in some villages. It seemed to us that the death of a cow may be of much greater significance to a poor family than the death of an infant. Why then should we not use our resources to help?

In collaboration with the British Veterinary Team in Sana'a, the Raymah Health Project therefore began a concerted campaign of immunization as soon as the outbreak was identified. At first the campaign encountered resistance on the part of the locals, but the benefits of immunization were so dramatic, immediate and clear-cut, that initial hostility was soon replaced with enthusiastic co-operation. Even the most superstitious peasant saw that a vaccinated animal survived, while in a non-vaccinated village a few metres away most of the cattle were dead within five days. This then enabled the team to vaccinate over 2000 cattle and halt the epidemic.

Other than the obvious beneficial effects this programme had on the domestic economy of Raymah, there were two additional side-effects of the intervention especially relevant to this chapter. Firstly, the work in the crisis amongst the cattle enhanced and widened the image of the Project in the eyes of the people. This greatly helped in many of the other efforts in the field of agriculture and veterinary work. These included small projects with vaccination of poultry for Newcastle disease, experimentation with vegetables and crops, and the setting up of a pilot goat dairy scheme (Underwood and Underwood, 1979).

The second benefit of the cattle programme was its unexpected influence on the vaccination programme amongst the children. This programme had floundered due to lack of interest. The local people could see no value in a painful injection, which in undernourished children often produced a nasty local infection and a significant period of ill-health. All this trouble, a Raymi might say, was for a theoretical condition which the child might never get, and if it did was anyway the result of some magical and fateful confluence. The idea of a vaccination seemed to most Raymis an uncomfortable impertinence. The needle was seen as desirable only as a part of cure. That is, it was desirable during the post-causation phase of illness when painful symptoms already existed. The Rinderpest programme manifestly changed this; the intervention was seen to prevent a disease. From then on the demand for immunization of the children exceeded the Project's capacity to provide it.

In our opinion, health workers, including auxiliaries, should be trained to possess some basic agricultural and veterinary skills, especially expertise in immunization of cattle and poultry, the diagnosis and treatment of common treatable diseases of animals and crops, and the principles of cultivation of nutritionally valuable foodstuffs such as pulses, legumes, and fruits.

These few examples support the view that medical work must be integrated with other aspects of development. Moreover the doctor and the members of the health team, if they are ready to move out of their limited if important roles as curers, are in an excellent position to play a part in those other fields which are probably more basic to development.

Let us finish by looking again at Dalton's impudent remark on doctors. In Dalton's time, and as we have shown in this paper in

Raymah today, even good doctors are worse than useless if their role is confined within the rigid straight-jacket of cure. It seems to us that the doctor who is prepared to study the culture and its illnesses will find avenues for change that are appropriate to it. While many of these avenues may not appear to have an obvious connection with orthodox medical work, and may themselves eventually require others with special training and gifts for their elaboration, we believe a doctor working in this way may be able after all to provide something rather better than nothing at all.

Acknowledgements

The Raymah Community Health Project is a combined project between the Catholic Institute of International Relations (CIIR) as part of the British Volunteer Programme, the Raymah Development Board and the Government of the Yemen Arab Republic. CIIR, 4 Cambridge Terrace, London NW14 JL, England, is an organization with volunteers in Third World countries, which works for an increased awareness of the real causes of underdevelopment. It is not a funding body, and we wish to gratefully acknowledge the support of the following organizations: Catholic Relief Services (CRS), EZE (West Germany), The Royal Dutch Government, and Oxfam (UK).

We would like to express our gratitude to Eric Lawson, Jill Lawson and Henry Schapper, for their help in the preparation of this chapter.

References

NOTE: The data on which this chapter is based are derived from the authors' work in Yemen, most of which is as yet unpublished. A series of papers are in preparation on patterns of morbidity in adults and children, on the growth and nutrition of children, and on the nature of local beliefs on illness. In addition to the reference quoted below (Underwood and Underwood, 1979) a full report on the Project has been completed but is available in only limited numbers from CIIR (Underwood, P. and Underwood, Z. (1979). "When Water is Better than Oil—An Account of the Setting up of a Community Health Project in Raymah (YAR)". CIIR, London).

Douglas, M. (1970). "Witchcraft—Confessions and Accusations". Tavistock, London.

George, S. (1976). "How the Other Half Dies: The Real Reasons for World Hunger". Penguin Books Harmondsworth.

Hamilton, A. (1974). The traditionally orientated community. *In* "Better

Health for Aborigines" (B. S. Hetzel, Ed.), Chapter 1.2. Univ. Queensland Press, St Lucia, Queensland.

Jelliffe, D. (1966). "The Nutritional Status of the Community". World Health Organization—Monograph Series No. 53. WHO, Geneva.

Jelliffe, D. and Jelliffe, E. (1975). Human milk, nutrition and the world resource crisis. *Science, N.Y.* **188**, 557–561.

Lawrence, P. (1964). "Road Belong Cargo". Manchester Univ. Press, Manchester.

Ministry of Development. (1976). "Statistical Year Book, YAR" Sana'a, YAR.

Morley, D. (1973). "Paediatric Priorities in the Developing World". Butterworth, London.

Ronart, S. and Ronart, N. (1959 and 1966). "Concise Encyclopaedia of Arabic Civilisation", Vols 1 and 2. Djambatan, Amsterdam.

Spooner, B. (1970). The Evil Eye in the Middle East. *In* "Witchcraft—Confessions and Accusations" (M. Douglas, Ed.), Chapter 15. Tavistock, London.

Underwood, P. and Underwood, Z. (1979). Bread instead of cake: an innovatory goat improvement scheme as part of a community health project in rural Yemen. *In* "Australian Goat Breeding, Husbandry, Science and Veterinary Practice: Proceedings of Second National Goat Breeders Conference". Goat Breeders Society of Australia, Roleystone, Western Australia.

17
The African Experience

S. Ofosu-Amaah
Department of Community Health, University of Ghana Medical School, Accra, Ghana

The disease burden in Africa is still very great

I. Introduction

This section deals with the experience of the peoples of Africa in terms of the factors and determinants which have affected their health status and have moulded their systems of health care. The focus will largely be on Africa south of the Sahara because the experience of that large segment of the continent has a coherence peculiar to itself, and in matters of health demonstrates the remorselessness of ecology and history to a degree hardly paralleled on other continents. Africa north of the Sahara has had essentially different experiences and has been largely influenced by Mediterranean and Middle Eastern factors (Boateng, 1978).

At present the continent of Africa has the worst health status in the world. The estimate for the expectation of life at birth is the lowest of any continent—45·8 years for males and 48·9 years for females; the world average respectively being 55·9 years (males) and 58·6 years (females). Crude death rates were estimated at 18 per 1000 persons in Africa as against a world average of 11·9 per 1000 for 1975–80 estimates (Nortman and Hofstatter, 1978). Infant mortality and 1–4 year age mortality rates are 150 per 1000 live births and 30 per 1000 respectively (World Health Organization, 1976a).

Kimble (1960) emphasized the fact that the average rural African "lives in thraldom to sickness", because of the poor state of his diet, housing, sanitation, health facilities and also because of his ignorance of the precepts of modern hygiene.

II. Major Health Determinants

A. Geography

Africa, the second largest continent, with an area of 30·32 million square km^2—a quarter of the earth's land surface—is unique in having the equator bisecting it into northern and southern halves, and therefore having a rather symmetrical arrangement of ecological zones (see Fig. 1). The northern half is much wider in its east–west dimension, but most of this is covered by the 10·4 million km^2 expanse of the Sahara Desert (Last, 1965; Boateng, 1978).

These features of the geography of the continent have significant implications for health. The distribution of the land mass about the

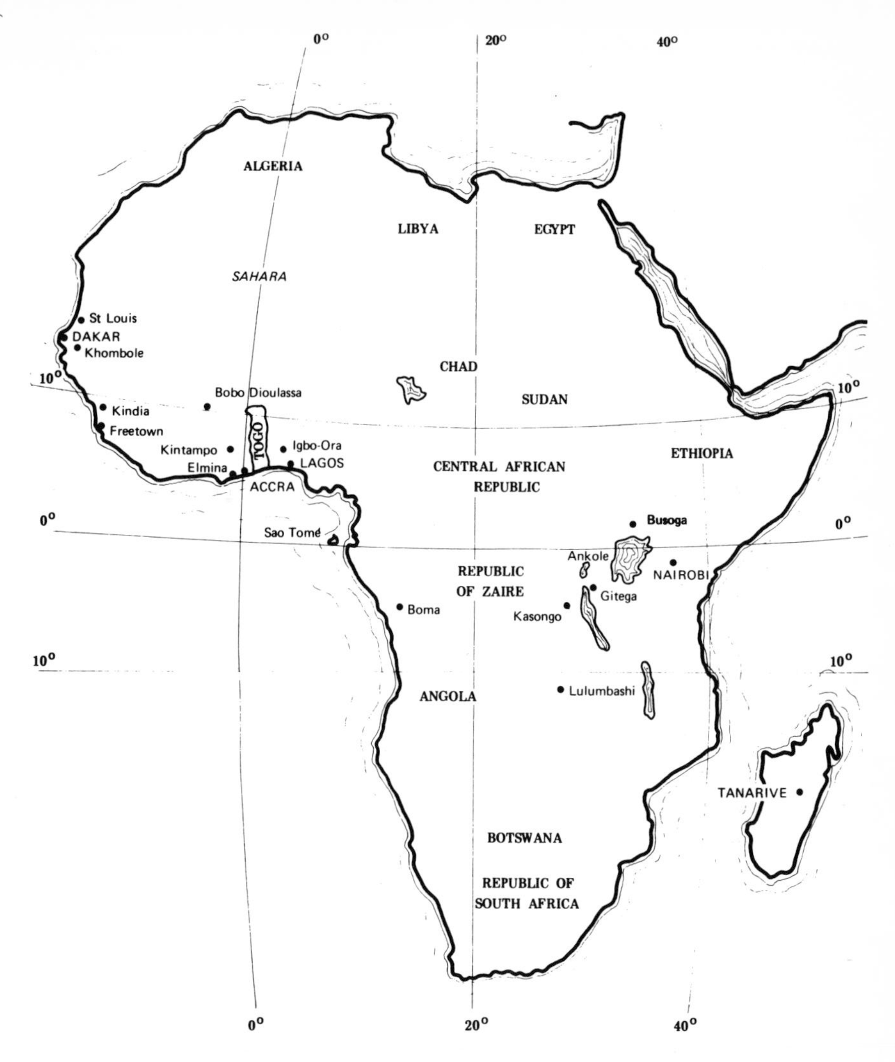

Fig. 1. Africa.

equator puts most of it between the tropics of Cancer and Capricorn and therefore temperatures are uniformly high; since most of Africa is plateau averaging over 500 m above sea level, oceanic influences on the temperatures are not marked. This implies that there is a year round flourishing of arthropod and other disease-bearing organisms, which are not subject to the inhibiting low temperatures of temperate zone winters.

On the other hand rainfall over most of the continent is seasonal and extremely variable with a tendency for years of great rains and floods and years of drought appearing in clusters (Dekker, 1965). One recalls to mind the major Sahelian drought of the early 1970s, and also the Ethiopian drought, both of which caused great havoc and famine to man and his animals. Besides, much of the rainfall of Africa occurs in tropical storms because of the position of the equator and the prevailing wind system. This, coupled with the nature of the soil, leads to severe erosion and also reduces the amount of ground water. The implications of these factors for water resource development, agriculture and nutrition are obvious.

The upwarping of the edges of the African plateaux means that many of the great rivers have rather narrow outlets, often through a series of rapids (ideal breeding sites for the Simulium fly vector of river-blindness) to the sea. Few rivers are navigable from the coast for great distances inland (Dekker, 1965).

The vegetation in the middle belt of Africa is tropical rain forest which is bordered north and south by grassland or savannah merging into desert through a drier interphase or sahel. Over the centuries this vegetation cover has been disturbed by the "slash and burn" shifting type of cultivation. Presently most of the tropical rain forest is secondarily derived; although luxuriant it does not generally support large numbers of livestock. It is therefore poor in animal protein foods. Arthropod life is also luxuriant and this means there is much vector-borne disease for most of the year, e.g. mosquitoes and malaria.

The savannah, which is grassland and wooded scrubland, has developed to its present extent mainly because of perennial burning for agriculture and overgrazing. The savannah is an ideal habitat for grazing animals and wild beasts, especially in East and Central Africa. It is also ideal for some arthropods such as *Glossina morsitans*, the vector of Rhodesian sleeping sickness.

It is also conceivable that the vastness of the Sahara and its bordering sahel may have been caused by both the activities of man and the changes of climate over the centuries (Last, 1965). On account of climate, 42% of the continent is arid or extremely arid, 22% semi-arid, and only 36% sub-arid or humid (Dekker, 1965). Climate and history have ensured that 20% of the population of the continent live in arid or very arid regions (annual rainfall less than 250 mm); 20% live where the annual rainfall is between 250–500 mm p.a.; 42% live where the rainfall is between 500–1500 mm p.a., and only 16% of the population live in regions with more than 1500 mm of rainfall p.a. Last (1965) also quoted Hance, who remarked that in Africa the force of the physical environment is tremendously important. The physical problems seem to be greater and more intransigent than in the temperate zones.

The aridity of most of the continent and the seasonality and variability of rainfall lead to frequent droughts and famine; in addition, there are the many poor agricultural practices in the face of poor soils and the constant threat of erosion; the high temperatures all the year round favour the survival of vectors and disease-causing pests. All these factors have been and are still a tremendous hindrance to the maintenance of human well-being in Africa.

B. History

The early history of most of the peoples of tropical Africa (negroid) is a history of small bands of hunters and food-gatherers moving generally from the north-east (Nubia or Cush) to the south and west to set up grassland states and driving the earlier indigenes into the tropical rain forest (Fage, 1964; see also Black, this volume).

It is thought that until quaternary times the Sahara was well-watered grassland abundant in fauna which was hunted equally by people of Mediterranean and Negro stock. The desertification of the Sahara led to movement into the Nile valley and the beginning of Egyptian civilization in the fourth millenium, and of the negroid stock into the Sudan or Nubia where developments were slower. By the eighth century B.C. the Nubians or the peoples of Cush were strong enough to conquer Egypt and establish the twenty-fifth Dynasty. The conquest of Egypt by the Assyrians in the seventh century B.C. was probably the beginning of the migration of the Negro (now Bantu-speaking groups all over sub-Saharan Africa) (Fage, 1964).

1 The Arabs

The Moslem religion was spread by conquest into the savannah states of Africa from the seventh to the fourteenth century A.D. This caused great population movements—some of which influenced trade for the better (gold, kola, salt)—and some for the worse—slaves, and the spread of diseases from the Middle East, e.g. urinary schistosomiasis and later syphilis. Arab civilization and medicine followed the trade routes across the Sahara and led to the adoption of Arabic concepts of treatment—cupping, cautery, cataract surgery, medicines and herbals and even to the establishment of Arab schools of medicine. Most of these Arab medical practices have either become embedded in African traditional medicine or have continued in coexistence with it.

Arab slave-raiding spread panic and confusion and largely destroyed the settled pastoral life of communities in East and Central Africa. Sultan Mansa Musa of the Mali Empire died of sleeping sickness in 1373 A.D., according to the Arab writer Al Qualquashaidi (Ackerknecht, 1965).

The autochthonous form of schistosomiasis in Africa was the bowel (*S. mansoni*) type, but the Arab penetration of Africa spread urinary schistosomiasis (*S. haematobium*) from a probable focus in the Sudan. It is interesting to note that in the northern half of Madagascar and the northern half of Rwanda, which came under Moslem influence, urinary schistosomiasis is predominant, and that in the southern halves of these two countries the bowel form is predominant (Simmons *et al.*, 1951).

2 The Europeans' Fifteenth Century

In causing the spread of disease, depopulation and disorganization (difficult and trying as it was to the indigenes of Africa), the Arab slave trade did not equal in intensity, in magnitude, or in the resultant disruption of African life the enormous holocaust of the European slave trade.

It is estimated that in the three centuries of the European slave trade, 13 million Africans were successfully transported, while probably 18–24 million persons died during the voyage. It is estimated that a total of about 33 million people were taken away (Condé, 1971). But this was only one aspect of the story. The slave trade debased life in Africa for over ten generations. In terms of total health it disrupted communal life, removed large numbers of able-bodied men and women at the reproductive age, increased mortality rates, caused a decline in birth rates and serious economic and social disarray.

Another aspect of the effect of the migrations and population movements especially of communities trying to escape slave raiding, warfare and other catastrophes has been that these people breached what German geographers term "*Grenzwildnis*", or "boundary wilderness", or even "epidemiological barriers", which were either zones of natural wilderness traditionally recognized as unsuitable for human exploitation or natural foci of infection (Ford, 1966). They perished from great epidemics such as sleeping sickness, yellow fever, malaria and other vector-borne diseases. Also the rather delicate balance of African food supplies was upset. The result was the depopulation and economic decline from which Africa has hardly recovered.

The European penetration also brought to Africa tuberculosis, measles, syphilis, but on the other hand allowed diseases such as yellow fever, and hookworm (*Necator americanus*) to spread to the New World (Ackerknecht, 1965).

The other important historical event was the partition and colonization of Africa by the states of Europe. This "scramble for Africa" started in the second half of the nineteenth century, but was intensified after the Berlin Conference of 1884 when the "rules for partition" were agreed to. By 1914 only Ethiopia and Liberia remained free of colonial rule. There were two distinct types of colony depending on climate and other conditions suitable for European life—the "colonies of settlement" mainly in Southern Central and Eastern Africa, and the "colonies of exploitation" to the north and west (Boateng, 1978).

The partition of Africa was not a peaceful taking over of a continent. There was resistance in many places and the European powers had to make alliances with indigenous States. The times were brutal and population movements continued with obviously undesirable effects on the health of those involved. "With the apparent partial exception of West Africa, the unhealthiest period in all African history was undoubtedly between 1890 and 1930" (Hartwig and Patterson, 1978).

3 Africa after Decolonization 1960–

The partition of Africa succeeded in creating over fifty-five national States with political boundaries hardly corresponding to natural ecological zones or even to ethnic and cultural boundaries. This has led to civil unrest and tremendous social and political upheavals. It has also led to the sudden movement of millions of rural Africans who were fleeing from their homelands and seeking refuge in adjoining neighbouring countries. It is estimated that at present there are about four million refugees in Africa (Komba, 1979). The sudden movement of peoples from their countries does not enhance their health status. There are many refugee camps in many parts of Africa where health conditions are very poor indeed.

One must of course mention the forces which are also working in the direction of uniting Africa in activities that enhance the development of the economic and social life of her people. These organizations also have direct health aims. Some of these are the Organization of African Unity (OAU) and United Nations bodies such as the World Health Organization (WHO), United Nations Children's Fund (UNICEF), Food and Agriculture Organization (FAO), etc. These have, over the years since their founding, played an active role in encouraging the development of health services and programmes that influence the health status of the peoples of Africa.

C. Demographic Factors

The study of African demography is a relatively recent phenomenon. Data before the second half of the twentieth century are scarce and not very reliable. The consensus among experts is that between the sixth and nineteenth centuries, from descriptions of visitors like the Arabs Ibn Batuta, and early European visitors, the population was in equilibrium but that this was subsequently disturbed by the slave trade and the European penetration of Africa. Kuczynski (1944) estimated that the sub-Saharan African population was the same as it was 200 years previously.

The dynamics of the population of Africa is now receiving considerable attention. The high morbidity and mortality rates relate to what McDermott (1969) termed the "core" pattern of diseases or the disease substrate related to poverty, ignorance in the "overly traditional society"—mainly affecting young children and mothers—and the "local overlay" of vector-borne and macroparasitic diseases, which in Africa among all the continents are of such dire consequences. The mortality in Africa today is higher than that experienced by Europe in the middle of the eighteenth century, i.e. just prior to the European industrial development (Condé, 1971).

The pattern and causes of death in Africa differ sharply from that of technically advanced societies. One-third of deaths in the African population in general are due to infective and parasitic diseases; but in children under five years of age, three-quarters of deaths are due to infections. Infant mortality rates of 150–200 per 1000 live births are still common, and mortality in children from 1–4 years may be 20 to 50 times higher than in the developed world. Of course there are differentials within the same region and even within the same countries which are tremendous. For instance, the infant mortality rate in northern Ghana in 1969 (Gaisie, 1969) was 208 per 1000 live births but it was only 52 in the urbanized capital, Accra.

Fertility rates in Africa are among the highest currently known, but again there are regional differences, the highest rates being found in West Africa, Sudan and Zambia (50 per 1000), the lower rates in Central Africa, with East Africa, South Africa and Madagascar in between. The differences in fertility rates have been ascribed by Bourgeois-Pichat (1965) to differences in what he termed the expectation of fertile life in African women.

In the past fifty years there has been a steady decline of mortality rates due mainly to the intervention of medical science but this has scarcely affected fertility rates in sub-Saharan Africa. Okonjo (1978) estimated that in 1975 the population of Africa was 400 million. It is expected that the rate of population growth will increase from an average of 2.77% (1975–80) to 2.88% (1985–90) and decline to 2.77% by the year 2000. This is because fertility is expected to remain high and will perhaps only fall to 39% by the year 2000. The African population will remain as young as it has been with about 45% under fifteen years of age, compared to a world average of 36%.

Another feature of the African population is the tremendous migratory pressure on the towns and cities. In 1975 24.4% of the African population lived in urban communities but this is expected to reach 37.7% by the year 2000, i.e. from 70 million urban dwellers to 208 million, a threefold increase in 25 years. The health problems of sprawling shanty towns are serious and increasing.

This is not surprising because of the failure to bring about equitable social and economic development in most African countries, which in health terms is signified by the great differential between rural and urban mortality—a reversal of the situation in Europe during the industrial revolution.

Another demographic problem important to health is the migration of able-bodied young men from impoverished countries to seek work as miners—in Southern and Central Africa—or as miners or farmers in West Africa.

D. Developments in Health

The encounter between Europe and Africa from the fifteenth century was generally traumatic to both European and African health.

Malaria and yellow fever, dysentery and other forms of febrile illness took a heavy toll of life. This was especially true of the West Coast of Africa which became known as the white man's grave with very good reason; what was not realized then was that it was and has largely remained the African child's grave as well.

The development of the response to African health problems may be divided into five major phases or aspects. Most of these overlap and they have each influenced the other phases in their evolution. These are:

The traditional phase of African medicine
The period of early traders, explorers and slavers
The Christian missionary phase
The colonial phase
The post-colonial phase

The evolution of medical services has depended on the discoveries of the medical and biological sciences, the development of new drugs and techniques of health care and the general social and economic changes which have occurred over the face of Africa, particularly in the past 100 years. There were also the differing political and social viewpoints of the European colonizing powers.

1 Traditional Medicine

The health beliefs, attitudes and practices of the peoples of Africa have of course had an immense influence on the health status of the continent. It is clear, however, that the large majority of the peoples of Africa have not been touched much by the major advances of science and technology that have influenced social and economic as well as health status developments in Europe or America over the past 500 years. Traditional African medicine and health care persists all over the continent today and there is a great need not only to intensify research into herbal medicine but also into the old systems of health care and the many types of health providers. Among these are herbalists and healers who deal with spirits (magic, juju), as well as bone-setters, blood-letters and inoculators of smallpox (noted by Mungo Park in the Gambia) (Schram, 1971).

In Swaziland there are herbalists and diviners. The herbalists give enemas, purges, poultices, steambaths, set limbs, chant spells and suck objects from the body. The diviners still hold seances to discover evildoers as they did in ancient times (Pielemeier, 1975).

In many parts of Africa healers recognized the connection between some insect vectors such as the tsetse fly and disease, the fact that smallpox was contagious, and that some areas of land were dangerous to the health of man. Smallpox was so feared that cults arose in western Africa, e.g. the Shopona cult of the Yoruba and Akotia cult in Accra (Schram, 1971). Whenever epidemics broke out supplications were made to the gods.

Sometimes the traditional remedies were brutal or dangerous—for instance the drinking of cow's urine in parts of Nigeria as a remedy for convulsions. This causes pulmonary congestion and death in many children.

In Ethiopia some harmful practices include uvulectomies, gum cutting and the pulling of back teeth of infants for the treatment of diarrhoea (Britanak *et al.*, 1974). The application of old butter to the umbilical cord of newborns frequently led to neonatal tetanus. Phillips (1965) reported the use of certain herbal eye remedies for treating measles eye infections, which on examination were found to be infected concoctions with pH 10.0.

In many African communities there is still a fatalism about illness, and in most rural communities patients might still consult traditional healers before visiting a modern clinic. As an aside one might note that the traditional explanation for mental illness, and the community's involvement with the mentally ill person might have been contributory to the relative efficiency of traditional therapy (Menes, 1976).

Traditional medicine has been rather resistant to European influences except perhaps in the field of midwifery in which for over the past fifty years there have been many and increasing attempts to bring the traditional birth attendant into the fold of modern midwifery. For the past ten years there has been an insistence among medical scientists and sociologists for a closer examination of the practice of traditional medicine with a view to its integration in its positive aspects with modern practice (World Health Organization, 1976b).

Traditional medical practice is still very alive and is actively accepted by about 70% of the African people—mainly those living in the rural sector. This is due in part to that group's remoteness from medical care.

2 The Early European Explorer and Trader Phase

In the fifteenth century European medicine was not much different from Arabic medicine as practised in old Mali. The aetiology of many diseases was a puzzle to most European physicians who ventured into Africa with the many explorers, traders or slavers.

Even before the turn of the fifteenth century European explorers were reporting the many dangerous febrile and dysenteric diseases which took a great toll of lives because foreigners had no resistance to them. Many of the early visits were made by naval personnel accompanied by surgeons, as well as by persons interested in trade of all types— gold, ivory, slaves. The Portugese came first under the exploratory and missionary zeal of Prince Henry the Navigator. By 1448 the Portugese had set up trading posts on Arquin Bay on the island of Sao Thome. In 1482 they had set up the famous trading fort, or castle, at Elmina, Ghana, for a lucrative trade in gold. Then of course many sailors from other countries in Europe followed—the English, the Dutch, the French, etc.

Of medical importance were the early descriptions of tropical fevers and other diseases by slave-trading doctors such as T. Aubrey (who published in 1729 "The Sea-Surgeon, or the "Guinea Man's Vade Mecum"), Paul Isert, 1783–87 in Ghana, Peter Thonning, 1799–1803;

both in the Danish Service (Schram, 1971). Among the most influential writers were Thomas Winterbottom in 1802—"Medical Directions for Use of Navigators and Settlers in Hot Climates"—and James Boyle, who published "A Practical Medico-Historical Account of the Western Coast of Africa" in 1831. Between 1822 and 1830, 1298 white troops out of 1658 who landed in West Africa died and all but 30 were invalided back to Britain.

Differing types of medical care were given to different classes of people—the best available at the time to the soldiers, explorers and traders whom the physicians accompanied; then a survival treatment to the slaves—who the slave doctors had to examine as to their fitness for travel; and lastly an altruistic/paternalistic treatment to Africans for whom many well-meaning doctors tried to care.

A positive effect of the contact with Europe after the discovery of America was the shipment of many types of food crops from Central America and other places to Africa (Dickson, 1969). These included sweet potatoes, guava, red pepper, groundnuts, maize, rice, yam, cocoyam, onions, pineapples, papaya, okra, eggs, tomatoes, and tobacco. The Portugese also brought pigeons, hens, pigs, sheep, and distributed bananas from the East Indies and other places. These were to have a profound effect on nutrition and the food trade in Africa.

3 The Christian Missionary Effort

Christian physicians came to Africa almost as early as the explorers and traders. The Christian missions wanted to spread Christianity and Western civilization in Africa and they realized immediately the need to treat the sick, to establish hospitals and to train Africans to work with them, as an essential part of their Christian strategy. The Catholic missionaries in 1504 founded a hospital on the island of Sao Thome, and in 1507 in Mozambique. Catholic missionary medical work spread to many parts of Africa—Algeria, Tunisia, Central Africa, the Congo, Mozambique, Uganda, West Africa and South Africa. By 1956 there were over 200 Catholic mission hospitals in Africa, and several orphanages, leprosaria, and dispensaries, all under the very active support of the papacy.

The protestant missions came later in the eighteenth century—starting principally in Southern Africa with the Swellendam Leprosarium (1756). The London Missionary Society also brought David Livingstone, who became the most influential of the missionary doctor-explorers in South, Central and East Africa from 1841 to 1873.

From 1840 the Church Missionary Society (CMS) had physicians who set up in Sierra Leone and ten years later in Nigeria. The Nigerian

Mission flourished—opening up hospitals, and dispensaries. The CMS also started medical work in East Africa, founding a fifty-bed hospital in Mombasa in 1893, and a leper colony soon after. In the Sudan the Mission started a hospital at Omdurman in 1900 (Squires, 1958).

The University Mission to Central Africa was a direct result of Livingstone's advocacy for work in the Shire Highlands in Central Africa. Baptist missionaries worked in the Belgian Congo, the Basel Mission in Ghana, and the Wesleyan Methodist Missionary Society founded Ilesha Hospital in 1912. In that year also, Dr Albert Schweitzer set up his world-famous hospital in Lambrene.

Another important aspect of the medical influence of the Christian missions is in the training of health workers. For obvious reasons, on-the-job training of Africans was inevitable at all the hospitals. At the Victoria Hospital at Lovedale, South Africa, which started in 1841, the dual objectives were the healing of the sick and the training of African nurses, attendants and dispensers (Hailey, 1957). In 1917, in Uganda, Sir Albert Cook and his brother started a medical school at Mengo Hospital. This faltered and after a second attempt was taken over by the Government to become the Medical School at Mulago. In 1918 Lady Cook started the first Ugandan Nursing School at Mengo Hospital (Foster, 1970).

In 1893 the CMS founded Livingstone Medical College in London for training lay missionaries in medical care and hygiene so that they could be more useful to the communities they were going to serve. This was a most practical step both in helping the indigenes and for survival in the often harsh environments.

The achievements of Christian missionary medical effort in Africa over the past 500 years in healing the sick, in the teaching of the precepts of hygiene, and in the training of Africans in health work is inestimable. This effort still continues in many African countries but inevitably the development of national health services has gradually overshadowed the size of their contribution.

4 The Colonial Medical Establishment

The European powers originally began by protecting their trading companies with military forces, and it was the military doctors who took care of the European traders and soldiers and later their African collaborators. As they settled down in particular communities by treaty or "pacification" the influence of the settlements extended. Gradually the parent governments in Europe formalized things and set up colonial governments.

Hospitals were set up and physicians were specially appointed to take care of the "natives". There were divergencies among the various European nationalities in the evolution of health systems. These policies depended upon the nature of the problems of the particular territories and the attitude of the colonizing power to the indigenes.

In general it can be said that the British concentrated on the building of hospitals though of course some public health measures were also undertaken. As soon as it was practicable civilian doctors took over from military surgeons. There was also much co-operation with the missionary medical workers.

The French on the other hand allowed army physicians to run the health service, although from 1905 the French Ministry of the Colonies tried unsuccessfully to turn over the health system to civilian physicians (Janssens, 1971). It was said that "the French tackled the battle for health as a military operation" (Menes, 1976). They maintained only a few strategically sited high-class hospitals, and used them as bases for taking curative and preventive medicine to the surrounding countryside. From this developed the mobile system of epidemic control, which most countries in Africa copied. Another point of difference with the British system was the French disregard for missionary medical collaboration, which impeded the development of missionary medicine in French Africa (Janssens, 1971).

The Belgian administration relied on hospitals and collaboration with the religious orders. Their system emphasized the intensive circumscribed investigation treatment of endemic diseases in successive areas of a country. The Government was also very interested in the health of labourers especially those working in the mining concerns and ensured that the companies provided good care. By the time of Zairean independence, Belgium had built up one of the most extensive health systems in Africa, but the fatal flaw was its heavy dependence on European health workers at practically all levels. The system collapsed at independence when the Belgians were forced to withdraw hastily in 1960. There was not a single Zairean physician trained (Lashman, 1975).

There was some degree of compulsion upon the indigenous populations in French and Belgian territories in the fight against epidemics, in respect of immunizations which were made compulsory, and in the issuing of passes for people moving from one part of a country to another.

The years from the end of the nineteenth century to the middle of the twentieth century (just before the independence of many African territories) were years of steady expansion in four main areas. These were:

The development of hospitals, clinics and dispensaries of all types
The intensification of research into endemic and parasitic diseases and the application of public health measures to contain them
The training of Africans in the various categories of health work
The development of efforts to change health habits among the population

III. The Fight Against Endemic and Epidemic Disease

Janssens (1971) is of the opinion that the origin of public health services coincided with the introduction of smallpox vaccination in these colonial territories. It is equally true that the most arresting disease problem which galvanized European medicine into a massive public health effort was the sleeping sickness epidemic of Busoga in Uganda in 1901 and in other African territories (Hailey, 1957). Pasteur's proposal of the germ theory of disease set in motion much fundamental research in microbiology and parasitology. Some of the greatest scientists of the day such as Dr R. Koch travelled to Africa to set up research stations (Scott, 1939).

The development of the production of vaccines was another impetus. The problems of transporting smallpox vaccine led to the setting up of vaccine institutes, particularly in French Africa. These were to develop into important research institutes, e.g. Institutes Pasteur at Boma (1894), Tananarive, Madagascar (1898), St Louis, Senegal (1897—moved to Dakar in 1913), Morocco (1911), Brazzaville (1911), Bamako (1907). Other research institutes were the South African Institute of Medical Research at Johannesburg (1912), and those at Lubumbashi (1913), Gitega (1920), Accra (1920), Freetown (1921), and Kindia (1922) (UNESCO, 1970).

Research by the colonizing powers was directed mainly to endemic and parasitic disease of the tropics. This led to the founding of schools or institutes of tropical medicine, e.g. those at Liverpool and London (1899), at Hamburg (1900), at Lisbon and Brussels (1961), and at Leiden, Amsterdam and Antwerp (1933) (Janssens, 1971). These schools trained physicians for work in the tropics, and carried out research in tropical diseases both in their schools and in the field through expeditions.

Scientific expeditions became very important, even fashionable, as daring scientists tried to grapple with the grave epidemic and endemic disease problems of Africa at the turn of the 19th century. The diseases which attracted the greatest notice at the time were trypanosomiasis (sleeping sickness), yellow fever, smallpox and malaria (Janssens, 1971).

"Sleeping sickness was to Africa what bubonic plague was to Europe" (Schram, 1971). The spread of this disease coincided with the opening up of the continent. It is estimated that 500 000 deaths occurred in the Congo and 200 000 in the Busoga epidemic of 1901–08 in Uganda (Hailey, 1957). The vector, the tsetse fly, is widely distributed in tropical Africa—in areas with well-watered vegetation but also in grassland areas not far from wooded land where there is game. May (1961) put the case most poignantly when he wrote: "This disease is of great importance and has played a considerable role in keeping Central Africa in its present state of backwardness." He also thought that it was entirely possible that the small contribution of the people of Africa towards the arts in general and literature in particular and their inability to raise their living standards above the most primitive level has been directly or indirectly related to their relationship with this parasite.

The disease decimated whole populations, lowered fertility rates and caused the migration of communities to safer areas which then became crowded and helped this and other diseases to spread. These migrations severly affected animal husbandry and agriculture—and hence the nutritional status of the people concerned.

The great concern about this disease led to the interest of the colonizing powers in public health measures, especially in epidemic disease control. In 1904 the French declared the existence of a "state of imminent danger" to public health (Hailey, 1957). This attitude influenced the development of health services in the countries under the French. Schram (1971) quotes a 1912 recommendation by Aubert and Heckenrodt proposing systematic medical touring of areas, and in 1916 the French Equatorial African Health Council organized mobile health services, to which the French Parliament responded by voting one million francs annually for medical assistance. This eventually led to the gradual containment of sleeping sickness and some other epidemic diseases. When a resurgence of sleeping sickness occurred in 1944 the French developed the Service Général d'Hygiene Mobile et de Prophylaxie (SGHMP) with headquarters in Bobo Dioulaso in Upper Volta. Between 1950 and 1952 10 366 680 persons were examined and 21 792 new cases of sleeping sickness found and treated (Hailey, 1957). Serious and arseno-resistant cases were sent to sleeping sickness hospitals or "hypnosaries". In 1948 there were eighty-two hypnosaries with 9568 patients in French West Africa and seven with 598 patients in Togo. From 1946 onwards, pentamidine became the main chemoprophylactic agent (Simmons *et al.*, 1951).

The Belgian Colonial Government did the same type of work, and, like the French, concentrated on case-finding, treatment and prophylaxis in endemic foci—"pentamidinization".

The British developed medical field units, but their bias was towards vector control. The most ambitious was the Anchau Scheme in Northern Nigeria in which 600 square miles of territory 60 to 70 miles in length was rendered tsetse-free and by 1946, 50 000 persons had been settled in an integrated development scheme (Hailey, 1957).

In the Volta River Basin of West Africa over one million people have onchocerciasis. Of these 70 000 are blind and another 30 000 have partial vision (Onchocerciasis Control Programme, 1973). Onchocerciasis or river blindness is a scourge of Sahelian West Africa. Since the riverine valleys are the more fertile, this disease competes with man, eventually driving him out to higher, less well-watered and less fertile terrain. The disease has wiped out many villages and caused people to flee to other parts of West Africa. This has led to untold suffering and greatly hindered agricultural progress and hence the economic development. The creation of irrigation canals has improved the breeding chances of the blackfly, where formerly there might have been a small focus. This happened dramatically in Loumana village in Upper Volta in 1955 when 15 km^2 of rice paddy were developed. Onchocerciasis increased rapidly, nearly obliterating the settlement. The use of insecticides prevented the worst from happening. DDT and other insecticides had been tried successfully in eradication at the more localized *Simulium naevi* foci in Kenya in the Kodera area of South Kavirondo. Insecticides were also effective in reducing the incidence of the disease in the Kinshasa area of Zaire by spraying breeding sites of *S. damnosum* by helicopter, twenty-five years ago (Williams, 1974).

Yellow fever caused thousands of deaths in both Africans and Europeans. In 1910 Sir Rupert Boyce was sent from London to help fight a serious epidemic in Sierra Leone and Ghana (Duff, 1933). The saga of the Rockefeller Yellow Fever Commission in Africa is well known. Hideyo Noguchi, the famous Japanese scientist, mistakenly thought yellow fever was caused by the *Leptospira icteriodes*; he died tragically of the disease in Accra in May 1928 (Scott, 1965). Now fifty years later the Japanese Government is establishing a medical research institute in Ghana in his memory. Yellow fever has been largely controlled through immunization, and through attempts to control the urban vector, the mosquito *Aedes aegypti*. Since it is a zoonotic disease in which the cycle is maintained in forest-living primates, men who work in these forests in various occupations are liable to contact the disease and spread it to human settlements (see also Stanley, this volume).

The major endemic diseases to which a great deal of attention has been paid by most sub-Saharan countries of Africa include schistosomiasis, smallpox, leprosy, yellow fever, malaria, yaws, and since 1971, cholera (El Tor). Like sleeping sickness and river blindness, these attempts initially have taken the vertical one disease approach and have yielded very good results except in the case of malaria.

Yaws was also controlled spectacularly in the 1950s through the use of penicillin; but its recent resurgence in parts of Africa indicates the basic weakness of the health care system in Africa—its lack of coverage, its shortage of resources, its relatively poor management procedures in the face of a population still woefully lacking in basic health knowledge.

Malaria is the most serious, pervasive and costly disease by far in Africa, particularly in tropical Africa. Over the centuries it has caused untold morbidity and mortality and is thought to be the ecological force behind the genetic change in haemoglobin, leading to the sickle cell and other haemoglobin diseases in an evolutionary effort in man in Africa to achieve a balanced polymorphism (Allison, 1975). It, and possibly the other major mosquito-borne disease, yellow fever, prevented any major colonization of West Africa by Europeans.

In the first two decades of this century Europeans in malarious districts in Africa reluctantly took to screens and mosquito netting when it was noted that most gametocytes (i.e. in the form that is sucked by the mosquito and undergoes the cycle of change in the mosquito) are prevalent in young children. European communities in Africa started segregating themselves from the indigenous population. African children were not allowed into the white areas.

By the end of the colonial era in Africa great gains had been made in the control of many endemic and parasitic diseases through the public health services. There was also modest to fairly substantive health infrastructural development in most African countries. Many of the doctors and senior health workers were from the metropolitan countries, although the more economically advanced states had increasing numbers of senior health personnel who were indigenes.

There was segregation of health facilities for whites, Asians and Africans. Kenya in 1953 (Hailey, 1957) had 101 hospitals with 7270 beds for Africans, 10 hospitals for Asians, and 12 for Africans. In the Belgian Congo in 1952 there were ninety-two European hospitals and 1916 hospitals, clinics and dispensaries for Africans, with 46 333 beds.

IV. Post-Colonial Health Developments

In general most of the new states formed in the 1960s tried to maintain the systems of health care bequeathed to them from the colonial era.

Factors that have influenced further developments of the health system and health status are related to economic and social developments and population growth. One must especially take into account the most massive rural to urban migration in the history of the continent.

Twenty years after independence it is clear that many African countries have not made much progress in economic terms. The GNP in most countries is still under US$400 but in many it is even less than US$200 *per capita*. Of the twenty-nine least developed countries in the world, sixteen were in the African region in 1976 (World Bank, 1978). The percentage of national budgets spent on health ranges from 4–14%. The *per capita* expenditure on health ranges from less than US$1 to US$10 p.a. (World Health Organization, 1974).

Although progress in education shows substantial gains, still only 20% of the population are literate. In many countries 20% or less of school-age children attend school. The gains made in many countries, however, have allowed a virtual explosion of personnel who can and are being trained in the health services. Unfortunately, with the substantial urban migration, most of the best-educated workers (70% of them) prefer to remain to cater to the needs of the 20% urban population. The progress made in health education and in changes in health behaviour have hardly touched the rural poor.

Another major factor is the inability of Africa to feed itself. FAO (1979) reported that from the records of forty-four countries in Africa, twenty-six countries in 1975 produced *per capita* less food than those countries produced in the years 1961–65. The situation has deteriorated since the 1960s. So Africa is a net importer of food—this in spite of the fact that 80% of the population are rural and 70% are engaged in agricultural pursuits. Bailey (1975) reported on the food and nutrition situation in Africa. He wrote that malnutrition was rampant because of famines (droughts) and seasonal food shortages as well as changing food habits especially in the large and growing urban slums in Africa; 30% of children were moderately underweight and 4% suffered from severe protein-energy malnutrition. It must be realized that he was writing of 60 million children, and six million children under five years of age respectively. Adults also undergo seasonal weight changes.

Deficiencies of iron and vitamin A and B groups are common and there is endemic goitre. Malnutrition in children adds substantially to their burdens of infection (see also Gracey, this volume).

Africa is also well behind in the provision of a clean water supply and hygienic excreta disposal. In the urban areas 27 million people or 66% have mains connections of water to their houses (37%) and the rest obtain water from public stand pipes. In rural Africa in 1975 only 21% (41 million) had access to clean water supplies. Seventy-five per cent of people in urban Africa (30 million) have adequate faecal disposal arrangements. Fifteen per cent have water closets. Only 28% or 55 million people in rural Africa have acceptable excreta disposal systems (World Health Organization, 1976c).

It is therefore not surprising that diarrhoeal diseases are among the major killers, in particular of children. In 1971 when El Tor cholera struck Africa, seventeen countries became rapidly affected and reported 42 866 cases. Presently El Tor cholera has assumed an endemic nature on the African continent—ready to assume epidemic status when national vigilance is lowered (World Health Organization, 1975). After independence the emphasis shifted to hospital construction in the urban areas in most countries. This increased health care costs without increasing coverage, and at the same time it upset programmes in preventive medicine. In 1971 the health worker population ratios were: doctors 1 : 17 500; nurses 1 : 6000; midwives 1 : 17 000; sanitarians 1 : 37 500; technicians 1 : 62 000; sanitary engineers 1 : 2 370 000 (World Health Organization, 1976a).

In the area of endemic and parasitic disease control, most of the progress made since independence in many countries has depended on outside bilateral or multilateral assistance—in the control of onchocerciasis, measles, malnutrition, smallpox—through agencies such as the WHO, UNICEF, World Bank, United States Agency for International Development (USAID), Swedish International Development Authority (SIDA), Canadian International Development Agency (CIDA), and of the former colonial powers.

Malaria continues to affect over 100 million persons causing 800 000 deaths p.a.—75% of which are in children under five years of age (see also Zulueta, this volume). Smallpox, on the other hand, is thought to have been eradicated from Africa through one of the most spectacular prophylactic programmes of health care of all time (see also Fenner, this volume). It is still considered necessary to remain vigilant towards a disease which has caused great mortality in Africa (Quenum, 1977). Since 1966 entomological research has been carried out by the inter-country organization—Organisation de Coopération contre les

Grandes Endemies (OCCGE)—in French West Africa. Encouraged by the preliminary results of the research, the World Bank, WHO and other agencies of the United Nations, USAID and the European Economic Community (EEC) have decided to spend at least US$120 000 000 in a twenty year programme of research and control of *Simulium damnosum* in the Volta Basin area covering 700 000 km^2 in seven countries in West Africa, initially (Mali, Upper Volta, Niger, Ivory Coast, Ghana, Togo and Dahomey) (Onchocerciasis Control Programme, 1973). This is the greatest one-disease control programme ever undertaken in Africa and it is hoped that it would be possible for the cost to repay itself many times over if successful.

Gradually the fact of population increase is being realized and a few countries have official programmes in family planning such as Kenya, Mauritius and Ghana, but many more countries are now allowing programmes in family planning. The health problems of mothers and children are being tackled more seriously than ever before, thanks mainly to help from international organizations.

Another significant development is in the area of manpower development. Before 1960 there were only four medical schools in sub-Saharan Africa. Now practically every country has a medical school, and some such as Nigeria have eight and are developing more. Other health-training institutions are being opened all over Africa to train nurses, midwives, sanitarians, pharmacists, radiographers and health auxiliaries.

There is great interest in medical research and since 1960 at least 30 medical research institutes or centres have been started in Africa with a view to studying endemic and other important local diseases. Interest in health services research is great and there are many pilot projects being run by medical schools and health agencies to study rural health problems, e.g. at Igbo-Ora in Nigeria; Khombole in Senegal; Ankole in Uganda; Kasongo in Zaire, and Kintampo and Danfa in Ghana. The WHO Special Programme in Research and Training in Tropical Disease (World Health Organization, 1976a) is reawakening interest in African medical schools in tropical diseases.

The major anxiety in African health thinking now is about how to reach the rural poor with appropriate health services in the face of near-stagnant economic growth and a population rapidly increasing in numbers (Quenum, 1979). At the WHO Regional Meeting in Kigali in 1978 it was stated that 290 million, or 80% of the African population lacked basic medical care, and that until recently the major thrust had been to imitate the high technology models of the industrialized countries (World Health Organization, 1978).

Many African countries are interested in changing direction in the provision of health services—towards increased coverage, increased community participation—through carefully made national health plans. Primary health care is the leading idea (World Health Organization, 1978).

Greater co-operation in health among the countries in the region gives hope that useful ideas gained from different countries will be more easily adopted in other African countries in contrast to the earlier attitude of looking to models from the developed world.

V. Conclusion

In this brief survey of some of the ecological and historical factors which have determined the experience of Africa in health, it is clear that there has been great progress, especially during the colonial era, in the overcoming of major epidemic and endemic diseases, but that the disease burden in Africa is still very great. Possibly more so than in any continent, medical science—both preventive and curative—has and can still play a very significant role in development of the social and economic well-being of the peoples of Africa.

References

Ackerknecht, E. H. (1965). "History and Geography of the Most Important Diseases". Hafner, New York.

Allison, A. C. (1975). *In* "Man-made Lakes and Human Health" (N. F. Stanley and M. P. Alpers, Eds), 401–426. Academic Press, London and New York.

Bailey, K. V. (1975). *Wld Hlth Org. Chron.* **29**, 354–364.

Boateng, E. A. (1978). "A Political Geography of Africa". Cambridge Univ. Press.

Bourgeois-Pichat, J. (1965). *In* "Man and Africa", (G. E. W. Wolstenholme and M. O'Connor, Eds), 65–97. Ciba Foundation Symposium. Churchill, London.

Britanak, R. A., Davies, J. H. and Daly, J. A. (1974).

"Syncrisis", Vol. VIII: "Ethiopia: The Dynamics of Health". US Department of Health, Education and Welfare, Washington, DC.

Condé, J. (1971). "The Demographic Transition as Applied to Tropical Africa". OECD, Paris.

Dekker, G. (1965). *In* "Man and Africa", G. E. W. Wolstenholme and M. O'Connor, Eds), 30–64. Ciba Foundation Symposium. Churchill, London.

Dickson, K. B. (1969). "A Historical Geography of Ghana" Cambridge Univ. Press.
Duff, D. (1933). "Annual Medical and Health Report". Government Printer, Gold Coast.
Fage, J. D. (1964). *In* "Encyclopaedia Britannica", Vol. I, 294–302. Univ. of Chicago Press.
Food and Agriculture Organization (1979). *In* "The State of Food and Agriculture 1978". FAO Agriculture Series No. 9, Rome.
Ford, J. (1966). *In* "Human Ecology in the Tropics" (J. P. Garlich and R. W. J. Keay, Eds), 81–97. Pergamon Press, Oxford.
Foster, W. D. (1970). "The Early History of Scientific Medicine in Uganda". East African Literature Bureau, Nairobi.
Gaisie, S. K. (1969). "Estimates of Vital Rates for Ghana", Population Studies, Vol. 23, No. 1, 21–42.
Hailey, W. M. (1957). "An African Survey". Oxford Univ. Press.
Hance, W. A. (1958). "African Economic Development". Harper, New York.
Hartwig, G. W. and Patterson, K. D. (Eds) (1978). "Disease in African History". Duke Univ. Press.
Janssens, P. G. (1971). *Trans. R. Soc. trop. Med. Hyg.* **65** Suppl., s2-s15.
Kimble, G. H. T. (1960). "Tropical Africa", Vol. II. Twentieth Century Fund, New York.
Komba, M. (1979). *Africa, London* **94**, 27–28.
Kuczyunski, R. R. (1944). "The Demographic Transition as Applied to Tropical Africa". OECD, Paris. Quoted by J. Condé (1971).
Lashman, K. E. (1975). "Syncrisis", Vol. XIV: "Zaire". US Department of Health, Education and Welfare, Washington, D.C.
Last, G. C. (1965). *In* "Man and Africa" (G. E. W. Wolstenholme and M. O'Connor, eds), pp. 6–23. Ciba Foundation Symposium. Churchill, London.
McDermott, W. (1969). *In* "Human Ecology and Public Health" (E. D. Kilbourne and W. G. Smillie, Eds), 4th edn, 7–28. Macmillan, London.
May, J. (1961). "Studies in Disease Ecology". Hafner, New York.
Menes, R. J. (1976). "Syncrisis", Vol. XIX: "Senegal". US Department of Health, Education and Welfare, Washington, DC.
Nortman, D. L. and Hofstatter, E. (1978). "Population and Family Planning Program", 9th edn. Population Council, New York.
Okonjo, C. (1978). *In* "The Physician and Population Change" (L. S. Block, Ed), 4–26. World Federation for Medical Education, Bethesda, Md.
Onchocerciasis Control Programme (1973). OCP/73.1. Onchocerciasis Control Programme, WHO, Geneva.
Phillips, C. M. (1965). *In* "Science and Medicine in Central Africa" (G. J. Snowball, Ed), 13–30. Pergamon Press, Oxford.
Pielemeir, N. R. (1975). "Syncrisis", Vol. XIII: "Botswana, Lesotho and Swaziland". U.S. Department of Health, Education and Welfare, Washington, D.C.

Quenum, C. A. A. (1977). Report of the Regional Director to the 27th Annual Meeting of the WHO Regional Committee for Africa. AFR/RC 27/3. Brazzaville.
Quenum, C. A. A. (1979). Report of the Regional Director to the 29th Annual Meeting of the WHO Regional Committee for Africa. AFR/RC 29/3. Brazzaville.
Schram, R. (1971). "A History of the Nigerian Health Services". Ibadan Univ. Press.
Scott, D. (1965). "Epidemic Disease in Ghana 1901–1960". Oxford Univ. Press.
Scott, H. H. (1939). "A History of Tropical Medicine", 2 vols. Arnold, London.
Simmons, J. S., Whayne, T. F., Anderson, G. W., Horack, H. M., Thomas, R. A. (associate author) and collaborators. (1951). "Global Epidemiology", Vol. 2. Lippincott, Philadelphia.
Squires, H. C. (1958). "The Sudan Medical Services". Heinemann, London.
United Nations Educational, Scientific and Cultural Organization (1970). "Survey on the Scientific and Technical Potential of Countries of Africa". UNESCO, Paris.
Williams, J. (1974). *The Geographical Magazine*, London **47**, 78–82.
World Bank (1978). "World Bank Atlas". Washington, DC.
World Health Organization (1974). "Demographic, Socio-economic and Health Situation in the African Region. Reference Data of July 1973". WHO AFR/VHS/53.
World Health Organization (1975). *Wld Hlth Org. Chron.* **29**, 29–30.
World Health Organization (1976a). *Wld Hlth Org. Chron.* **30**, 2–42.
World Health Organization (1976b). "African Traditional Medicine". Afro Technical Report Series No. 1, Brazzaville.
World Health Organization (1976c). "World Health Statistics Report", Vol. 29, No. 10.
World Health Organization (1978). *Wld Hlth Org. Chron.* **32**, 409–447.

18

The Inverse Care Law in Papua New Guinea

Anthony J. Radford
Department of Primary Care and Community Medicine, Flinders University of South Australia, Adelaide, Australia

Authorities who are responsible for the provision of services in developing countries frequently take little notice of differences between providers and users.

I. Introduction

In 1971 Tudor Hart used "The Inverse Care Law" to describe the relationship between the degree of real need for health services and the provision and availability of such services (See Figs 1 and 2).

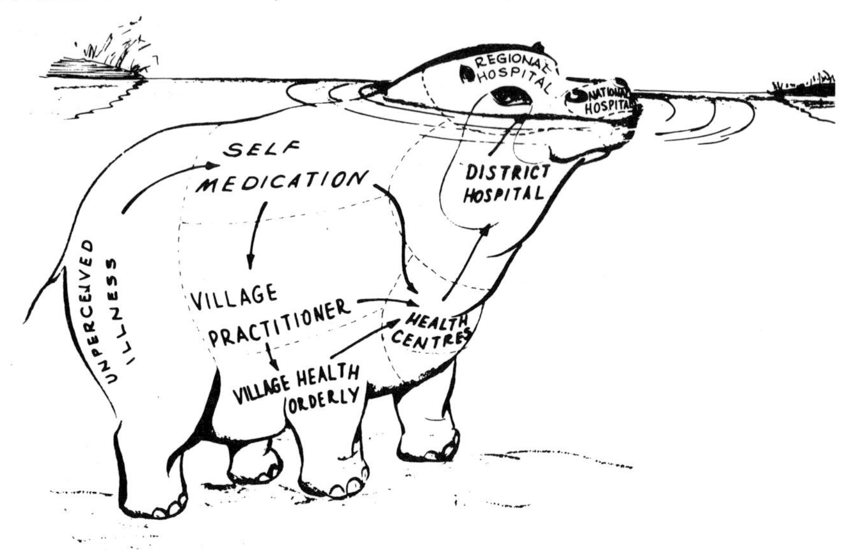

Fig. 1. Distribution of illness. (From Radford, 1978.)

The factors which determine what services a community receives are related not only to geographical features such as distance, but also to the social environments of political demand and expediency, professional pressures, customs and beliefs as well as the nature of the development process. These factors also determine variations in disease patterns (see Table I).

TABLE I. *Difference in Hospital Mortality by Region in Papua New Guinea*

Highlands	Islands
Pneumonia	Cancer
Gastroenteritis	Tuberculosis
Meningitis	Pneumonia
Digestive system	Circulatory system disease
Nutritional deficiency	Injuries and accidents

(Source: Bell, 1973)

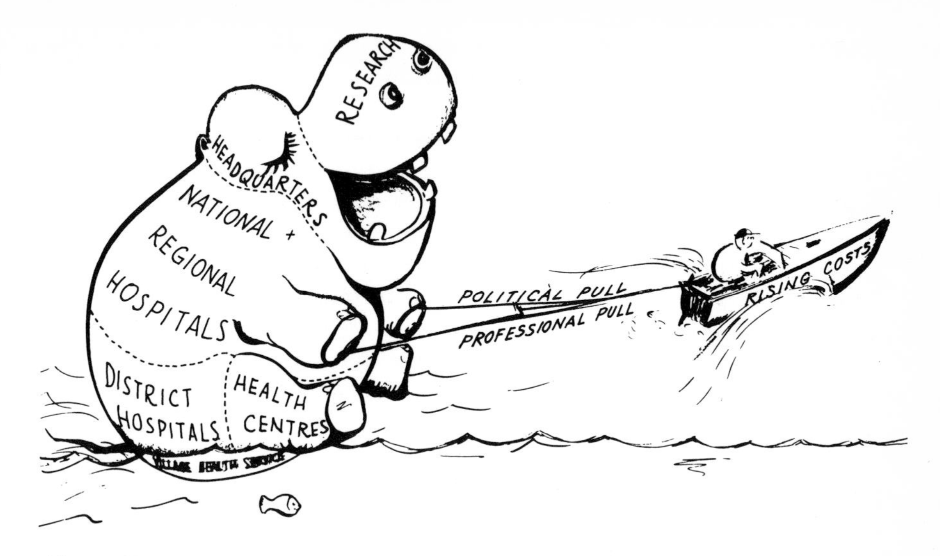

Fig. 2. Distribution and determinants of resource allocation. (From Radford, 1978.)

In 1966 King illustrated different levels in the provision of care by drawing "isocares" around health centres. The exponential fall in the usage of services in relation to distance from a static facility has been described in many places, e.g. in Uganda by King (1966), in India by Frederiksen (1971), in New Guinea by Radford (1972) and in the United States by Geiger (1968). The isocare concept is helpful because distance is perhaps the most significant determinant of health care provision and utilization.

Authorities who are responsible for the provision of services in developing countries frequently take little notice of differences between providers and users, thereby increasing the likelihood of passive avoidance, if not rejection, of most health care transplants. In New Guinea, as in most colonies, services were initially established to protect and care for intruding foreigners, and only later were extended to the indigenous people who settled near the centres of administration. Lastly, for altruistic or, more commonly, for economic reasons, they considered the health needs of the population at large (Essai, 1961; Firth, 1978; Maddocks, 1978). After independence, when nationals take over both medical training and the conduct of services, there has rarely been any attempt to integrate traditional medicine, which most of the population use before consulting the Western-based system. China is a notable exception.

This chapter explores the aetiological factors which the social environments play in disease patterns and service provision in Papua New Guinea.

The bird-shaped island of New Guinea (see Fig. 3) lies between the northern tip of Australia and the equator, and is exceeded in size only by the island continent beneath it and Greenland. A central cordillera of mountains forms an axial skeleton which, until well into this century, locked the most densely populated and largely malaria-free communities of the island from contact with the outside world. The nature of its varied geography has favoured the development of an intense communality, one illustration of which is that more than a quarter of the world's known languages are spoken among its four million inhabitants.

Highland population densities reach up to 700 per km^2. Sweet potatoes and green vegetables form the basis of their diet. Lowland areas include swamps and sinuous river systems populated with sago- and fish-eating people who are settled as sparsely as 1 per km^2. Other coastal and inland areas support yam-, sago- and taro-eating communities with varying degrees of malarial endemicity and with population densities between 50 and 100 per km^2. Although some island complexes include small groups of Micronesians, Polynesians and negritos, the majority of the people are Melanesian. While a small number are foraging rain-forest nomads and a number of the highlanders live in scattered homestead settlements, most live in 15 000 hamlets or villages in groups varying in number from under twenty to over 500. Urbanization is essentially a post-1945 phenomenon and, although growing at between 5% and 10% per annum in recent years, still accounts for under 15% of the total population.

New Guinea's modern political divisions reflect the accidents of international politics in an almost identical fashion to those of the Camerouns in West Africa. The western half was "unified" under the Dutch from 1828 until 1962 when the United Nations held it as a Trust Authority for a few months before it was established as the easternmost Indonesian province of Irian Barat. This chapter is concerned only with the eastern half of the island which in 1884 was divided into north-eastern German New Guinea and southern British New Guinea. The British sector became Australian Papua in 1906. After the Pacific war these two areas were jointly administered by the Australian Government until 1973 when self-government was granted. Independence followed in 1975.

The people of Papua New Guinea have more or less successfully married their essentially animistic approach to life, intimately related

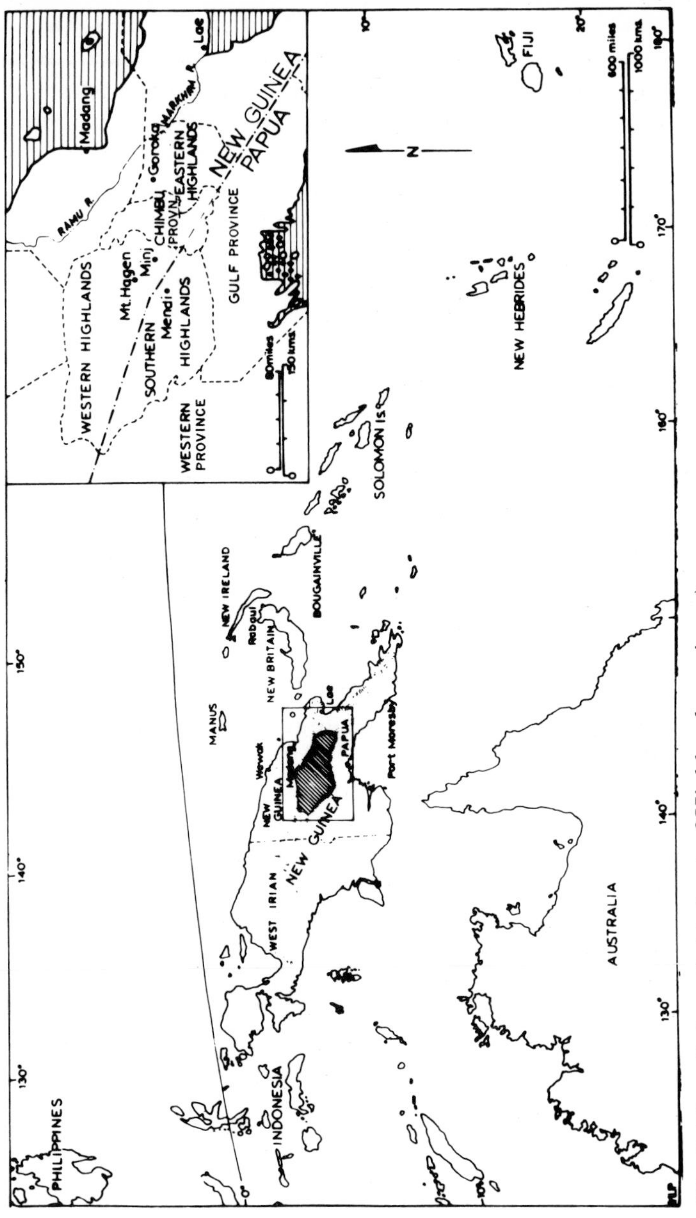

Fig. 3. New Guinea (with inset of Highland provinces).

as it is to the natural and physical environments in which they live, to one or more of the plethora of the Christian denominations. Illness is most commonly believed to be related to disharmony between individuals, with or without the malevolent intervention of an intermediary, or between a person and the supernatural. Some diseases, such as measles, influenza and gonorrhoea, are recognized as concomitants of European contact.

II. Transcultural and Developmental Aspects of Illness and Health

There have been few attempts in New Guinea to recognize traditional care practices or to involve them in the new order of care (for one example see Zigas, 1978) and the result is often a delay or denial of access to effective care. There are two aspects of denial of traditional processes which are particularly unfortunate. The first aspect is that the majority of the causes of illness and death (see Table II) are readily preventable and/or are easily cured with prompt treatment. The second is the lack of recognition that the accepted indigenous practitioner is better able to resolve any interpersonal dysequilibria than is the modern practitioner, be he foreigner or national.

There are extensive home remedy and traditional systems of care throughout Papua New Guinea, although both have been only infrequently described (see bibliography in Hornabrook and Skeldon, 1977; Lewis, 1975). It is usual to obtain access to either or both of these systems before or while seeking more modern care. Occasional pleas to explore ways of integrating traditional concepts with modern approaches to health care delivery have occurred (Watson, 1968; Radford, 1973), and while a ministerial pronouncement was made in 1973 permitting traditional practitioners access to patients in hospitals, few attempts have been made to effect either of these approaches. Nevertheless varying degrees of inpatient contact with traditional healing practices has occurred pari passu with modern medicine, although such ministrations have usually gone on unknown to the majority of expatriate nurses and doctors who staffed the services.

It has sometimes been possible to override or provide an acceptable alternative to traditional processes. The miraculous effects of a single injection of penicillin (and for years before that arsenicals and bismuth) against yaws facilitated the acceptance of injections for immunizations and other therapies. One example of this was the immunization of

TABLE II. *A Comparison of the Leading Causes of Death in Papua New Guinea*[a] *with the United States*[b]

Papua New Guinea 1961/62	USA 1900	USA 1960
1. Pneumonia	Pneumonia	Diseases of the heart
2. Tuberculosis	Tuberculosis	Cancer
3. Nutrition	Diarrhoea	Cerebral haemorrhage
4. Diarrhoea	Diseases of the heart	Accidents
5. Meningitis	Cerebral haemorrhage	Diseases of early infancy
6. Cancer	Nephritis	Pneumonia
7. Malaria	Accidents	Arteriosclerosis
8. Diseases of early infancy	Diseases of early infancy	Diabetes mellitus
9. Accidents	Diphtheria	Congenital malformation
10. Diseases of the heart	Meningitis	Cirrhosis of liver
11. Nephritis		

[a] Selected hospitals, Government Annual Reports.
[b] Hanlon, J. J. (1964). "Principles of Public Health Administration," 4th edn, Mosby, St Louis.

pregnant mothers to preclude neonatal tetanus—a technique which was pioneered in New Guinea (Schofield *et al*., 1961).

An acceptable alternative to traditional taboos against giving fresh meat to children and pregnant women has occurred through the introduction of processed meat and fish. Unfortunately, concentration on expensive and sophisticated technocratic approaches to the preparation of largely unpalatable vegetable protein was temporarily promoted in New Guinea, as it has been elsewhere, rather than seeking ways to increase readily available, cheap and acceptable protein sources such as green-leaved vegetables and soya bean.

The dietary changes of modernization with increased fat intake, decrease in exercise and increase in salt consumption may well see the emergence of coronary heart disease and essential hypertension which have been virtually absent from rural communities (Maddocks and Rovin, 1965; Maddocks, 1967; Sinnett, 1975). The introduction of salt in its non-iodized form led to several thousand cases of goitre and many hundreds of cases endemic cretinism (see review in Hetzel and

Pharoah, 1971). While depot injections of iodized oil enables eradication and prevention of these diseases, and has been a milestone in New Guinea's medical history, the preclusion of importation of non-iodized salt (as is now the case for bulk salt) would have been cheaper, quicker, more extensive and equally effective.

Although the development process brought a considerable increase in services through a breakdown in isolation, development of an improved level of cohesion among some groups, education, agriculture and modern health care, it also has been responsible for the rapid spread of yaws (Radford, 1979), then malaria (Radford *et al.*, 1976), tuberculosis, endemic cretinism (Pharoah and Hornabrook, 1974) venereal disease (Rhodes and Anderson, 1970; Hart, 1974), road accidents, episodic alcoholism and, in towns, new forms of malnutrition. The rapid growth of transport facilities has enabled considerable expansion of cash-cropping and the stocking of stores with large amounts of palatable protein. It is believed that the considerable decline in severe protein-energy malnutrition which occurred in the highlands in the 1960s was more related to this than to specific health education about food crops and diets. Similarly a concentration of school and village nutrition education based on a thorough knowledge of traditional food beliefs and concepts, acceptable introduced new nutrients and working with senior village women is more likely to be effective than those centralized and expensive units being established at the base hospitals for the few that get there.

Research is another area where the Inverse Care Law has been applied. A large number of research projects have been conducted which are of little likely benefit to the inhabitants and which were often of an intrusive nature. More importantly, although an institute for medical research was established in the late 1960s, perusal of its bibliography reveals that, while of great scientific interest, less than 20% of its publications relate to major causes of illness and death. A committee with national representation to vet all research projects was established just before independence and more recently the Institute's programmes have been directed to the more major causes of morbidity and mortality (Pharoah *et al* 1971; Lawrence *et al.*, 1979).

III. Health Services

Health care in Papua New Guinea is sought along any of the lines of access illustrated in Fig. 4. Papua New Guinea has been fortunate in comparison with other Third World countries in its allocation for

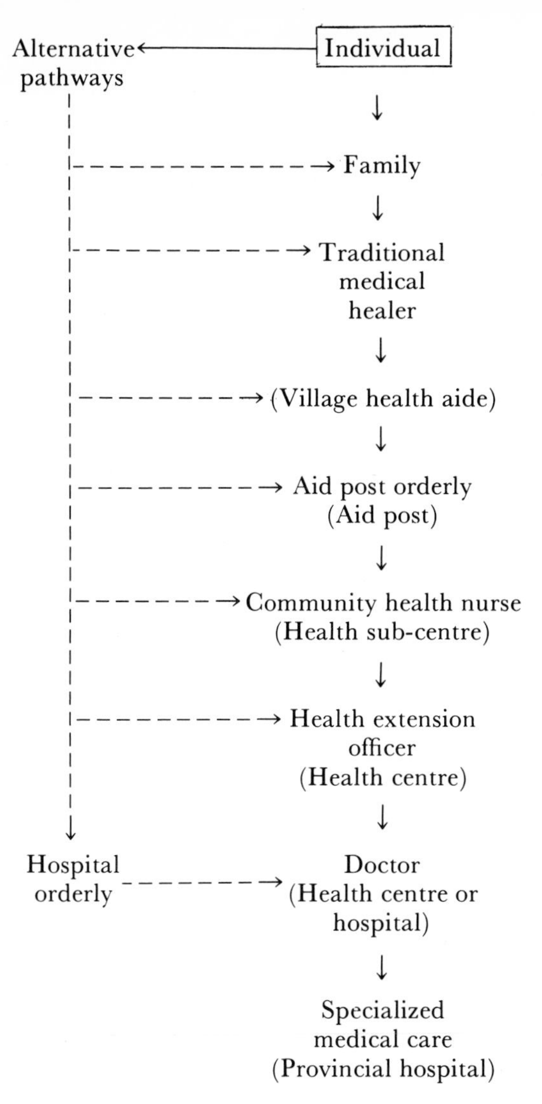

Fig. 4. Lines of access to care in Papua New Guinea.

health services with a high of 20% of the government budget soon after the Second World War, dropping to 8% in the early 1970s. This was equivalent to 3% of the GNP and represented between around $10 per head in 1974, rising to $15 per head per year in 1979.

Two-thirds of the 230 doctors in practice*— the same number as five

*in 1978.

years ago—are expatriate. They are in government service (175); with the university (20); in private practice (16); with the missions (16) and with the defence forces (6). Nursing graduates have increased 50% since 1974 and, except in rural areas, very few are expatriate. Of the 400 mission nurses, whose services are almost exclusively rural, over two-thirds are still expatriate. Health extension officers, New Guinea's peripherally based medical assistants, have increased in numbers by 70% since independence but have only exceeded the numbers of centrally situated doctors in the last two years. Unlike most developing countries there is in Papua New Guinea the infrastructure for a complete and comprehensive rural health care service, but its activity pattern has not enabled it to function as such. In 1971 care cost $8–$10 per day at a base hospital, $2–$4 at a rural hospital and 25–30 cents at an aid post.

The emphasis on expensive hospital buildings in the late 1960s and early 1970s has left the country with an unfortunate legacy. It is not that such structures were not required but that the type of structure built has enforced a crippling, recurrent expenditure for services which are provided to only a minority of the population. A small rural province with, say, $4 per head per year for all its health services, when provided with a $500 000 hospital for a population of 50 000 people incurs an annual maintenance cost of $150 000, or $3 per head, leaving $1 per head for all other services. Conversely, if such a structure had been built for $150 000 with costs around $50 000 a year to maintain then $3 a head could have been available for the rural services for the majority.

Figure 5 illustrates the dictum that health services are most utilized when placed close to the people for whom they are intended (King, 1966). In the highland area described there is an extensive road system which, in 1971, enabled 71% of the inpatients of that area access to hospital by vehicle (including 12% by ambulance). The majority of the country is not so fortunately serviced. Furthermore, the outer third of the area which is more deprived, less developed and with higher morbidity provides only 13% of the inpatients. The policy of concentrating resources in centralized facilities, characteristic of most health services, denies access to the most needy and is perhaps the most sentinel example of the Inverse Care Law.

In developing countries around 50% of mortality occurs before the age of five years and the bulk of this is in infants. There is little evidence that modern hospitals are able significantly to lower infant and child morbidity or mortality rates, especially in Papua New Guinea, where only about one-in-ten die in hospital. Despite this, over 50% of the

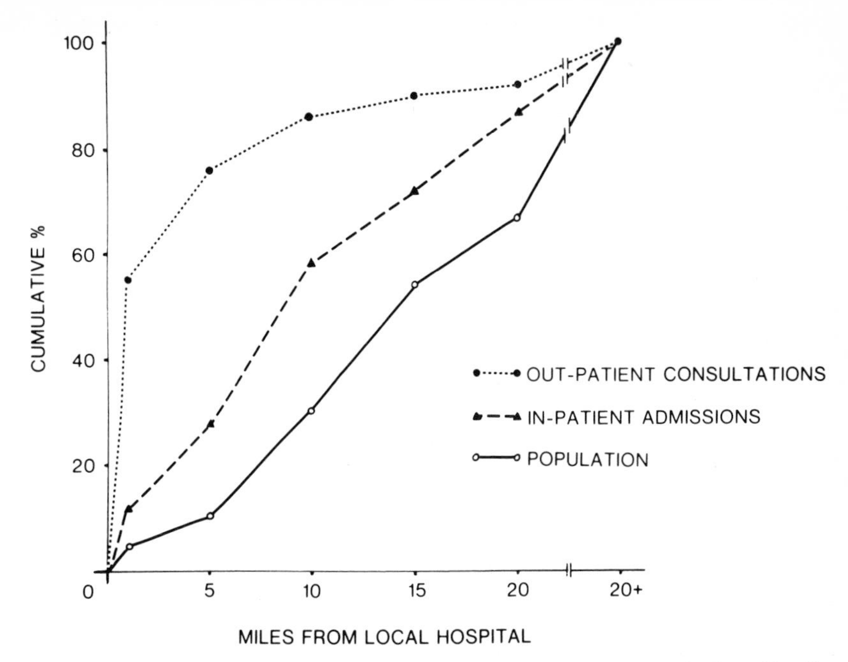

Fig. 5. Utilization data for a rural hospital in relation to population distribution.

health budget has been channelled into base hospital construction and maintenance or into high cost technology units such as the radiotherapy unit at Lae. As so often happens, this unit, part provided as an inappropriate gift (with a recurrent maintenance component) from an industrial nation, provides but a few extra months of life for a few people with usually advanced stages of cancer brought great distances to a service in cultural isolation from their families. "There is little relationship between the cost and size of a medical unit with its therapeutic efficiency" (King 1966). This story is unfortunately reproduced in almost every country, but it is the developing countries who can least afford it (see Dumont, 1968).

A schematic representation of the health services and the interrelationship of health workers is shown in Figs 6 and 7.

IV. Health Workers

Doctors consume the largest proportion of resources through a cost in excess of $10 000 per year of training and then in the salaries, equipment

Facility	Aid post	Health centre	Provincial hospital	Provincial Health Office Regional base hospital
Population covered	500 – 3000	10 000 – 50 000	50 000 – 250 000	
Activities	Primary care ⇄ referral ⇄	Primary care ⇄ referral ⇄ secondary care ⇄ referral ⇄	Primary care secondary care ⇄ referral ⇄ tertiary care ⇄ referral ⇄	
	Ambulatory care of Tb/leprosy mobile clinics ←	referred back — ← referred back ← community nursing (under Fives, antenatal, family planning, school health)	Tb/leprosy diagnosis	
	Village water supply, aid post, clinic houses ←	community health projects (with local council)		

Staff	Aid post orderly	Health extension officer (medical assistant) 2 Community nurses 1–2 Nurse aids 1 Aid post orderly supervisor 2–20 Orderlies according to inpatient/outpatient load	1–6 Doctors 2–10 Nurses 10–30 Orderlies Health extension officers for specialized units for Tb/leprosy Provincial health educator Provincial health officer Provincial malaria officer Health inspector	
	←	Supervision ←	Supervision ←	Headquarters Port Moresby

Fig. 6. Schematic representation of existing health services in Papua New Guinea.

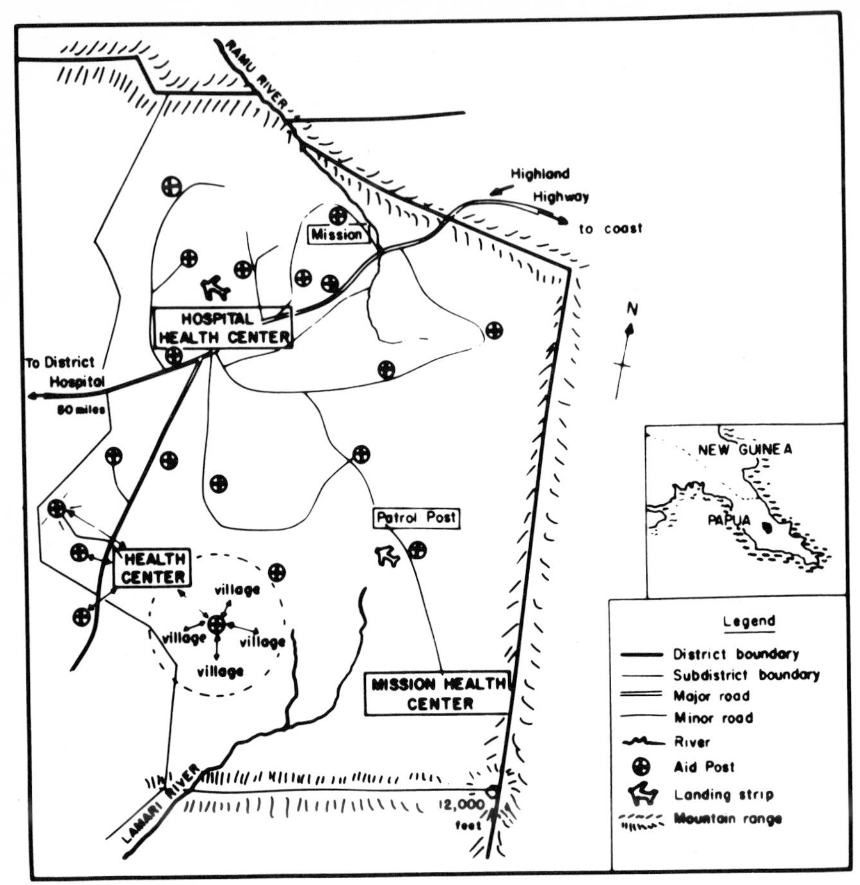

Fig. 7. Diagrammatic representation of or provision of rural care.

and supporting staff they demand afterwards. In Papua New Guinea there is no bonding of graduates either in terms of a given number of years of service or in any period of practice required in rural areas. They may go into private practice, where their cost benefit is minimal, whenever they wish and are now beginning to do so. In early 1979 not a single registered national doctor was employed in any of the highland provinces where 40% of the population lives.

Young graduates often undertake specialized training without any rural experience and are therefore less likely to develop natural empathy with, and an understanding of, the rural situation or of the conditions of most of the country's health workers who may seek their advice and from whom they receive referrals. Their undergraduate experience provides only a limited and decreasing experience outside the national capital and there are moves to reduce it further as most of the medical faculty, few of whom have any peripheral experience, do not perceive such training as warranting a high priority. A three month rural internship is no longer a prerequisite to registration. Until recently, quarters for such training, and those of the health extension officers, have been of such poor quality compared to those of any centralized tertiary institution that any rural training was in some measure a negative conditioning process. These factors, together with the lure of the towns, fear for their safety, or perhaps a perceived career in politics together with the lack of a national ideology has resulted in a marked maldistribution of doctors (Table III). Three years in a community-based national health service for each graduate following

TABLE III. *Doctor : Population Ratios in Papua New Guinea*

		1974		1978	
	Population	Doctors	Approx. ratio	Doctors	Approx. ratio
Central Province	7%	40%	<1 : 2000	36%	1 : 2000
Highland Province	40%	19%	>1 : 20000	15%	1 : 30000

internship would staff the sixty rural hospitals and health centres which could justify a doctor in the health team (Radford, 1972).

The Aid post is the smallest and most peripheral health care unit—it is a primary health subunit with a small ward. The pattern of rural morbidity is such that an adequately trained and motivated Aid Post Orderly (APO) can deal with three-quarters of all potentially fatal illness, initiate therapy for most of the other diseases and arrange transport to a larger centre (Sturt and Stanhope, 1968; Scragg, 1969; Becroft, Stanhope and Burchett, 1969; Dowell and Stanhope, 1970; Vines, 1970). Peripheral care units using APOs and maternal and child health services can be most effective.

In a highly malarious area of the East Sepik Province where no general development (road system, cash cropping, etc.) had occurred Sturt (1972) showed a progressive fall in infant mortality from over 160 per 1000 live births to almost 60 per 1000 over an eight year period. A major key to this success was the regular, supportive supervision by an expatriate doctor or nurse, but they had much better than national average staff to population ratios.

Until recently, the APOs' education never exceeded completion of primary school. Now up to two-thirds of some intakes have varying levels of secondary schooling and there is danger that their level of education may preclude their willingness to work at a village level. Their medical training consists of a basic one year programme and, more recently, a number have been required to undertake a "post-graduate" internship of up to one year.

This training should enable them to:

1. maintain an aid post and provide simple curative treatments for the commonly occurring diseases;
2. recognize complications which require further treatment at a health centre or hospital, initiate first aid and referral;
3. conduct domiciliary treatment for endemic diseases such as leprosy and tuberculosis;
4. regularly patrol a group of villages, usually three to ten, recognizing and managing obvious illness as well as poor hygiene such as polluted water supply, poor latrine, and inadequate refuse disposal;
5. assist various medical patrols such as malaria eradication, anti-tuberculosis and maternal child health clinics, and,
6. report epidemics such as gastroenteritis, whooping cough, malaria or deaths of an unusual nature in his area (Radford 1972).

Only since 1976 have APOs been employed full-time and the allocated health budget has risen from less than 6% in 1975 to 8% in 1979. They are exclusively male (except for a few mission-trained workers) which, in a country where the male/female dichotomy is so marked, must lead to marked underutilization of services. This eurocentric approach has been unfortunate as they are the potential providers of primary care for 90% of the population and see an average of twenty patients per day. There is now an average of one orderly per 1640 of the population but three-quarters of the population still live more than an hour's walk from an aid post.

Despite Health Department claims that the aid post orderly was "the backbone of the rural health services" and would "continue to be so for many years to come", the policy throughout the 1960s was, except in those areas where services were administered by Christian missions, to slow down APO training until it finally ceased in 1966. Repeated attempts by district health officers failed to get this policy changed. Eventually as the political process with an indigenous majority in parliament began to work, the Health Department was directed to recommence APO training in 1972. There are now eight training schools, six of which are conducted by various mission agencies who can produce graduates at a fraction of the cost of government institutions.

The axiom that "health workers work as well as the amount of regular supportive supervision they receive" (Radford, 1978) has not been well applied. Orderlies are often left without support from the health extension officers, just as the staff of the health centres are often denied supportive supervision from doctors or senior health extension officers, few of whom are trained or motivated to supervise. Aid posts or health centres have been without a supervisory visit for six, twelve, or more months at a time. Thus their potential is often greatly under-realized. As with the system of village health orderlies initiated by the German administration in New Guinea before the First World War, they tend to be "effective in proportion to their traditional status and personality" (Rowley, 1957), which after the Second World War was often of a relatively low order due in part to their younger age and also to their being "foreigners to the areas to which they were commonly sent". This is not always a limiting factor if they speak the language of the area, as intertribal suspicion is often greatest between nearest neighbours. Two illustrations of this are the aid post serving five villages where each had built a "twenty-bed ward" and the hospital which was little used by one area because the majority of orderlies were from a group with whom they were at enmity and they feared sorcery at their hands. Community participation in selection of candidates for village service would help ensure greater access to care which needs to be "of the village rather than of the Health Department" (Maddocks, 1978). In 1976, an earlier suggestion (Speer, 1972) was implemented and training of both male and female village aides for work within a given village commenced, with candidates often being selected by the villagers themselves. There are, however, still less than 100 such aides in service.

Community health nurses currently spend large amounts of time, often several hours a day, in expensive vehicle travel with little opportunity to develop effective community relationships and with consequent poor attendances at clinics. Such clinics are often conducted in a mechanistic manner with little attention to appropriate health education, follow-up or to evaluation, which often results in those most in need of care not getting it. A survey of twenty-five non-attenders enrolled at one clinic produced seven children whose conditions justified hospitalization. Participation of village women in the organization and conduct of such services is virtually non-existent. The "restless posting syndrome", whereby officers rarely serve more than one year in a given area, is endemic in government middle level management and precludes the easy development of effective working relationships between providers and users. Much more effective relationships are developed by mission services with consequent greater attendances and higher completed immunization rates.

Male hospital nurses were, until 1968, trained in almost equal numbers to females, but in subsequent years male trainees were actively discouraged. This conservative view of recruitment left hospitals and health centres with minimal male staff as the older hospital orderly category was being phased out. Rural employment of trained female nurses is largely on an ad hoc basis as they come and go with their husband's postings and intermittent pregnancies. While females have an especially important role in obstetrics, child care and education, as with males their participation has cultural limitations. Thus a reverse situation from the male-dominated aid post staffing was developing in hospitals. In the last two years the proportion of male nurse graduates has risen significantly.

Although between half and two-thirds of all pregnant women receive some antenatal care from the maternal and child health service, rural maternal mortality is still of the order of 1% (Johnson, 1971). And although rural infant mortality has fallen from levels as high as 350 per 1000 to around 100 per 1000, and possibly lower, urban levels are now under 30 per 1000 in some towns (Bell, 1973). As with traditional healers, minimal or non-existent recognition, support or involvement of village midwives has developed.

The acceptability of desired, community-initiated family planning has been demonstrated in Papua New Guinea (Watson *et al.*, 1972) and it has been shown that services can be delivered in villages as well as from town centres (Christie *et al.*, 1972). However, in 1973 family planning still received only a fraction of one tenth of 1% of the health budget despite the socioeconomic as well as health benefits which derive from reduced fertility (Jones, 1969).

V. Conclusion

The greatest deficiency of twentieth century medicine is not the lack of resources to develop new high cost technology. It is the failure to distribute the simple, effective methodologies of prevention and cure that are available based on an appropriate cultural template, together with the failure to concentrate on health promotion activities as part of a general development plan. In Papua New Guinea a copy of the Australian approach to medical services has been produced.

Emphasis has usually been placed on policies which express professional or political security rather than those based on the actual needs of the population. This holds, even conceding that the more highly educated and vocal city dwellers will demand and get a differentially greater proportion of health and other resources compared with their poorer rural cousins or the "septic fringe" dwellers on the edges of towns.

The potential defect of any national health plan, and Papua New Guinea is one of the few countries to have developed one (Dept Health, 1974), is that if the strategies, and especially if the tactics, for their implementation are devised in too much detail centrally they may not be readily, or indeed appropriately, applicable in a given province or district. The tremendous variability within and between the provinces of Papua New Guinea highlights this issue. Each province is now developing its own health plan. The greatly increased numbers of peripheral health workers compared to doctors in the last five years is evidence of fulfilling one national plan guideline which will help to reverse the Inverse Care Law of the past. Failure to derive and implement tactics to achieve its guidelines will result in the majority of the population remaining isolated from the health and medical services they need, be they island-bound, locked in highland valleys, or housed in squatter settlements.

There is little evidence that curative services ever result in any great rise in productivity but there is evidence that a rise in the socioeconomic standards of a community will result in a marked improvement in health and is likely to do more to improve the health of Papua New Guineans than centralized investigative and treatment services. The real object of national development must be to make the country a better place to live in and the first end in achieving this is the "promotion of well-being of the rural majority" (Fisk, 1972).

References

Becroft, T. C., Stanhope, J. M. and Burchett, P. M. (1969). *Papua N. Guinea med. J.* **12**, 48–55.

Bell, C. O. (1973). *In* "The Diseases and Health Services of Papua New Guinea" (C. O. Bell, Ed.). Department of Public Health, Port Moresby, 134–172.

Christie, J., Christie, D. and Radford, A. J. (1972). *Papua N. Guinea Med. J.* **15**, 28; 165–167; and 281.

Department of Health (1974). *Papua New Guinea National Health Plan 1947–78*, Konedobu.

Dowell, M. and Stanhope, J. M. (1970). *Papua N. Guinea Med. J.* **13**, 132–136.

Dumont, R. (1968). "False Start in Africa". Sphere Books in association with Deutsch, London.
Essai, B. (1961). "Papua and New Guinea: A Contemporary Survey", 199–226, Oxford Univ. Press, Melbourne.
Fisk, E. K. (1972). *In* "Change and Development in Melanesia" (M. Ward, Ed.), 9–23. Fifth Waigani Seminar. Australian National Univ. Press. Canberra.
Firth, S. (1978). *In* "Papua New Guinea Portraits" J. Griffin (Ed.), 28–47, Australian National Univ. Press, Canberra.
Frederiksen, H. (1971). "Epidemographic Surveillance". Carolina Population Centre Monograph. Univ. North Carolina Press, Chapel Hill.
Geiger, J. H. (1968). "Health and Social Change: The Urban Crisis". Lowell Institute Series, Boston.
Hart, G. (1974). *Br. J. ven. Dis.* **50**, 453–458.
Hetzel, B. S. and Pharoah, P. O. D. (Eds) (1971). "Endemic Cretinism". Papua New Guinea Institute of Medical Research, Monograph Series No. 2.
Hornabrook, R. W. and Skeldon, G. H. F. (Eds) (1977). "A Bibliography of Medicine and Human Biology of Papua New Guinea". Institute of Medical Research Monograph Series No. 5, Classey, Faringdon.
Johnson, D. G. (1971). *Papua N. Guinea med. J.* **14**, 133–135.
Jones, G. W. (1969). "The Economic Effect of Declining Fertility in Less Developed Countries". An Occasional Paper of the Population Council, New York. W. M. Fell, Philadelphia.
King, M. (1966). *In* "Medical Care in Developing Countries" (M. King, Ed.), 2–8, 168. Oxford Univ. Press, Nairobi.
Lawrence, G., Shann, F., Freestone, D. S. and Walker, P. D. (1979). *Lancet* i, 227–230.
Lewis, G. (1975). "Knowledge of Illness in a Sepik Society: A study of the Gnau, New Guinea". London School of Economics, Monographs on Social Anthropology. Athlone, London.
Maddocks, I. (1967). *Med. J. Aust.* **1**, 1123–1126.
Maddocks, I. (1978). *In* "Basic Health Care in Developing Countries: An Epidemiological Perspective" (B. S. Hetzel, Ed.), 23. Oxford Univ. Press.
Maddocks, I. and Rovin, L. (1965). *Papua N. Guinea med. J.* **8**, 17–21.
Pharoah, P. O. D. Butterfield, I. H. and Hetzel, B. S. (1971). *Lancet* i, 308–310.
Pharoah, P. O. D. and Hornabrook, R. W. (1974). *Lancet* ii, 1038–1400.
Radford, A. J. (1972). *In* "Change and Development in Melanesia" (M. Ward, Ed.) 250–279. Fifth Waigani Seminar. Australian National Univ. Press, Canberra.
Radford, A. J. (1973). *In* "Priorities in Melanesian Development", (R. J. May, Ed.), 145–150. Sixth Waigani Seminar. Australian National Univ. Press, Canberra.
Radford, A. J. (1978). *In* "Basic Health Care in Developing Countries: An Epidemiological Perspective" (B. S. Hetzel, Ed.), 149. Oxford Univ. Press.

Radford, A. J., van Leeuwen, H. and Christian, S. H. (1976). *Ann. trop. Med. Parasit.* **70**, 11–23.
Radford, R. (1979). "Highlanders and Foreigners in the Upper Ramu: the Kainantu Area 1919–1942", 211. M. A. Thesis. Univ. Papua New Guinea.
Rhodes, F. A. and Anderson, S. E. J. (1970). *Papua N. Guinea med. J.* **13**, 49–52.
Rowley, C. (1957). *S. Pacific* **9**, 391–399.
Schofield, F. D., Tucker, V. M. and Westbrook, G. R. (1961). *B. med. J.* ii, 785–789.
Scragg, R. F. R. (1969). *Papua N. Guinea med. J.*, **12**, 73–83.
Sinnett, P. F. (1975). "The People of Murapin". Papua New Guinea Institute of Medical Research, Monograph Series No. 4. Classey, Faringdon.
Speer, B. (1972). Quoted in Radford (1972).
Sturt, J. (1972). *Papua N. Guinea med. J.* **15**, 215–220.
Sturt, R. T. and Stanhope, J. M. (1968). *Papua N. Guinea med. J.* **11**, 111–117.
Tudor Hart, J. (1971). *Lancet* i, 405–412.
Watson, E. J. (1968). *Papua N. Guinea med. J.* **11**, 130–132.
Watson, E. J., Read, D. A. and Radford, A. J. (1972). *Papua N. Guinea med. J.* **14**, 133–135.
Vines, A. P. (1970) "An Epidemiological Sample Survey of the Highlands, Mainland and Islands Regions of the Territory of Papua and New Guinea". Department of Public Health. Government Printer, Port Moresby.
Zigas, V. (1978). "Auscultation in Two Worlds". Vantage, New York.

19

Health Care in the USSR

I. D. Ladnyi*

World Health Organization, Geneva, Switzerland

The main principle of the USSR public health is its state nature and the public health development plan is part of the general state national economic plan.

* Assistant Director-General.

I. Territory and Population

The USSR covers an area of 24 400 000 km^2. From east to west its territory extends for over 9000 km and from north to south 4500 km. The total population according to the 1979 census was 262 442 000, giving a population density of 10·8 per km^2. However, the density of the population varies greatly from one area to another. Territory and distribution of population by republics is given in Table I. Most of the country has a continental climate with a cold subarctic climate in the north and subtropical climate in the south.

The country is inhabited by over 100 different nationalities and ethnic groups. The USSR is composed of fifteen Union Republics: The Russian Soviet Federative Socialist Republic; Ukrainian; Byelorussian; Uzbek; Kazakh; Georgian; Azerbaijan; Lithuanian; Moldavian;

TABLE I. *Territory and Population of the USSR (by Republics)*

	Territory in thousand km^2	Population × 10^3 in the Years				
		1913	1940	1959	1970	1979[a]
RSFSR[b]	17 075·4	89 902	110 098	117 534	130 079	137 552
Ukrainian SSR	603·7	35 210	41 340	41 869	47 126	49 757
Byelorussian SSR	207·6	6 899	9 046	8 056	9 002	9 559
Uzbek SSR	447·4	4 334	6 551	8 119	11 800	15 391
Kazakh SSR	2 717·3	5 597	6 148	9 295	13 009	14 685
Georgian SSR	69·7	2 601	3 612	4 044	4 686	5 016
Azerbaijan SSR	86·6	2 339	3 274	3 698	5 117	6 028
Lithuanian SSR	65·2	2 828	2 925	2 711	3 128	3 399
Moldavian SSR	33·7	2 056	2 468	2 885	3 569	3 948
Latvian SSR	63·7	2 493	1 886	2 093	2 364	2 521
Kirghiz SSR	198·5	864	1 528	2 066	2 933	3 529
Tajik SSR	143·1	1 034	1 525	1 981	2 900	3 801
Armenian SSR	29·8	1 000	1 320	1 763	2 492	3 031
Turkmen SSR	488·1	1 042	1 302	1 516	2 159	2 759
Estonian SSR	45·1	954	1 054	1 197	1 356	1 466
USSR Total	22 402·2[c]	159 153	194 077	208 827	241 720	262 442

[a] On 17 January 1979.
[b] Russian Soviet Federative Socialist Republic.
[c] Including territories of the White Sea (90 000 km^2) and Azov sea (37 300 km^2) which are not included in any of the Union Republics.

Latvian; Kirghiz; Tajik; Armenian; Turkmen; and Estonian Soviet Socialist Republic. The majority of the republics are divided for administrative purposes into regions which comprise districts with an average population of from 20 000 to over 100 000 people. The Union Republics also contain twenty autonomous republics, ten autonomous regions (oblasts) and ten national okrugs—administrative entities, based on the presence of a large concentration of a particular national or ethnic group. The majority of the population live in towns and cities. The rural population accounts for 38% of the total according to the 1979 census. The proportion of the population reaching the age of sixty years and over in 1939 was 6·8% of the total; in 1959, 9·4%; and in 1970, 11·8%. The average life expectancy was seventy years in 1971/72 (see Table II). The USSR has a vital interest in increasing its population

TABLE II. *Average Life Expectancy in Pre-revolutionary Russia and the USSR*

	Average life span in years		
	Males	Females	Both sexes
1896–1897[a]	31	33	32
1926–1927[b]	42	47	44
1938–1939	44	50	47
1955–1956	64	72	69
1971–1972	64	74	70

[a] In 50 provinces of European part of Russia.
[b] In European part of the USSR

and, in view of this, birth control measures have never been encouraged and the demographic policy of the State is aimed at increasing the birth rate.

II. The Health of the Population and Health Services in Pre-revolutionary Russia.

There was no organizing centre in pre-revolutionary Russia to deal with public health problems on a nationwide scale. Practically each government department and ministry had its own medical section. Besides, the various charitable, religious and public organizations had a number of medical institutions in their charge.

Only in some areas was medical care under the control of institutions of local administrations ("*Zemstvo*"),* which functioned in thirty-four out of eighty-nine provinces. In 1913 there were 28 000 doctors for the whole country with a population of 159·2 million, i.e. one doctor for about 5700. In many areas there was not a single doctor while in some areas of the country there was one doctor for scores of thousands of population.

In rural areas for example, inhabited by 130·7 million people, there were 4975 doctors (i.e. approximately one doctor per 26 200), while in what are now the Central Asian Republics there was only one doctor for 35 000 to 50 000. There was an acute shortage of hospitals and other medical institutions. The total number of registered hospital beds for the whole country was 208 000, i.e. 1·3 hospital beds per 1000 population. About 35% of towns had no hospitals at all.

It was very difficult to maintain specialized medical care since 25% of all hospitals had less than five beds. In 1913 there were only 7500 beds for expectant mothers and post-partum women. Russia had nine outpatient mother and child centres and a few small hospitals for children and outpatient departments belonging to the medical faculties. Only about 5% of all deliveries were medically assisted. As a result over 30 000 young women died annually of post-natal sepsis. Russia had no state sanitary or epidemiological services. There were only a few score sanitary inspectors. In 1913, which was a peak year for government spending on public health, the total expenditure per capita of the population was 91 kopeks, yet only 5 kopeks out of this total was spent on sanitary and epidemiological measures which at the time were especially urgent.

In 1913, the year before Russia entered the First World War, infant mortality was 269 per 1000 live births, that is over a quarter of infants died of disease and deformity before reaching one year of age, and a total of 43% of children died before reaching the age of five. The general mortality rate in the country was 29·1 per 1000 (see Table III) and according to the 1896/1897 census the average expectation of life was thirty-two years only.

The deplorable sanitary conditions that were so much a feature of pre-revolutionary Russia were responsible for the high incidence of infectious and parasitic diseases including cholera, smallpox, plague and typhus. According to statistics over 1 million adults and 2 million children died each year due to infectious and parasitic diseases. Every year from 5–7 million people suffered from malaria, and from 1907–11,

*"*Zemstvo*"—elective local council designated to cater for the rural population in pre-revolutionary Russia. Their functions included maintenance of schools, rural hospitals and dispensaries.

TABLE III. *Birth Rate and Mortality in Pre-revolutionary Russia and the USSR*

Year	Per 1000 population		
	Births	Deaths	Natural increase
1913	45·5	29·4	16·4
1940	31·2	18·0	13·2
1950	26·7	9·7	17·0
1955	25·7	8·2	17·5
1960	24·9	7·1	17·8
1965	18·4	7·3	11·1
1966	18·2	7·3	10·9
1967	17·3	7·6	9·7
1968	17·2	7·7	9·5
1969	17·0	8·1	8·9
1970	17·4	8·2	9·2
1971	17·8	8·2	9·6
1972	17·8	8·5	9·3
1973	17·6	8·7	8·9
1974	18·0	8·7	9·3
1975	18·1	9·3	8·8
1976	18·4	9·5	8·9

2·8 million cases of cholera were registered, out of which 443 000 died. It is worth noting that out of every 1000 persons examined by physicians during that time, thirty were found to have syphilis and gonorrhoea. Medical examination of young people drafted for military service indicated that 50–100 out of every 1000 suffered from tuberculosis, a startling discovery when one considers that the young draftees were among the most healthy of the population. These gloomy statistics reflected the wretched conditions in which the majority of prerevolutionary Russia's population lived.

III. Basic Principles of the Health Services in the USSR

After gaining political power in 1917, the Communist Party of the Soviet Union placed the questions of public health protection as the most important tasks of state. The prevention of disease was defined as the main direction of public health protection. At all stages of development of the Soviet State the interests of public health protection were taken into account in the solution of all national economic tasks. (The methodological basis underlying the principles of Soviet public health protection are built on Marxist concepts of the social conditionality of health, the dependence of health and the organizational principles and forms for public health systems upon the method of producing material values and the level of development of the productive forces of society.)

The main principle of the USSR public health is its state nature and the public health development plan is part of the general state national economic plan. All basic public health measures carried out in the USSR are financed by the state. One of the general principles of public health planning is to combine centralized planned management and active participation of the working masses in drawing up plans. In practice all medical establishments and public health administration bodies, from rural hospitals to the Ministry of Health, take part in working out current and long-term plans. The state character of public health in the USSR is an expression of socialist democracy which guarantees the right of the people and guarantees their realization. The State-run health service is one of the functions of the Soviet State and its duty to ensure each Soviet citizen's right to health also implies that the health of each citizen is regarded not only as his personal right, but as part of the national wealth. Medical care is freely available to the entire population of the country, regardless of social, political, economic, racial or any other factors.

The funds are provided out of the national budget for medical care and the development of public health services and institutions are growing constantly. Table IV gives some idea of the budget allocations for public health in USSR. In addition to these allocations from the State budget, hospitals and other medical institutions receive over two billion roubles per year from industrial enterprises, collective farms and other establishments. Apart from the allocations for public health mentioned above, the State expenditure for the development of medical

TABLE IV. *State Budget for Public Health (in comparable prices)*

Year	Budget allocations (in billion roubles)	*Per capita* expenditure
1913	145·4	0·9
1940	903·5	4·7
1950	2 162·6	11·6
1960	4 841·0	22·6
1970	9 300·0	38·2
1975	11 469·9	43·8

science and medical education is not included in the public health item of the national budget, but comes under science and education expenditure. The State social policy coupled with a government-run public health service gives a guarantee to Soviet citizens, one of their basic social rights—the right to health care. The USSR Constitution contains a special clause to this effect and reads:

> Citizens of the USSR have the right to health protection. This right is ensured by free, qualified medical care provided by state health institutions; by extension of the network of therapeutic and health-building institutions; by the development and improvement of safety and hygiene in industry; by carrying out broad prophylactic measures; by measures to improve the environment; by special care for the health of the rising generation, including prohibition of child labour, excluding the work done by children as part of the school curriculum; and by developing research to prevent and reduce the incidence of disease and ensure citizens a long and active life. (Article 42)

It has already been noted that before the October Revolution, Russia was at the bottom of the list of countries in terms of the number of medical personnel, hospital beds, and medical institutions. In 1913, for example, Russia had an average of 1·8 doctors and 13 hospital beds per 10 000 population. According to statistics for 1977 the USSR had an average of 34·4 doctors and 121 hospital beds per 10 000 population. The number of health workers with a secondary medical education reached over 2·5 million. At present even the remotest towns and villages throughout the USSR have their own hospitals, polyclinics, pharmacies and other medical institutions.

Table V summarizes main indicators of development and present status of health services in the USSR.

The USSR has a single system of health services, subordinate to the USSR Ministry of Health. All public health institutions from the smallest medical units staffed by paramedical personnel to the largest city hosptials and medical research institutes are administered by the USSR Ministry of Health, which controls the activities of all the services and plans all measures relating to the prophylactic and curative services in the country. The unified nature of Soviet public health implies unity of aims, methods of work, principles guiding trained medical personnel in their activities, as well as unified principles of administration and management of health services.

The planned development of public health implies that being an integral part of the Soviet economy it is subject to the laws of planned development. There are current plans and long-term plans laying down guidelines for the future development of health care over a period of several years as regards basic indices such as improvement of the

TABLE V. *Main Indices of the Development of the Public Health System (in thousands)*

	1913	1917	1940	1965	1970	1975	1976	1977
Total number of physicians in all specialities	28·1	16·5	155·3	554·2	668·4	834·1	864·6	893·0
Total number of physicians per 10 000 population	1·8		7·9	23·9	27·4	32·6	33·5	34·4
Total number of medical personnel with secondary special education	46	24	472	1692	2123	2515	2586	
Number of hospital beds for inpatients	208	119	791	2226	2663	3009	3076	3144
Number of hospital beds per 10 000 population	13		40	96	109	118	119	121
Number of medical establishments providing outpatient treatment for the population	5·7		36·8	36·7	37·4	35·6	35·7	
Number of women's consultation centres, children's outpatient clinics (independent and components of large medical establishments)	0·009	0·06	8·6	19·3	21·0	22·1	22·3	22·5
Number of beds (therapeutic and obstetric) for pregnant women and women in childbirth	7·5	5·9	147·0	227·0	224·0	223·0	223·0	223·0
Number of sanitary and epidemiological stations	1		1943			4754		

people's health, expansion and modernizing of medical institutions, training of medical personnel, production of medical supplies and equipment. Five-year plans for the development of the national economy automatically covered public health and the country's medical industry. It is worth noting that each health level beginning from rural hosptials to the Ministry of Health, takes part in producing current and long-term plans. Health care development plans emphasize the future development of specialized medical services as a major means of improving the quality of health care. Constant efforts to expand, improve and modernize the technical and economic basis of the country's public health system are aimed at improving the health standards of the population, at more effective control of disease, and at improving physical well-being generally. The plan also determines the most important long-term trends in medical research. The basic guidelines for the development of the country's economy are laid down and co-ordinated by the State Planning Committee of the USSR. Following approval by a session of the USSR Supreme Soviet, the economic development plan becomes law.

IV. The Organization of the Public Health Services in the USSR

A. Structure of Public Health Services in the USSR

The Ministry of Health of the USSR is the supreme and central body in the administration of public health and is responsible for all activities and services of public health in the country. The Ministry is headed by the Minister of Health, who is appointed by the USSR Supreme Soviet.

Every constituent and autonomous republic has its own public health ministry which comes under the USSR Ministry of Health. Also coming under the jurisdiction of the USSR Ministry of Health are the Academy of Medical Sciences and the leading medical research institutes. The health ministries of constituent and autonomous republics represent the second highest level of administration of public health, being in charge of health care in their respective republics.

The USSR Ministry of Health and the health ministries of the constituent republics direct the various health services through the agency of public health departments attached to regional, city and district executives of the Soviets of People's Deputies (i.e. through local government bodies). Regional public health departments supervise the work of the medical and sanitary institutions of all the departments located within the region or territory concerned. They draw up and implement public health programmes and plans for their particular region or territory. Regional public health departments represent the third level of administration of health care, while city and district public health departments represent the fourth level. District public health departments in towns with an administrative division by district come under the city public health department.

City and district public health departments are in charge of all public health matters in the town or district concerned, supervising directly all curative and prophylactic institutions within their jurisdiction, providing trained medical personnel, finance and medical supplies.

The administration of the provision of health services in rural areas is the responsibility of the head doctors of central district hospitals, who are simultaneously the chief surgeons of the districts concerned. They report to the regional public health departments.

The specific features of health care for the employees of a number of ministries have necessitated the creation of a network of the so-called departmental medical and sanitary institutions controlled by the department concerned. However, the existence of such institutions does not violate the paramount principles of the planned and unified nature of the Soviet public health system as overall administration of all medical services is in the hands of the USSR Ministry of Health.

All types of sanitary and anti-epidemic work in the country at the district level and higher are carried out by the sanitary and epidemiological stations operating in each district, region and territory. The State Sanitary Inspectorate is headed by the Chief Governmental Sanitary Doctor, who is a deputy of the Minister of Health of the USSR. The Chief Governmental Sanitary Doctor has under him the chief sanitary doctors of constituent republics, the head doctors of regional, city and district sanitary and epidemiological stations. The decisions of chief sanitary doctors can be overruled only by a higher-level superior sanitary body.

All central public health bodies come under the USSR Council of Ministers and the Council of Ministers of a constituent or autonomous republic, while local public health bodies report to the corresponding Soviet of People's Deputies and their executives. Central and local public health bodies at all levels are in charge of all matters relating to the improvement of the provision of curative and prophylactic assistance to the population, disease control and treatment, sanitary inspection of the housing, public utilities and industrial enterprises, sanitary and prophylactic measures to safeguard and improve the health of all population groups, mother and child care, sanitary education, pharmaceutic industry, and medical research. Public health bodies and institutions are guided in their day-to-day activities by the Fundamental Principles of the Health Legislation of the USSR and of the Union Republics and by other legislative acts, by the sanitary legislation on environmental protection and amelioration and on labour protection, by government decisions on the development of health services and medical science and by the decisions of Party organs relating to the protection and improvement of the people's health.

B. Sanitary and Epidemiological Services

Before the October Revolution sanitary and epidemiological services were practically non-existent. Only in some cities were there sanitary inspectors and epidemiologists. In 1922 the Government issued a specific decree on sanitary bodies which defined tasks facing the State control and supervisory bodies. The functions of sanitary inspectors in supervising the sanitary conditions of housing and controlling the observance of sanitary standards in the production, transportation and storage of food products were clearly defined. In 1932, countrywide sanitary and epidemiological stations were started.

Preventive and current sanitary supervision is the main trend in the activities of the country's sanitary and epidemiological services. In 1975 the USSR had about 4800 sanitary and epidemiological stations staffed by 50 000 doctors (epidemiologists, bacteriologists, virologists and sanitary doctors).

The country's sanitary and epidemiological service employs sanitary doctors of many different specialities, including industrial hygiene, occupational diseases, food hygiene, communal hygiene, etc. In addition, there are over 150 000 medical assistants and disinfection instructors working in close contact with the sanitary doctors and epidemiologists. The head doctor of a local sanitary and epidemiological station is simultaneously chief sanitary doctor of the district, town or city. The number of staff members of the sanitary and epidemiological station varies according to the population of the corresponding administrative territorial unit.

The sanitary and epidemiological stations handle a tremendous amount of work. Thus in 1974 over 1·5 million houses, 1 million foodstores, restaurants, dining rooms and similar establishments, 168 000 industrial enterprises, 391 000 schools, nurseries, kindergartens and other establishments were covered by regular sanitary inspection and supervision. A total of 12 million sanitary surveys were conducted and 14 million sanitary bacteriological and 8 million sanitary chemical tests were carried out.

As mentioned earlier, the sanitary and epidemiological station, the basic unit of the country's sanitary and epidemiological service, organizes all sanitary and anti-epidemic measures in its particular area (district, town, etc.), and exercises sanitary supervision, that is to say, sees that all sanitary regulations and standards are strictly observed by all organizations and institutions. The sanitary epidemiological service has been granted the right to control the observance of sanitary and hygienic norms and rules in planning the construction and reconstruction of establishments. These agencies enjoy broad powers up to imposing a fine, or even closing down offending enterprises.

C. Curative and Prophylactic Institutions

Hospitals, polyclinics and treatment and disease prevention centres form the backbone of the network of medical institutions in the USSR. General hospitals, in addition to inpatient departments, usually contain a polyclinic for outpatients. Such hospitals vary in size and capacity depending on the character and size of the area they serve. There is a tendency to enlarge existing hospitals since highly qualified and specialist medical care can be provided only by medical institutions containing all the main well-equipped specialized units and staffed by highly qualified specialists in a variety of medical branches. Between 1971 and 1974, for example, the average number of beds at central district hospitals serving rural areas increased from 165 to 196 and at regional hospitals from 597 to 698. There are a number of large urban hospitals with 800 to 1200 beds or more in big cities. An incorporated hospital has an inpatient department, which depending on its capacity has several units—therapeutic, surgical, obstetric and gynaecological, among others. Large general hospitals have in addition departments of neurosurgery, nephrology, cardiology, pulmonary physiology, gastroenterology and others. An integral part of the incorporated hospital is the polyclinic, i.e. the outpatient department. There are also some polyclinics which are not attached to hospitals. These polyclinics make diagnoses, offer treatment by various specialists and carry out prophylaxis. A feature of polyclinics in the USSR is that they are centres of therapy and prophylaxis for the areas they serve. For this reason most polyclinics, especially in urban areas, serve as district polyclinics and they serve a particular administrative part of the city. In small towns and villages they cater for the entire population.

Outpatient care is ensured by a widespread network of outpatient polyclinics, outpatient departments of dispensaries and other primary health care establishments, combining general and specialized treatment in their activities. Primary health care administered by outpatient establishments is organized on the principle of localities according to which the territory served by the establishment is divided into localities with a definite number of inhabitants. The main ones are the therapeutic localities designated in towns for serving an average of 2000 adults, and paediatric localities, organized in towns and cities with 800 to 1000 children under fifteen years of age. The principle of giving primary health care according to territorial localities is also extended to physicians of other specialities; obstetricians and gynaecologists, oncologists, ophthalmologists, general surgeons and other specialists. The division into localities allows regular follow-up for people living in the area and ensures immediate treatment at the clinic or at their home.

In 1977 there were more than 35 000 outpatient establishments in the country. In 1976 the outpatient establishments of the system of the USSR Ministry of Health alone registered 2·3 billion calls on doctors, including house calls, as compared to 1·8 billion calls in 1970 and 1·1 billion calls in 1960. In the period from 1971 to 1977 the development of outpatient care was accomplished by organizing and building large outpatient clinics, registering 800 to 1200 visits by patients during every shift.

Under the Ninth Five-year Economic Development Plan (1971–75), the number of endocrinological units within polyclinics increased by 23% to reach a total of 3200; the number of urological units increased by 14% to reach a total of 3000; cardiorheumatological units by 12% to reach 3550. In this period 269 allergy units were created.

In addition to small specialized units, treatment and disease-prevention centres and other institutions, providing highly skilled medical aid to the population in a number of narrow fields, large specialized medical centres are also being set up in the USSR. There are centres for cardiovascular surgery, children's surgery, chest diseases, neuro-oncology, nephrology, kidney transplantation, treatment of myocardial infarction cases, etc. Such centres are usually planned on the basis of large medical research institutes and provide qualified medical aid to the population of several regions and even republics.

A summary of the work of outpatient establishments is shown in Tables VI and VII and gives the average number of visits per citizen according to the Union Republic.

Expansion of the network of inpatient establishments has been envisaged by the national economic plan. In 1976 there were 24 000 inpatient hospitals in the Soviet Union with 3 076 000 hospital beds (119·3 per 10 000 population as compared to 80·4 in 1960 and 40·2 in 1940). In 1976 in the hospitals of the USSR Ministry of Health alone 56·3 million inpatients were treated as compared to 38·5 million in 1960 and 15·2 million in 1940.

Table VIII indicates the trend in the increase of the number of hospital beds and the provision of the population with hospital beds according to Union Republics. It is planned to increase the total number of hospital beds to 3·3 million by 1980 to reach a goal of 125 beds per 10 000 population.

TABLE VI. *Outpatient Medical Service for the Population (System of USSR Ministry of Health)*

	Average number of visits per citizen								
	Urban dwellers			Rural dwellers[a]					
	To physicians			To physicians			To doctors' assistants, nurses		
	1970	1975	1976	1970	1975	1976	1970	1975	1976
USSR	10·7	11·3	11·6	3·4	4·3	4·5	4·0	4·3	4·4
RSFSR	10·5	11·1	11·4	3·3	4·3	4·4	4·2	4·7	4·9
Ukrainian SSR	11·9	12·0	12·4	3·9	4·7	5·0	4·5	4·4	4·4
Byelorussian SSR	12·4	13·0	13·3	3·7	4·8	4·9	3·3	3·7	3·8
Uzbek SSR	10·2	11·7	11·7	2·6	3·9	4·2	4·8	4·1	4·1
Kazakh SSR	8·4	9·6	10·0	2·7	3·7	4·0	3·3	4·5	3·6
Georgian SSR	12·0	12·9	13·1	4·6	4·7	4·8	1·6	1·6	1·7
Azerbaijan SSR	11·4	11·6	11·9	2·2	2·9	3·2	3·0	2·6	2·8
Lithuanian SSR	12·4	13·9	14·1	4·7	6·2	6·5	2·4	2·3	2·2
Moldavian SSR	10·1	11·4	11·6	2·7	3·5	3·7		5·3	5·2
Latvian SSR	11·9	12·8	13·0	4·5	5·3	5·6	2·3	2·4	2·4
Kirghiz SSR	10·5	11·4	11·7	3·2	3·9	4·0	3·5	3·8	4·0
Tajik SSR	8·5	10·8	11·6	1·8	2·8	3·0	4·4	6·0	6·3
Armenian SSR	8·7	9·6	9·5	3·7	4·6	4·3	3·7	3·8	3·1
Turkmen SSR	8·6	9·2	9·6	2·9	3·5	3·7	4·4	5·3	4·8
Estonian SSR	10·3	11·1	11·4	4·7	5·7	6·0	2·0	2·1	2·2
Average for USSR	10·7	11·3	11·6	3·4	4·3	4·5	4·0[b]	4·3	4·4

[a] Including visits made by rural dwellers to urban medical establishments.
[b] Except the Moldavian SSR.

In the USSR hospitals both with and without outpatient departments, are divided into general and specialized ones. The same applies to children's hospitals. Specialized hospitals are those caring for cases of tuberculosis, infectious diseases and patients suffering from mental illness. Most clinical hospitals are highly specialized units or general hospital complexes with specialist sections.

A general hospital provides facilities for the training of medical personnel and for advanced and refresher training. Treatment and disease prevention centres of various kinds, disease prevention institutions and those providing specialist medical aid to the sufferers of a number of specific diseases also form part of the basic health institu-

TABLE VII. *Work of Outpatient Medical Establishments (System of USSR Ministry of Health)*

	1960	1965	1970	1975	1976
Number of applications for aid to curative and prophylactic outpatient medical establishments (in millions)					
Visits to doctors	1 044·3	1 349·3	1 633·3	1 969·5	2 205·6
House calls for doctors	84·9	115·0	135·4	138·8	151·4
Number of applications for aid to doctors, doctors' assistants and nurses at outpatient medical establishments in rural areas					
Visits to doctors' assistants and nurses working independently	201·3	230·2	274·5	289·1	292·2
House calls for doctors' assistants and nurses	82·8	107·0	146·4[a]	138·1	138·1
Number of patients served by ambulance and emergency aid teams	23·2	34·4	51·8	71·0	74·1

[a] With the exception of the Moldavian SSR.

tions in the USSR. There are centres for dermatology and venereal diseases, tuberculosis, oncology, neuropsychiatry, cardiorheumatology, thyroid gland disease, and remedial gymnastics centres. These institutions, some of which have inpatient departments of their own, are integrated into a system to provide a wide range of inpatient and outpatient services by methods peculiar to them. These institutions are called upon to complement the disease-prevention services to the population made available by all the other public health services in the country. The treatment and disease-prevention centres concentrate their efforts on the early detection of disease and on keeping careful health records of specific groups as well as on treatment and the provision of social hygiene and, if necessary, timely home-visiting services. Among their functions is help to patients in finding suitable employment, and evaluation of disability pension qualifications as well as the provision of a wide range of advice and consultation services to curative and prophylactic institutions. Treatment and disease prevention centres work in close contact with polyclinics and hospitals, and in

TABLE VIII. *Number of Hospital Beds and the Provision of the Population with Hospital Beds According to Union Republics*

	Number of hospital beds (in thousands)					Number of hospital beds per 10 000 population				
	1940	1965	1970	1975	1976	1940	1965	1970	1975	1976
USSR	790·9	2 225·5	2 663·2	3 009·2	3 076·0	40·2	95·8	109·2	117·8	119·3
RSFSR	482·0	1 241·1	1 469·2	1 649·2	1 682·8	43·3	97·6	112·4	122·5	124·1
Ukrainian SSR	157·6	428·2	511·0	578·3	589·7	37·7	94·0	107·6	117·8	119·6
Byelorussian SSR	29·6	80·0	94·2	107·0	111·2	32·6	92·4	103·8	114·2	118·1
Uzbek SSR	20·3	96·0	123·5	145·6	151·2	30·1	92·4	101·8	103·4	104·5
Kazakh SSR	25·4	123·6	156·4	178·6	182·2	39·5	102·6	118·2	124·6	125·6
Georgian SSR	13·3	38·2	43·1	48·0	49·6	36·0	84·8	91·0	96·9	99·3
Azerbaijan SSR	12·6	39·8	48·8	54·8	55·8	37·8	85·7	93·5	96·3	96·6
Lithuanian SSR	8·9	26·6	32·4	36·9	37·7	30·0	88·9	102·2	111·2	112·7
Moldavian SSR	6·1	30·1	35·8	42·0	43·1	24·6	89·4	99·1	109·2	110·9
Latvian SSR	12·0	26·2	28·1	31·7	32·1	63·0	115·1	117·9	126·9	127·8
Kirghiz SSR	3·8	23·8	31·9	37·4	38·8	24·1	91·1	106·3	111·2	112·6
Tajik SSR	4·5	22·4	29·2	33·5	34·6	28·6	87·8	97·9	96·0	96·4
Armenian SSR	4·1	17·8	21·9	24·4	24·5	30·1	79·4	86·0	86·0	84·8
Turkmen SSR	5·6	17·4	22·6	25·8	26·4	41·6	90·6	101·8	100·0	99·6
Estonian SSR	5·1	14·3	15·1	16·0	16·3	47·7	110·1	110·2	111·3	112·8

so doing expand the range of medical services provided to specific groups of patients.

The network of medical establishments rendering inpatient treatment is shown in Table IX.

TABLE IX. *Network of Medical Establishments Rendering Inpatient Medical Treatment (The System of the USSR Ministry of Health)*

	1960	1965	1970	1975	1976
Total number of medical establishments including	25 682	25 377	25 369	23 397	23 063
Regional hospitals	160	182	185	181	180
Town hospitals	4 185	4 067	3 990	3 842	3 791
Central district and district hospitals of rural areas	3 184	3 461	3 664	3 721	3 728
Local hospitals	12 941	11 684	11 263	9 899	9 640
Inpatient dispensaries	2 300	2 684	2 955	2 183	2 168
Maternity homes	775	721	693	645	633
Mental and neuropsychiatric hospitals	320	389	408	447	456
Other hospital institutions	1 817	2 189	2 211	2 479	2 467

D. Medical Care for Industrial Workers

As mentioned earlier, curative and prophylactic institutions in urban and rural areas of the USSR provide medical care to the population of the localities they cater for. In addition there are medical services which are set up with due regard to some specific features of certain occupational groups. Such services complement the overall system of medical institutions and include those designed to provide medical assistance to the workers in industrial enterprises. A typical medical and sanitary centre of a large factory or plant is a conglomeration of all medical units and institutions operating at a particular industrial enterprise including an inpatient department, a polyclinic, medical posts (established at individual workshops) as well as what is known as a prophylactorium, i.e. an overnight sanatorium in which workers and office employees of a factory or plant requiring treatment and constant medical observation stay overnight. At the same medical and sanitary centre, a nursery, kindergarten, pharmacy and some other units are provided.

A medical post is set up directly in the workshop and staffed either by paramedical personnel or by doctors, assisted by nurses. The personnel of a medical post administer aid directly to those working in a workshop, perform various prophylactic functions, and supervise the observance of industrial safety rules and hygiene standards. In all cases requiring specific medical attention a medical post refers its patients to the polyclinic of the medical and sanitary centre which in their turn, if necessary, send them to the inpatient department of a medical and sanitary centre or to a city hospital.

Table X gives some idea of the health institutions of industrial

TABLE X. *Health Institutions Maintained by the USSR Ministry of Health at Industrial Enterprises*

Types of institution	1975
Medical and sanitary centres	1 405
Inpatient departments	989
Number of hospital beds contained	205 047
Medical posts	33 814
Those staffed by doctors	2 648
Those staffed by doctors' assistants	31 166
Workshop therapeutic units	14 158

enterprises. Medical care for industrial workers is not limited to health institutions only. As an example in Table XI figures are given on the expenditure for labour protection, i.e. prevention of occupational injuries. Besides this the State allocates about 1·5 billion roubles annually for the manufacture of special clothing, footwear and other items of individual protection. The State allocated 15·4 billion roubles for the improvement of working conditions in the ninth five-year period (1971–75). Compared with 1970, occupational injuries decreased by 18% according to statistics for 1976.

TABLE XI. *Expenditure for Labour Protection (millions of roubles)*

1970	1971	1972	1973	1974	1975	1976
1 292	1 394	1 494	1 631	1 795	1 892	2 025

E. Medical Care in Rural Areas

The principles underlying the organization of therapeutic and prophylactic care, including primary health care, for urban and rural populations, are standard for the entire country. However, the great variety of geographic and economic conditions, the character of rural settlements and other entities of rural life determine the specific features of organizing health care there. Briefly the rural public health system created in the USSR is based on step-by-step medical service for the village population.

Due to the vast territory of the Soviet Union the main task is to locate medical institutions close to places of residence of rural dwellers. Primary medical centres set up on state farms bring primary health care considerably closer to the rural population. These primary medical centres usually have several rooms with two to three beds each and are staffed by a doctor's assistant, a midwife and a nurse. Usually such primary medical centres are created in villages with a population of 300 to 900 people. They are thus able to administer medical aid to the inhabitants not only of the given village, but also, as is often the case, to those of neighbouring villages. The primary health centre with a doctor's assistant in charge provides primary health care for the rural population, under the supervision of the physician of the local rural hospital, who makes regular scheduled rounds to all the medical centres in their locality.

The personnel of the medical centre take an active part in organizing medical examinations of the rural population by physicians, and helps to select persons who are to be kept under dispensary care. These persons are prescribed treatment by the physician when they attend the primary medical centre.

A major function of the primary medical centre is to provide outpatient services to the population. In cases when the professional knowledge of the doctor's assistant is inadequate, the patient is referred to a doctor at the nearest hospital.

Prophylaxis and improvement of local sanitary and hygienic standards are important functions of these medical centres. The doctors' assistants, midwives and nurses are duty bound to give the local inhabitants health instructions and to train some of them as voluntary sanitary inspectors to assist in supervising basic hygienic and sanitary standards locally, and work to improve the environment.

The number of primary medical centres in rural areas is growing. In 1975 there were 92 000, and they were staffed by more than 195 000 doctors' assistants and midwives.

The main establishment of the doctor's locality in the rural areas for rendering primary health care is the outpatient department of the rural district hospital or an independent outpatient department. On an average 5000 to 7000 people live in the rural doctor's locality, within a service radius of from 5 to 10 km. Physicians of the hospital receive adults and children at the hospital, visit patients on house calls and provide emergency aid.

The outpatient department of the rural doctor's locality is concerned with the early detection of disease and their timely treatment; sending patients to hospital when the case merits inpatient care; the selection of persons who need dispensary care, and regular examination and application of preventive measures.

Specialized medical aid for outpatients at every rural doctor's locality is provided by the following: internists, paediatricians, general surgeons, obstetricians and gynaecologists. Ambulance services for the population of the rural locality are provided by the central district hospital.

A mobile ambulatory unit may be created with the status of a separate structural subdivision of the local hospital. This type of primary health care is of great importance in territory with a wide service radius.

The head doctor of a rural hospital assisted by his staff is also responsible for the work of primary medical centres in his area staffed by doctor's assistants and midwives. There were about 10 000 such hospitals in the USSR in 1977.

The second level is the district hospital where qualified medical aid is administered by specialists (ten to twelve different specialists). The average handling capacity of district hospitals is about 200 inpatients, and many are being expanded to accommodate 250–400 and more inpatients. A central district hospital is also the administrative centre co-ordinating and controlling the work of all public health institutions in the rural districts. Its head doctor is at the same time the chief surgeon of the district with all head doctors of rural hospitals and other curative and prophylactic institutions reporting to him. About 50% of patients from rural areas receive inpatient care there. In 1972 there were more than 3700 central district and district hospitals.

The third stage is the regional (territorial republican medical establishment, where rural populations can receive complete outpatient and inpatient specialized treatment. In 1977 there were 180 regional hospitals in the USSR. These are usually large general hospitals with 600 or more beds, including a polyclinic where doctors administer outpatient aid to rural dwellers referred to them from district hospitals and sometimes directly from rural hospitals, and an inpatient department with a full range of specialized sections.

Regional hospitals, being centres of highly skilled specialist medical services for the rural population, provide facilities for the advanced retraining at refresher courses of doctors working in the medical institutions of the regions, particularly in rural and district hospitals, and as a training centre for secondary medical schools graduating medium medical personnel. All regional hospitals have conventional ambulance services and many of them have air ambulance services.

The district and regional inpatient hospitals cater to an estimated 60% of all patients in rural areas. The remaining 40% are taken care of by rural hospitals and curative and prophylactic institutions in the towns. A considerable proportion of the rural population receive treatment in inpatient urban curative and prophylactic institutions (over 25% of all patients from rural areas). Differences in the provision of medical assistance to the urban and rural populations of the USSR are gradually disappearing. This is reflected in the continuing levelling out of the proportion of urban and rural patients receiving hospital treatment.

F. Mother and Child Care

The health services for women and children, like those for the rest of the population, follow the area principle. For every 800–1000 children of an urban district there is a paediatrician in the local children's polyclinic who acts as a family doctor, giving professional advice and administering medical asssistance, consultation and preventive aid to children. His immediate assistants are nurses on the staff of children's polyclinics who visit the children in their homes not only to help the doctor in the administration of treatment, but also to train the mother and other members of the family in child care, to give them general health instruction, etc.

All infants during the first year of life are periodically visited (without being called) by a paediatrician. They are examined by a psychoneurologist, an orthopaedist, eye specialist and an ear, nose and throat specialist. A child in its second year is examined by a dentist and a specialist in the treatment of speech defects.

The main establishments rendering primary health care to women are women's consultation centres, which are part of maternity homes, outpatient polyclinics or medical centres of an industral enterprise. The women's consultation centre is a therapeutic and prophylactic establishement offering primary obstetric and gynaecological care, providing visiting nurse services, carrying on health education, social and legal work. The leading method in the work of women's consultation centres is dispensary care; all women are registered for surveillance in the early periods of pregnancy, physicians of various specialities conduct follow-up care, a wide range of laboratory tests are made. Planned prophylactic surveys of the female population are carried out for the purpose of the early diagnosis of gynaecological disease.

On visits to the women's consultation centre the pregnant woman is given recommendations by the physician regarding personal hygiene, regimens of work and leisure, diet, etc. In the post-partum period active follow-up care is continued. When a woman fails to attend the post-partum clinic, a visiting nurse is sent to her home.

Women's consultation centres or obstetric and gynaecological offices which are part of the medical centres of industrial enterprises have the same round of therapeutic and prophylactic duties as territorial women's consultation centres but function according to the principles of production-shop sectors.

In rural areas primary obstetric and gynaecological care is provided by the outpatient departments of central district and local hospitals and by obstetric and gynaecological offices of outpatient polyclinics in line with the principles of the urban areas.

Thus these mother and child institutions ensure continuous medical observation and supervision of the health of mothers and children thereby carrying into effect the prophylactic principle underlying the entire system of public health in the USSR. This system is supplemented by pre-school children's institutions, nurseries and kindergartens, some of which have been integrated into nursery-cum-kindergarten complexes. In the nurseries and kindergartens the children are kept under constant medical observation by staff paediatricians. In addition to the area paediatricians and those working at pre-school children's institutions, there are also school doctors who keep under medical observation the health and physical development of all the pupils, paying particular attention to prophylactic measures such as health education, control of vaccinations and other sanitary measures.

Children with poor health are sent to schools situated out of town which are known as "forest schools". These are unique educational and medical institutions which provide excellent conditions for normal study and medical supervision by highly skilled specialists. There are also special institutions for expectant mothers where they can rest under constant medical observation.

Table XII indicates the trend in the increase of the number of mother and child care institutions as well as in the number of paediatricians, obstetricians and gynaecologists. As the table shows, the number of specialists employed in mother and child care has increased fivefold. Today practically all women give birth under qualified medical supervision and 90% do so in maternity homes.

During the period 1965–75 the number of pre-school institutions increased by 70%. In 1975 there were over 115 000 nurseries, kindergartens and nursery-cum-kindergarten complexes accommodating over 11.5 million children (see Table XIII).

TABLE XII. *Mother and Child Care Institutions*

	1940	1950	1965	1970	1975
Maternity consultation clinics, children's polyclinics (independent and attached to other medical institutions)	8 600	11 300	19 300	21 000	22 079
Beds for pregnant and post-partum women	147 100	143 000	227 000	224 000	223 000
Number of paediatricians	19 400	32 100	71 700	79 000	96 300
Number of obstetricians and gynaecologists	10 600	16 600	35 400	40 500	49 600

TABLE XIII. *Pre-School Establishments (in thousands)*

	1913	1940	1965	1970	1975	1976
Number of permanent pre-school establishments including	0·2	46·0	91·9	102·7	115·2	117·6
Kindergartens	0·2	24·0	39·0	35·4	34·1	33·9
Crèche-kindergartens	–	–	28·5	47·7	65·3	68·7
Crèches	0·0	22·0	24·4	19·6	15·8	15·0
Number of infants in permanent pre-school establishments	5·4	1 953	7 673	9 281	11 523	12 108
Including those in kindergartens	4·0	1 172	3 281	2 791	2 591	2 559
Crèche-kindergartens	–	–	2 926	5 309	7 879	8 533
Including infants of crèche age (up to three years)	–	–	953	1 398	2 067	2 228
In crèches	1·4	781	1 466	1 181	1 053	1 016

There are laws according to which all working women are entitled to 112 days of fully paid maternity leave. In cases of multiple birth or childbirth complications the leave is automatically extended. After childbirth a woman may not work for a full year, during which time she retains her job and a continuous work record. Nursing mothers are entitled to additional rest and breaks during the working day.

Apart from these and other privileges and benefits there are allowances to mothers of large families and unmarried mothers, to children of low-income families, etc.

G. Ambulance Services

The ambulance service, as one of the most important kinds of primary health care is represented by a network of special establishments, stations, hospitals or departments. The ambulances are specially equipped and most have radio telephones to keep in touch with ambulance stations. There are also ambulances manned by specialized teams, and equipped to give emergency medical care including reanimation and care of victims of poisoning and heart failure.

Until recently there were two types of emergency medical services, the ambulance service and an emergency aid service provided by town outpatient clinics. These two services have now been merged with resultant reduction of time needed to reach patients.

As mentioned in Section E, ambulance services in the rural areas are provided by special units attached to central district hospitals and to regional hospitals. Many large regional hospitals also maintain an air ambulance service to rush qualified aid to accident victims and seriously ill patients in areas of difficult access, or where a patient needs urgent transportation to a specialized hospital.

Air ambulance services are essential in the vast territories of the Central Asian Republics, Kazakhstan and eastern areas of the Soviet Union.

The establishment of the unified emergency service in town and rural areas provides emergency on-the-spot medical aid in cases of sudden illness or accidents and maintains treatment of patients during transportation to inpatient establishments. This service also supplies vehicles for conveying persons in need to emergency treatment to inpatient hospitals at the request of medical establishments. The rule of the ambulance services in the USSR is to never refuse aid.

The intensive development of specialized types of emergency services began in 1965, and now there are specialized teams and units in resuscitation, cardiological, neurologic, toxicologic, paediatric among others.

In 1976, for example, ambulance services in the USSR comprised 4051 stations and units staffed by 30 000 physicians and over 70 000 medical workers with a secondary medical education, who dealt with over 71 million emergency calls.

There are three medical research institutes located in Moscow, Leningrad and Kharkov devoted to research on urgent problems of ambulance and emergency services.

H. Participation of the Population in Public Health Work

In the Soviet Union many different forms of participation by the general public in health work have developed. The population takes an active part on a voluntary basis in some aspects of the provision of medical aid, sanitation and other public health activities.

Public councils attached to many curative and prophylactic institutions are now very popular in the USSR. Among their members are representatives of public organizations, workers of industrial enterprises, collective farmers or tenants of nearby blocks of flats, including pensioners and housewives. These public councils help local public health institutions in their activities.

The Red Cross and Red Crescent societies are mass public organizations who also assist public health bodies and institutions in the discharge of their functions. These societies have membership of over 90 million. They organize training in first-aid methods, set up sanitary posts at industrial enterprises, collective farms and offices to see that work places are kept in a satisfactory sanitary condition and also to assist trained medical workers.

These societies train nurses who look after lonely, sick and aged people in their homes on a voluntary basis, and without remuneration. Members of these societies act as public sanitary inspectors, that is to say they see that streets and backyards are kept in a satistactory condition. The inhabitants of towns and villages, on their part, guided by medical workers, carry out various campaigns to improve the sanitary standards of their towns and villages. It is a tradition now to lay out public gardens and parks, to give lectures and talks on medical and sanitary subjects.

All local Soviets of People's Deputies (regional, city and district) also have public commissions composed of their deputies. The basic responsibility of these commissions is to help the local public health bodies and institutions to improve the functioning of all the health services. These commissions have broad powers and they use them effectively as they exercise control over many medical institutions and have the right to demand accounts from public health administrators. They have direct links with various public organizations and with all sections of the population, workers, office employees, and collective and state farmers whose interests they represent.

References

Relevant references for further study are listed as follows.

Burenkov, S. P. (1977). The main goals of the Soviet public health and the decisions of the 25th CPSU Congress. *Sovetskaya medicina* **1**, 3–10.

Burenkov, S. P. (1977). 'The great conquest of the October Revolution. *Sovetskoye zdravoohraneniye* **11**, 372.

Burenkov, S. P. (1978). A complex programme for further development of public health. *Sovetskoye zdravoohraneniye* **3**, 3–11.

Burenkov, S. P. (1978). Tasks of improving the public health services. *Sovetskoye zdravoohraneniye* **9**, 3–10.

Burgasov, P. N. (1973). "Country's Sanitary Defence", 64. Znanije, Moscow.

Chebotarev, D. F. (1977). Medicosocial aspects of the population's ageing. *Sovetskoye zdravoohraneniye,* **6**, 8–13.

Lidov, I. P., Stochik, A. M. and Tserkovny, G. F. (1978), "Soviet Public

Health and Organization of Primary Health Care for the Population of the USSR" 175. Mir Publishers, Moscow.
Lisitsin, Yu.P. (Ed.) (1967). "The System of Public Health Services in the USSR", 138, Moscow.
Novikova, E. (1975). "Children Get All the Best", 61. Maternal and Child Health Care in the USSR. Znanije, Moscow.
Petrovsky, B. V. (1971). "Health of the People as the Most Important Gain of the Socialist Society" 104. Medicina Publishers, Moscow.
Petrovsky, B. V. (1976). "The Achievements of the Soviet Public Health within the Framework of the 9th five-year Plan", 160. Medicina Publishers, Moscow.
Petrovsky, B. V. (Ed.) (1977). "Sixty Years of the Soviet Public Health", 416. Medicina Publishers, Moscow.
Petrovsky, B. V. (1978). Sixty years of the Soviet public health (achievements and way of future progress). *Sovetskoye zdravoohraneniye* **7**, 3–9.
Romanenko, A. E. (1977). Health protection of toilers in the villages. *Sovetskoye zdravoohraneniye* **11**, 23–29.
Romanenko, A. E. (1979) Organization of specialized medical aid for the population of an industrial city. *Sovetskoye zdravoohraneniye* **3**, 3–12.
Safonov, A. G. (1977). Levelling of the health care for urban and rural populations. *Sovetskoye zdravoohraneniye* **1**, 14–22.
Sharmanov, T. S. (1979). The significance and place of primary health care in the public health of Kazakhstan. *Sovetskoye zdravoohraneniye* **1**, 3–6.
Timakov, V. D. (1972). "Man, Medicine, Technical and Scientific Revolution", 61. Znanije, Moscow.
Trofimov, V. V. (1967). "Fifty Years of Public Health Care in the Russian Federation", 332. Medicina Publishers, Moscow.
Venediktov, D. D. (1977) "Problems of International Health", 376. Medicina Publishers, Moscow.
USSR Statistics for 1977 (brief statistics annual), 238. Statistical Publishers, Moscow.

20

Changing Patterns of Health Care in Western Countries

Anthony Hordern*
Sydney, Australia

No Western nation has yet developed an optimal method of satisfying the public, the health care providers and the government.

---

* Honorary Psychiatrist, Sydney Hospital.

Developed nations particularly have experienced an accelerating rate of change since 1945. Advances in technology have transformed the Western World into a vast technosociety characterized from a health standpoint by alterations in disease profiles, changes in social institutions, increased stresses on individuals, higher expectations of doctors, and soaring health care costs. The last of these phenomena especially has compelled Western medicine, traditionally patient-centred, antidotal— and largely anecdotal—to recognize the desirability of supplementing this with a society-centred, preventive, scientific approach. This chapter, after discussing these topics, briefly reviews health care systems in three major developed nations: the United States, the United Kingdom and Australia.

I. Health Problems of the Technosociety

Whereas in developing countries the infective diseases, especially in the very young, aggravated by poverty, malnutrition and adverse social conditions, are the main causes of mortality and morbidity, their counterparts in the developed nations are the ageing and degenerative disorders which occur in middle and later life in settings of affluence, superabundant calories and adequate social support systems. These "diseases of affluence" (Kemp, 1967) and "diseases of civilization" (Burkitt, 1973)—coronary heart disease, obesity and diabetes, alcoholism, bronchial carcinoma, and so forth—have ramified throughout Western society and within it even those who do not overindulge in food, alcohol or nicotine frequently court ill-health by consuming a diet inadequate in roughage with too much milk, fat, sugar, salt and red meat and—arguably—too many chemical additives (Hordern, 1976; Segall, 1977). Furthermore, the spectrum of disease has widened in recent years, because many social and emotional problems have become "medicalized" (Fry, 1972; Sax, 1974).

In recent years many formerly revered social institutions have lost their capacity to evoke respect and/or to inspire. The American presidency, post-Watergate, under the remorseless scrutiny of television, has failed to regain its former status; organized religions (especially the Roman Catholic Church because of its inflexible opposition to "artificial" conception control, divorce and other modern trends), are losing their adherents; the American Army post-Vietnam has encountered problems of morale and purpose; and police forces everywhere, made to enforce unpopular laws, have come to be regarded, especially by the young, with suspicion and hostility. The technosociety, furthermore, is characterized by increasing social equality, the working class having acquired money and clout, and the professional and managerial classes having had to share both affluence and influence. Professional individuals are less respected than formerly; their expertise is now more frequently questioned, and the Protestant ethic of hard work, thrift, morality and the making of personal financial provision for the future (through savings, insurances and so forth) has been replaced by an hedonistic, leisure-centred ethic in which, it is believed, the State, as an universal "milch cow", should and will provide if illness, calamities or age supervene. "Permissivity" in dress, behaviour, communication and liberal legislation has become widespread, and non-medicinal tranquillisers such as alcohol, cigarettes and marijuana, have become increasingly popular.

Many aspects of life in the technosociety exert pressure on individuals, the two greatest areas of stress, according to Eyer (1975), being the disruption of social communities and the rise to hierarchically controlled, time-pressured work. Families have become "fractured", as Toffler (1973) has observed, and as they have dwindled in numerical size, with the growing enthusiasm for co-habitation, the waning popularity of marriage, the increasing recourse to divorce, and the rise of one-parent families (usually headed by the mother), the nuclear family, which replaced the extended family, is also passing into obsolescence. Marriage, nonetheless, as the cornerstone of the family, has long been recognized to exert a protective effect on health (Lynch, 1977; Somers, 1979) and many individuals who lack families and who lead lonely, isolated lives are too vulnerable to survive in good health without readily accessible social support. In this situtation, lack of education is the most critical disadvantage, for those belonging to society's unskilled 10% "underclass"are insufficiently knowledgeable to obtain assistance from community agencies and other support systems (Morris, 1979). Individuals of both sexes and all ages have come under pressure, but those affected most severely have probably been the elderly, women of mature years, and youngsters under the age of eighteen (Hordern 1976). At a time of striking medical progress in the conquest of infectious and other diseases, advances in medical technology, a decline in the ethic of self-sufficiency and of acceptance of suffering, lack of support from family, community and church, and the mounting pressures of an increasingly complex environment, it is understandable that public expectations of doctors are higher than ever (Office of Health Economics, 1972). The latter are besieged by near-insatiable demands and stressed by incessant pressures on their time (Mawardi, 1979). It is hardly surprising therefore that role strain and other factors produce high rates of alcoholism, drug abuse and suicide amongst medical practitioners (Ellard, 1974).

Because of the steady increase in the number of old people, the continuance of scientific and technical advances, and cultural progress (EEC Plenary Assembly—*British Medical Journal*, 1979), as well as inflation and other factors, health costs soared in the mid-1970s, and seem destined to rise still further, perhaps to as high as 10% of a developed country's gross national product (GNP). Modern medicine is predominantly hospital-orientated, and large general hospitals, especially teaching institutions, are enormously expensive to build, equip and operate, taking the lion's share of health care funds. Highly skilled staff, many of whom have to provide 24-hour coverage, are costly to employ—salaries take up to 75% of hospital budgets. Sophisticated diagnostic devices—CAT scanners, automated laboratory equipment, laser "knives" and so on—and specialized treatment units and programmes—intensive care units, facilities for organ transplants, renal dialysis programmes—also swallow funds with alarming rapidity. Patients, unaware of the true costs incurred, want Rolls-Royce care at Ford Popular prices; physicians, largely oblivious of economic considerations, often attempt to give it to them. Many governments, by fostering the expectations of patients and by denying physicians the wherewithal to satisfy them, place the latter in an invidious position (Cox, 1977).

It is unfortunate that, mainly due to television and other media, the Western public's image of contemporary medical practice is based largely on dramatic cures in a few patients treated effectively in high-energy, high-technology, high-cost hospital environments; such illnesses, such forms of treatment and such environments receive a disproportionately high share of health funds as well as the greatest emphasis in teaching. The bulk of health problems, however, comprises two much larger groups of ailments: (i) chronic, often irreversible, diseases, such as circulatory disorders, chronic bronchitis, obesity, arthritis, chronic alcoholism and psychiatric illnesses; and (ii) minor, self-limiting disorders such as upper respiratory infections, allergies and stress reactions such as tension headaches, dyspepsia and anxiety states (Furnass, 1976). Provision must be made, therefore, for these conditions to be treated efficiently and economically, as well as for the more expensive types of treatment sometimes necessary.

Traditional antidotal patient-centred medical care—a "salvage" operation concerned with "illth", i.e. illness, the opposite of health (Furnass, 1976)—has, it has become clear, not only been ineffective in promoting health and longevity, but also has become exorbitantly expensive both for individuals and for third parties (insurance companies, employers, governments and so on) (Carlson, 1975). Because an "engineering" approach to medicine has prevailed until recently, pathogenic factors in the environment—low social status, substandard housing, adverse working conditions, unemployment stresses and economic insecurity—have not been accorded their appropriate importance as contributors to ill-health. The modern approach therefore is preventive rather than antidotal, and is focused on society as well as the sick individual, a disease being regarded not merely as a process taking place in the latter, but as the product of an interaction between an individual and his or her environment.

The links in the causal chain leading to such common major illnesses as ischaemic heart disease, cancer, strokes, and other ailments, Powles (1977) has suggested, comprise macrosocioeconomic health determinants (a nation's economic development and organization, its labour market, its consumption patterns and their inculcation, and the hygienic quality of its natural and artificial environment), microsocioeconomic health determinants (notably marriage, and the individual's integration into the social order) and personal determinants of health (individual consumption patterns and life styles). Whilst educating individuals to avoid harmful practices and to become more stoical, more self-reliant and more prepared to regulate their own medical care, as proposed by Illich (1975), would obviously be advantageous, most people are unable to diagnose and treat themselves appropriately, as shown for example by the renal conditions produced by abuse of analgesics (Duggan and Nanta, 1976). The primary care physician is thus more essential than ever in the technosociety of today, not only in healing and, where necessary, referring patients for specialist treatment, but also in acting as guide, confidant, counsellor and friend in matters pertaining to health in its broadest sense.

II. Health Care in the United States of America

In July 1976, the United States, with an area of 3 537 000 square miles had a population of 214 659 000 with 49 815 000 white and 6 572 000 Negro families (88.7% and 11.3%) (*CBS News Almanac*, 1978). Over half (51.2%) of the population was female: the average length of life for white females was 77.2 years and for females of other races was 72.3 years; the corresponding figures for white males was 69.4 years and for males of other races was 63.6 years. The overall mortality rate was 8.9 per

1000 population, heart disease accounting for 38% of all deaths (American Medical Association, 1978).

In 1976 the United States had 409 446 medical practitioners, 22 117 of which were inactive. Patient-care activities were carried out by 79.5 per cent of all physicians, 68.0 per cent of whom were office based. In 1976 there were 189 physicians per 100 000 population (1 for every 529 people) versus 142 per 100 000 (1 for every 702) in 1960. There were an estimated 1 450 000 registered and practical nurses and, in toto, some 5 088 950 individuals were employed in the health care industry, which was the third largest employer in the US economy. Hospitals in the United States in 1976 numbered 7082, with 1 434 000 beds; practically 60% were short-term general community hospitals with fewer than 200 beds. The cost of health care by 1978 had risen to about $US 180 billion annually, 8.8 per cent of the GNP, with hospital costs, at 40–45% of health expenditure, constituting the largest item (*Newsweek*, 1979).

The health care delivery system in the United States, private in the main but supplemented by a public sector at the local (city and county), state and federal levels, reflects the private enterprise ethos of the nation. The public sector is designed to fill the needs the private sector does not cover, i.e. health care for the poor, public health and environmental programmes, laboratory facilities, treatment for the chronically sick, medical care for special groups (veterans, merchant seamen, American Indians, migrant workers, mothers and children and so on), funds to develop health resources (research; manpower; hospital construction) and funds to improve particular aspects of health care (Regional Medical Programs for cancer, heart, stroke and kidney disease; health planning; experimental community health delivery systems and a variety of other programmes (Duval, 1976).

Private medical care is notable for the paucity of primary care practitioners, especially in isolated rural areas and in impoverished city centres, and for the multiplicity of subspecialists or specialoids. The average American therefore has to refer himself as an insured patient to the appropriate specialist or subspecialist who, in conformity with his training, customarily practises at or near a well-equipped general hospital. The poor and the dissolute, devoid of insurance, frequently seek treatment at hospital Accident Rooms. Rich and poor alike are thus propelled towards the hospital, usually a highly technological, surgically and diagnostically orientated acute specialist unit, unnecessarily expensive for the provision of most medical care. The fact that 79% of Americans held hospital insurance coverage in 1975 versus 60 per cent with coverage for physician's office and home visits (now quite rare), indicates the average individual's scale of priorities (American Medical Association, 1978).

The American public now expects "miracle cures" for many conditions and feels frustrated when these are not forthcoming. Resentment towards its doctors—many of them conspicuously wealthy after earlier indebtedness—has grown as, despite mounting fees, access to them has become increasingly difficult. Though most patients like their doctors, malpraxis suits have, facilitated by the contingency principle, become increasingly common. Such enormous sums have been awarded recently that malpraxis insurance, especially for specialists such as orthopaedic surgeons, has become increasingly expensive and almost impossible to obtain.

Concern for the over-65s and for the indigent led the US Federal Government to enact Medicare (for the aged) and Medicaid (for the poor) in 1965. These programmes have proved extremely expensive: between 1967 and 1978 the cost of Medicare rose from $US 3 billion to $US 24 billion, and that of Medicaid from $US 2.2 billion to $US 18 billion. Health Maintenance Organizations (HMOs, prepaid medical and hospital care plans) were signed into law in December 1973 in an attempt to cut health costs, and Professional Standards Review Organizations (PSROs) were later established also, 185 being in existence by early 1979. From the mid-1970s onwards, furthermore, despite opposition from the American Medical Association, fearful of the looming spectre of governmental control, soaring health care costs and difficulty of access to physicians produced increasing pressures on the US Government to enact some form of universal health insurance coverage. By mid-1979, two and a half years after the Democrats came into power, both President Carter and his rival, Senator Edward Kennedy, had presented plans for comprehensive National Health Insurance coverage (*Newsweek*, 1979). These proposals, coming at a time when the established national health insurance plans of many countries—Britain, Australia, Sweden and so forth—were being thrown into reverse or otherwise modified because of the rapid, serious cost increase that had attended them (despite their control of physicians' incomes) seemed quite remarkable to non-American observers (*Lancet*, 1979).

III. Health Care in the United Kingdom

In 1976 the United Kingdom (England, Wales, Scotland and Northern Ireland), a nation with an area of 94 222 square miles, had a population of 55 928 000 with some 12.5 million two-parent and 1.2 million one-parent families; approximately 1 691 000 individuals were of New Commonwealth or Pakistani ethnic origin (HMSO, 1977; Central Statistical Office, 1978). Over half (51.3%) of the UK population was female; the average length of life for women was 75.5 years and for men 69.2 years. The overall death rates were 11.4 per thousand population for women and 12.3 per thousand for men; 31.5 per cent of male deaths and 24.0 per cent of female deaths were due to coronary artery disease.

Comprehensive universal health care for the UK population—and utilized by 98% of it—has been provided by the National Health Service (NHS) since 1948. Some 24 500 general practitioners were working in the NHS in 1976; each was allowed a list of 3500 patients, but the average doctor had 2400. Apart from general practitioners, 36 770 physicians and surgeons, including over 13 600 consultants, were then employed in the 2770 NHS hospitals which contained 498 000 beds and were staffed by 258 000 full-time and 170 000 part-time nurses and midwives. Most of these hospitals had been built in the nineteenth century, but many had been improved and extended, and some new hospitals have been constructed (HMSO, 1977). Government expenditure on the NHS had risen to 6.9 per cent of the GNP by 1976/77, hospitals absorbing about 56% of the total NHS costs (Snaith, 1979).

It is a striking fact that, next to the Royal Family, the NHS has always been the most popular of British institutions (Klein, 1979). Central taxation meets most (88%) of its cost, the remainder being covered by National Insurance contributions and by charges paid by individuals for prescriptions, dentures, spectacles and other services. Throughout the life of the NHS Labour governments have made repeated attempts for doctrinaire reasons to squeeze private practice out of it, though by 1974 only 4 500 NHS beds—less than 1% of the total—were private.

The original organization of the NHS utilized the fact that prior to its inception specialization in medicine in Great Britain had not gone as far as in the United States so that a division had developed between hospital-based specialism and community-based generalism (Godber, 1978). A tripartite structure was therefore established (hospital and consultant services, general practitioner services, and local authority services) which was administered in fourteen hospital regions in England and Wales, five in Scotland, and one in Northern Ireland, by regional health boards under the central supervision of the Ministry of Health (teaching hospitals were administered separately by boards of governors coming directly under the Ministry of Health). Junior hospital doctors were paid full-time salaries while senior staff—consultants—were in the main left free to choose between full-time and part-time sessional payments, the latter permitting them limited private practice. General practitioners were remunerated on the basis of a capitation fee for each patient on their lists, supplemented by additional dues and allowances.

Sickness, at the time the NHS was established, was thought of largely in acute medical and acute surgical terms. The hope and expectation was that when better, more accessible care was made generally available, the nation's health would improve, the pool of illness would be mopped up, and health costs would gradually be reduced. The dream was never realized. Although deaths from tuberculosis, infective diseases and so forth dropped, mortality and morbidity from the "diseases of affluence" and psychomedical disorders rose, and costs soared, for though the number of general practitioners increased only slightly between 1951 and 1968, prescriptions rose by 25%, radiography by 50%, pathological tests by over 200%, and the number of consultants by almost 400% (Cochrane, 1972). From an estimated cost of £110 million in 1948, the NHS budget rose to £384 million in 1951–52 and £6234 million in 1976–77.

Although the NHS embodied a noble ideal and functioned effectively for many years, particularly in the cases of patients with acute and severe illnesses, problems became apparent, many of them related to chronic underfinancing, and, in the early 1970s especially, widespread dissatisfaction with pay, working conditions and career prospects was expressed by general practitioners and hospital medical staff. The fact that NHS payment levels were not related either to quantity or quality of work performed irked and de-incentivated some practitioners, and among junior hospital doctors especially the triad of low pay, uncertain prospects and poor facilities impelled a constant 20% to 30% of British medical graduates to emigrate. Most went to Canada, the United States, Australia or New Zealand, the positions they left being filled by foreign medical graduates, mainly from India and Pakistan.

Since many of the problems of the NHS were attributed to its tripartite organization, the Health Service was reorganized from April 1974, each of the fourteen former hospital regions in England (for example) each being placed under a Regional Health Authority which exercised planning, co-ordinating, supervisory and executive functions over a number of Area Health Authorities. The latter, ninety in all, were subdivided into 230 Districts, each controlled by a District Management Team. In addition, Joint Consultative Committees, appointed by local and by health authorities, and Community Health Councils, designed to represent the interests of the consumer, were created (McKeown and Lowe, 1974).

The period following the NHS reorganization nevertheless proved exceptionally difficult. In the summer of 1974, threatened or actual strikes by nurses, ancillary hospital workers, local government officials, pharmacists and radiographers took place, to be followed in 1976, 1977 and 1978 by disputes by unions representing ancillary hospital staff. The main problems underlying the latter disputes, according to Bosanquet and Healy (1979), were pay, the absence of a developed industrial relations system, and incident-prone districts. At its thirtieth anniversary in July 1978, the Labour Government and most of the general public seemed satisfied with the NHS despite its shortcomings, but a substantial proportion of the medical profession considered itself exploited and under-rewarded, and was concerned about uneven hospital care and substandard facilities.

IV. Health Care in Australia

In 1977 Australia with an area of 2 968 000 square miles had a population of some 14 074 000, one-fifth of which was foreign-born, with approximately equal numbers of males and females. The average expectation of life at birth was 68.9 years for men and 75.9 for women. The crude death rate was 7.91 per 1000, heart disease accounting for 35.6% of all deaths (Cameron, 1978).

Australia had some 21 600 medical practitioners in 1977, one for every 644 persons. In 1977–78 it had approximately 188 812 registered nurses and 35 620 nursing aides caring for patients in 87 946 beds in 1068 approved hospitals, 735 of them public and 333 private. The cost of health care had by then reached $A7151 million annually, 7·89% of the GNP, with hospital costs, at 60% of health expenditure, constituting by far the largest item (*AMA Gazette*, 1979a).

The health care delivery system in Australia in many ways is midway between that of the United States (predominantly free-enterprise private care with some governmental support) and that of the United Kingdom (predominantly state-financed, state-run health care with a small private component). As in the United States, the patient in the open fee-for-service medical market can go to the doctor(s) of his choice, his costs being defrayed partly through state and private insurance and partly from his own pocket. In Australia as in the United Kingdom, however, the average individual has a general practitioner whom he (or she) regards as his (or her) personal doctor though, unlike his UK counterpart, the Australian GP is usually willing to tackle a wide range of problems (sometimes even major surgery) and so is less inclined to transfer patients to specialist care.

The health responsibilities of the Federal (Commonwealth) Government extended only to quarantine until 1946, but thereafter it became more active, establishing a Pharmaceutical Benefits Scheme in 1950 and a Pensioner Medical Scheme in 1951. From 1953 onwards, the National Health Acts enabled non-profit health insurance funds to be created, contributors to which were automatically entitled to government benefits. By 1962, 78% of Australians had health insurance cover and the proportion reached 88% in early 1975. Under the Health Benefits Plan, which started to operate in 1970, the "gap" between the patient's insurance cover and the doctor's "most common fee", the maximum amount for which the patient was legally responsible, was fixed at $A5·00 (Lovell, 1976).

The rise in health costs that occurred in the early 1970s generated a demand for governmentally supervised health care. Accordingly Gough Whitlam's Labour administration, which came into power in 1972, initiated a comprehensive universal health insurance scheme, despite vigorous opposition from the Australian Medical Association (AMA) and other bodies. The Health Insurance Commission, "Medibank", became operational in July 1975, financed by a 1·35% levy on taxable income up to $A150 annually, and by contributions from other Commonwealth sources. It provided *inter alia*: (i) medical care from general practitioners remunerated on a fee-for-service basis by Medibank, which also paid specialists (on a different scale); (ii) standard accommodation for all, irrespective of means, in public hospitals; and (iii) help for individual States by sharing hospital running costs on a fifty-fifty basis. Private medical and hospital care remained available as alternative options (Munro, 1976).

Under the new scheme doctors could be paid by individual patients (helped by Medibank or a private fund) or could "bulk-bill" Medibank for 85% of their scheduled fees. With the data thus generated the Medibank computers, later provided with additional material from the private funds, were able to build up, doctor by doctor, a profile of patients seen, services rendered and amounts charged. The findings showed *inter alia* that in the months after Medibank was instituted the number of patients consulting doctors rose by only 2 % and that those who were bulk-billed, contrary to expectation, on average claimed fewer services than their non-bulk-billed counterparts (Hicks, 1978a; *Choice*, 1978).

In October, 1976, the new Liberal Government under Malcolm

Fraser, despite its pre-election promise not to change Medibank, modified it to "Medibank II" by raising the levy to 2·5%, thus encouraging people to opt for private care. Health costs, however, continued to rise, albeit at a slower rate (36·6% in 1974/75, 27·1% in 1975/76, and 19·7% in 1976/77), the main factor not being an increase in doctors' services per person (which rose from 4·7 in 1973/74 to 5·9 in 1975/76) or in doctors' fees (which rose 31% in 1974/75, 20·5% in 1975/76 and 7·5% in 1976/77), but an increase in doctor-initiated tests, procedures and referrals, together with a rise in hospital costs and inflation (*Choice*, 1978). In May 1978, therefore, at the suggestion of the Federal Minister of Health, the Australian Medical Association committed itself to the concept of peer review. In planning a series of clinical audits, however, the Australian Medical Association was thinking primarily in terms of quality of patient care, whilst the Government was thinking principally of cost. The two goals were almost diametrically opposed (Arnold, 1979).

Continuing its efforts to shift the expense of health insurance back onto the private sector, the Liberal Government, in July 1978, unveiled Medibank III, under which patients paid more towards the cost of a consultation, the maximum patient contribution for any one-scheduled-fee service being increased from $A5·00 to $A10·00. In November, 1978, the Government abolished the levy completely and with it ended Medibank Standard (though Medibank Private, a health care fund like eighty-odd other health funds, survived). Funding from consolidated revenue was introduced, with a 40% refund on doctors' fees up to $A20·00. In May 1979, the rebate on the first $A20·00 of the doctor's fee was removed also (85% of doctors' fees were under this amount). Since hospital charges were to rise 25% in September 1979, and doctors' fees (after a 22-month freeze) by 13·5% two months later the year seemed likely to be expensive for the health care consumer whether he continued with the by now very costly (about $A700 annually per family in New South Wales) health insurance, or whether he met the new charges out of his own pocket (Bromby, 1979).

In conclusion, three aspects of health care delivery in Australia in the late 1970s were noteworthy: hospitals, surgical operations and medical manpower. Hospitals were in oversupply: their average bed occupancy was only 68%, and hospitalization was 30% higher than in the USA, and twice as high as in the UK. Because these practices were costly and inefficient, avoidance of unnecessary hospitalization, shorter stays and a rationalization of hospital services with a reduction in the number of beds were advocated by a team of Commonwealth investigators (*AMA Gazette*, 1979b). The team also drew attention to the abnormally large number of operations, many of them relatively non-essential such as tonsillectomy, hysterectomy and cosmetic procedures, performed in some areas presumably as a result of overservicing by an excess of surgeons. Finally Australia, like other developed nations, was acquiring too many doctors because overseas medical migrants were adding to the number of its own medical graduates. It was calculated that, if the 1978 rate of increase was maintained, there would be 165 doctors per 100 000 population by 1981 or 1982 (against the World Health Organization's recommended level of 150 per 100 000) and an excess of 3500 doctors by 1991 (Hicks, 1978b).

V. Summary

Faced with essentially similar challenges—a changed and widened profile of illnesses many of them related to life-style, changes in society, increased pressures on individuals, ever-higher expectations of doctors and soaring health costs—the United States, the United Kingdom and Australia have developed different, but not totally dissimilar, health care delivery systems, each of which has proved increasingly expensive and each of which has exhibited individual strengths and weaknesses. American health care, hospital-centred, multispecialty orientated, sophisticated and highly technological, is handicapped by maldistribution of resources, shortage of primary care physicians and difficulty of access to doctors: as a consequence a move towards governmentally supervised national health insurance has become evident, greeted with concern by the medical profession. Great Britain's National Health Service provides free access, general practitioner medical treatment supported by adequate specialist and hospital care, but though the NHS is popular with the public, numerous hospitals are outdated, staff and equipment shortages present problems, and many doctors and health care personnel are disenchanted and dissatisfied. The Australian plan for comprehensive health insurance coverage, Medibank, engrafted onto a pattern of health care approximately halfway between the systems of the United States and the United Kingdom, underwent repeated modifications and was eventually terminated in less than four years, creating problems for the public, the health care providers, and the Government. Clearly no Western nation has yet devised an optimal method of satisfying all three parties.

References

AMA Gazette (1979a). In brief. AMA Gaz. **224**, 3.
AMA Gazette (1979b). Summary. Hospitals document bears heavily on medical practice. *AMA Gaz.* **224**, 27–28.
American Medical Association (1978). "Socioeconomic Issues of Health 1978." American Medical Association, Monroe, Wisconsin.
Arnold, P. C. (1979). Crises down under. *Br. Med. J.* i, 107–108.
Bosanquet, N. and Healy, G. (1979). Is the NHS really torn by strife? *New Society* **48**, 328–329.
British Medical Journal (1979). EEC Plenary Assembly. Declaration on health costs. *Br. Med. J.* i, Supplement, 65.
Bromby, R. (1979). The health scheme mess. *National Times* 16 June.
Burkitt, D. P. (1973) "Some diseases characteristic of Western Civilization". *Br. med. J.* i, 274–278.
Cameron, R. J. (1978). "Year Book Australia, 1977–78". Australian Bureau of Statistics, Canberra.
CBS News Almanac (1978). Hammond Almanac Inc., Maplewood, New Jersey.
Carlson, R. J. (1975). "The End of Medicine". John Wiley, New York.
Central Statistical Office (1978). "Facts in Focus", 4th edn. Penguin, Harmondsworth.
Choice (1978). Review. The new health policy: a misdiagnosis of the ailment? *Choice* **19**, 358–362.
Cochrane, A. L. (1972). "Effectiveness and Efficiency: Random Reflections on Health Services". Nuffield Provincial Hospitals Trust, London.
Cox, K. R. (1977). Who owns the problem of health care costs? *Med. J. Aust.* **2**, 727–730.
Duggan, J. M. and Nanra, R. S. (1976). Analgesic addiction of a nation. *In* "The Magic Bullet". Society for Social Responsibility in Science, Canberra.
Duval, M. K. (1976). The national pattern of health care and delivery in the United States and its effect on the education, recruitment and migration of physicians". *In* "International Aspects of the Provision of Medical Care" (P. W. Kent, Ed.). Oriel, London.
Eyer, J. (1975). Hypertension as a disease of modern society. *Int. J. Hlth Services*, **5**, 539–558.
Ellard, J. (1974). The disease of being a doctor. *Med J. Aust.* **2**, 318–323.
Fry, J. (1972). Medicine and the society of man. *In* "International Medical Care" (J. Fry and W. A. J. Farndale, Eds). Medical and Technical Publ. Oxford.
Furnass, B. (1976). Changing patterns of health and disease. *In* "The Magic Bullet". Society for Social Responsibility in Science, Canberra.
Godber, G. (1978). The effect of specialization on the practice of medicine. *Lancet* ii, 257–259.
Her Majesty's Stationery Office (1977). "Britain 1977. An Official Handbook". HMSO, London.

Hicks, R. (1978a). Medi stampede "a myth". *The Australian*, 23 February.
Hicks, R. (1978b). Doctors must learn to cut costs". *The Australian* 24 July.
Hordern, A. (1976). "Tranquillity Denied". Rigby, Adelaide.
Illich, I. (1975). "Medical Nemesis". Calder and Boyars, London.
Kemp, R. (1967). Morbidity and social class. *Lancet* i, 1316–1318.
Klein, R. (1979). Public opinion and the National Health Service. *Br. med. J.* i, 1296–1297.
Lancet (1979). Round the world. United States: the President's plans for health care. *Lancet* i, 543–544.
Lovell, R. R. H. (1976). Aspects of the provision of medical care in Australia: the tyranny of history. *In* "International Aspects of the Provision of Medical Care" (P. W. Kent, Ed.). Oriel, London.
Lynch, J. J. (1977). "The Broken Heart". Basic Books, New York.
McKeown, T. and Lowe, C. R. (1974). "An Introduction to Social Medicine". Blackwell, Oxford.
Mawardi, B. H. (1979). Satisfactions, dissatisfactions, and causes of stress in medical practice. *J. Am. Med. Ass.* **241**, 1483–1486.
Morris, J. N. (1979). Social inequalities undiminished. *Lancet* i, 87–90.
Munro, I. (1976). In Australia now. *Lancet* i, 467–470, 525–529.
Newsweek (1979). US Affairs. Health care battle. *Newsweek* 28 May, 32–38.
Office of Health Economics (1972). "Medicine and Society". OHE, London.
Powles, J. (1977). Socioeconomic health determinants in working-age males. *In* "The Impact of Environment and Life-Style on Human Health". Society for Social Responsibility in Science, Canberra.
Sax, S. (1974). Bureaucracy and medical care. *Med. J. Aust.* **2**, 349–352.
Segall, J. J. (1977). Is milk a coronary health hazard? *Br. J. prevent. soc. Med.* **31**, 81–85.
Snaith, A. H. (1979). Supply and demand in the NHS. *Br. med. J.* ii, 1159–1160.
Somers, A. R. (1979). Marital status, health, and use of health services. *J. Am. Med. Ass.* **241**, 1818–1822.
Toffler, A. (1973). "Future Shock". Pan, London.

Part IV

Problems of Development and Urbanization

Introduction

Progressive urbanization and changes in technology and the distribution of resources and production have altered disease patterns throughout the world. The political and economic separation of nations into "developed" and "underdeveloped", or "developing", countries is reflected in changes in demography and in morbidity and mortality, so that the health problems of the two groups are very different.

The underdeveloped countries are facing problems due to disruption of traditional life styles, poverty, urbanization and rapid, usually unchecked, population increase. These were mentioned in Part III and are discussed further in the first two chapters of this section. Dr Maddocks surveys some problems associated with the transition of Papua New Guinea from a tribal society to a nation with cities and a recently developed technology. Dr Michael Gracey considers the next phase, that of massive rapid increases in the numbers of people, and their movement from rural to urban life. This is occurring in many parts of the world—Africa, South America, Asia and the Pacific region. The results are both tangible—a rise in infectious disease and undernutrition with a high infant mortality in large semi-urban shanty towns—and intangible—a loss of faith and the slow dissolution of family and group coherence leading to crime and violence.

These problems are discussed in a contemporary world, but they are not new. They are an apparently inevitable stage in the evolution of human society. The present developed nations have survived this phase in moving to a new life-style—that of urban technology.

Industrialization and urbanization lead to different health problems, and these are discussed in the remaining chapters in this section. They result from changes in the environment as well as in life-styles and nutrition. These include pollution, considered in part by Dr de Koning and Dr Higginson, as well as man-made hazards such as the motor car, the subject of the following chapter by Dr Ryan.

This new environment, the provision of plenty, and increasing longevity are the causes of the new patterns of disease, considered in the final chapters of this section. Dr Armstrong and Dr McMichael describe overnutrition, and Professor McCall shows that this is one factor in the present epidemic of cardiovascular disease. Finally, Dr Lefroy surveys a new phenomenon—the geriatric revolution, when for the first time in human history the aged form a significant proportion of living people.

21

Economic Demography of the Twentieth Century

R. T. Appleyard

Department of Economic History, University of Western Australia, Perth, Australia

---

Economic, social and political changes in this century. . . have by any reasonable criterion been dramatic.

The earth is presently inhabited by approximately 4000 million human beings. By the end of the millenium the number will have probably increased to 6000 million (Fig. 1b). I say "approximately 4000 million" because, despite a marked improvement in the accuracy and coverage of census and related data during recent years, estimates of many national populations are still subject to considerable error. And I say "will have probably increased to 6000 million" because of inherent uncertainties and difficulties associated with world population projections.

Accuracy of projections for economically developed countries will depend especially on the projector's judgement concerning likely attitudes of young people towards the number and spacing of their children. Unexpected downward changes in fertility of couples during the last few decades have emphasized the rapidity with which attitudes can alter concerning marriage, childbearing and desirable family size. Accuracy of projections for economically underdeveloped countries will depend especially on changes in rates of economic growth and on the distribution of wealth in these countries and between developed and developing countries. Overall recent high levels of fertility have produced very "young" populations whose potential for high rates of demographic growth is considerable. Over 40% of the populations of many developing countries are under fifteen years of age, so there will need to be a dramatic decline in the size of families of couples during the next twenty years if population growth is to be reduced significantly. A more likely trend is that completed family size will, at best, decline only slowly and that the proportion of the world's population in developing countries will therefore increase.

Spengler has estimated that on the basis of present demographic structures, growth in Third World countries is likely to continue at a high rate, perhaps slowing to 2% per annum by the year 2000, whereas the rate of growth in developed countries will be about 0·8%, "if that". As a result, by the end of the millenium the population of the Third World may be 5000 million or more whereas the developed world may have fewer than 1500 million persons. This would raise the Third World's share of global population to about 77%, up from 68% in 1965.[1]

Differential rates of economic and demographic growth between developed and developing nations during the last few decades have been a function of each nation's capacity and willingness to initiate appropriate policies. By and large, developed countries have been successful in retaining their positions at the top end of the international economic ladder, and their people's ready access to effective methods of population control has allowed them to achieve their objectives

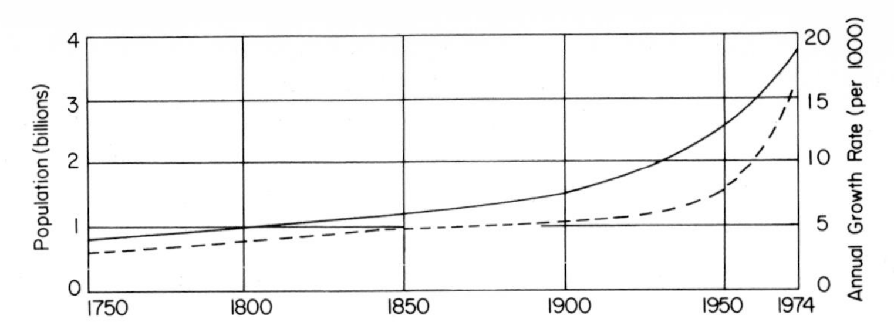

Fig. 1a. Growth of world population, 1750–1974. (Source: A. J. Coale (1974). *Scientific American* Sept., 42.)

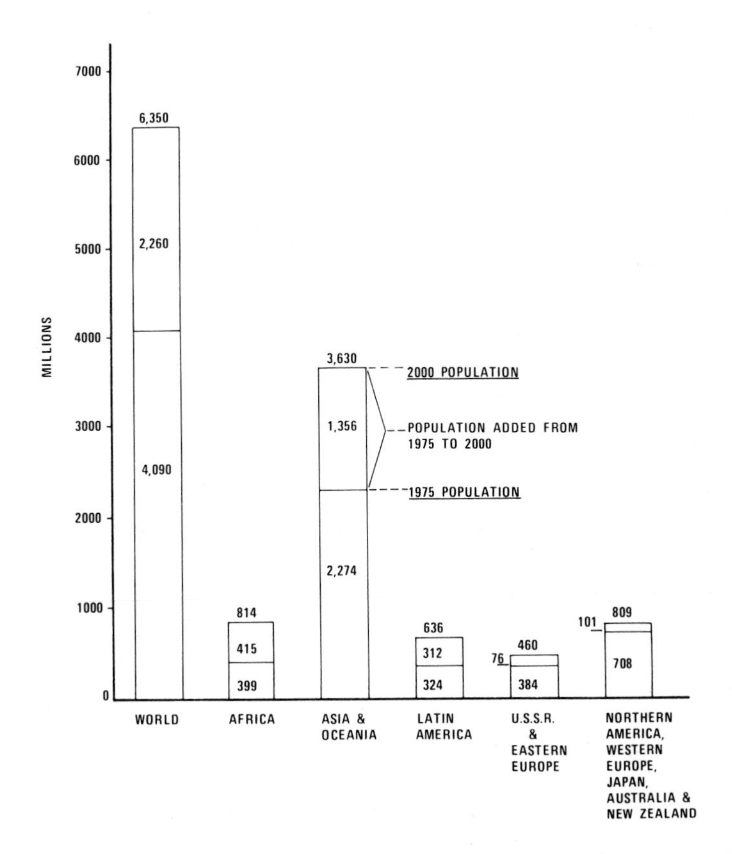

Fig. 1b. Total population of the world and major regions for 1975 and 2000 (medium projections).

concerning numbers and spacing of children. Most developing countries, on the other hand, have not been politically strong enough to greatly alter the distribution of world wealth in their favour. While they have achieved significant improvements in death rates by controlling diseases which previously contributed to high mortality because the means of control was available at little cost, they have been nowhere near as successful in achieving significant declines in birth rates. Dissemination of effective birth control information and devices has been difficult in some countries and, as will be shown, there has been a lack of willingness on the part of large proportions of developing country populations to reduce fertility.

While it is true that several countries, only recently classified as developing, or underdeveloped, have achieved favourable rates of economic and demographic growth (e.g. Singapore, Hong Kong Taiwan and Korea), their success has been in part due to the fact that developed countries found it convenient to utilize the large and relatively cheap labour forces in these countries through investment in their manufacturing and tertiary sectors, and partly because the recipient countries, through strong leadership and few religious or cultural constraints, have implemented effective programmes of population control. But the number of such nations relative to the total number of developing countries is small. The typical developing country (India, Bangladesh, Indonesia), though also a recipient of some economic assistance through overseas aid and investment, and having implemented family planning programmes, has not been notably successful in raising real income per capita, or in redistributing wealth more equitably, or in reducing rates of population growth. Governments have typically been willing but their capacity to achieve, and hence achievement itself, has been modest.

The "population problem" as we understand it today is of fairly recent origin and refers mainly to economically undeveloped countries (see Fig. 1). Developed countries are seen as having made the long transition from sustained periods of high fertility and mortality (which kept population growth to modest levels) to low fertility and mortality. The transition process in countries such as Great Britain is still debated by historical demographers, although there is little disagreement that population growth increased substantially during the late eighteenth century. Borrie, for instance did not attribute declining mortality during this period to any real "breakthrough to higher expectations of life", but rather to the absence of great killing diseases such as the plagues of earlier centuries.[2] And Krause[3] convincingly argued that fertility was affected by a complex of variables: decline in the age of marriage as a result of improved economic conditions as the industrial revolution gained momentum, the weakening of restrictions regarding apprenticeship, the weakening of sexual mores during the (Napoleonic) wars, and the extension of poor relief. Lower age at marriage exposed women to the risk of childbearing for longer periods, and in the absence of effective contraception contributed to higher fertility. Increased illegitimacy also contributed. While fertility fluctuated, claimed Krause, mortality did not decline until after 1820 mainly because of the dislocation and distress caused by war amongst the poorest classes.[3] The advancement of medical techniques and practice also contributed to declining mortality, but only slowly. There was little improvement in our knowledge of the transmission of diseases in the eighteenth century, hospitals were few and far between, amputation and other surgery invariably led to death, and midwifery was primitive, mother and child being at high risk of death.

As both medical practice and standards of living gradually improved, so rates of population growth increased. From the mid to the end of the nineteenth century the population of England and Wales almost doubled. In addition, emigration to countries of the New World, sparsely populated by hunters and gatherers, provided a demographic safety valve. These countries also provided the raw materials necessary to sustain the momentum of economic growth. By the mid-twentieth century, birth rates and death rates in most European-type countries had declined to levels where replacement was barely being achieved, and despite a "baby boom" in the post-war period, birth rates have recently declined again to the point where zero growth, a radical and to many an unachievable goal in the 1960s, is now almost a reality for most developed countries. Control over mortality and fertility in developed countries is much tighter than control in developing countries, and though man must die, if he lives in the developing world the cause of his death is more likely to be coronary heart disease, cancer or stroke, but not infectious diseases.[4] Furthermore, length of life in countries such as Australia has risen to seventy-five years for females and sixty-nine for males. Developed countries may experience population problems but these bear little resemblance to the nature and magnitude of the population problems of developing countries.

Explanation of the reasons why the population problem is so different in developed and developing countries is conveyed by the demographic theory of transition. The pattern described above is by and large the pattern that has been followed by most western countries. As death rates decline, so urbanization and industrialization increase; this in turn increases social and occupational mobility and living standards.

Advances in science and technology further increase control over fertility so that by the twentieth century the "typical" married woman in a developed country would have had three pregnancies compared with six or more by her forebears in the pre-industrial stage of her country's development.[5] This pattern of change has invariably been identified as the long-term path which developing countries must also follow. But while there is much relevance in the experience of developed countries during the eighteenth and nineteenth centuries, the ready availability of medical and contraceptive knowledge and equipment to present-day developing countries has clearly "dislocated" the long-term process of transition, especially because it has not been matched by redistribution of wealth through aid, trade and other income-equating devices. Twentieth-century man's ability to control birth and death rates has thus not been matched by his willingness to redistribute income.

For example, international action during the late 1940s and early 1950s led to the spraying of insecticides over huge areas of the developing world, and also to widespread distribution of medicines to control diseases which previously had caused high mortality, especially infant mortality. These campaigns were arguably the most successful and far-reaching in world history. Malaria, a killer and debilitator in large areas of the developing world was controlled in some areas by spraying insecticides on the breeding grounds of mosquitoes. Yellow fever and other diseases which typically killed humans in great pain were largely controlled by widespread vaccination. Antibiotics, only recently available, became a major "weapon" in both the control of disease and also in prolonging life. The impact of these campaigns, headed by the World Health Organization and other specialized agencies of the United Nations, can be readily observed in charts on death rates in developing countries (Fig. 2). The rapidity and magnitude of decline in mortality within a few years was due to the fruits of medical research being readily and cheaply available to most developing countries.

Population growth is a function of natural increase (births less deaths) and international migration (immigration less emigration). In any year, the difference between numbers of births and deaths, plus the difference between gain through immigration and loss through emigration, determines a country's increase (or decrease) in population. In developing countries, population increase is determined mainly by natural increase, net migration generally being small because the countries do not require immigrants (aside from a few selected skilled/professional workers). Thus when death rates decline as steeply as in India (see Fig. 2), rates of population increase rise sharply because there is no corresponding decline in birth rates. Campaigns in develop-

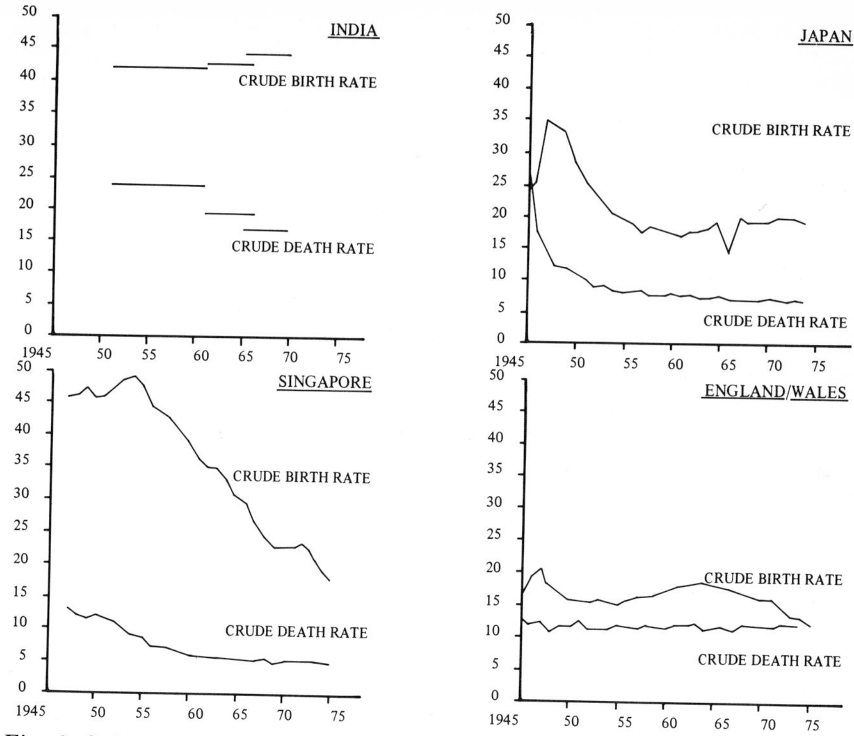

Fig. 2. Selected crude birth and death rates. (Source: *UN Demographic Year Books.*)

ing countries to reduce birth rates have been nowhere near as successful as the campaigns to reduce death rates, partly because the determinants of fertility are more complex, depending upon social, cultural and economic variables. Techniques of fertility control are known in these countries and dissemination is not difficult, but unlike information and techniques for the control of mortality, they are not so readily or so widely practised.

Acceptance of effective family planning by large numbers of people in the developing world is thwarted by religious beliefs and by perceptions concerning labour (children) as a partial substitute for capital. One church has persistently opposed the use by its believers of the most effective family planning techniques (the contraceptive pill, intrauterine devices (IUDs) and abortion) and instead encouraged the unreliable rhythm method of contraception. Religion aside, however, willingness to accept effective techniques invariably depends on social class and income, and though the correlation is by no means unity, there is overwhelming evidence that the better educated and wealthier people in developing countries are more apt to limit their completed family size to two or three children than are the uneducated and poor. The sad fact about developing countries is that a large majority of their population is in the latter category, and in the absence of a large middle class, overall birth rates have therefore not declined. Peasant farmers, who comprise over 70% of the populations of many developing countries, lack equipment to efficiently till their small farms. Children are typically considered by parents as both "hands in the field" from early ages, and "supporters" during their old age. A recent survey in a town in Indonesia showed the extent to which children are employed: At average age 7·9 years they care for chickens/ducks; at 8 care for younger children; at 8·8 fetch water; at 9·3 care for goats/cattle; at 9·5 cut fodder; at 9·7 harvest rice; at 9·9 transplant rice; at 12·9 work for wages; and at 13·0 they hoe the fields.[6] Many demographers and economists now believe that lack of incentive, rather than ineffective dissemination of information on fertility control, has been the main reason for insignificant reductions in fertility. Thus while intentional human action has exacerbated the population problem in developing countries, it must also be acknowledged that the action was logical for persons within the socioeconomic milieu of the rural sector within a low per capita income developing country.

Existing knowledge of the functional relationship between population growth and per capita income suggests complexity not easily unravelled. In many ways the dilemma at the microcosmic level, described above, is also the dilemma facing governments. Savings from subsistence incomes are small or negligible and many peasants, in debt to money-lenders, have no expectations of early release. Lacking the captial, and credit, necessary to purchase equipment which would increase productivity, they are forced to employ family labour, which partly explains why they continue to have large families. The government of a typical developing, non-industrial country therefore collects insufficient revenue to extend and improve infrastructure. Much export income, typically dependent on world prices for primary products which in the past have tended to fluctuate widely, is siphoned off to service overseas loans. Thus both individual farmers and their governments make only small contributions to productivity and therefore have limited capacity to raise per capita income. In addition, population growth rates may equal or be only slightly lower than rates of growth in GNP which further exacerbates growth of per capita income.

Population growth rates in many low-income developing countries are unlikely to decline in the near future. High fertility and relatively low mortality for a generation have assured high birth rates for the next twenty years. As already noted, reduction in death rates (especially reduction in infant mortality), combined with sustained high birth rates, have created populations with over 40% under fifteen years of age. As marriage rates are generally high in developing countries, and average age at marriage is low, the more numerous fecund women now in present populations are exposed to the risk of pregnancy for longer periods than were their mothers (and certainly longer than their grandmothers). In the absence of incentives to use effective methods of contraception, for reasons already noted, the demographic "potential" of such populations is enormous. It was on the basis of these demographic conditions, and attitudes, that Spengler concluded that the proportion of the world's population in developing countries will increase to 77% by the end of the century. His judgement is supported by most demographers. Caldwell, for example, claims that programmes of population control over the last fifteen years have clearly demonstrated that high fertility in developing countries cannot be quickly reduced and that "global population numbers will inevitably rise to far above their present numbers before either stationary or acceptably slow worldwide population growth can be achieved".[7]

High rates of population growth, together with high levels of unemployment and underemployment in the rural areas of developing countries, have also been mainly responsible for the migration of large numbers of persons from rural to urban areas. During the last few decades, millions of workers (and their families) living at subsistence levels in rural areas have moved to towns and cities where they expected to find employment and better living conditions. Rural families are often separated by this mobility: husband moves alone to the city; wife and children remain in the village. Internal migration of this kind has not only increased the populations of cities many fold, but health, sewerage and other services, never comprehensive or totally efficient, are now unable to cope with the additional demands. Lacking adequate funds to maintain and extend social overheads governments have been powerless to prevent serious erosion of both the standard and coverage of such services. Also, typical of these cities are large shanty towns on their outskirts in which hundreds of thousands of migrants live in physical conditions much worse than those in the rural villages whence they came.

"Developing" is, of course, a relative concept and rates of economic growth in countries so classified are diverse. Achievement depends on so many things: the magnitude of resources (both renewable and non-renewable); the level of education and skills of the population;

success in attracting overseas investment, which usually depends upon the magnitude of resources; the level of internal savings from income; political leadership, organization and stability. . . . City-type states such as Hong Kong and Singapore, and small countries such as South Korea and Taiwan have clearly had, or have developed, the key components necessary for economic growth. Larger countries such as Pakistan, India and Indonesia have been largely thwarted in their efforts to raise GNP per capita because they lack the key components and also because their populations are so large. The success of Hong Kong and Singapore, both predominantly Chinese populations, has been facilitated by widespread and effective family planning clinics which their people have used because they perceived the advantages of raising small families. Couples in the larger, poorer countries have not perceived the advantages despite the availability of appropriate information and devices for effective family planning.

High, sustained birth rates in many developing countries have been the root of their population problems. Aside from the unwillingness of families to reduce family size, there has also been reluctance to adopt rigorous and effective methods of population control. Japan, though hardly a "developing" country, is nonetheless a salutory example of how the application of effective methods can reduce fertility. At war's end, Japan's economy had been devastated by widespread bombing by allied planes. Both death and birth rates were high (see Fig. 2), but the former declined rapidly once infrastructure had been repaired and improved and medical supplies became readily available. Birth rates, however, did not decline until the early 1950s, thus causing high rates of population growth, exacerbated by the return to Japan of 8 million demobilized military personnel and repatriates. The genesis of striking reductions in the birth rate was an amendment in 1949 to the Eugenic Protection Law of 1948 which permitted a woman to undergo an abortion for economic reasons.[8] The amendment led to a remarkable increase in the number of abortions: from 246 104 abortions in 1949 to 1·17 million in 1955. Even by 1968 the number of abortions was 757 000 but by then Japanese women, like their Western sisters, were, in addition, adopting less drastic but nonetheless efficient measures of family planning. Though its economy had been devastated during the war Japan, like Germany, had been a major industrial power and even though reconstruction required great national effort and sacrifice, it was essentially an exercise of repair not, as for developing countries, a journey into new territory. Having all the "components" for economic growth, Japan's achievements during the 1950s and 1960s were no surprise to other nations. Today, unlike developing countries where a generation of high birth and relatively low death rates has caused demographic structures favourable to continued high population growth, Japan has all the hallmarks of a Western-type, stationary, ageing population. Its manufacturing sector is capital-intensive, and many companies which produce commodities requiring labour-intensive operations have moved their factories to nearby developing countries where labour is relatively cheap and plentiful. The benefits of this mobility to both Japan and the developing countries are obvious.

Transition from a state of underdevelopment to development is basically an economic/demographic process: a low per capita income/feeble infrastructure/essentially rural-oriented economy becomes a high per capita income/industrial-based/large service-sector economy. Demographic changes facilitate, and in turn are facilitated by the process. In the case of Great Britain, where the process took at least two centuries, there occurred great changes in the distribution of labour between rural and urban areas as well as between the primary, secondary and tertiary sectors of the economy. Even though distribution of wealth remained uneven (a large proportion of the population earning low, subsistence incomes) the country's capacity to control fertility and mortality gradually increased.

Having passed through the transition, developed countries now have populations with the desire and capacity to control both fertility and mortality. Poverty, while it still exists, is not severe or widespread enough to lead those suffering from it to produce large families. The demographic and economic profile of a Western family is two children born fairly soon after marriage, which on average occurred at age twenty-one years for women and at twenty-six for men. By the time the wife reaches thirty years of age her youngest child will have begun school and she will probably return to the workforce, especially if she had acquired professional skills before marriage, or she may never have left the workforce except during confinements. The couple's ownership of consumer durables is high, especially of such goods as vehicles and refrigerators, which they may consider "essential". Their health will normally be good and each can expect to live for three score years and ten; their control over fertility and the spacing of children will be almost complete. Thus their "intentional human action", made possible by significant changes in economic conditions, and the ready availability of health care which also increases longevity, is in striking contrast to the economic/demographic profiles of families in developing countries.

Economic, social and political changes in this century, and especially since 1945, have by any reasonable criterion, been dramatic. The growth of population, and especially the growth of urban populations, the unprecedented exploitation of resources to service man's ever-increasing demand for goods and services, especially in developed countries, has in many ways outstripped his concern and his capacity to prevent a marked deterioration in his physical environment. In his rush to proliferate new industrial plants and extend existing ones to meet the demands of larger populations earning higher incomes; in his drift towards cities where both the manufacturing and service sectors have been established; and in his seeming insatiable demand for the earth's agricultural and mineral resources, man has been a very tardy custodian of his physical environment. His concern for physical damage, and for the consequences of air, noise and visual pollution caused largely by his massive demand for resources, has generally lagged well behind his propensity to repair the damage he has caused. Indeed, full recognition of the environmental problem was slow, articulated in the first instance by small groups of protestors whose campaigns then gained widespread support and forced industry and governments to exercise controls on production and exploitation which recognized the importance of protecting the environment. Together with resolving problems caused by the present uneven distribution of the world's wealth, and problems posed by relatively high rates of population growth in developing countries, the most demanding challenge for man in the remaining years of the twentieth century will be to protect the "fragile nest" in which he lives and to preserve endangered species of flora and fauna.

References

1. Spengler, J. J. (1978). "Facing Zero Population Growth". Duke Univ. Press.
2. Borrie, W. D. (1970). "The Growth and Control of World Population", 61–70. London.
3. Krause, J. T. (19—). Changes in English fertility and mortality, 1781–1850. *Econ. Hist. Rev.* 2nd Series, **11**, 52–70; Some implications of recent work in historical demography. *Comp. Studies Society History* **1**, 164–188; Some neglected factors in the English Industrial Revolution. *J. econ. Hist.* **19**, 528–540. Other scholars who have made significant contributions to the debate are H. J. Habakkuk, T. McKeown, R. G. Brown and A. M. Carr-Saunders.
4. McCall, M. G. (1969). Man and medicine. A chapter *In* "Man and His Environment", (R. T. Appleyard, Ed.). Nedlands.
5. Borrie, W. D. (1970). "The Growth and Control of World Population", 13. London.

6. International Year of the Child (1979) "Today's Children". Source of information was *Development and Cooperation* **4**, 1978.
7. Caldwell, J. C. (1976). "The world population outlook", a paper delivered to the Australian and New Zealand Association for the Advancement of Science (ANZAAS), Hobart, 1976. Unpublished.
8. United Nations, Economic Commission for Asia and the Pacific (1978). "*The Development of Family Planning in Japan with Industrial Involvement*". Population Studies Translation Series No. 2, New York.

22

The Impoverishment of Community Life and the Need for Community Health

Ian Maddocks*
Adelaide, Australia

Community is hard work, not only in its building but also in its maintenance.

* Visiting Senior Specialist, Flinders Medical Centre.

I. Introduction

Ninety-nine per cent of the history of man and his immediate evolutionary ancestors was spent by the riverbank in communities of about forty to sixty hunters and gatherers, and for most of the remaining 1% humans grouped in small villages. The human genotype, we might argue, is given most "naturally" to life in small intimate communities, held together by kinship and custom.

Yet we find ourselves grouping more and more into larger and larger conurbations. The city has a power to fascinate, excite and attract. In evolutionary terms it has been likened to the archipelago for the way in which it promotes diversity and accelerates change. The city gathers together people of different languages, skills and cultures, and in that setting cross-fertilization, stimulus and opportunity speed the creativity and technology which we count as progress. We accept that the city has allowed the greatest flowering of human ingenuity and achievement.

However, cities have proved very uncomfortable for many of their inhabitants. Early city life was frankly unhealthy, with contagion, contamination and pollution ever present. In those cities which were able to afford them, sanitary reforms and planning regulations largely eliminated the threat of infectious disease, but even where the physical environment is relatively favourable, city life seems to be demanding and stressful, promoting physical and psychological discomfort.

A common way of describing the problem of living in cities is to say "We have lost our sense of community." Unease and sickness in modern society is attributed to the disruption of a coherence which previous societies possessed. The structures of cities deprive people of supports which in earlier ages they could take for granted. "Community" here conjures an ideal image from the past, an atavistic recall of pre-industrial society. Only in traditional village life, where it survives in a few untrammelled corners of the globe, can this dimly grasped tribal memory be clearly seen, and we find it compellingly attractive.

II. A Traditional Community

For six years I studied a Papuan village close to Port Moresby (Hetzel, 1978). Pari was a village of about 100 houses and 1000 people, its simple dwellings clustered closely along a short length of beach, some over the sea and some on the land. The village was arranged in thirteen distinct descent groups, but for many purposes it functioned as a single huge extended family. Its members remembered a common history, recited through at least seven generations, and shared a rich culture of legend and ritual, song and dance. They knew in great detail the features of sea and land, reef and garden, which constituted their compact universe. Each person knew every other person, knew stories about him, had years of remembered personal and public family relationships to guide attitudes towards him.

The social institutions of Pari confirmed and extended an intricate network of obligation and exchange. Family and peer groups were welded by engaging in competitions of display and achievement. Traditional enterprises such as fishing expeditions or trading ventures were undertaken by groups within which the balance of responsibility and return was carefully maintained. Individual status was won by displays of largesse, but every "gift" involved some obligation, and there was no word for "thank you".

There was necessary ritual and customary procedure for the performance of any significant activity. The spirits of the ancestors were known to be close in attendance, interested participants in village affairs. Failure to adhere to customary rules or to maintain the social harmony would upset the ancestors and lead to trouble—poor harvests, sickness, empty fishing nets.

The anthropologist Murray Groves (1957) has related how, at another village of the Motu language group (to which Pari belongs), he encountered a man singing songs as he wrapped young bunches of bananas to protect them. Groves questioned him about the songs, and was told, "The songs that I sing are my ancestors' songs. My forebears have always sung them and their gardens have always prospered. Therefore I always sing these songs. It is the way of the ancestors; it is *helaga*."

Those practices which made for coherence in the community; which celebrated the close association of the people with the sea and the earth; which remembered and invoked the support of the ancestors; which blessed co-operation in working to exploit the resources of that little world, were, in Motu, *helaga*. *Helaga* governed all important activities. It may be translated "holy", "proper", "correct". It offered meaning, and it also offered a powerful conviction of control for it provided direction and instruction about ways to avoid misfortune, to overcome danger, to counter distress.

For the people of Pari there was no "bad luck". Every happening had a cause and a reason, and called forth an appropriate response. For any serious illness, for example, the family would gather to review their situation—who had made some wrong action, who had shown or caused anger. Perhaps a woman had unwisely flirted, perhaps a bride price had been unfairly distributed. These circumstances could be aired and redressed, since the surest way to health for a sick person was to re-establish harmony, just as it was the surest way to ensure success in fishing.

III. Three Expressions of Community

Life in Pari village incorporated three aspects of "community".

1. There was a *spatial* expression. The village was a close arrangement of dwellings clearly set apart from other habitations, a distinct and well-defined entity which the eye might encompass with a single view from some point of vantage.
2. There was a *social* expression of community. For its people, life centred in the village. The political and social structures, and the rituals and language employed in Pari were those of the Motu people, but always with a peculiar local flavour. In speech the Pari people, alone among nearby villages, dropped their "h's". Only Pari had the important annual season of tuna fishing with a wealth of legend, ritual and taboo. Virtually all the exchanges which oiled the social machinery of the village took place between its own descent groups and families.
3. Pari was a place of *communion*, of shared values and close human relationships. Through marriage and descent, each person could claim kinship with every other person. From infancy to old age, people knew each other in extended families and in peer groups as few siblings know each other in Australian families. They also knew the ancestors, whose spirits stayed close to the hearths where once they had gathered. A complex network of human sharing was reinforced by a common understanding of *helaga*, and of the significance which attached to interpersonal harmony.

The coexistence of these three expressions of community in village life is what gives it such powerful and romantic appeal. It is tempting to suggest that this is how human life "ought" to be, that each of us has a right to the physical and emotional security which that stable little world seems to offer, and to the supportive web of kinship and friendship which is apparent there.

Two warnings should temper our romanticism. Firstly, the community life of Pari demanded a tremendous amount of effort from all members of the village. The busy tide of exchange and support which flowed along the village street night and day made living in Pari a full time job. Community is hard work, not only in its building but also in its maintenance. Secondly, it is well to remember that in most parts of the world rural life has been brutish and hard, with hunger and sudden death never far away. Members of rural villages seize with alacrity any opportunity to leave the security and stability of their traditonal lot in favour of the uncertainty and excitement and individual opportunity of the city. This is as true for Pari as for anywhere else in the world.

IV. The City

Few centres of habitation now combine the three features of community seen in Pari village. In towns and cities spatial arrangement, social pattern and kinship linkages are rarely congruent. Neighbours are neither workmates nor friends; relatives are scattered widely; institutions draw their members sparsely from a wide range of places and classes. The values and mores of the city are those of competitive growth and success. They spill over into the country, and the centripetal pull of the city, exercised through its centralized political power, its diverse opportunities and the narrow urban focus of the ubiquitous media, continues to depopulate the villages and to mould the towns to pale images of the metropolis.

Cities are divisive. They gather large numbers of people together, yet separate them, segregate them and isolate them. Physical setting, historical, economic and social forces combine to make one suburb a desirable location for the estates of the rich, while another houses the grimy tenements of the poor. Collingwood, an inner suburb of Melbourne, began as a swampy hollow by the River Yarra and attracted trades and industries of a noxious kind because land was cheap and water handy. Inevitably, therefore, it became a poor area of inferior housing (Barrett, 1971).

Children are stratified by schooling into a hierarchy of achievement which determines their future employment. Families are scattered by the restless mobility which relocates individuals and households every few years. Work is specialized, and the territory of each skill is defended by unionist or professional.

The very load of human numbers around them limits what people can offer to others, and they come to expect little for themselves. City dwellers come into contact with vast numbers of people each day and are forced to conserve their energy by allotting less time to each contact, by ignoring many of them, by withdrawing or screening off large areas of potential contact, by cultivating superficial forms of involvement and by handing over to specialized institutions the responsibility for undertaking those sorts of contact which make the greatest demands (Milgram, 1970). Inevitably some who have great needs receive little attention from society, while others, seem unduly privileged. Cities promote a wide spectrum of advantage and disadvantage. Disadvantaged people are unfavoured in many ways: living in poor environments, forced to expose themselves to dangerous occupations, they are less articulate, lack political power, suffer more sickness and have limited access to health care. The so-called "Inverse Care Law" has been described for many places. Disadvantage, disease and poor medical care are closely linked, though casual relationships are difficult to demonstrate.

Conventional wisdom and statistics both suggest that in modern cities there has been an increase in violent crime, vandalism, depression, youthful alcoholism, drug addiction and attempted suicide. These problems are regarded as indicators of societal stress and they have been much studied. But their origins remain complex and elusive. Poverty, overcrowding, rapid change and psychological overload may all be important, but studies which take a global view of urban stress rarely show useful associations, it seems. Fischer (1973) found no evidence to support the common contention that aggregation of large numbers of diverse people creates powerlessness and isolation: he concluded that "personalities are shaped in smaller social contexts", and found that powerlessness was reported more often when subjects had no contact with immediate neighbours. The absence of close personal support was also shown to be important in the origins of depression (Brown and Harris, 1978). Psychiatric disorder was more common in women in London than in a rural population, and in the London population working-class women were four times more likely than middle-class women to develop a depressive disorder when they experienced a severe personal threat (usually a major loss or disappointment). This class difference was not due to a different incidence in threatening life events, but to a greater exposure of working-class women to what were called "vulnerability factors". These included having small children in the home, loss of mother before the age of eleven and unemployment. By far the most significant factor was the absence of a confiding tie with husband or boyfriend.

Brown and Harris (1978) were cautious in interpreting their findings. But their work suggests that the intimate personal environment of individuals is critical for their coping. The Dean of Theology at

Yale recently remarked, when discussing community, "For me, one good friend is enough". Lacking the supportive environment of the village, we depend upon key individual relationships. There are no tidy little villages hidden within the complex and chaotic fabric of the city. The city is its own peculiar mess. So when we use the word "community" today, we are giving it meanings other than that of a clearly indentifiable stable locality.

V. Community Health

"Community" may be a synonym for "society"—"the good of the whole community". It may refer to a political institution—the European Economic Community. It can be used to indicate certain categories of people who share certain characteristics or interests or training. So we might refer to a church community or the medical community.

In the field of social work, "community" is much used as an adjective in such phrases as community care, community involvement, community development. It is not a descriptive adjective in the usual sense. It conveys no concrete image, but rather affirms an intention or an emotion, an interest or an obligation.

The same usage gives us "community health". This phrase reflects a popular and political awareness of the unease and sickness which can be attributed to modern urban living, and the failure of conventional individual health care to tackle it effectively. Booming economic growth in the Western world has not significantly ameliorated either sickness or disadvantage in its urban societies. Widespread misgivings have led to substantial funding by governments of special community health programmes. These have been firmly within the long tradition of public initiative which in earlier generations introduced public hospitals, infant welfare clinics, free immunizations and infectious disease control. The instigators of the community health programmes saw that urban health problems were complex, and that the traditional narrow medical focus of existing institutions offered no prospect of improving health. They deployed professionals from many disciplines, aiming to cleanse and purify the urban ghettos and raise health standards generally through quality primary care, health education and preventive medicine.

Community health was to be aware of the environmental and social causes of disease and to work to prevent them; was to understand the corporate and family associations of individual distress and mobilize appropriate responses; was to recognize the great needs of disadvantaged groups and individuals and seek to provide special programmes to redress their particular problems.

Community health assumed values such as equity and health care as a universal right. It asserted that the well and the advantaged have an obligation to assist the sick and the needy. It assumed that its initiatives would be implemented by professional staff who were highly trained in new and specialized aspects of health care delivery.

The volume "Community Health in Australia" (Walpole, 1979) was an anthology of contributions from the newly appointed Professors of Community Medicine in virtually all the medical schools of Australia. In general, their evangelism ran along familiar lines:

- social environments determine health, and we must change life-styles rather than expend more on therapy;
- health teams are the best way to deliver health care, and they must concentrate on health education;
- health workers must see the whole community as their responsibility, working together not only with other professionals but also with volunteers and community representatives.

Most of the contributors failed to define their use of the word "community", and they seemed to pay little heed to the historical, cultural and social determinants of disadvantage. The health care they proposed for Australian cities was a variation on "more of the same"—more doctors, more nurses, more social workers, more volunteers, more meetings, more money, more transport, more clinics, more intervention. Four contributors were less assertive and more cautious in their hopes. Hicks noted that for all the rhetoric expended on this theme, experience suggests that real reform does not occur, and that professionals cannot help dominating their clients and serving their own ends; Gordon gave a wise old-stager's advice that big talk is easy but small changes are realistic, and long, slow revolutions are best. Lickiss hinted at the politics of health care when she described the doctor as potentially as "liberator"; and Opit argued that community health must be seen as "essentially subversive action which runs counter to the history of medical care development during the last 200 years". "Subversive" community health, according to Opit, requires a profound change in the values of professionals, a radical change in methods of financing health services, and a fundamental change in public expectations of the roles of doctors and other health professionals. Is this really "subversive"? Changes which depend upon what doctors and administrators initiate will almost certainly perpetuate for community health the established *helaga*, the powerful values of the city—central organization, global planning, growth, specialization and professional dominance. These are the very values which underlie the divisive and stressful discomforts of the city.

Community health requires a different *helaga*, an alternative understanding of meaning and control in the city, a new framework of community. This will grow from outside of conventional institutions. Some observers are optimistic that new cultural developments among young people will provide a lead: "Perhaps the culture just now being developed by the new generation—the new emphasis upon imagination, the senses, community and the self—is the first real choice made by any Western people since the end of the Middle Ages" (Reich, 1970). A movement to community is happening in many places, and though it is hesitant, fragile and disintegrated, it recalls some features of that tribal memory that any of us might recognize. Households gather around a disenchantment with what is, and a vaguely articulated ideology of non-consumerism, voluntary simplicity, self-help and "down-to-earth". To some extent, frugal life-styles and mutual dependence are enforced by limited resources, since many participants are young and unemployed, but the movement is also fed by a variety of meditation and self-actualization techniques and expressions of religion. Membership of households or adherence to specific spiritual commitments may be transitory, but a common bond of understanding is usually apparent which allows individuals to regroup and to continue their exploration of radical alternatives.

This is not to suggest that the future can be left to groupies with green thumbs. But as energy costs rise and economic growth continues to be slow, we must expect less mobility in urban life and a greater emphasis on localities. This could have very positive social effects, though it may at first be seen as retrogression or decay. It may lead to a restoration of processess for internalizing norms of behaviour which we have steadily been losing—neighbourliness, sociability and a sense of public responsibility. Clunies-Ross (1977) has suggested institutional changes which could take advantage of this trend. He envisaged a system of "neighbourhood assemblies, each covering a small number of households (say forty to eighty), assemblies which every resident of the neighbourhood (of the age of, say, fourteen years or more) would be able to attend as a speaking and voting member". Such assemblies could be given incentives to accept responsibility for the care of their local environment and for certain aspects of social welfare. One or several assemblies could form the field of action for basic health services—the area to be served by a community health nurse, for example. That is not a far cry from the successful Chinese deployment throughout urban localities of health workers nominated by their neighbourhoods and responsible to them.

The values which are expressed most clearly within the alternatives movement have begun to influence a wide range of fellow-travellers, and have been important in a number of experiments in health care:

Community Child Care is a people-based movement which has been highly successful in arming ordinary people to fulfil their responsibilities as parents and as sharing members of human groups (McCaughey and Sebastian, 1977). This movement recognizes that children commonly lose not only a sense of personal identity and worth, but also a sense of belonging and commitment to their people and their place. It sees the roots of this unease in the wider environment within which families operate, and defines "community" in these terms: "That process of interaction between people knowing and being known, caring and being cared for, sharing, exchanging, trading and so on. The geographical context in which this process can occur most easily in the field of child care is that of the immediate neighbourhood and then the municipality."

Women's health centres are not tied to a small geographical context, but they have evolved a process of interaction and sharing which is quite different from the usual one-way relationship of professional to client seen in sickness consultations. When I visited the Christmas party at the Women's Health Centre in Hindmarsh, Adelaide, I felt an intruder not only as a male, but also as a doctor. It was the only such occasion I had seen in a health institution which was not dominated by professionals. Indeed, it seemed to have been organized by the clients, whose vigorous dancing and feasting celebrated their feelings of involvement and participation in the work of the Centre.

Self-help movements in psychiatry and drug rehabilitation have gained ground in recent years. The efficacy of Alcoholics Anonymous has long been recognized. In Hamburg, Germany, the Release Organization, started by drug addicts, seeks to allow each individual to achieve a personal experience of success. In Australia, experience has been growing with therapeutic households for psychiatric care. These are run as participatory democracies, and have shown the value of allowing people who would otherwise be classified as dependent patients, the opportunity to accept responsibility for contributing to a supportive environment and for working through crises with each other.*

Each of these examples embodies features of community which were apparent in Pari village—a small human focus, its size limited by

* See several articles in *Social Alternatives*, 1978, Vol. 1, No 2. Quarterly published by the Department of External Studies, University of Queensland.

geography or commitment; a sharing of knowledge, obligation and responsibility; and *helaga*, a common ideology, and agreed emphasis on priorities, beliefs or rituals.

No universal manifesto is possible for this approach to community health. It is a process which is continually evolving, and which varies from place to place and from time to time in response to local direction. It works small and slow. It is essentially subversive in that it bypasses established structures, keeps professionals at bay, and encourages people to liberate themselves from the demands of disease, disadvantage and dependency.

VI. Conclusion

Urban life is chaotic and barely comprehensible. The word "community" has had little relevance to the city. Community has to be built, and that is a process which is painful, small and slow. Wherever community is achieved it risks conflict with established central structures.

The meaning of disease and the control of sickness situations have become the province of the professional health workers. The doctors and their acolytes control the health *helaga*. But health is more than optimal individual functioning. It is a sharing, and an exchange of knowledge and power between people who appreciate each other within a common understanding of the order and significance of the universe.

Community health happens where there is community. It needs to draw upon sophisticated expertise and technology, but it cannot be applied to human groups by professionals, and so the role of health professionals in health care needs to be redefined. Community health is the process of restoring the health *helaga* to Everyman, and it begins where tiny social groupings find significance, knowledge and power for themselves.

References

Barrett, B. (1971). "The Inner Suburbs: The Evolution of an Industrial Area". Melbourne Univ. Press.

Brown, G. W. and Harris, T. (1978). "Social Origins of Depression". Tavistock, London.

Clunies-Ross, A. (1977). (Book Reviews) *J. econ. Studies* **4**, 179.

Fischer, C. S. (1973). *Am. Soc. Rev.* **38**, 311.

Groves, M. (1957). *Quadrant* **1**, 39.

Hetzel, B. S. (Ed.) (1978). "Basic Health care in Developing Countries". IEA-WHO Handbook. Oxford Univ. Press.

McCaughey, W. and Sebastian, P. (1977). "Community Child Care". Greenhouse Publications, Melbourne. (See also *Ripple*, the Community Child Care Quarterly, 1979, No. 16, published by Community Child Care, Fitzroy, Victoria.)

Milgram, S. (1970). *Science, NY* **167**, 1461.

Reich, C. (1970). "The Greening of America". Random House, New York.

Walpole, R. (1979). "Community Health in Australia". Penguin Books, Ringwood, Victoria.

23

Malnutrition

Michael Gracey

Gastroenterological Research Unit, Princess Margaret Children's Medical Research Foundation, Subiaco, Western Australia

. . . Hundreds of millions of children throughout the world are malnourished and a large proportion of them become enmeshed in the "malnutrition/gastroenteritis" vicious circle.

I. The Upsurge of Urbanization

One of the most significant changes affecting mankind in the twentieth century has been the rapid growth of urbanization. This has outstripped total population growth to such an extent that the world's total population has doubled in that time while the numbers living in cities have increased fivefold. This has led to unmanageable stresses on many urban administrations and has put many millions of families under immense personal pressures; understandably, the poor have suffered most. This problem has become so pressing that a new term has been introduced to describe these people, "New Urban Families". Their plight was considered by an International Workshop of the International Paediatric Association immediately before its Congress in Vienna in 1971 (Vahlquist *et al.*, 1973).

This tendency towards rapid urbanization is complex in its origins and far-reaching in its consequences. Details about this demographic shift are outside the scope of this chapter but some pertinent facts are worthy of mention. It is important, for example, to realize that more than 70% of the world's population live in the so-called developing or less developed countries which, collectively, account for almost 90% of the world's total present population growth. By the year 2000 A.D. about three-quarters of the world's inhabitants will live in these countries. This rapid population growth in these countries partly reflects the revolution in medicine and public health that has occurred since the last century. The decline in mortality which is occurring in less developed countries stems in part from their generally younger age structures (Fig. 1) which, in turn, are boosted by declining mortality which applies largely to infants and children. In many such countries almost 50% of their population are under fifteen years of age while in most developed countries less than 30% are in this age group. It is often not recognized that the biggest populations of less developed countries are in Asia and that five of these, China, India, Indonesia, Pakistan and Bangladesh, contain more than half of the entire population of the Third World.

Cities in the Third World are being flooded by an apparently uncontrollable wave of humanity from rural areas which is subjecting them to a much worse urban crisis than that experienced by today's developed countries during their main period of urban growth. The larger cities are growing faster and cities with current populations over 5 million growing fastest of all. Calcutta, for example, is already grossly overcrowded yet is expected to increase its population to more than 15

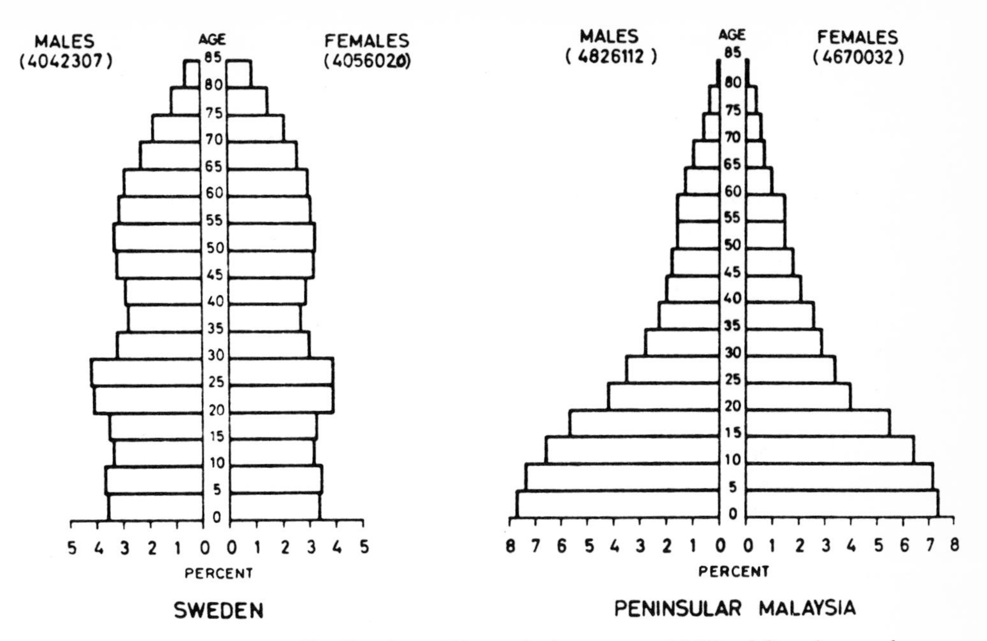

Fig. 1. Age and sex distributions ("population pyramids") of Sweden and Malaysia showing the relatively younger population of a developing country when compared to an industrialized country. (Reprinted from "Paediatric Problems in Tropical Countries" (M. J. Robinson and E. L. Lee, Eds) by permission of the publisher, Churchill Livingstone.)

million by 1980. In this overcrowded, blighted cities like this, a very significant proportion of the population is made up of squatters who have been unable to make a successful adjustment to the shift from a rural to an urban environment. What starts out as a "halfway house" between these two environments eventually turns out to be little better than a shift from underemployment in a rural setting to unemployment in a megalopolis with a collection of unfamiliar pressures and patterns of living.

The growth of cities around the world and the drift of population from rural to urban areas is of such magnitude it can be thought of as the equivalent of an "urban avalanche". This population change has had dramatic consequences. In many instances newly arrived families find themselves caught up in an inextricable set of circumstances: the father unemployed, the children unschooled and the mother facing unfamiliar social pressures which often lead, amongst other things, to a decline of breast feeding and a lack of family cohesion and support in times of need. All these changes are complicated by unavailability of homegrown foods, higher costs and lack of understanding of shopping and this usually occurs along with housing difficulties and unsanitary conditions. All these and other interrelated factors adversely affect the health and nutrition of the most vulnerable part of the family, the younger children and the mother. These are some of the factors which make malnutrition one of the three main diseases of children in developing countries (Jelliffe, 1974). Diarrhoeal diseases, often termed "gastroenteritis", along with malnutrition are the main causes of death of infants and children in these countries and each year collectively account for millions of deaths, especially before the age of two years.

For the past several years we have conducted a joint research programme into the problem of diarrhoeal disease in malnourished children in collaboration with paediatricians in Indonesia. Much of what follows stems from the experience gained from that programme and because of our involvement there, many of the comments relate to Indonesia. Obviously conditions in different developing countries vary but many of the problems occurring in Indonesia have similarities in other developing countries.

In many ways the stresses experienced by the developing world's New Urban Families are exemplified by what is happening today in Jakarta, the rapidly sprawling capital of the Republic of Indonesia, one of the most heavily populated countries in the world. This is of particular significance to Australia, and especially to Western Australia, its wealthy sparsely populated neighbour to the south. The contrasts in population density become dramatic when we consider that the total population of Western Australia, which covers the western third of the continent and extends over 2.5 million km^2, is only 1.2 million (see Fig. 2) while Indonesia has a land area of 1.9 million km^2 and its 1979 population was estimated at 145 million. Forty-four per cent of Indonesia's population are under fifteen years of age (see Fig. 3). Furthermore, its population continues to grow very rapidly (Fig. 4), approximately 2.5% to 2.8% annually. The population pressures are greatest on the relatively small island of Java (Fig. 5) and in Jakarta, the seat of Government and the commercial and administrative centre for the Republic (Fig. 6). These estimated growth rates are disturbing enough but the discrepancy between urban and rural areas is cause for even greater concern and the expectation is that the problems facing New Urban Families in Jakarta show no signs of diminishing in the foreseeable future. In the decade 1971–81 the estimated growth rate for Indonesia as a whole is 26% and for Jakarta itself an alarming 71%. Other cities are growing even faster with Bandung, also on the over-

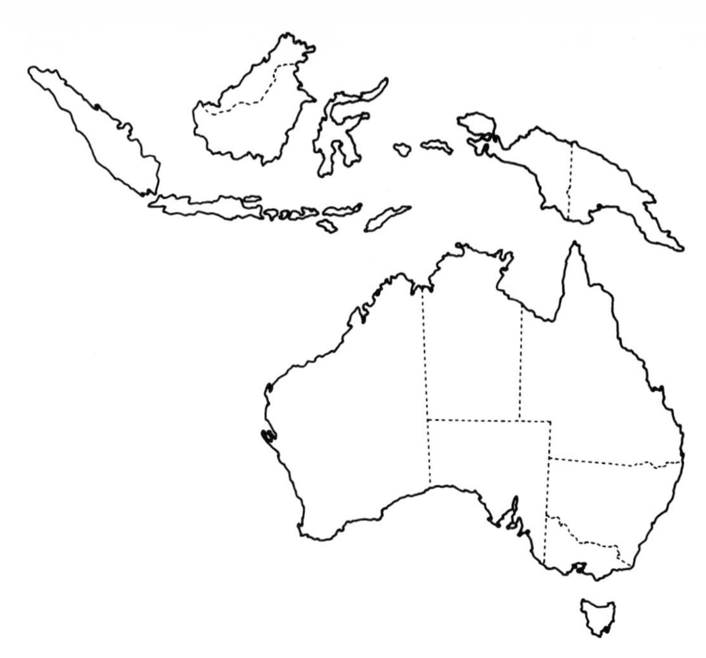

Fig. 2. Map showing Australia and its closest northern neighbours, Papua New Guinea in the east bordering Irian Jaya the easternmost province of the Republic of Indonesia which extends from its outer islands westward to Java and Sumatra.

crowded island of Java, expected to grow by 242% in the fifteen year period from 1970 to 1985. In other parts of the world cities are also showing double digit growth rates per annum; for example, Dacca (Bangladesh) 16.2%, Guadalajara 12.2%, Lima 11.8%, Kinshasha 11.2% and Seoul 10.8% per year (Dwyer, 1978).

II. The Decline of Subsistence

The situation in the rural areas also shows danger signs. For example, in overcrowded Java, about half the rural households, over 30 million people, are virtually landless and this does not include small-holders or tenants who have lost out with the increasing modernization of rice production and who have largely been reduced to the equivalent of landless labourers. About three-quarters of Java's farming families do not own enough land for their subsistence needs and, overall, their aggregate per capita food production and income are dangerously low.

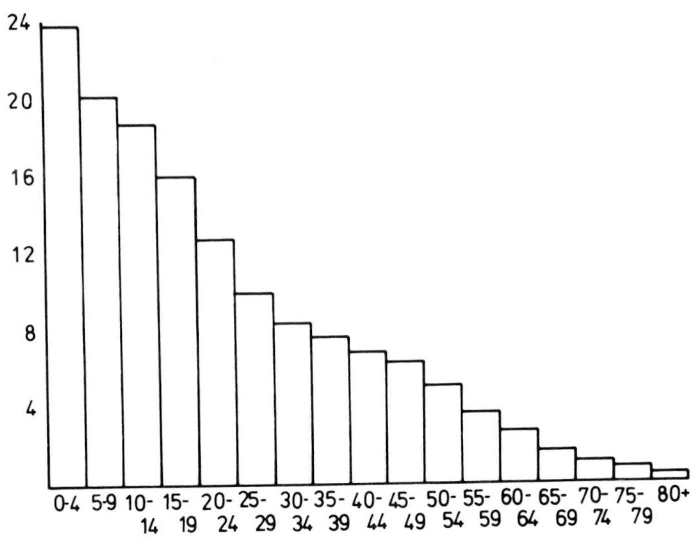

Fig. 3. Estimated percentage distribution of population in Indonesia showing that more than half the population is less than fifteen years of age. (Biro Pusat Statistik, Republik Indonesia, 1978.)

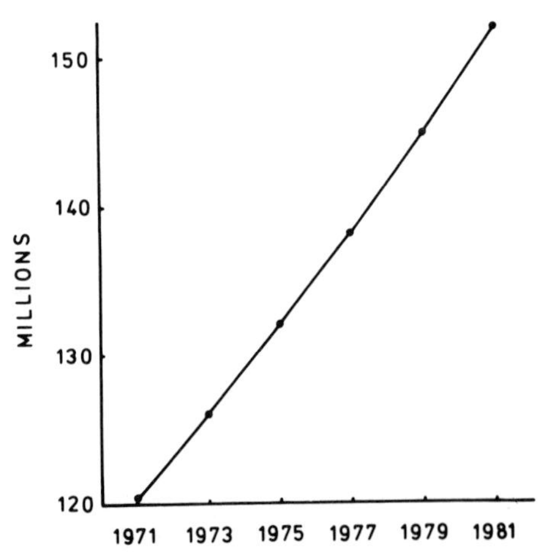

Fig. 4. Estimated population growth in Indonesia. (Biro Pusat Statistik, Republik Indonesia, 1978.).

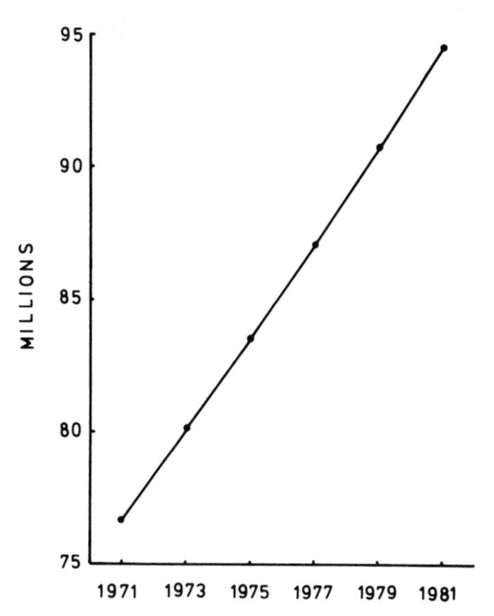

Fig. 5. Estimated population growth in the neighbouring Indonesian islands of Java and Madura. (Biro Pusat Statistik, Republik Indonesia, 1978.)

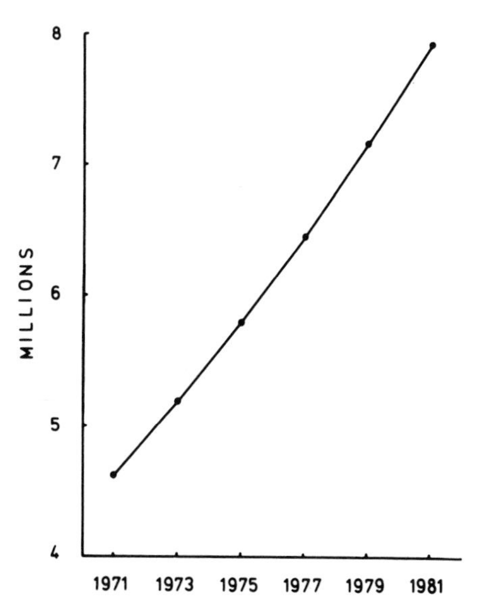

Fig. 6. Estimated population growth of Jakarta, the capital of Indonesia, for the decade 1971–81. (Biro Pusat Statistik, Republik Indonesia, 1978.)

For a detailed account of the process of ecological change and "agricultural involution" in Indonesia the reader is referred to Geertz (1963).

III. Malnutrition and Its Accompaniments

It is on this background of severe social and economic pressures that malnutrition becomes a major problem. Although precise information is not available, hundreds of millions of children throughout the world are malnourished and a large proportion of them become enmeshed in the "malnutrition/gastroenteritis" vicious circle (Jelliffe, 1974). This situation is typical of the millions of poor in Indonesia, and the disease patterns seen in infants and young children reflect this with gastrointestinal infections and infestations being prominent health hazards. Indeed, these diseases rather than chronic starvation or malnutrition *per se* are the main determinants of morbidity and mortality patterns. Before 1969, information about health problems prevailing in Indonesia was scarce and vital statistics, therefore, inaccurate. With the implementation of the five-year Development Plan in that year an epidemiological surveillance system was introduced which produced some important information. It showed that the crude death rate (CDR) and infant mortality rate (IMR) are still very high by international standards with the CDR 20 per 1000 per year and the IMR 150 per 1000 per year (Central Bureau of Statistics, Jakarta, 1975) while 50% of all deaths occur in the under five age group (Bahwari *et al.*, 1976). Most of these deaths are due to diarrhoeal diseases and other infectious diseases, often complicated by malnutrition.

The precise extent of these diseases is unknown and very difficult to document. A prospective study in a community of almost 3500 people in Ujung Pandang, Sulawesi, gives some idea of the extent of the problem (Brotowasisto, 1975). As can be seen in Table I, infants

TABLE I. *Estimated annual diarrhoeal episode attack rate in Ujung Pandang, Sulawesi. (Brotowasisto, 1975)*

Age group	Estimated annual attack rate
0–1 year	98·5%
1–4 years	163%
5–9 years	40%
10–14 years	16%

and young children are specially prone to diarrhoeal episodes which have very significant morbidity and mortality in developing countries.

The childhood diarrhoeal disease problem is important in terms of usage of scarce hospital facilities as well; almost 30% of admissions to the large children's ward of the Main General Hospital in Jakarta are for "gastroenteritis". Our joint research programme has been based in the Department of Child Health in the University of Indonesia who staff that busy children's ward in that hospital. The aim of the projects has been to document important factors responsible for causing childhood diarrhoea in order to plan more effective strategies for prevention, diagnosis and treatment. As will be shown, the results indicate that environmental factors are very important in determining these disease patterns which are bound to persist until general standards of living, nutrition and hygiene are improved.

IV. Causes of "Gastroenteritis" in Malnutrition

In most reported studies the rates of isolation of enteric pathogens from faecal or rectal swab specimens of patients with "gastroenteritis" are quite low. For example, Cramblett and his colleagues (1971) made a ten-year long study of this from reports from North America and Europe and found that in two-thirds of patients with diarrhoea investigated recognized pathogens were not found. In their own study of children in Columbus, Ohio, no aetiological agent was found in three-quarters of 270 patients investigated. Among the bacterial pathogens found, enteropathogenic *Escherichia coli* appeared to be very important and a large range of serotypes were implicated. However, the situation in developing countries seems to be quite different. In Indonesia, the reported rates of isolation of enteropathogenic *E. coli* are extremely high; Dewanto *et al.*, (1968) found various pathogens in 70% of 448 children with diarrhoea under two years investigated in the General Hospital in Bandung, Java. In a survey of 746 outpatients without diarrhoea under four years of age in Kampala, Uganda, 8% of the children had enteropathogens, mostly *E. coli*, isolated from their stools (Büttner and Lalo-Kenyi, 1973). In studies of patients with diarrhoea in developing countries rates of isolation of enteric pathogens are even higher. In our own investigation of infants and children with acute diarrhoea in Jakarta enteropathogens were isolated from specimens from most patients (Table II). Guerrant *et al.*,(1975) found potential pathogens in thirty-one out of forty consecutive children studied with

TABLE II. *Rate of isolation of recognized enteric pathogens in faecal specimens from twenty-six Indonesian infants and children with acute diarrhoea*

	Isolations of enteropathogenic *Escherichia coli*	Isolations of *Klebsiella* spp.	Isolations of *Salmonella* spp.
Outpatients (10)	7	4	4
Children's ward (9)	7	3	3
Neonatal ward (7)	2	3	1

diarrhoea in Brazil. Toxigenic *E. coli* were found in twenty patients (50%), invasive *E. coli* or *Salmonella* sp. in four (10%) and both toxigenic and invasive microorganisms in seven patients. In a study of 176 men with acute, watery diarrhoea studied in the Cholera Research Hospital in Dacca, Bangladesh, enterotoxigenic strains of *E. coli* were isolated from 109 patients (62%) (Merson *et al*., 1979).

The whole question of the real pathogenic role of various microorganisms in causing diarrhoeal diseases in malnourished children is still unresolved and requires much more research, especially collaborative research between groups of investigators with different technical skills and access to different types of clinical problems around the world. The complexity of the problem can be exemplified by a recent, brief report from central Java (Sebodo *et al*., 1977) in which enteropathogenic or enterotoxigenic *E. coli* were found not uncommonly in symptomless children as well as children with diarrhoea; other potential pathogens including viruses and yeasts were found too.

The speed of developments in technical aspects of this field makes it important also to realize that the spectrum of microorganisms, bacterial and viral, which are capable of causing diarrhoeal disease may be considerably wider than suggested by currently held views about enteropathogenicity. For example, strains of *E. coli* which cause diarrhoea but do not produce heat-labile or heat-stable enterotoxins and do not invade the intestinal mucosa have recently been reported (Levine *et al*., 1978). We have preliminary information that yeasts may also contribute to diarrhoeal disease in malnourished children (Thelen *et al*., 1978) and that this effect may be toxin-mediated (unpublished observations).

The frequent gastrointestinal infections and infestations which so commonly occur in malnutrition, have a damaging effect on the lining mucosa of the upper gastrointestinal tract. In the tropics the intestinal villi are shorter and wider than in Western subjects, the enterocytes are more irregular and there is an increase in the numbers of inflammatory cells in the underlying lamina propria (Baker *et al.*, 1962; Spring *et al.*, 1962). The duodenojejunal morphology is altered as early as three months of age in apparently healthy Guatemalan infants although fetuses in that country have normal, tall, finger-like villi (Viteri and Schneider, 1974). In malnourished children quite marked histological abnormalities occur in the proximal small intestinal epithelium (Burman, 1965) as the result of the combined effects of malnutrition and repeated gut infections and parasitic infestations which prevent the mucosa achieving its normal process of regeneration of the intestinal villi. This is of immense practical importance since it depresses the activity of the intestinal digestive and absorptive mechanisms which normally reside in the intestinal villi. Of greatest practical importance is depression of the activity of the enzyme lactase responsible for digestion of lactose (sugar of milk) before its absorption. This form of secondary lactase deficiency causes an osmotic type of diarrhoea producing dehydration which can be serious in malnourished children. This, in combination with the high frequency of hypolactasia, perhaps genetic in origin, in certain populations including Asians and Africans (Cook and Kajubi, 1966; Chung and McGill, 1968) has to be borne in mind when devising feeding schedules and nutritional rehabilitation programmes for malnourished people, especially children. This has important implications, frequently overlooked in the past, for international food relief programmes which often include milk powders.

Of all the common childhood illnesses, diarrhoeal diseases have the greatest ill effect on nutrition, mainly because of associated poor appetite and the common practice of withholding food from children with diarrhoea. Recent studies have shown that when fluid replacement by mouth is coupled with education about proper dietary feeding practices during and after diarrhoea there is an improvement of appetite and increased weight gain. This is a crucial aspect with long-term nutritional significance for children with diarrhoeal disorders. Another important aspect in maintaining nutrition is the promotion of uninterrupted breast feeding and the continuation of feeding the usual foods during diarrhoeal episodes as soon as the child can eat.

V. The Upper Intestinal Microflora in Malnutrition

There are also important alterations in the upper intestinal microflora in malnutrition. In well-nourished adults and children the upper intestine normally harbours a relatively sparse microflora.

Up till recently, few studies were available of the upper gastrointestinal microflora in children with malnutrition. In Guatemala, it had been found some years ago that malnourished children with diarrhoeal illnesses had very large numbers of bacteria in jejunal contents but that malnourished children without diarrhoea had a normal, relatively sparse flora (Dammin, 1965). Unfortunately, these results came from post-mortem specimens obtained some hours after death, so their validity was somewhat doubtful. More recently microbial overgrowth in the upper gut was found in life in malnourished young Australian Aborigines (Gracey and Stone, 1972) and in Guatemala (Mata *et al.*, 1972).

Similar findings have now been made in children in Africa (Heyworth and Brown, 1975; Rowland and McCollum, 1977). The clinical significance of these observations is not yet clear but there is some experimental evidence to suggest that the presence of a heterogeneous bacterial overgrowth (or "mixed bacterial soup") in the upper intestine in this situation may contribute to diarrhoea and fluid loss, which are characteristic of childhood malnutrition, by interfering with the intestinal absorption of nutrients and fluid and electrolytes (Thelen *et al.*, 1978).

VI. Environmental Contamination

Another interesting observation is that malnourished children frequently have faecal microorganisms in their mouth and throat secretions where they are not normally present (Gracey *et al.*, 1973). This is probably a reflection of the degree of faecal contamination of the environment in which malnourished children live and their impaired capacity to resist potentially pathogenic microorganisms from establishing themselves on mucous membranes. This seems supported by our observations in ninety-two Australian Aboriginal children over two years of age, from remote parts of Western Australia, 60% of whom had faecal microorganisms in their oropharyngeal secretions compared with only 5% of fifty-nine non-Aboriginal children of similar ages in Perth (Gracey *et al.*, 1979b).

The potential contribution of faecal contamination of the environment to this overall problem of the "gastroenteritis-malnutrition" complex is difficult to document. Certainly we have found faecal contamination of food, drink and eating and drinking utensils, especially of dirty baby's bottles, to be a significant problem in remote, fringe-dwelling Aborigines living in very unsatisfactory accommodation on cattle stations, missions and in country towns (see Fig. 7a and b). The risk of diarrhoeal disease from contaminated weaning foods and water supplies has been mentioned in two recent publications from the Medical Research Council Laboratory in Keneba, the Gambia (Rowland and McCollum, 1977; Rowland *et al.*, 1978) and one from Nigeria

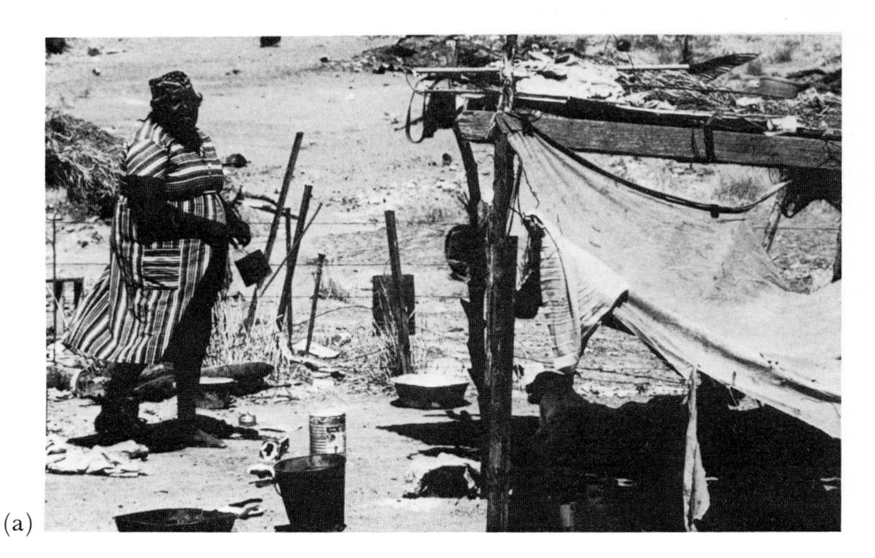

(a)

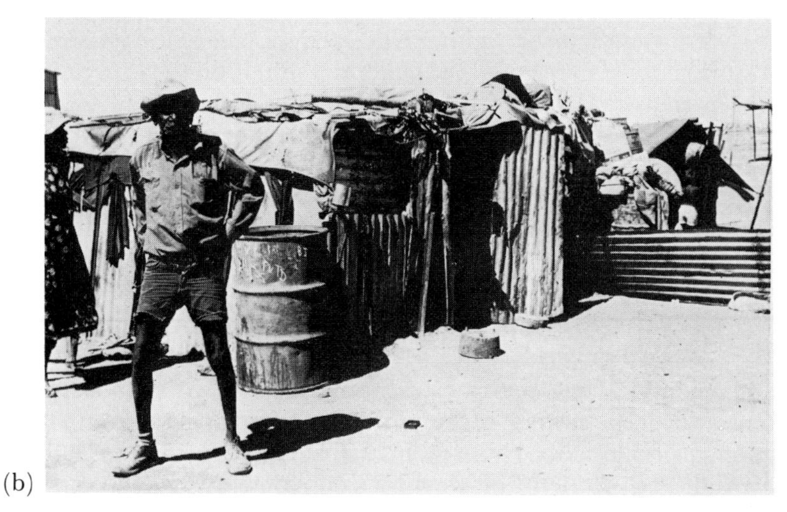

(b)

Fig. 7 (a) and (b). Examples of unsatisfactory living conditions for Aborigines living in the remote far northern Kimberley district of Western Australia. (Reproduced with permission of the Editor, *Medical Journal of Australia*.)

(Tomkins *et al.*, 1978). Environmental contamination as a potential cause of infections in malnourished children appears also to be a major problem in Jakarta. We found a high degree of faecal pollution of surface waters used for various domestic purposes, including food preparation, by the poorer sections of the community (Gracey *et al.*, 1976). *Salmonella* were isolated from ten out of twenty-one (48%) of water samples, and twelve out of nineteen of aquatic sediments tested (Gracey *et al.*, 1979a). Altogether fourteen serotypes and thirty-seven isolations were recorded. It must be appreciated that the Ciliwung River and criss-crossing canals from where these samples were taken are an integral part of the life of the city of Jakarta and a reminder of its past colonial designers. This is particularly important for the poorer sections of its population many of whom live in very inadequate squatter settlements near these surface waters (Fig. 8) and especially for the children who customarily walk barefooted through streets and alleys heavily contaminated with human and animal excreta and who play and swim in the city's rivers and canals.

The finding of *Salmonella* sp. so frequently in these water sources in Jakarta prompted an investigation of the Salmonella carrier rate in a sample of 464 apparently healthy subjects, adults and children, selected at random from within and around the General Hospital in the centre of that city. Many of these subjects were relatives and other visitors to the hospital, some were paper sellers, food-stall vendors and car drivers, others were hospital employees. Thirty-nine subjects (8·4%) were found to be Salmonella carriers, suggesting there is a substantial pool of carriers in the general population to perpetuate the "gastroenteritis-malnutrition" complex.

These findings reveal a public health problem of major proportion in modern Jakarta, a problem likely to be repeated in many other overcrowded, inadequately serviced, dirty and rapidly expanding cities throughout the Third World.

VII. How Can the Problem be Overcome?

This disturbing and complex background is obviously important in causing and perpetuating malnutrition and its constant companion, infection, in millions of children in the developing countries and in underprivileged sections of wealthy countries, such as Australia's Aborigines (Gracey, 1978). What can be done about this, one of the major health problems facing mankind (Scrimshaw *et al.*, 1968)? It is interesting to note the comments in a recent report from Nigeria

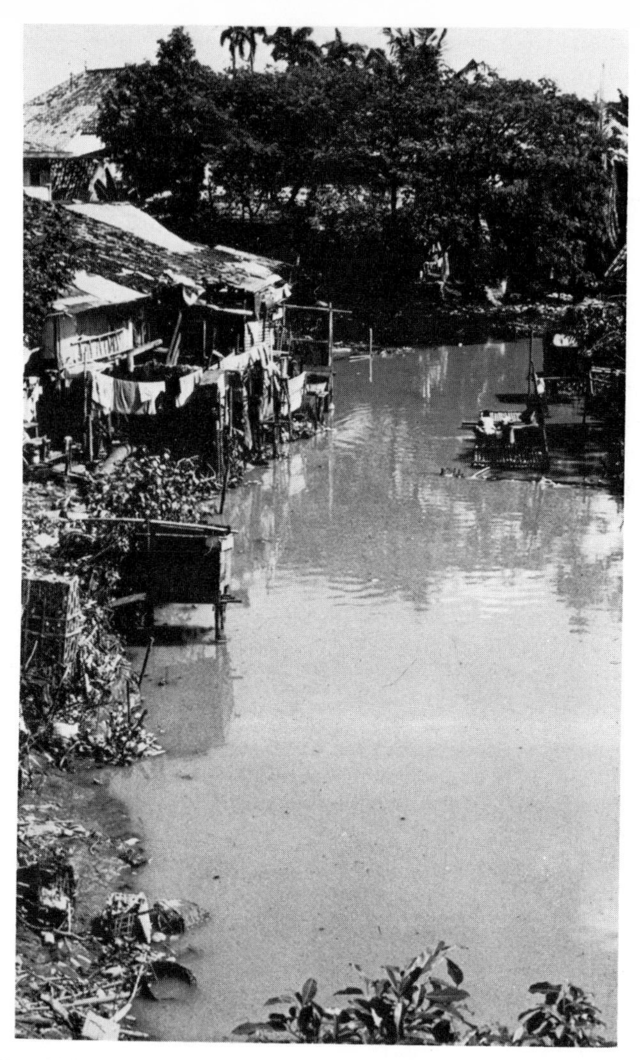

Fig. 8. The Ciliwung River, Jakarta, about 200 m from the Main General Hospital. The river is lined by makeshift squatter settlements; in the left foreground is an open rubbish dump and a crude communal privy. On the right in the middle distance is a floating pontoon used for washing clothes and washing fruit and vegetables. (Reproduced with permission of the Editor, *Transactions of the Royal Society of Tropical Medicine and Hygiene.*)

(Tomkins *et al.*, 1978); they say "until this cycle of upper bowel colonization and protracted diarrhoea is broken, a diet-based nutrition programme cannot be expected to function effectively". An editorial in the *Lancet* (1978) called for a "vigorous research effort" into this subject and for it "to be given special emphasis in 1979, when the Year of the Child coincided with the United Nations Conference on the Application of Science and Technology". Where such unsatisfactory conditions exist and are likely to persist, the importance of breast feeding and supplying nutritious and clean food for infants in the early months of life must be recognized and the early introduction of other foods or bottle feeding must be discouraged because of the high risk of exposure to gastrointestinal infections. This is probably the most important, short-term measure which can be implemented, without the need for advanced or expensive technology to help lessen this problem. Apart from its medically related significance, breast feeding is of very great economic importance to developing countries and, therefore, internationally. For example, Jon Rohde (1974) reckoned that the cost of dietary raw materials for the lactating mother to produce her own breast milk is less than 30% of the market value of the milk and, on that basis, estimated that continued breast feeding nationwide in Indonesia through the second year of life would save that country US$62 million in 1974.

It should be stressed that infants, children and fertile, pregnant or lactating mothers often constitute about three-quarters of total populations in developing countries. Apart from their numerical importance, these individuals are usually less influential economically, politically and socially and therefore more vulnerable to the stresses imposed by the pressures related above. These factors are often overlooked and need much more emphasis in planning health care programmes in developing countries. These remarks apply right across the board including the allocation of time and staff in training doctors and nurses and in their deployment in urban and rural areas.

Control of population growth in a very important aspect to be considered to help overcome these massive disease problems. High birth rates are characteristic of less developed countries and in many exceed 40 per 1000 per annum. Some developing countries like Hong Kong, Malaysia, Singapore and Sri Lanka are already experiencing a decline in fertility rates and in some the birth rates have dropped to less than 30 per 1000. Many other governments including those of China, India, the Philippines and Indonesia are making serious attempts to lower their birth rates. Personal, religious, family and society's attitudes to family planning vary from place to place and often prevent effective implementation of desired controls. Progress has been much less effective in Africa and Latin America than in Asia.

There is a risk of identifying all developing countries as a homogeneous unit where superficially similar problems will respond to similar control measures. This is not true and programmes have to be devised according to differing local conditions. There is no doubt that these countries are going through a phase of rapid demographic change and there are already changes occurring in morbidity and mortality patterns and it is anticipated that there will be further declines in fertility. Without such a trend the prospect remains for population growth to continue or increase because of the capacity to lower mortality rates even further. This disturbing prospect must be kept in mind when planning strategies for development programmes in these countries.

Obviously there are many other strategies which can and are being taken. These include nutrition rehabilitation programmes to help improve the nutritional status of pregnant and lactating women in vulnerable areas and community-based food supplementation programmes. The encouragement of indigenous food production and traditional food preparation and eating practices within the framework of food production for the poor in developing countries is also very important. Earlier detection of milder degrees of malnutrition in village settings can also be useful, particularly where community identity is strong. Earlier recognition of diarrhoeal disease in undernourished infants and children is emerging as an important factor and simple schemes for prevention and treatment of dehydration due to diarrhoea using simple salt and sugar solutions to be made up with local utensils or simple measures and then given by mouth are providing encouraging results in many countries including India, Indonesia, Bangladesh and the Philippines. The continuation of normal feeding as soon as the child can eat is also important to prevent unnecessary starvation and to maintain nutrition. Nutrition education appropriate to local conditions and customs is, of course, of great importance.

The background on which malnutrition flourishes is of such complexity and has such important social, cultural, economic and political ramifications that its eradication must depend on the involvement of individuals, groups and institutions from diverse disciplines. Governments and international agencies obviously have a key role to play. The problem is of great magnitude and urgency and shows no signs of decreasing in the foreseeable future. For children growing up in developing countries more has to be done, tomorrow is too late. . . "his name is today".

References

Bahwari, Setiady, Adhyatma and Sudarto (1976). *In* "Proceedings of Second Asian Congress of Paediatrics" 111–121. Indonesian Paediatric Association, Jakarta.

Baker, S. J., Ignatius, M., Mathan, V. I., Vaish, S. K. and Chacko, C. C. (1962). *In* "Intestinal Biopsy" (G. E. W. Wolstenholme and M. P. Cameron, Eds), 84. Little Brown, Boston.

Brotowasisto (1975). *In* "Diare, Masalah dan Penanggulangannya", 20–26. Departemen Kesehatan, Republik Indonesia.

Burman, D. (1965). *Arch Dis. Child.* **40**, 526–531.

Büttner, D. W. and Lalo-Kenyi, A. (1973). *Ze. Tropenmed. Parasit.* **24**, 259–264.

Chung, M. H. and McGill, D. B. (1968). *Gastroenterology* **54**, 225–226.

Cook, G. C. and Kajubi, S. K. (1966). *Lancet* i, 725–730.

Cramblett, H. G., Azimi, P. and Haynes, R. E. (1971). *Ann. N.Y. Acad. Sci.* **176**, 80–92.

Dammin, G. J. (1965). *Fedn Proc. Fedn Am. Socs exp. Biol.* **24**, 35–38.

Dewanto, O., Alisjahbana, A., Suratman, E. and Sugiri (1968). *Paediat. Indon.* **8**, 45–60.

Dwyer, D. J. (1978). *Geogrl Mag.* Vol. L, **5**, 519–522.

Geertz, C. (1963). "Agricultural Involution. The Processes of Ecological Change in Indonesia". Univ. California Press, Berkeley, and London.

Gracey, M. (1978). *Med. J. Aust.* **1**, 202–205.

Gracey, M. and Stone, D. E. (1972). *Aust. N.Z. J. Med.* **3**, 215–219.

Gracey, M., Stone, D. E., Suharjono and Sunoto (1973). *Aust. paediat. J.* **9**, 260–262.

Gracey, M., Stone, D. E., Sutoto and Sutejo (1976). *Envir. chld Hlth* **22**, 18–23.

Gracey, M., Ostergaard, P., Adnan, S. W. and Iveson, J. B. (1979a). *Trans. R. Soc. trop. Med. Hyg.* **73**, 306–308.

Gracey, M., Ostergaard, P. and Beaman, J. (1979b). *Med. J. Aust.* **2**, 212–214.

Guerrant, R. L., Moore, R. A., Kirschenfeld, P. M. and Sande, M. A. (1975). *New Engl, J. Med.* **293**, 567–573.

Heyworth, B. and Brown, J. (1975). *Arch Dis. Child.* **50**, 27–33.

Jelliffe, D. B. (1974). *In* "Medicine in the Tropics" (A. W. Woodruff, Ed.), 391–419. Churchill Livingstone, Edinburgh and London.

Levine, M. M., Bergquist, E. J., Nalin, D. R., Waterman, D. H., Hornick, R. B., Young, C. R., Sotman, S. and Rowe, B. (1978). *Lancet* i, 1119–1122.

Mata, L. J., Jiminez, F., Cordon, M., Rosales, R., Prera, E., Schneider, R. E. and Viteri, F. (1972). *Am. J. clin. Nutr.* **25**, 1118–1126.

Merson, M. H., Ørskov, F., Ørskov, I., Sack, R. B., Huq, I. and Koster, F. T. (1979). *Infect. Immun.* **23**, 325–329.

Rohde, J. E. (1974). *Paediatrica Indon.* **14**, 198–207.

Rowland, M. G. M. and McCollum, J. P. K. (1977). *Trans. R. Soc. trop. Med. Hyg.* **71**, 199–203.

Rowland, M. G. M., Barrell, R. A. E. and Whitehead, R. G. (1978). *Lancet* i, 136–138.
Scrimshaw, N. S., Taylor, C. E. and Gordon, J. E. (1968). *Wld Hlth Org. Monogr. Ser.* No. 57, Geneva.
Sebodo, T., Soenarto, Y., Rohde, J. E., Ryan, N. J., Taylor, B. J. Luke, R. J. K., Bishop, R. F., Barnes, G. L., Holmes, I. H. and Ruck, B. J. (1977). *Lancet* i, 490–491.
Spring, H., Scribchadh, R., Gangarosa, B. J., Benajati, C., Kundel, D. and Halstead, S. (1962). *Am. J. clin. Path.* **38**, 43–51.
Thelen, P., Burke, V. and Gracey, M. (1978). *J. med. Microbiol.* **11**, 463–470.
Tomkins, A. M., Drasar, B. S., Bradley, A. K. and Williamson, W. A. (1978). *Trans. R. Soc. trop. Med. Hyg.* **72**, 239–243.
Vahlquist, B., Stapleton, T. and Béhar, M. (1973). *Aust. paediat. J.* **9**, 45–47.
Viteri, F. and Schneider, R. E. (1974). *Med. clins N. Am.* **58**, 1487–1505.

Acknowledgement: To P. C. Y. Chen and S. T. Chen for permission to use Figure 1.

24

Air Pollution and Human Health

H. W. de Koning

Division of Environmental Health, World Health Organization, Geneva, Switzerland

The health of man can be directly affected by breathing polluted air.

I. Air As a Resource

The air around us in one of our most valuable resources. The average male, for example, exchanges about 15 kg of air a day, compared to less than 1·5 kg of food or about 2·5 kg of water (World Health Organization, 1972). Our atmosphere also acts as a window to space, allowing sunlight to reach the earth's surface while forming an opaque ozone screen (in the stratosphere) to filter out much of the deadly ultraviolet rays. The atmosphere also acts like a greenhouse, passing short-wave radiant energy, but absorbing long-wave heat energy reflected from the earth's surface: thus shielding the earth against excessive losses of heat radiation from the surface to space, thereby warming the layer of air close to the earth's surface (World Meteorological Organization, 1979).

Air pollution can interfere with all of these phenomena. The health of man can be directly affected by breathing polluted air. Man's health and well-being can also be indirectly affected when the delicate energy balance in the atmosphere is disturbed, or when possible climate modification takes place.

Unpolluted air is a concept only, that is, the composition of the air if man and his resultant effects did not exist on earth. Table I gives an approximation of the composition of unpolluted air, determined by measurement at remote places—the middle of the sea, the poles and the mountains.

II. Air Pollution, Natural and Man-made

Ambient air is more than a mixture of these gases. When sampled close to the ground, it contains other gases, vapours and particulate matter derived from either natural sources such as volcanoes, sea spray, forest fires, or erosion by the wind from the beach, desert, soil and rock, or from man's activities. Some components such as spores, seeds, and pollen grains, for example, are not pollutants; they are natural constituents frequently found in the atmosphere. Air pollution is the result of the discharge into the atmosphere of foreign gases, vapours, droplets and particles, or of excessive amounts of normal constituents such as carbon dioxide and suspended particulate matter by the burning of fossil fuels.

The major air pollutants emitted into the atmosphere are listed in Table II.

TABLE I. *Gaseous Composition of Dry Unpolluted Air*

Constituent	Molecular formula	Volume fraction
Nitrogen	N_2	78·09%
Oxygen	O_2	20.94%
Water*	H_2O	
Argon	Ar	0.93%
Carbon dioxide	CO_2	0.0318%
Neon	Ne	18 ppm
Helium	He	5.2 ppm
Methane	CH_4	1.0–1.2 ppm
Krypton	Kr	1.1 ppm
Nitrous oxide	N_2O	0·5 ppm
Hydrogen	H_2	0·5 ppm
Carbon monoxide	CO	0.1 ppm
Xenon	Xe	0.09 ppm
Ozone	O_3	0.02 ppm
Organic vapours	—	~ 0.02 ppm
Sulphur dioxide	SO_2	~ 0.001 ppm
Nitrogen dioxide	NO_2	~ 0.001 ppm
Ammonia	NH_3	~ 0.001 ppm

* In the usual range of absolute humidities, water vapour adds another 1 to 3% by volume.

Of the pollutants listed in Table II, some are directly emitted into the atmosphere as a result of man's activities; these are so-called primary pollutants. The others, called secondary pollutants, are generated as a result of atmospheric reactions (e.g. photochemical reactions, catalytic oxidation, hydrolysis, etc.). Particles emitted to the atmosphere may be organic or inorganic in composition, and may participate in the formation of secondary particulate pollutants. Some particles are also formed from gaseous pollutants as a result of chemical reactions. In most cases, particulate matter is analysed for specific substances of interest. If health effects are being considered, the chemical composition of the respirable fraction ($0{\cdot}01 - \approx 10\mu m$) is most important.

III. Air Quality in Urban and Rural areas

Table III gives an example of the comparison of the number of particles in a rural and urban atmosphere.

TABLE II. *Major Primary and Secondary Air Pollutants*

Gases	Suspended particulate matter
Inorganic	*Inorganic*
Sulphur oxides (SO_2, SO_3)	Metals (Pb, Cd, Be, Hg, etc.)
Nitrogen oxides (NO, NO_2)	Fluorides
Ozone (O_3)	Nitrates, sulphates, phosphates
Carbon monoxide (CO)	Asbestos
Hydrogen sulphide (H_2S)	Mineral dusts (silicates, silica, etc.)
HCl, Cl_2, fluorides, etc.	
Ammonium compounds (NH_3, etc.)	
Carbon dioxide (CO_2)	
Organic	*Organic*
Hydrocarbons (paraffins, olefins, aromatics)	Polycyclic organics (benzo [a] pyrene, etc.)
Oxygenated compounds (aldehydes, ketones)	Oxygenated compounds
Sulphur-containing compounds (mercaptans, etc.)	Pesticides
Nitrogen-containing compounds (peroxyacetyl nitrate (PAN), etc.)	
Halogenated compounds	

TABLE III. *Number of Particulates in 100 ml of Air*

	Number of particles		
Particle size	Rural atmosphere	Stuttgart	New York
0·3	1000	20 000	20 000
0·4	400	8 000	8 000
0·5	300	3 000	3 000
1·0	40	300	30
2·0	10	30	2
3·0	4	10	6
4·0	2	10	3

Air pollutants are emitted either from mobile (automobiles, airplanes) or from stationary sources. The latter include large single sources, point sources, such as power stations, cement plants, refineries, etc., or area sources such as residential areas with individual domestic heating systems in each dwelling. After the pollutant is emitted into the air, it is transported and diffused in the atmosphere by the air movement. Depending upon the meteorological conditions, the pollutant may be dispersed, thus gradually reducing the concentration or, in the absence of air movement, its concentration may rapidly increase to levels that are dangerous to human health. There are a number of incidents recorded where pollutant concentrations rose to levels that caused a number of excess deaths (World Health Organization, 1972).

Characteristic background and urban concentrations (annual mean) of selected air pollutants are given in Table IV. The table shows

TABLE IV. *Average Levels of Air Pollution*

	Background concentration (ppm)	Urban concentrations (ppm)
Sulphur dioxide	0·0002–0·0004	0·03
Nitrogen dioxide	0·001–0·003	0·05
Ozone	0·01	0·03
Carbon monoxide	0·1	4
Carbon dioxide	335	355
Hydrocarbons	—	—
Methane	1–1·5	2
Non-methane	0·001	0·5
Suspended particulate matter[a]	1–30	100

[a] $\mu g/m^3$.

that urban concentrations generally have higher levels of air pollution and are therefore of most immediate concern for man's health.

IV. General Effects of Air Pollution

The effects of pollutants on man can be classed as either general or specific. Examples of general effects include the general deterioration of building materials and ornamental features such as statues, marble structures, etc. There is also the general nuisance of soiling of the outdoors, including clothes-lines, park benches, etc. Other effects include reduced visibility because of smoke or haziness, or in extreme cases, a reduction of sky light. On a global scale, somewhat more significant phenomena involve the possible modification of climatic variables (World Meteorological Organization, 1979) in particular:

(a) The amount of ultraviolet light that reaches the earth is increasing because the ozone layer in the stratosphere is being depleted through reaction with halogens released by man, mainly from stratospheric flight and the photo dissociation of freon gas (various chorofluoromethane substances used as the propellant in spray bombs). An increase in ultraviolet light reaching the earth would cause increased incidence of skin cancer.

(b) The increased rate of combustion of fossil fuels (which produce CO_2), coupled with an increased rate of deforestation (forests consume CO_2), has led to a gradual increase of the level of CO_2 in the atmosphere. Since CO_2 absorbs the long-wave heat radiation reflected from the earth's surface, an increase means a warming of the atmosphere (the so-called greenhouse effect). Aerosols, including dust, can produce a warming or a cooling of the atmosphere, depending upon their absorption properties and the reflectivity of the ground surface. The most immediate impact of such changes would be in a shift of agricultural zones with the overall possibility of lower productivity.

(c) Increased acidity of precipitation near industrial areas with possible effects on soil fertility, vegetation and aquatic biology in lakes and rivers.

(d) Increase in condensation nuclei with a possible effect on cloudiness and precipitation processes.

All of these effects concern man and indeed his ability to survive on this earth. They are the subject of much research and scientific debate. Both the World Health Organization and the World Meteorological Organization, together with the United Nations Environment Programme, are instituting monitoring and research projects to clarify the issues involved and to promote measures to prevent further deterioration of our environmental and climatic conditions.

V. Specific Effects of Air Pollution on Man

Interpretation of health reactions to air pollution depend upon evidence obtained from two types of studies: epidemiological and toxicological. Epidemiological studies are concerned with the effects occurring in human populations exposed under natural conditions. Toxicological studies are carried out on man and animals, during which the level, the duration and the conditions of exposure are under control of the investigator. Both types of evidence are needed to form a reasonable judgement on the effects of air pollution on human health. When they lead to divergent conclusions, it would seem prudent to rely somewhat more on epidemiological evidence.

The effects on human health of exposure to air pollution may be either short-lived and reversible or permanent. Acute and chronic effects may occur after a short-term or single exposure to a hazardous substance at high concentration, or may result from low-level long-term exposures, whether continuous or repeated intermittently. Classical toxicological studies on animals are generally designed to detect only the acute effects of short-term exposures. Epidemiological studies of natural living populations, on the other hand, tend to focus on chronic effects of long-term exposures.

A number of factors affect the sensitivity of the population. These include age, sex, general state of health and nutrition, concurrent exposures, pre-existing disease, and temperature and humidity at the time of exposure. In general, older persons, the very young, those in poor health, cigarette smokers, the occupationally exposed, and those with pre-existing bronchitis, coronary heart disease and asthma, are more vulnerable to air pollution exposures.

The World Health Organization has for many years been involved in health effects research through collaboration with national institutes. An integrated and expanded programme on the assessment of health effects of environmental conditions was initiated in 1973, with financial support of the United Nations Environment Programme, under the title of WHO Environmental Health Criteria Programme (World Health Organization, 1974, 1976). The main objectives of this programme are (i) to assess existing information on the relationship between exposure to environmental pollutants and man's health and to provide guidelines for setting exposure limits consistent with health protection, and (ii) to identify gaps in knowledge concerning the health effects of recognized or potential pollutants, and to stimulate and promote research in areas where information is inadequate.

The list of chemicals and physical hazards dealt with under the programme is regularly reviewed. To date, about twelve criteria documents have been issued and many more are in preparation. The list of documents that have been completed includes Mercury, Polychlorinated biphenyls, Lead, Nitrogen oxides, Nitrates, Nitrites and *N*-nitroso compounds, Principles and Methods for Evaluating Toxicity of Chemicals (Part 1), Photochemical oxidants, Sulphur oxides and Suspended particulate matter, DDT, Carbon disulphide, Mycotoxins, Noise and Carbon monoxide. Each of these documents, in addition to reviewing chemical and physical properties, analytical methods, environmental concentrations and epidemiological and clinical studies of effects, includes a chapter on the evaluation of health risks to man. The latter, where applicable, includes sections on relative contributions to the total dose from air, food, water, and other exposures. Whenever possible, guidelines on exposure or dose limits are given.

The International Agency for Research on Cancer (IARC) is conducting a separate programme for the evaluation of potentially carcinogenic chemicals in the environment (IARC, 1978). Up until September 1978. nineteen volumes in the series of IARC Monographs on the Evaluation of the Carcinogenic Risk of Chemicals to Humans were published or in press. In these a total of 420 chemicals have been evaluated. For twenty-six chemicals a positive association was established between exposure and the occurrence of cancer in humans (see Table V). The type of exposure for which the association was found was occupational for seventeen chemicals, iatrogenic for eight, and dietary for one; however, the general population may also be exposed to most of these chemicals. For the other chemicals, information was mostly insufficient to permit a clear-cut evaluation of their potential to cause cancer in humans (see also Higginson, this volume).

Table VI presents a breakdown of the categories of chemicals included in the IARC programme.

VI. Measures to Protect Human Health from the Effects of Air Pollution

When public concern about air pollution and its effects becomes strong enough, it usually results in the passage of air pollution control legislation and the setting up of an administrative apparatus for its enforcement. The types of legislation adopted may vary in different countries according to their constitutional framework. Also the development of legislative measures has undergone considerable change in the last ten years from the specific types of control legislation for air, for water, for solid waste, and so on, to more integrated forms of legislation. Lately, this has even progressed further with the introduction of almost completely integrated programmes such as on impact assessment and on land-use planning in which air, water and solid-waste control are components of the overall planning and development schemes.

TABLE V. *Chemicals or Industrial Processes Associated with the Induction of Cancer in Humans (Compiled from Volumes 1–19 of IARC Monographs on the Evaluation of the Carcinogenic Risk of Chemicals to Humans)*[a]

1. Aflatoxins
2. 4-Aminobiphenyl
3. Arsenic compounds
4. Asbestos
5. Auramine (manufacture of)
6. Benzene
7. Benzidine
8. *N*, *N*-bis (2-Chloroethyl)-2-naphthylamine
9. bis (chloromethyl) ether
10. Cadmium-using industries (possibly cadmium oxide)
11. Chloroamphenicol
12. Chloromethyl methyl ether (possibly associated with bis (chloromethyl) ether)
13. Chromium (chromate-producing industries)
14. Cyclophosphamide
15. Diethylstilboestrol
16. Haematite mining (radon?)
17. Isopropyl oils
18. Melphalan
19. Mustard gas
20. 2-Naphthylamine
21. Nickel (nickel refinning)
22. Oxymetholone (?)
23. Phenacetin
24. Phynytoin
25. Soot, tars and oils
26. Vinyl chloride

[a] The list of twenty-six chemicals or industrial processes given above should not be taken as a thorough compilation of chemicals known to induce cancer in humans. It reflects only those chemicals or industrial processes which have been evaluated in the programme up to now (IARC Monographs, Volumes 1–19). Other agents have been designated as human carcinogens: tobacco smoking and, among others, betel-nut chewing, wood dust, certain mineral oils, and so on. Some of these have been scheduled for future consideration.

In air pollution, basically two approaches for the control and prevention of harmful effects are used: (1) air quality management and (2) best practicable means. *Air quality management* aims at the preservation of environmental quality by prescribing the degree of pollution which shall be tolerated, leaving it to the local authorities and to the polluters themselves to devise and implement actions which will assure that the prescribed degree of pollution will not be exceeded. Ambient air quality standards for different pollutants are typical examples of this type of legislation. Such legislation is difficult to enforce and is nowadays usually supplemented by additional legislation prescribing how the standards are to be achieved and maintained. The *best practicable means* approach stresses that the air pollutant emissions should be kept to a minimum. Emission standards are used to define the best practicable means for single sources of air pollution. This type of legislation requires that there must be an authority to decide for each industry on the best means to control the emission of a particular air pollutant.

TABLE VI. *Major Use-exposure Categories for the Chemicals or Industrial processes Evaluated in Volumes 1–19 of the IARC Monographs on the Evaluation of the Carcinogenic Risk of Chemicals to Humans*

Major use or exposure category	Number of chemicals
Industrial chemicals[a]	213
Pharmaceutical preparations and/or veterinary drugs	84
Naturally occurring substances (environmental and food contaminants)	42
Pesticides	34
Food additives or cosmetic ingredients	31
Miscellaneous chemicals and analogues	7
Industrial processes	5
Industrial byproducts and contaminants	4
Total	420

[a] Although the major exposures or uses of these compounds are industrial, environmental contamination and subsequent exposure of the general population may occur, particularly following industrial accidents or because of environmental pollution.

The "air quality management" approach and the "best practicable means" approach differ widely in details concerned with enforcement and cost/benefit and there exist numerous possibilities for combining the two approaches. It is thought, however, that the "best practicable means" approach has the greater potential as the chief instrument for air pollution control in the future.

References

International Agency for Research on Cancer (1978). Annual Report. IARC, WHO, Lyon.

World Health Organization (1972). "Hazards of the Human Environment". WHO, Geneva.

World Health Organization (1974). "Health Aspects of Environmental Pollution Control: Planning and Implementation of National Programmes". Report of a WHO Expert Committee, TRS 554. Geneva.

World Health Organization (1976). "Environmental Health Criteria 1, Mercury" Background and Purpose of WHO Environmental Health Criteria Programme. Geneva.
World Meteorological Organization (1979). "World Climate," a Conference of Experts on Climate and Mankind. Geneva.

25

Cancer and the Environment

John Higginson

International Agency for Research on Cancer, World Health Organization, Lyon, France

---

Cancer is now the cause of almost one fourth of all deaths in industrial states. . . . It is necessary to develop a balanced and commonsense approach.

I. Introduction

In the eighteenth and early nineteenth centuries cancer was considered relatively unimportant, and furthermore to be hereditary in origin or an inevitable accompaniment of ageing. Accordingly, few people believed in the possibilities of prevention and elimination through environmental control. Today, following the virtual disappearance of those infectious diseases which killed so many in early life, cancer is now the cause of almost one-fourth of all deaths in industrial states. It is usually regarded by the public as the most important disease due to environmental pollution.

In 1775, Percivall Pott, a London surgeon, suggested that cancer of the scrotum in chimney sweeps was caused by soot, and that this could be prevented by improved hygiene. For several reasons this view was accepted only slowly, but since then many other occupational cancers have been demonstrated such as lung cancer in pitchblende miners and bladder cancer in dye workers, thus confirming that chemicals in the work environment could produce cancer. At the same time, medical missionaries such as David Livingstone and Albert Schweitzer reported that cancer was rare or non-existent in black Africans but unfortunately they failed to appreciate the biases introduced by a skewed population distribution. Thus historical recognition of the importance of the industrial environment has had considerable influence on scientific thought. This influence was further emphasized by the fact that early experimental studies were largely concentrated on synthetic chemicals. Nevertheless, Stern in Verona, in 1834 emphatically disagreed that cancer frequency could be related only to "civilization". By mid-century, cancer had been demonstrated in communities at all stages of industrial development, although the distribution by anatomic site varied widely. Thus cancer of the liver is common in Africa, but cancer of the large intestine is rare, whereas the converse is true in North America and Europe (Clemmesen, 1965). Moreover, it gradually became clear that other environmental related factors were important in cancer causation, including behavioural, cultural and dietary patterns (Clemmesen, 1950).

Much of the recent controversy on environmental cancer, however, has resulted from a failure to appreciate these earlier studies on the above factors, and a mistaken limitation by many ecologists of the term as applying only to industrial carcinogens. This chapter attempts to review and summarize recent developments in environmental carcinogenesis and their implications for control (Higginson, 1979).

II. The Concept of the Environment

A. Chemical Environment

For centuries, man has been exposed in the ambient environment to numerous carcinogens (cancer-producing stimuli), arising from burnt organic matter, fungal contamination of foods, etc. Moreover, since the end of the nineteenth century, the number of synthetic chemicals entering the environment has increased considerably. In 1977, Chemical Abstract Service listed over 4 million distinct entities (a number increasing by about 4000 to 6000 per week), of which about 63 000 are estimated to be in common use. The biological effects of the majority have never been investigated and, due to the immense logistic problems involved, full studies are unlikely to be carried out for most compounds within the foreseeable future. Such evaluations are complex, and are dependent on both experimental studies and *in vivo* systems complemented by epidemiological data where available. Exposure to potential carcinogens in high doses may occur in the workplace, as a result of drug therapy or through such cultural habits as cigarette smoking. Most other exposures occur at low levels in the general environment, e.g. water, air and food. The role of chemicals is very complex, however, since they must be considered not only in terms of carcinogenic potential, or toxic action, but also in their ability to inhibit or enhance tumour formation. Further, chemicals which are themselves harmless may interact within the body to form carcinogens, whereas in other cases a carcinogen may be detoxified. Thus, unlike radiation, the dose of a chemical at the target cell cannot be easily estimated. These facts illustrate some of the issues that are involved in research on the chemical environment, and explain why it is not possible to extrapolate easily and directly from animals or *in vivo* systems to man.

B. Physical Environment

Solar radiation is the major cause of cancer of the skin. Recent changes in cultural habits, e.g. dress and longer vacations, have increased exposure in many populations, often unprotected by natural pigmentation. Although exposure to background ionizing radiation is universal, the most important added exposures come from diagnostic medical sources. So far, additional exposures in the general population from nuclear power sources, although subject to intense controversy, appear very low.

C. Biological Environment

It was assumed, until recently, that as in animals, viruses were major causal factors in human cancer, but to date no tumour in man has been shown unequivocally to be due only to a virus. However, there is supportive evidence for a role by viruses in Burkitt's lymphona, a rare tumour in African children, nasopharyngeal cancer in Chinese and liver cancer in Africa.

Schistosomiasis, a parasitic disease widespread in the Middle East, Africa and Asia, causes cancer of the bladder, and *Clonorchis sinensis*, a liver fluke, cancer of the liver in South-East Asia. Infestation by such parasites reflects local cultural and agricultural practices.

D. Cultural and Behavioural Environment

The most important step towards control of human cancer over the last fifty years has been the recognition of cancer hazards related to certain cultural habits, notably cigarette smoking. Moreover, excessive drinking is also an important factor in many populations. In India betel chewing is responsible for cancer of the mouth and upper digestive system.

Certain types of behaviour have been implicated as risk factors in tumours of the breasts, uterus, ovary and these include "age at first pregnancy or marriage", "number of children" and frequency of and age at intercourse. The mechanisms whereby such behavioural habits modify cancer incidence are imperfectly understood, but may be linked to subtle biochemical changes which involve the hormonal status of an individual, of metabolizing enzymes in the liver and other organs, DNA repair, etc. (Higginson and Muir, 1976; Wynder *et al.*, 1978)

E. Dietary Environment

Although dietary patterns may be imposed by regional practices in developing countries, in cash societies there is a greater variety. Diet is often considered only in terms of food additives, mycotoxins, pesticides, etc. However, the relationship between diet and cancer is much more complex, and thus obesity, fat intake, calorie intake, etc. have been shown to be important factors in certain cancers. The interaction between diet and cultural habits is at present poorly understood and is a subject of intensive research.

In the discussion below, a convenient distinction is made between obviously discrete chemical or physical environmental factors which may cause cancer, and those related to behaviour or diet which may be better described as "carcinogenic risk indices". It is now increasingly apparent that these latter will be eventually measurable according to biochemical and physiological changes. At present this is only possible for a few parameters, e.g. hormones, faecal flora, fibre, etc.

III. Distribution of Human Cancer and its Relation to the Environment

Cancer incidence is usually expressed as morbidity, number of new cases, or mortality, number of deaths, per 100 000 per year. In making comparison between countries it is necessary to correct for age structure. In Table I cancer incidences are summarized for a number of populations representative of both the industrial and non-industrial world. This table illustrates that while overall cancer frequency may vary by a factor of 3, cancer for individual sites may vary up to a 100-fold. Such variations are believed to be largely environmental. However, there is no obvious pattern common to any particular culture or environment. Furthermore, even within the same country groups of high and low cancer frequency may live in close proximity; thus differences have been frequently described between urban and rural dwellers. In Iran for example, the incidence of oesophageal cancer may vary over thirtyfold within a distance of 500 km. Reference, however, should be made to more extensive publications for further discussion of geographic and other differences (Higginson and Muir, 1976; Waterhouse *et al.*, 1976).

More is known about the causation of human cancer than is generally realized. Although usually several factors may influence cancer development, a single factor may be predominant in the sense that in its absence that specific cancer would not occur. Thus general air pollution seems to increase the effects of cigarette smoking, but no effect can be demonstrated in non-smokers.

For convenience, cancers can be classified into three categories: (i) cancers for which specific causal factors have been described; (ii) cancers for which the evidence of environmental origin represents the most rational interpretation of the available data; (iii) cancers for which no aetiological hypothesis can be put forward.

TABLE IA. *Cancer Incidence Rates*[a] *for Selected Sites and Registries—1968–72: Males*

	Site of cancer										
	Buccal cavity	Naso-pharynx	Oesopha-gus	Stomach	Large intestine	Liver	Lung	Prostate	Skin[b]	Leuka-emia	All sites[c]
Africa											
Nigeria, Ibadan	1·8	0·7	1·5	7·2	2·5	10·4	0·8	10·0	1·2	4·0	79·5
South America											
Brazil, Sao Paulo	12·7	0·6	13·1	49·5	15·6	1·4	25·0	16·3	41·4	4·2	230·6
North America											
Canada, Manitoba	3·4	0·5	3·3	16·3	34·4	1·4	44·2	37·6	54·9	10·8	255·0
USA, Bay area											
White	7·4	0·7	4·0	11·4	43·5	2·8	60·8	44·6		9·8	298·4
Black	6·9	1·1	15·2	22·6	34·8	4·2	72·9	77·0		8·1	344·4
Chinese	5·8	19·1	9·2	12·0	43·0	21·1	60·0	18·2		7·2	259·2
Asia											
India, Bombay	19·3	0·4	15·2	9·3	9·0	1·4	13·5	8·0	2·1	3·3	141·0
Japan, Miyagi	1·1	0·3	12·9	84·6	12·4	1·8	20·0	2·7	1·3	4·6	184.7
Singapore											
Chinese	4·0	18·7	21·0	44·3	21·9	34·2	56·9	3·6	6·6	4·5	254·1
Malay	5·1	4·8	2·0	9·2	8·1	14·6	13·9	4·8	4·6	4·5	91·4
Indian	12·7	0·9	5·6	25·8	11·4	11·4	10·0	4·0	2·7	5·6	129·9
Europe											
Norway	2·1	0·4	2·8	24·6	22·8	1·5	22·2	33·1		7·7	195·8
Switzerland, Geneva	5·9	0·4	8·5	18·1	32·7	9·4	60·4	29·9	24·9	9·2	278·1
UK, Birmingham	2·5	0·4	5·0	23·3	32·6	1·0	77·1	17·7	29·8	6·1	240·2

[a] All incidence rates are age-adjusted to the "world" standard population being expressed per 100 000 per annum.
[b] Excludes malignant melanoma.
[c] This represents the total incidence per 100 000 (age-adjusted) for all sites but excludes skin.

TABLE IB *Cancer Incidence Rates*[a] *for Selected Sites and Registries–1968–72: Females*

	Site of Cancer												
	Buccal cavity	Naso-pharynx	Oesoph-agus	Stomach	Large intestine	Liver	Lung	Breast	Cervix uteri	Corpus uteri	Skin[b]	Leuka-emia	All sites[c]
Africa													
Nigeria, Ibadan	1·3	0·3	1·1	6·4	3·2	3·9	0·8	15·4	21·6	1·6	1·6	3·9	107·0
South America													
Brazil, Sao Paulo	2·2	0·3	2·2	21·5	17·8	0·6	5·1	47·3	27·5	8·5	37·4	3·7	199·0
North America													
Canada, Manitoba	1·8	0·1	1·2	7·6	29·4	1·1	8·0	64·2	18·6	14·2	39·3	6·8	226·6
USA, Bay Area													
White	3·9	0·3	1·9	5·8	34·4	1·4	19·1	79·9	12·1	29·9		6·1	275·5
Black	2·9	0·3	3·7	6·6	29·0	1·4	18·5	57·9	25·8	13·3		5·6	231·9
Chinese	1·8	6·4	1·8	9·8	23·2	4·5	22·2	44·0	16·0	16·1		6·3	203·9
Asia													
India, Bombay	8·5	0·3	10·8	5·8	5·9	0·6	3·1	20·1	23·2	1·3	1·2	2·4	120·5
Japan, Miyagi	0·9	0·1	4·1	40·1	10·4	0·6	7·0	13·0	13·8	1·3	1·3	3·7	127·7
Singapore													
Chinese	1·1	7·1	6·4	18·0	16·5	8·0	17·3	19·4	18·6	4·9	4·9	4·1	153·1
Malay	1·1	0·6	3·7	9·7	5·8	6·8	7·5	17·6	11·6	3·8	3·3	2·4	96·4
Indian	20·7	0·0	5·9	21·5	18·3	6·9	7·9	25·5	29·8	2·9	4·8	3·9	179·0
Europe													
Norway	1·1	0·2	0·7	12·7	20·1	0·8	4·7	44·4	18·1	9·7		4·7	183·4
Switzerland, Geneva	1·3	0·2	1·3	10·0	21·5	1·4	7·5	70·6	16·1	16·3	14·7	7·1	214·9
UK, Birmingham	0·9	0·2	2·7	10·6	23·7	0·5	11·5	53·0	12·6	8·5	18·8	4·3	182·9

[a] All incidence rates are age-adjusted to the "world" standard population being expressed per 100 000 per annum.
[b] Excludes malignant melanoma.
[c] This represents the total incidence per 100 000 (age-adjusted) for all sites but excludes skin.

IV. Cancers of Defined Aetiology

A. Cultural Habits

For a number of cancers the causal factors have been identified with some certainty. Of these the most important is cigarette smoking, which in addition to cancer of the lung has been implicated in tumours of the mouth, larynx, pharynx, oesophagus, stomach, bladder and pancreas. The habit is calculated to be the cause of about 85% of all lung cancers in the United Kingdom and about 35% of all cancers in males in North America, England and Japan. In India, cigarettes are less important but the betel quid, which usually contains tobacco, causes cancers of the buccal cavity and upper oesophagus, which form about one-third of all cancers (Table II, and Figs 1 to 6).

Excessive indulgence in alcoholic beverages is also responsible for cancers of the mouth, larynx, pharynx and oesophagus and is important in enhancing the effect of cigarette smoking. Although the pernicious effects of cigarette smoking are now clearly recognized, the habit is unfortunately expanding in many developing countries where tobacco growing is an important cash crop.

B. Cancers in the Work Environment

Cancer-producing chemicals in the workplace are important not only as occupational hazards but also in view of their possible escape into the general environment (Table III). While legislation governing such hazards exists in many countries in North America and Europe, workplace hazards are of increasing importance in developing countries, especially those with artisanal industries where preventive measures may be often non-existent.

Most important of all workplace hazards discovered is that of asbestos. In view of its valuable properties asbestos has been increasingly used over the last fifty years. At first only considered to give rise to a fibrosing disease of the lung, it has been demonstrated not only to produce lung cancer but also to strongly enhance the carcinogenic effect of cigarette smoking in asbestos workers, and further, cause cancers of the lung covering (mesothelioma). While modern methods have significantly reduced such hazards in the workplace, and while it would not appear as yet to have given rise to a public health problem in the general population, its use in numerous situations, e.g. asbestos cement, thermal insulation, etc., requires that it be used with adequate control, especially in many developing countries.

TABLE II. *Major Identified Aetiological Factors for Common Male Cancers in Selected Industrialized and Non-Industrialized States*

Site of cancer	Industrialized states		Non-Industrialized states	
	Factor	Approximate proportion believed due to factors	Factor	Approximate proportion believed due to factors
Buccal cavity and pharynx	Alcohol, tobacco	90%	Betel quid chewing, smoking	95%
Oesophagus	Alcohol, tobacco	90%	Betel quid chewing, smoking	80%
Liver	Alcohol	85%	Aflatoxin, hepatitis	90%
Larynx	Alcohol, tobacco	90%	Betel quid chewing, smoking	90%
Lung	Tobacco	85%	Tobacco	85%
	Occupation	10%		
Penis	Non-circumcision	90%	Non-circumcision	90%
Bladder	Tobacco, occupation	60%	Tobacco, schistosomiasis	80%
Malignant melanoma	Ultraviolet radiation	60%		
Skin	Ultraviolet radiation	90%	Burn scar, tropical ulcer	70%
	Occupation	2%		

Figures 1–6. Histograms illustrating the role of different environmental•factors in cancer in the United Kingdom, India and Southern Africa.

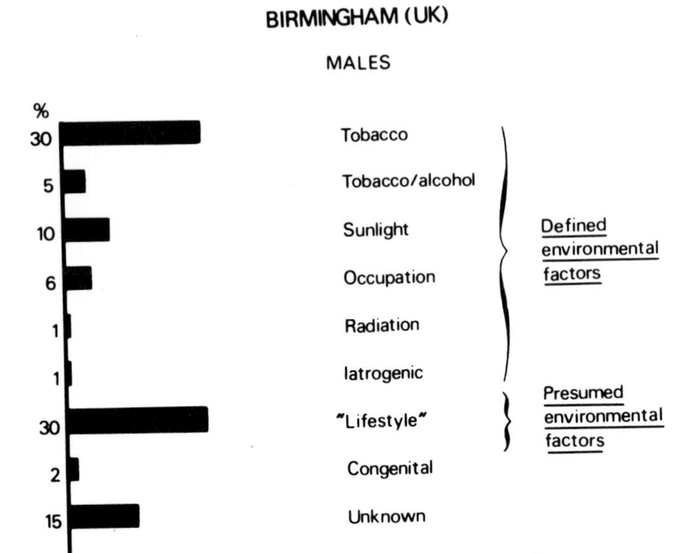

Fig. 1

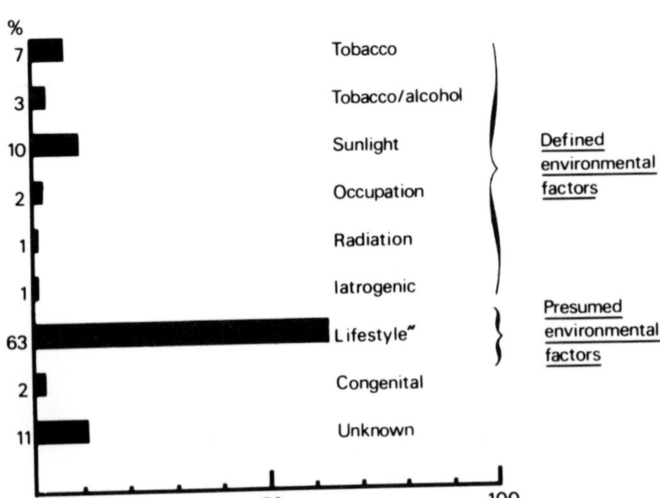

Fig. 2

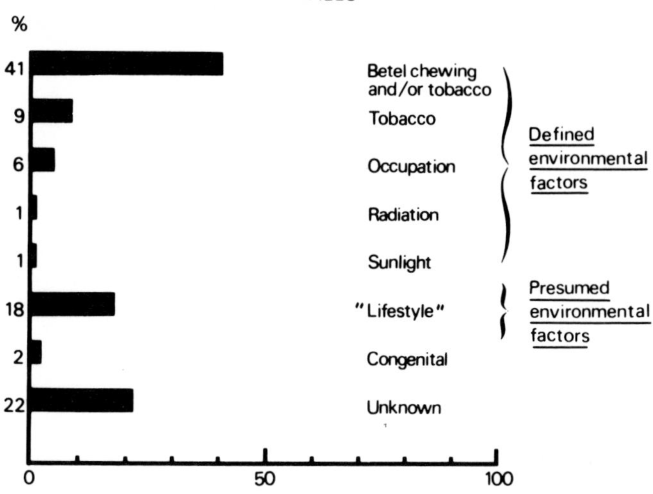
BOMBAY
MALES
%
41
9
6
1
1
18
2
22
Betel chewing and/or tobacco
Tobacco
Occupation
Radiation
Sunlight
"Lifestyle"
Congenital
Unknown
Defined environmental factors
Presumed environmental factors
0
50
100

Fig. 3

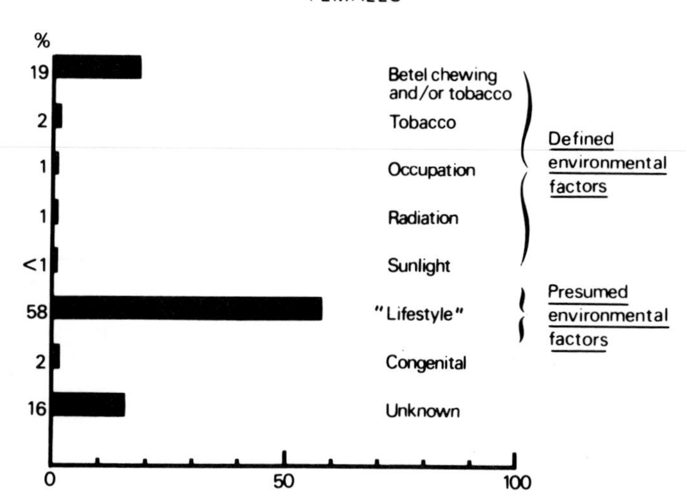
BOMBAY
FEMALES
%
19
2
1
1
<1
58
2
16
Betel chewing and/or tobacco
Tobacco
Occupation
Radiation
Sunlight
"Lifestyle"
Congenital
Unknown
Defined environmental factors
Presumed environmental factors
0
50
100

Fig. 4

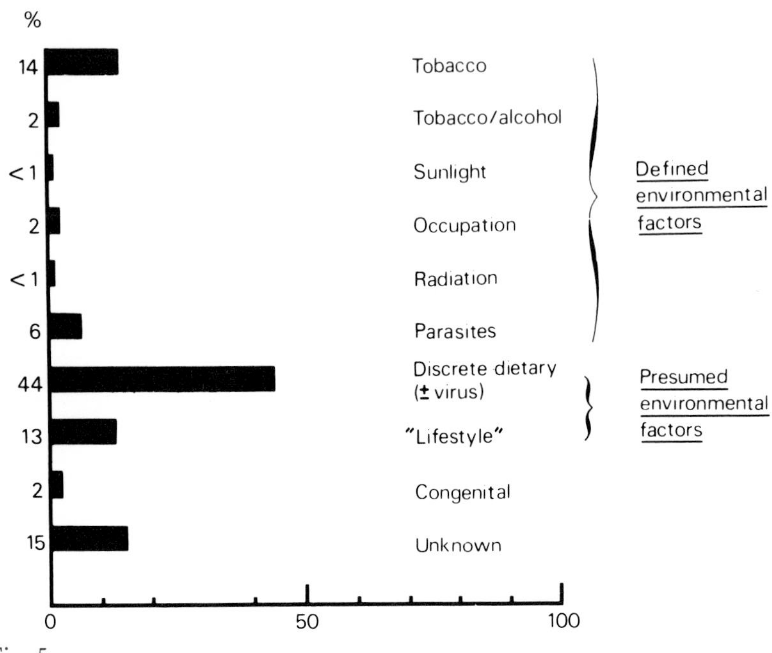

Fig. 5

C. Workplace-Associated Cancers and the Social Environment

Cancer in the workplace has been the subject of a recent report from the United Kingdom (Office of Population Censuses and Surveys, 1978), which indicates that much of the differences between occupations are due to the consequences of the social life-style of the population from which the workforce is drawn. For example, cancer of the oesophagus in barmen is a job-associated cancer related to the excessive drinking and smoking occurring in that occupation, as is high lung cancer in transport workers who also smoke heavily. This is a finding of considerable importance as it implies that a much greater part of cancer in the workforce due to environmental influences other than direct occupational exposures.

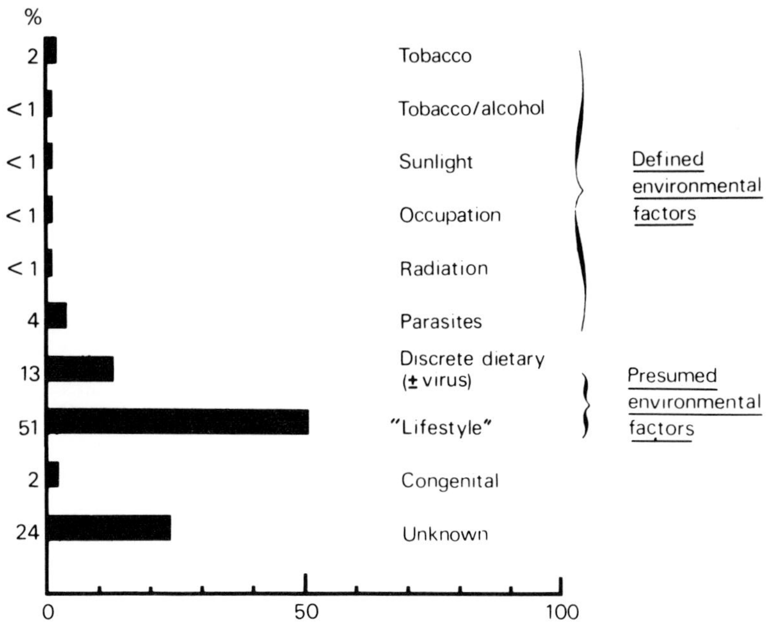

Fig. 6

V. Cancers of Suspected Environmental Aetiology

Cancers in this group arise largely in the breast, ovary, uterus, prostate, stomach and large intestine. They form approximately 60% of cancer in females and 40% in males. There are two major hypotheses regarding their causation. First that they represent the summated effect of multiple carcinogenic chemicals in the general environment at low doses, each carcinogen being assumed to add to the total cancer risk. Others believe that they are largely multifactorial in origin, being dependent on an interplay of various life-style factors which are described above in terms of behavioural or dietary patterns. Direct evidence as to these two hypotheses is difficult to obtain, but some inferences can be drawn from epidemiological studies based on geographical, residential and migrant variations (Higginson, 1979).

TABLE III. *Compounds Reported Carcinogenic to Man*

Chemical	Target organ(s)	Source
Aflatoxin	Liver	Diet
4-Aminobiphenyl	Bladder	Occupation
Arsenic compounds	Skin, lung(?), liver	Diet, Drugs Occupation
Asbestos	Lung, serosa, intestine	Occupation
Auramine	Bladder	Occupation
Benzene	Bone marrow	Occupation
Benzidine	Bladder	Occupation
Bis (chloromethyl) ether	Lung	Occupation
Cadmium oxide (and sulphate)	Prostate (?), lung	Occupation General pollutant
Chloramphenicol	Bone marrow	Therapy
Chromium compounds	Lung	Occupation
Haematite (mining)	Lung	Occupation
Melphalan	Bone marrow	Therapy
Mustard gas	Lung	Therapy, occupation
2-Naphthylamine	Bladder	Occupation
Nickel compounds	Nasal cavity, lung	Occupation
N,N-bis (2-chloroethyl)-2-naphthylamine	Bladder	Therapy
Soot and tars (also some polycyclic aromatic hydrocarbons)	Skin, lung	Occupation
Diethylstilboestrol	Vagina, uterus	Therapy
Vinyl chloride	Liver, lung, brain	Occupation

A. General Pollution

While the effects of high exposures are well recognized there is little agreement regarding the role of general ambient environmental pollution. There is evidence, however, that populations inhabiting industrial and urban areas are more likely to be exposed to chemical pollutants than rural communities, although agricultural use of chemicals is increasing throughout the world. Despite long-standing pollution and industrialization associated with the growth of the petrochemical industry, the data from Europe and North America show that, with some exceptions, cancer rates have remained relatively stable if tumours related to alcohol or tobacco exposures are excluded (Devesa and Silverman,

1978). Attempts have been made to correlate cancer patterns with population density, urban/rural environments, etc., especially in the United States, but results have been inconsistent (Haenszel *et al.*, 1962; Haenszel and Taeuber, 1964). Cancer of the prostate in blacks in the United States is twenty to thirty times more frequent than in industrial Japan, and several times higher than in the industralized United Kingdom.

B. Water and Air Pollution

No cancer has been demonstrated unequivocally to be related to water pollution. Air pollution, a frequent index of industrialization in terms of fossil fuels, apparently is not a cause of cancer *per se*, but may potentiate the effects of cigarette smoking.

In conclusion, although the cancer patterns in North America and Europe with high frequencies of cancers of the lung, large intestine, breast and uterus suggest a common environmental background, as compared to the very different patterns seen in Africa and Asia, there is little to support the hypothesis that such cancers are due to general industrial pollution. The possibility cannot of course be excluded that some so-called idiopathic cancers may be dependent on general pollution as is possibly the case for background radiation. It is also possible, indeed probable, that new carcinogens of industrial origin will enter the environment and be recognized in the future. However, for most cancers today of unknown but suspected environmental aetiology, it is necessary to seek alternative explanations. These comments in no way diminish the necessity to reduce pollution of the general or limited environment for other reasons related to health or quality of life.

C. Life-style

Apart from such obvious cultural habits as cigarette smoking and alcohol, life-style is a poorly defined term used to describe the cultural, behavioural and dietary environments outlined above, and which are not yet defined in objective biochemical or physiological terms. Thus early age at first pregnancy protects against cancer of the breast, while in contrast early and frequent intercourse is related to an increase in tumours of the cervix. The problem is made more complex due to the close interrelationship between behavioural patterns and the dietary environment. A consistent relationship has been shown between a low level of dietary fibre which reflects the local dietary culture, and a high frequency of cancer of the colon. Further, relationships have been demonstrated between dietary fat, calories, meat intake, etc. and cancer of the bowel, uterus and colon, all of which cancers are also related to behavioural patterns. Diet should not be considered only in terms of defined carcinogens, but also in less specific terms, such as its effect on age of menopause and fertility. Obesity which is dependent on calorie intake leads to increased oestrogen formation in the body, which would explain its relationship to cancer of the endometrium. Until these risk indices can be more definitively described, it is better to use the term "carcinogenic risk factors", while recognizing that they represent the effects of important underlying biochemical and modulating influences. Evidence indicating the importance of life-style factors has been further strengthened by observations on Mormons and Seventh Day Adventists in the United States. In both these groups there is a lower incidence of non-tobacco and non-alcohol related tumours, than in the general American population. Some of the numerous life-style risk indices that have been found to be related to the onset of cancer are presented in Table IV.

VI. Proportion of Cancers due to Environmental Factors

Although cancer is a multifactorial disease, it is important to evaluate the relative importance of various environmental factors, since the removal of predominant agents may have significant impact in terms of preventive strategy. The histograms in Figs 1 and 6 refer to such calculations, which have been made on a United Kingdom industrial population, an industrialized population in the Bombay area of India, and an urban population in Africa. The basis for these calculations is discussed elsewhere (Higginson and Muir, 1979). The proportions in these histograms are approximations. Nonetheless, they indicate the various strategies that must be adopted by public health authorities to effect control.

VII. Implications for Cancer Control

There is a widespread assumption that most cancers of environmental origin can be controlled by simple legislative action controlling industrial chemicals within the ambient or work environment. As shown above, while certain cancers can clearly be related to such exposures, for most cancers there is no evidence of such a relationship, and only a proportion of the total cancer patterns can be so attributed even in

TABLE IV. *Life-style carcinogenic risk indices*

1. *Behavioural patterns*
Age at first pregnancy
Age at first marriage
Parity
Age at menarche
Age at menopause
Number of sex partners
Cigarettes
Residence
2. *Dietary factors*
Protein
Fat
Calories
Malnutrition
Meat
Fish
Dairy produce
Vegetables
Vitamins
Alcoholic beverages
Nitrates
Obesity
Underweight
Fibre
Pollutants
3. *Other factors*
Occupation
Air pollution
Water pollution

sophisticated industrialized states. Thus strategies for cancer control should be established both in terms of individual and community respectively (Higginson, 1976).

A. Individual Responsibility

The difficulty of controlling cancer caused by voluntary cultural habits is well recognized, and should not be underestimated. Thus many individuals, especially those with relatively boring or frustrated lives, consider the pleasures of present smoking or drinking more important than the reduction of a theoretical risk of cancer later. Further, the powerful effects of the local cultural environment in cigarette smoking, etc., tend to be ignored. These factors are compounded by the unwillingness of governments to control a habit which is an important source of revenue. Thus, although levelling off of smoking habits is occurring in North America and Europe, it is rising in many non-industrialized countries. Lastly, apart from avoiding overeating, little can be suggested in terms of behavioural and dietary changes.

B. Community Responsibility

It has proved easier to get society to accept the concept of control of iatrogenic and industrial hazards where the individual does not perceive personal involvement, even though the effects may be relatively limited in terms of the total problem. Countries vary widely in their legislative approach to the control of carcinogenic hazards, and distinctions must be made between control within the workplace or situations where high risk exposures take place, and control of the ambient environment where there is some controversy as to the degree of risk. While all agree on the necessity to control industrial hazards, the relative influence of industrial chemicals in the general environment, may be less than that produced by modification of life-style factors, now an area of active research. Accordingly, while animal experimentation and other tests may provide help in preventing the widespread use of new, potentially carcinogenic hazards, it is unlikely that they will identify many of the major factors which are responsible for present cancer patterns.

Cancer control is thus highly complex, and can only be discussed in terms of principles as distinct from absolute criteria since objectives will vary from country to country. Thus, for example, although DDT is a carcinogen to experimental animals there is no evidence that it has caused cancer in man. So, while on the one hand its use in industrialized states might be considered undesirable, considerable health hazards have already occurred in a number of Asian countries, with numerous deaths, as a result of it being banned.

Similar problems of control arise with general life-style factors, where our knowledge at present remains insufficient to justify definite legislative action. There is little possibility in the immediate future of making effective suggestions as to changes in behavioural or dietary patterns. In most industrialized states it may be argued that reduction in calories and fat, with an increase in fibre may be beneficial. On the other hand, there are potent reasons for improving nutrition in terms of calories and fat in Africa and Asia. However, there is no evidence that such action will affect cancer patterns, and in fact overnutrition rather than undernutrition is associated with increased cancer. Moreover, it should be noted that the Finnish diet which carries a low risk of large bowel cancer is associated with a high risk of cardiovascular disease.

VIII. Conclusion

An attempt has been made to illustrate the complex problems of environmental cancer and associated public health problems, as well as the high degree of scientific incertitude in several fields. It is further emphasized that cancer should not be considered only in terms of the chemical environment. In controlling carcinogenic exposures it should be remembered that decisions are not the prerogative of scientists but reflect a high proportion of political and governmental influence (Ashby, 1976). These decisions should be based on the availability of an effective and objective evaluation of scientific data. Unfortunately, in recent years, the complexities of solving these problems have been exacerbated by an increase in confrontation and emotional reactions in different social groups and by groups with negligible scientific background or understanding. Moreover, the concept of life-style has proved difficult to accept in many circles. The problem is further compounded by the fact that extrapolation from animals to man remains problematic. Nevertheless, such models provide the only available method to protect against the entrance of new hazards. However, application of information from animal tests and mutagenic assays without regard to local needs and conditions may unnecessarily deprive less privileged societies of socio-economic benefits already enjoyed by industrial societies. In a period of lack of adequate scientific data, it is necessary to develop a balanced and commonsense approach to complex problems and ensure that they are dealt with in the least emotional fashion possible.

References

Ashby, the Rt Hon Lord (1976). *Proc. R. Soc. Med.* **69**, 721–730.

Clemmesen, J. (Ed.) (1950). "Symposium on Geographical Pathology and Demography of Cancer". Council for International Organizations of Medical Sciences, Oxford and Paris.

Clemmesen, J. (1965). "Statistical Studies in the Etiology of Malignant Neoplasms. I: Review and Results". Munksgaard, Copenhagen.

Devesa, S. S. and Silverman, D. T. (1978). *J. natn. Cancer Inst.* **60**, 545–571.

Haenszel, W., Loveland, D. B. and Sirkin, M. G. (1962). *J. natn. Cancer Inst.* **28**, 947–1001.

Haenszel, W. and Taeuber, K. E. (1964). *J. natn. Cancer Inst.* **32**, 803–838.

Higginson, J. (1976). *Am. J. publ. Hlth* **66**, 359–366.

Higginson, J. (1979). *In* "Carcinogens: Identification and Mechanisms of Action" (A. C. Griffin and C. R. Shaw, Eds), 187–208. Raven Press, New York.

Higginson, J. and Muir, C. S. (1976). *In* "The Physiopathology of Cancer: Diagnosis, Treatment, Prevention" (F. Homburger, Ed.), Vol. 2, 300–322. Karger, Basel.

Higginson, J. and Muir, C. S. (1979). Environmental carcinogenesis: misconceptions and limitations to cancer control. *J. natn. Cancer Inst.* **63**, 1291–1298.

Office of Population Censuses and Surveys (1978). "Occupational Mortality. The Registrar General's Decennial Supplement for England and Wales, 1970–1972". Series DS No 1. HMSO, London.

Waterhouse, J., Muir, C. S., Correa, P. *et al.* (Eds) (1976). "Cancer Incidence in Five Continents", Vol 3. IARC Scientific Publications No 15, Lyon.

Wynder, E. L., Hoffman, D., McCoy, D. *et al.* (1978). *In* "Carcinogenesis: A Comprehensive Survey" (T. J. Slaga, A. Sivak and R. K. Boutwell, Eds), Vol. 2, 59–77. Raven Press, New York.

26

The Automobile and Human Health

G. Anthony Ryan

Department of Social and Preventive Medicine, Monash University, Melbourne, Australia

---

The community pays a high and largely hidden cost for the convenience [of the automobile] in injuries and ill health.

I. Introduction

It is now almost 100 years since Benz made his first motor car in 1885. For the next thirty years or so the automobile was a plaything of the rich since cars were expensive and made in small numbers. With the advent of mass production in the 1920s cars became much cheaper and much more readily available. The immense personal mobility and freedom to travel at will that the motor car offers has almost universal appeal, shown by the growth in the numbers of cars.

The automobile has become intricately woven into the fabric of our society. It has profoundly influenced the shape of towns and cities, its manufacture consumes a substantial proportion of the output of the steel, rubber, glass and plastics industries, and the regulation of its use supports several government departments. Road, highway, and bridge construction is a major industry, as is the provision of fuel and lubricating oils. The automobile has also had social effects influencing patterns of use of leisure time, in travel to and from work and as a status symbol (Allen *et al.*, 1957).

In the most heavily motorized countries, the United States, Canada, Australia, there is one car for every two or three people (Borkenstein 1979). With vehicle densities such as this, the benefits of the car are being lost. Paradoxically, the popularity of the car, with its promise of freedom and mobility, leads to loss of mobility through traffic congestion as every other vehicle owner attempts to experience his own freedom and mobility. With increasing numbers of cars the other costs or dys-benefits become more obvious—deaths and injuries from collisions, air pollution from vehicle emissions, disruption of domestic life by traffic noise. The intrusion of cars, both moving and parked, also disrupts enjoyment of many scenic attractions, both rural and urban. This is another paradox, where the car provides easy access to such sites, but in so doing can destroy the very reason for visiting the site. These paradoxes and their implications for continued growth are examined at some length by Hirsch (1977). In this chapter I consider some of the identifiable costs to human health of the use of the automobile.

II. Crash Injury

The first recorded collision occurred in Paris in 1892 when the Baron de Zuylen drove his horseless carriage into Count De Dion's motor brake

(*The News*, 1965). The first recorded death in the USA was a pedestrian in New York in 1895 (*Guinness Book of Superlatives*, 1956). In England, the first death occurred in 1899 when a wheel of a Daimler motor car collapsed and the occupants were thrown out (Rolt, 1956).

From these early beginnings the number of deaths and injuries from motor vehicle accidents has increased dramatically until now in most industrialized nations, motor vehicle accidents form almost half of all deaths from accidents, poisonings and violence, and this latter group generally ranks fourth after heart disease, cancer and strokes (WHO, 1977). Motor vehicle crashes have replaced war as a cause of death and injury. In Australia, more people were killed or injured in road crashes between 1939 and 1969 than in warfare during the same period (Robertson, 1969).

The rates for each country are influenced by a number of factors, of which the most important appear to be the degree of motorization, i.e. the ratio of people to cars, and possibly the length of time motor vehicles have been present at an appreciable density. Countries with large numbers of vehicles compared to the population and in which cars have been present for a long time tend to have lower mortality rates, e.g. USA, Australia, New Zealand. Less well-developed countries in Africa and Asia tend to have higher rates, perhaps a function of learning to live with the automobile and its hazards (Smeed and Jeffcoate, 1969).

The two largest groups of road users killed are car occupants and pedestrians. The numbers of motor cyclists and pedal cyclists killed are very much smaller. The relative sizes of each group depends on the local cultural conditions within each country concerned. In the USA, where car ownership is almost universal, pedestrians comprise a relatively small percentage of total deaths (National Safety Council, 1976). This contrasts with the United Kingdom where until the 1950s pedestrian deaths outnumbered those of car occupants (O'Flaherty, 1973). As the rate of car ownership has increased in the UK, the relative proportion of car occupants killed has increased, but pedestrian deaths still form about 40% of deaths compared with less than 20% in the USA. Australia, with pedestrians forming about 20% of deaths from motor vehicles, lies closer to USA than UK (Australian Bureau of Statistics, 1978).

The majority of car collisions occur in urban areas, at intersections, at relatively low speeds. There are daily peaks in crash occurrence corresponding to the evening peak flow of traffic, and the nocturnal drinking habits of the driving population (Robertson *et al.*, 1966; Jamieson *et al.*, 1971; Ryan *et al.*, 1978). There are proportionately more alcohol-affected drivers involved in crashes at night and on weekend nights especially (Ryan and Salter, 1977). The presence of alcohol has been clearly documented in increasing frequency as the severity of crashes increases from property damage only, to fatal crashes (US Department of Transportation, 1968). Two groups of persons are commonly involved as pedestrians, the young i.e. children under ten years, and the old, those over sixty-five years. These two groups are not able to cope successfully with the task of crossing roadways in busy streets, the younger group because they have not yet learnt the required skills of judging speed and distance, and the older group because abilities are declining with age and infirmity. A third, smaller, group of males aged forty years and over who have a high blood alcohol concentration, tend to overlap with the older group. The alcohol in this case provides the degrading influence (Robertson *et al.*, 1966).

Studies of the causative factors of car crashes suggest that in all cases multiple factors can be identified as having a causal role in a particular crash. Human factors, i.e. factors relating to driver perceptions, hazard recognition, and information processing characteristics, have been identified as important. Interactions of these qualities with vehicle characteristics and environmental conditions are very common, e.g. a driver's attention and motor skills may be degraded by an elevated blood alcohol level, which, together with incorrectly inflated tyres, rain, a wet road with reverse camber on a deceptive corner, leads to a car skidding off the road into a pole. In this case driver, vehicle, and environmental factors all played a part, all were in some degree causative. There is a chain of causation, not a single "cause" of accidents (Mackay, 1966; Indiana University, 1973). Foldvary (1978) has shown that there are significant interactions between driver age, sex, time of day, day of week, power of car and a number of other factors.

The patterns of injury received are characteristic for each type of road user, but the most important characteristic of road trauma is that of injury to multiple body areas. In industrial trauma only one body area is involved, e.g. the foot or the hand. In car crashes it is usual for more than one area to be injured, the head and legs together being the most frequent combination, followed by head, chest and limbs (Jamieson and Tait, 1966). In Australia the patterns of injury of car occupants have been altered recently by the compulsory wearing of seat belts. Belt wearers tend to have less severe head, face and chest injuries than those not wearing belts (Nelson, 1974). However, front seat passengers are still injured more often and more severely than drivers or rear seat passengers (Robertson *et al.*, 1966; Jamieson *et al.*, 1971). Since, due to social custom, the front seat occupants of cars involved in crashes tend to be young females, and the most frequent injuries to front seat occupants are lacerations to the face, this group of road users are at considerably more risk of disfiguring injuries than their (commonly) male companions (Ryan, 1967).

Motor cycles are commonly involved in crashes when a car turns in front of them, the car driver not seeing the motorcycle. Motor cyclists suffer multiple injuries from their multiple impacts with the other vehicle and the road and roadside objects (Robertson *et al.*, 1966). Helmets are effective in reducing the severity of injuries sustained (Foldvary and Lane, 1964).

Pedal cyclists are injured when they turn in front of an oncoming vehicle without warning. They also suffer multiple injuries from multiple impacts from the striking vehicle and the road (Robertson *et al.*, 1966).

Pedestrians are not "run over" but are "run under". They are struck by the front of the car, their feet knocked from under them with their head striking the bonnet, windscreen, or roof of the car depending on its impact velocity. From there the pedestrian falls to the road suffering multiple impacts and multiple injuries (Robertson *et al.*, 1966; Ryan 1967; Jamieson *et al.*, 1971). In the light of the above information, it is not surprising that these unprotected road users contribute disproportionately to the caseload of severe injuries presenting at accident and casualty departments (Ryan *et al.*, 1978).

About half of car occupants involved in car crashes receive no injuries, one-third receive minor injuries, about one-sixth receive moderate to life-threatening injuries and less than 1% receive fatal injuries. In a recent on-scene study in Melbourne, one-third of all persons involved in a sample of traffic accidents were taken to hosptial for treatment, and of these, one-third were admitted for at least twenty-four hours. The activity restriction of one-third of those brought to hospital lasted longer than 30 days, indicating that there is a considerable morbidity resulting from injuries suffered in motor car accidents (Ryan *et al.*, 1978). There are some data to suggest that injuries to the lower limb and pelvis produce the longest stays in hospital (Nelson, 1974) and that about 8% of those who come to hospital end up with permanent disability (Gordon, 1976).

This brief outline indicates that injury from motor car accidents is largely a disease of the young male. While the risk of death from such injuries is very low, the large number of collisions occurring means that there are a considerable number of young males dying through use of the motor vehicle. There has been a disproportionate increase in deaths from external violence of young males in Australia since 1911, almost certainly due to motor vehicle accidents (Woodruff, 1963). This loss of the "breeding stock" of the human population must have some effect on the evolution of the human race, if only by eliminating those who are unable to cope with the triple and interrelated tasks of learning to drive a car, learning to drink alcohol, and finding a comfortable role identity.

For young males, one may speculate that the car provides a haven of privacy and mobility, the one part of the environment under direct control. The car then becomes an instrument for displaying one's skill, courage, and aggression in undertaking hazardous manoeuvres and showing one's defiance of the established order. Almost everyone will have, at some time, driven faster than usual after an angry exchange, so this behaviour is understandable. The car also provides a private retreat for meeting the opposite sex, and for consuming alcohol. All these activities involve an element of risk. (As an aside, the author estimated that in the USA in 1968 about 5000 unborn children died when their pregnant mothers were involved in crashes. This loss may perhaps be compensated for by an unknown number of conceptions taking place in cars.)

The car provides a convenient method for committing suicide, either by carbon monoxide poisoning or by deliberate crashes. Whitlock (1971) reviewed this subject briefly. In an on-scene study in Adelaide, at least three of 408 crashes involved suicidal intent, two were crashes into stationary objects, and one was a pedestrian stepping in front of a truck (Robertson *et al.*, 1966). It seems that a small, but definite proportion of motor vehicle crashes involve some suicidal intent. An unknown number may involve some homicidal intent.

The number of deaths of motor vehicle occupants in Victoria, and to a lesser extent in Australia as a whole, has shown a consistent downward trend since 1970 when the wearing of seat belts became compulsory (Vulcan, 1978) (Fig. 1). Before this time the trend had been upwards. Besides seat belts, other preventive measures having an effect in Victoria are, the rural speed limit reduced to 100 kph, the right of way rule changed to a priority road system, the compulsory taking of blood samples for testing for alcohol level from those brought to hospitals after road crashes, random breath testing of drivers, and the increasing effect of the Australian Design Rules which govern vehicle construction and safety performance. These latter reduce injury by requiring that vehicle components such as steering columns, doors and windscreens produce a minimum of injury and that brakes and tyres reach a minimum level of performance. The individual effect of these measures has not been quantified but together they have produced a marked fall in deaths of car occupants. The local newspapers through

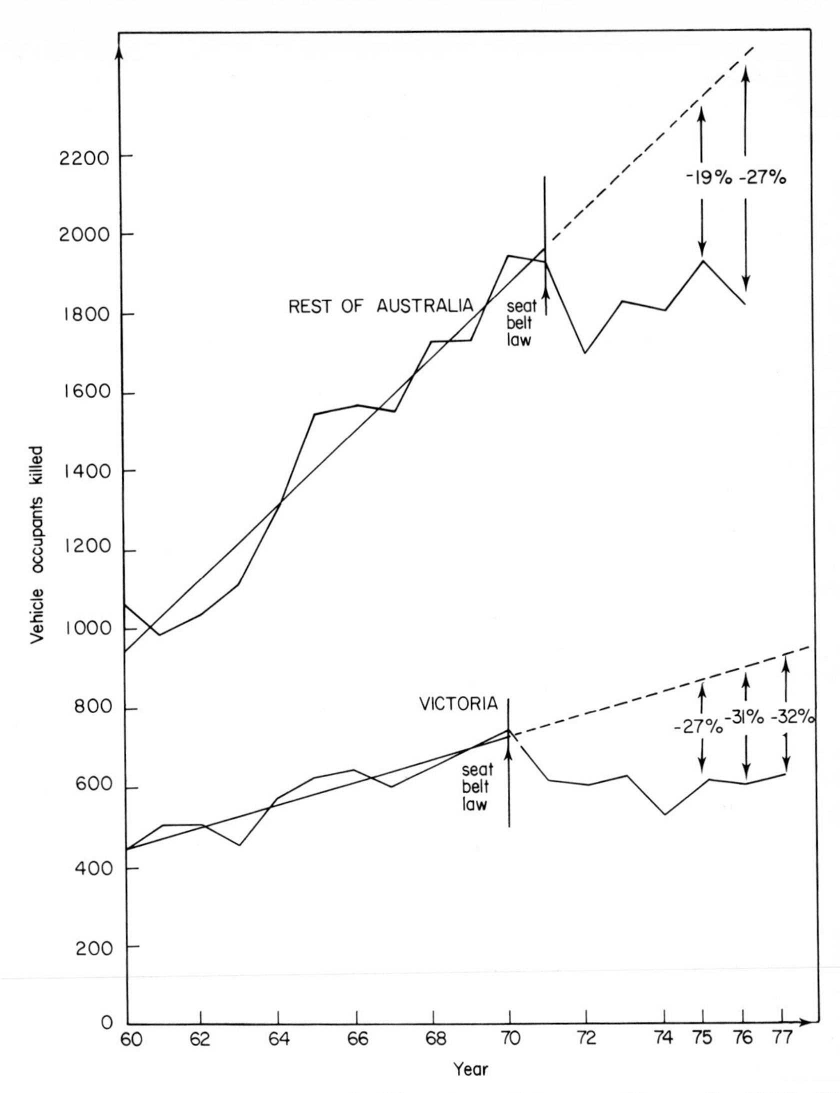

Fig. 1. Vehicle occupants killed in Victoria, and the rest of Australia, 1960–77. (From Vulcan, 1978.)

their safety campaigns have generated an awareness of the "road toll" which has played an undetermined part in ensuring the implementation of these measures.

The conclusion to be drawn from the above illustration is that there are effective countermeasures readily available which will reduce the numbers of deaths and injuries from motor vehicles. To implement them requires government action in the form of legislation, together with favourable community attitudes.

III. Vehicle Emissions

Internal combustion engines, both petrol and diesel, produce potentially dangerous substances in their exhaust—notably carbon monoxide (CO), various oxides of nitrogen (NO_x), hydrocarbons (HC) and lead, as well as particulates or smoke. Unburnt fuel also evaporates from tanks and carburettors as well as being blown out of the exhaust. Other substances entering the atmosphere which derive from the motor vehicle are asbestos fibres ground off the clutch and brake linings, and rubber particles from tyres.

A. Exhaust Emissions

Each of the constituents of motor vehicle exhaust gases has been shown to be harmful to human health in laboratory studies when tested alone and in sufficient concentrations. There is also evidence that some of these pollutants produce acute effects at the levels commonly found in the streets. What is not clear are the long term effects of living in an atmosphere with relatively low levels of these pollutants.

Theoretically, if combustion were perfect, the only exhaust products would be carbon dioxide and water. However, combustion is never perfect, so pollutants result. The proportions of CO, NO_x and HC emitted by an internal combustion engine vary with the mode of operation. For example, the greatest output of CO occurs when the engine is idling, of NO_x when accelerating and of HC when decelerating. An air/fuel ratio of 14·6:1 should ensure complete combustion. A mixture with more fuel gives more power, but more CO and HC. A leaner mixture, with less fuel reduces the CO and HC but increases the NO_x and reduces the power. Therefore, to keep pollutant levels at a minimum the optimum air–fuel mixture must be maintained as much as possible (Ministry of Transport, 1967). This is a complex technical problem in which there has been considerable progress, but a satisfactory result has not yet been achieved. The diesel engine produces generally lower levels of emissions, and particularly, very little CO, but otherwise it suffers from the same disadvantages as the petrol engine.

The automobile is the chief source of CO, HC and NO_x found in the atmosphere and produces only minor amounts of sulphur dioxide and particulates (Table I).

TABLE I. *Contribution of the Automobile to Air Pollution*

	% of total emission of each pollutant					
	Carbon monoxide	Sulphur oxides	Hydro-carbons	Nitrogen oxides	Partic-ulates	Total
USA 1965[a]	92	4	63	46	8	60
Port Phillip region 1976[b]	82	13	48	78	1	58

[a] From Hickey, 1971.
[b] Environment Protection Authority of Victoria, 1979.

1 Carbon Monoxide

The petrol internal combustion engine is the main source of CO in areas where the burning of coal and coke is not prevalent. Levels of CO measured in streets in urban areas show peaks corresponding to the morning and, to a lesser extent, the evening traffic peak. Concentrations are highest where there are large numbers of slow moving vehicles, i.e. in urban centres. Instantaneous peaks of over 200 ppm have been measured on sidewalks in these situations, with hourly averages of 10–30 ppm being not uncommon (Brief *et al.*, 1960; Dinman, 1971; Godin *et al.*, 1972). The meteorological conditions, the width of the roadway and height of adjacent buildings influence the actual concentrations of CO reached (Klemer and Spengler, 1976).

Carbon monoxide combines with haemoglobin in the blood to form carboxyhaemoglobin (COHb), which reduces the oxygen-combining capacity of the remainder of the haemoglobin. COHb levels of less than 2% are not associated with any measurable health effects, while at 5% COHb there is some slight reduction of physiological function. Above this level there is marked reduction in physiological function. Light to moderate smokers have COHb levels between 5% and 10%. There is marked individual variation and some degree of adaptation to elevated COHb levels. Persons with reduced cardiac capacity are more susceptible to higher levels than others (Dinman 1971).

Impairment of physiologic functioning as shown by a decrease in auditory discrimination has been shown to occur following exposures to levels of CO which raised blood COHb levels by about 2% (Beard and Wertheim 1967). Such an increase might occur during a one-hour car drive on a very congested day in a city, or during a day's work as a parking inspector, traffic policemen, or toll booth operator, all situations close to many motor vehicles with idling engines. Fortunately, the time taken to eliminate half of the CO present in the blood is about four hours, so that most of the CO absorbed in the morning's drive to work is eliminated during the rest of the day. Godin *et al.* (1972) suggest that the city dweller is always close to the postulated point of impaired psychomotor performance, even though the general atmospheric level is below the accepted danger point. Smokers and those working in congested places are further at risk. There is also evidence that current levels of CO can produce increased mortality among persons with severe heart conditions (Cohen *et al.*, 1970).

2 Nitrogen Oxides

No ill effects have been demonstrated for exposure to nitric oxide (NO) even at high concentrations. Nitrogen dioxide (NO_2), however, does have a significant effect on human health. Inhalation at concentrations such as may be found in fires or industrial accidents leads to chronic lung damage. At levels slightly higher than those usually found in the urban environment decreases in lung function have been found in exposed children, associated with an increased incidence of respiratory infection. A synergistic effect has also been noted between nitrogen dioxide with ozone and other oxidants produced in photochemical smog. Nitrogen dioxide is the one gaseous pollutant which betrays its presence, by causing the brownish tinge found in smog (Battigelli, 1971).

3 Oxidants

In a complex series of reactions involving energy from sunlight, oxides of nitrogen and hydrocarbons from internal conbustion engine exhaust gases combine to produce ozone (O_3), nitric acid, peroxides, aldehydes, peroxyacetyl nitrate and other chemically active components. This reaction first became obvious in Los Angeles where temperature inversions trap automobile emissions in a vast saucer and the plentiful sunlight produces the typical brownish "smog". This "oxidizing" smog is commonly found where the same conditions hold, i.e. still air, large numbers of cars, and sunlight; in July 1970 severe smogs were reported in New York, Tokyo, Rome and Sydney (Hickey 1971). This "oxidizing" smog is different from the "reducing" smog of such places as London, which consists largely of sulphur dioxides and particulates from the burning of coal. The effects of "reducing" smog on producing acute and chronic respiratory disease have been well documented (Reid, 1964; Winkelstein *et al.*, 1967).

However, apart from the acute effects of eye irritation, and inflammation of the nose and throat (Durham, 1974; Hammer *et al.*, 1974) no long-term respiratory effects have been documented for oxidizing smog (Cohen *et al.*, 1972). Several reasons are suggested for this. Among these are: (1) The pollutants might not be harmful. This is unlikely in view of the deleterious effect of these substances in low concentrations on rubber, foam, dyes, plants and their irritating effect on human eyes. (2) The measurement techniques in use are not sensitive enough to detect the effects present. (3) There has not been enough time elapsed for the full effects to develop. (4) The mean level of pollution may be more important than the peak levels which are usually used in these studies.

Another factor of some importance is the large individual variation in tolerance to oxidant pollution. In one laboratory study, "Sensitive" individuals experienced symptoms at levels of O_3 which were only one-half of those at which "normal" individuals experienced symptoms. The levels involved (0·75 ppm and 0·5 ppm,) were at the upper end of the values experienced in Los Angeles and other urban areas (Hackney *et al.*, 1975a, b).

The long-term effects of oxidant pollution have not been established but it seems reasonable to assume that there are effects, if not yet measured, which would appear most readily in children, the elderly and those with chronic respiratory disease. These effects may relate more to the long-term base level of pollution rather than the peak values reached from time to time.

4 Hydrocarbons

The hydrocarbons found in exhaust gases, in addition to their involvement with oxides of nitrogen in producing oxidant pollution, have a possible health effect. The polycyclic hydrocarbons form a group of potential carcinogens. Benz(d)pyrene (BP), which is a potent carcinogen when painted on the skin of mice, is found in the smoke of cigarettes and in automobile exhausts. The instillation of BP into the trachea of Syrian hamsters, together with particulates such as haematite, readily produces a high incidence of pulmonary cancer (Coffin, 1971). Epidemiological studies have shown an association between residence in urban areas and increased incidence of mortality from lung cancer. One study showed a direct correlation between BP levels and an increase of lung cancer mortality in urban areas (Curnow and Meier, 1973). It is postulated that the effect of the BP present in urban air is enhanced by the increased levels of particulate matter also found there. In Japan, an association was found between traffic volume and incidence of lung cancer for residents of urban streets (Aoki and Shimizu, 1977).

5 Lead

Lead, as tetraethyl lead, has been added to petrol for many years to improve its "anti-knock" properties. This lead is then dispersed into the atmosphere in automobile exhaust gases, in particle sizes sufficiently small to penetrate the deeper parts of the lung. A small proportion of atmospheric lead comes from lead-processing operations, i.e. smelting and manufacture of storage batteries, but the automobile exhaust is the major contribution to air-borne lead levels. Studies of lead levels in Greenland snow layers show a dramatic increase from about 1750, at the beginning of the Industrial Revolution, and a sharp upward trend after 1940. In 1965 the lead concentration in Greenland snow was 400 times the natural level present in 800 B.C. (Lin Fu, 1979).

The toxic effects of lead are well known, with elaborate safeguards and monitoring systems being used to protect workers in occupational situations. It accumulates in the body mostly in the bone and is only slightly excreted. There is some controversy as to the relative contributions of the dietary and respiratory routes of ingestion to the total body burden of lead. Adults and children living close to freeways have higher blood lead levels than those living further away (Thomas *et al.*, 1967; Caprio *et al.*, 1974). The concentration of lead in air in or near freeways is higher than at sites more distant.

However, there is considerable controversy regarding the possible ill effects of present levels of lead in the atmosphere and their effects on the non-occupational body burden of lead. The epidemiological evidence was well reviewed by Goldsmith (1969) and rebutted by Stopps (1969), thus neatly illustrating the controversy.

Although there have been no reports of toxic effects of air-borne lead present at current levels of pollution, as the quantity of lead in the atmosphere increases with continued use of leaded gasoline and the emitted and absorbed lead accumulates in body tissues, it is reasonable to assume some symptoms will appear firstly in more sensitive population groups such as children. There is some recent evidence to suggest that children with relatively high lead levels in their teeth have some intellectual deficits and possible behavioural changes (Needleman *et al.*, 1979).

B. Asbestos

Asbestos fibres have been demonstrated to be present in the air of towns and cities. The likely sources are from manufacture of asbestos-containing building materials, the installation of insulation materials, and from the brake linings of motor vehicles. Asbestos is an important constituent of the lining materials which are subject to considerable wear leading to the release of asbestos fibres. Asbestos fibres identical to those found in brake linings have been detected in air sampled from the side of a busy freeway. The concentration of fibres was one-tenth of the then occupational limit of 5×10^6 fibres per m^3 (Alste *et al.*, 1976).

Asbestos fibres have been found in the lungs in routine autopsies in urban dwellers in several countries. These asbestos bodies tend to be short fibres rather than the long fibres found in occupational exposure. Exposure to asbestos dust in mining, processing, and by living in the same household as an asbestos worker, or near a mine or factory is associated with very high rates of pulmonary fibrosis, cancer and pleural mesothelioma, after a latent period of 15–20 years (Selikoff *et al.*, 1972). There is now some evidence of an association of lung cancer with increased levels of asbestos bodies, in persons who have not been associated with the asbestos industry (Warnock and Churg, 1975). The implication is that low levels of asbestos exposure are associated with an increased risk of cancer occurrence. Some of this low level of atmospheric asbestos must be derived from the brake linings of motor vehicles.

C. Discussion

The health effects of automobile emissions may be summarized as follows.

Carbon monoxide. Levels present in congested urban areas can produce COHb levels sufficient to cause significant degradation in psychophysiologic functions, if exposure is continued long enough. There is some evidence to suggest that continued exposure to low levels can cause an increase in mortality in those with severe cardiac disease.

Nitrogen dioxide has toxic effects on lungs in acute exposures, while chronic exposure to low levels causes a decrease in pulmonary function and increased susceptibility to respiratory infection in children.

Oxidants. Acute effects are mainly eye irritation and nose and throat inflammation. No long-term effects have yet been measured.

Hydrocarbons. An association is noted between the elevated benzpyrene levels found in urban areas and increased incidence of lung cancer.

Lead. The source and significance of the not inconsiderable body burden of lead found in urban man is a matter of some controversy, as yet unresolved. It seems reasonable that such a toxic substance as lead would have deleterious effects in the long term, which are as yet unmeasured. There are indications that these effects may well appear first in children.

Asbestos. Wear of brake and clutch linings contributes to atmospheric asbestos levels. Asbestos is a well known carcinogen in occupational and near-occupational settings. It is probable that asbestos from cars contributes to the incidence of lung cancer in urban areas.

While the acute effects of oxidants and nitrogen dioxide are unmistakable, and of carbon monoxide insidious, the long-term, carcinogenic or neurologic effects of hydrocarbons, asbestos and lead as yet are only tentatively documented. One estimate infers that automobile emissions contribute one-quarter of 1% of the total urban health hazard from air pollution. In the USA this represents a total of about 4000 deaths and 4 million illness-restricted days per year. The 4000 deaths is about one-eighth of the deaths from bronchitis, asthma and emphysema combined, or one-twelfth of deaths from automobile accidents. Four million days of illness is nearly equivalent to one-tenth of the total number of days lost from work each year because of respiratory illness (National Academy of Sciences, 1974).

IV. Noise

Motor traffic is the major source of noise in the urban environment. A survey in London in 1961 showed that at over four-fifths of the points measured the predominant noise was from road traffic (Ministry of Transport, 1967). On main roads at peak traffic periods sound levels at the side of the road were about 90 dB(A) and in side streets the level exceeded 75 dB(A) for 10% of the time. Table II shows typical noise levels for different urban environments. Night-time levels in residential areas in Adelaide, California and Los Angeles were about 7 dB(A) lower than London (Australian Academy of Science, 1976).

The decibel scale is logarithmic so a change of 10 dB represents a doubling of intensity. The (A) scale is a weighting scale which represents the characteristics of human hearing. At levels above 80 dB(A) an increasing percentage of the exposed population will suffer permanent loss of hearing with continued exposure.

There is some evidence to suggest that the falling off of hearing acuity with age is at least accentuated by traffic noise. Older members of the Mabaan tribe in the Sudan have better hearing than persons of the same age in cities in USA and Western Europe, or members of the same tribe who moved to Khartoum years before. The Mabaan live in surroundings where the average sound level is about 30 dB (Rossi, 1976).

Various studies have shown that although there is considerable

TABLE II. *Existing External Noise Climates*[a] *(London, 1961)*

Group	Location	Noise climate dB(A)[b] Day 8 am – 6 pm	Night 1 am – 6 am
A	Arterial roads with many heavy vehicles and buses (kerbside)	80 – 68	75 – 50
B	1. Major road with heavy traffic and buses	75 – 63	61 – 49
	2. Side roads within 45 – 60 ft of roads in Groups A or B1 above	75 – 63	61 – 49
C	1. Main residential roads	70 – 60	55 – 44
	2. Side roads within 60 – 150 ft of heavy traffic routes	70 – 60	55 – 44
	3. Courtyards or blocks of flats, screened from direct view of heavy traffic	70 – 60	55 – 44
D	Residential roads with local traffic only	65 – 56	63 – 45

[a] From O'Flaherty, 1973.
[b] Noise climate is the range of noise level recorded for 80% of the time. The level exceeds the higher figure for 10% of the time and is less than the lower figure for 10% of the time.

variation, an increasing proportion of the population exposed suffers disturbance of the duration and depth of sleep above levels of 30–40 dB(A). Intermittent and unexpected noise well above the background noise is more disturbing than a louder continuous noise (Australian Academy of Science, 1976; Rossi, 1976).

Perceived lack of control over the source of noise appears to be an important characteristic leading to adverse effects. Road traffic noise is not controllable by its recipient and its composition usually unexpected. One authoritative review states: "Uncontrollable noise, even at non-damaging levels, has a short-term stress effect and very likely, a long-term stress effect on behaviour." The authors further quote a study in which it was found that the verbal and auditory skills of children living in a multistorey building alongside an expressway decreased with increasing intensity of traffic noise at the level at which they lived, after accounting for differences in social class levels. The authors conclude: "Noise does affect human mental functioning. In the short term, loud noise fairly quickly causes over-arousal and interferes with performance. More critically, uncontrollable noise, even at fairly low levels produces a short-term stress after-effect. In the long-term, non-injurious noise seems to affect auditory ability in the developing person and may well be a source of general stress in the exposed population as a whole" (Australian Academy of Science, 1976).

There is no doubt, then, that road traffic noise, at least on main roads, reaches levels sufficient to produce both short- and long-term effects on those exposed.

Tests on vehicles in the UK showed that about one-quarter of cars exceeded the proposed limit of 85 dB (A), one-half of motor cycles exceeded their limit of 90 dB (A) and two-thirds of trucks exceeded their limit of 87 dB (A) (Ministry of Transport 1967). This suggests that only a minority of cars but a majority of trucks need to have their noise level reduced to achieve a satisfactory community level.

A UK study recommended that the sound level inside buildings should not exceed 50 dB(A) (Ministry of Transport 1967). The insulating effect of closed windows is about 20 dB(A) so that traffic noise externally should not exceed 70 dB(A). From Table II it can be seen that this level is exceeded for 10% of the time in residential areas and for much more of the time on and near traffic routes.

Noise from traffic disturbs conversation and listening to radio and television in those exposed. There are indications that at least a proportion of the population shows short- and long-term effects, on performance, auditory development, and general health.

V. The Automobile and Exercise Patterns

In the fifty or so years since mass production made cars readily available, the car has played an important part in changing the shape of cities. The spread of cities began about the time of the industrial revolution. Before this, towns were generally restricted in size to a maximum radius of about three-quarters of an hour travel time from these centres (O'Flaherty, 1973). Whereas this may have been 3–4 km when walking was the most available means, the same time allocation can mean 20–30 km at the present because of the availability of buses, trams and, of course, cars.

The point being made here is that the car has changed exercise patterns considerably. The urban dweller, at least in some countries, spends a considerable part of his time sitting behind the wheel of a car, travelling. Before these changes occurred, presumably urban dwellers spent roughly the same amount of time travelling, but used means with a higher expenditure of energy, e.g. walking, bicycling, or riding in trams and trains.

In the UK it has been estimated that men spend from 60–90 min each day driving, with similar figures being found for men and women in Adelaide (Carruthers and Murray, 1977; Sedgwick *et al*., 1979). Table III is derived from an international study of time usage in towns of roughly the same population in countries of Eastern and Western Europe and North and South America (Szalai, 1972). There is an association between widely dispersed areas (% population more than 20 km from town centres), high rates of car ownership, and predominance of the car as a means of travel to work. The USA samples are high in all these characteristics, Belgium, France and West Germany, and Peru are intermediate, while Bulgaria, Czechoslovakia, Hungary, East Germany, Poland, USSR and Yugoslavia are low on these indices. In the latter group the percentage of persons walking to work ranges from 22·2% in East Germany to 77·3% in a town in Yugoslavia. The time spent in walking to and from work is about 45 min, and is roughly the same time spent travelling by car to and from work in the other two groups. In the absence of historical data, this cross-cultural comparison suggests that there is substitution, culturally dependent, of a less, for a more, personally energetic means of transport.

Data from the UK show that there has been very little change in energy consumption in the diet over the past seventy years. It seems reasonable to suppose that this change in mode of travel has played some part in reducing the level of physical activity and thus increasing the incidence of obesity and ischaemic heart disease (Department of Health and Social Security, 1974).

VI. Indirect Effects

In addition to the direct effects of the use of the automobile, i.e. injuries, pollutants, noise, mobility, there are a number of indirect effects. The repair and maintenance of motor vehicles is a considerable industry. There is evidence to show that mechanics involved in brake lining repair are exposed to levels of asbestos fibres far in excess of accepted occupational limits, (Rohl *et al*., 1976). Also, the levels in the blood of metals such as lead, chromium and other heavy metals have been found to be elevated in persons working in mechanical workshops. The source of the lead appears to be from greases and oils, as well as the petrol exhaust fumes. A number of these workers also had elevated carbon monoxide blood levels (Clausen and Rastogi, 1977a, b).

TABLE III. *Cross-cultural Comparison of Travel to Work (adapted from Szalai, 1972)*

	44 cities in USA	Jackson, Michigan	Belgium	France, six cities	West Germany: Osnabruck	Peru: Lima, Callao	Bulgaria: Kazanlik	Czechoslovakia: Olomouc	GDR: Hoyerswerda	Hungary: Gyor	Poland: Torun	USSR: Pskov	Yugoslavia: Kragujevac	Yugoslavia: Maribor
% respondents living 20+ km from centre	29·8	13·8	3·9	0	0	0·1	0	0·2	0	10·9	0	0	0·4	0·1
% with car	88·5	97·3	55·2	20·7	16·0	6·1	3·8	15·7	14·0	3·1	4·3	1·9	8·0	18·2
% travelling to work by walking	5·0	5·5	21·2	27·0	29·2	18·8	38·6	44·7	22·2	29·2	41·7	62·5	77·3	42·5
bicycle	0·2	0	14·3	9·6	22·6	1·1	34·8	6·7	15·3	29·5	1·7	1·1	3·4	24·5
car	80·1	92·3	32·2	33·9	26·4	12·7	1·7	1·9	1·5	1·2	3·4	0·1	4·8	4·9
Time (min) to and from work walking	30	34	52	44	46	48	47	46	30	40	41	32	47	40
by car	46	39	55	46	41	93	73	62	66	48	50	–	53	44

Looking further afield, the manufacture of motor vehicles undoubtedly produces its toll of injuries, exposure to toxic chemicals, lead, asbestos, and damaging noise levels. The manufacture of tyres has been shown to produce an excess morbidity and mortality among certain classes of rubber workers (McMichael *et al.*, 1976a, b). All these manufacturing establishments will also contribute their own pollutants to their local environment adding to the burden of air, water and noise pollution.

VII. Discussion and Conclusions

The automobile is firmly embedded in the culture of industrial man. It is a much prized indication of income and status, as well as a very convenient and swift means of personal transport. It plays an important part in courtship rituals, extramarital affairs and other occasions when privacy and mobility are essential. The car can also be a convenient means of acting out aggressive, murderous and suicidal impulses. An elevated blood alcohol level in its operator considerably increases the risk of crash and subsequent injury. The automobile has shaped our cities and towns, and it seems that, if unchecked, will destroy the pleasure of the city through congestion, noise and fumes.

Use of the automobile for transport exacts an unmistakable cost in terms of lives and limbs from crashes. The evidence suggests that there are long-term effects on human health from air-borne pollutants, such as lead, CO, oxidants, as well as noise, but the exact nature of these effects has yet to be determined.

The technology to reduce the injuries and pollutants is known and available, but the institution of these measures requires governmental intervention. The reduction of deaths of motor vehicle occupants in Victoria since 1970 has resulted from governmental initiatives requiring the installation and wearing of seat belts, the lowering of speed limits to 100 kph, the introduction of legislation regarding testing for blood alcohol in hospitals and random breath tests on the road; and the construction of vehicles to meet the Australian Design Rules which govern the safety performance of vehicles.

The cost of the deleterious effects of the use of the car are borne by the community in general and they are not readily visible, therefore the cost of antipollution and anti-injury measures appears to be an added burden to the purchaser, without any apparent, immediate benefit.

It is fortunate that town planning measures which ensure a smooth, free flow of traffic, separating vulnerable areas, such as schools and residential areas from through traffic and shopping areas, also reduce the risk of crashes and reduce emissions. By and large, the risk potential for car crashes is built into the road layout of an urban area. Substantial reductions in crashes can be achieved by converting a grid system into one of T-junctions and cul-de-sacs. Such changes also reduce the through traffic carried by all except designated streets, thus reducing the noise and atmospheric pollution of the remainder (South Australian Government Committee of Enquiry, 1970).

In summary, the car has provided man with a means of personal transport of unprecedented mobility. This mobility is associated with the development of dispersed towns and cities where possession of a car is no longer an option, but a necessity. The car has social and psychological functions which together with the inappropriate use of alcohol contribute to the production of crashes and collisions. These collisions have definite patterns in time and space, and the resulting injuries are also well defined, affecting mainly the young males and to a lesser extent females. A small percentage of the injuries results in long-term disabilities. The exhaust products include carbon monoxide which in urban areas on still, congested days reaches levels which cause decrements in performance in exposed persons. Long-term effects may occur in those with chronic heart and lung disease. The oxides of nitrogen and hydrocarbons under the influence of sunlight produce oxidants of which ozone is the most important. Again, in the right conditions, levels of these substances are reached which affect the sensitive proportion of the population. Long-term effects are probable but have not been measured. Air-borne lead levels are correlated with traffic density, and elevated blood levels with residence close to main traffic routes. Long-term effects of the low levels found in children may include defects in mental functioning. Asbestos fibres, known carcinogens, are found in and near heavily used roads, the effects of the low levels present are as yet not ascertained. Traffic noise at the intensity found near main roads can have acute effects on hearing and sleep patterns and long-term deleterious effects on auditory and verbal skills in children. Use of the automobile in preference to walking or bicycling has contributed to the reduction in physical exercising of motorized societies, with a consequent increased risk of ischaemic heart disease. Persons repairing and maintaining motor vehicles are at risk from elevated levels of CO, lead and the heavy metals, and asbestos, in their workplaces. Factories manufacturing motor vehicles and their components contribute to injuries and ill health in their workers and pollutants to the environment.

All told, the motor car provides a swift personal means of transport for its user. However, the community pays a high and largely hidden cost for the convenience in injuries and ill health.

References

Allen, F. R., Hart, H., Miller, D. C., Ogburn, W. F. and Nimkoff, M. F. (1957). "Technology and Social Change". Appleton-Century-Crofts, New York.

Alste, J., Watson, D. and Bagg, J. (1976). *Atmos. Environment* **10**, 583–589.

Aoki, K. and Shimizu, H. (1977). *Cancer Inst. Monogr.* **47**, 17–22.

Australian Academy of Science (1976). "Report of a Committee on the Problem of Noise". Report No. 20, Canberra.

Australian Bureau Statistics (1977/78). "Year Book of Australia", No. 62, Canberra.

Battigelli, M. C. (1971). "Medical Aspects of Air Pollution". Paper No. 710298. Society of Automotive Engineers, New York.

Beard, R. R. and Wertheim, G. A. (1967). *Am. J. publ. Hlth* **57**, 2012–2022.

Borkenstein, R. F. (1979). *In* "Proceedings of the Seventh International Conference on Alcohol, Drugs and Traffic Safety". Australian Government Publishing Service, Canberra.

Brief, R. S., Jones, A. R. and Yoder, J. D. (1960). *J. Air Poll. Control Ass.* **10**, 384–388.

Caprio, R. J., Margulis, H. L. and Joselow, M. M. (1974). *Archs environ. Hlth* **28**, 195–197.

Carruthers, M. and Murray, A. (1977). "Fitness in Forty Minutes a Week". Fortuna publications, London.

Clausen, J. and Rastogi, S. C. (1977a). *Br. J. indust. Med.* **34**, 208–215.

Clausen, J. and Rastogi, S. C. (1977b). *Br. J. indust. Med.* **34**, 216–220.

Coffin, F. L. (1971). *In* "Medical Aspects of Air Pollution". Society of Automotive Engineers, Paper No. 710301. New York.

Cohen, S. I., Dean, M. and Goldsmith, J. F. (1970) *Archs environ. Hlth* **19**, 510–517.

Cohen, C. A., Hudson, A. R., Clausen, J. L. and Knelson, J. H. (1972). *Am. Rev. resp. Dis.* **105**, 251–261.

Curnow, B. W. and Meier, P. (1973) *Archs environ. Hlth* **27**, 207–218.

Department of Health and Social Security. (1974). "Diet and Coronary Heart Disease". Report on Health and Social Subjects No. 7. HMSO, London.

Dinman, B. D. (1971). *In* "Medical Aspects of Air Pollution". Society of Automotive Engineers, Paper No. 710300. New York.

Durham, W. H. (1974). *Archs environ. Hlth* **28**, 241–254.

Environment Protection Authority of Victoria (1979). "Draft State Environment Protection Policy for the Air Environment of Victoria and Explanatory Document". Melbourne.

Foldvary, L. A. (1978). *Accid. Prev. Anal.* **10**, 143–176.
Foldvary, L. A. and Lane, J. C. (1964) *Aust. Road Res.* **2**, 7–25.
Godin, G., Wright, G., Shephard, R. J. (1972). *Archs environ. Hlth* **25**, 305–313.
Goldsmith, J. R. (1969). *J. air Poll. Control Ass.* **19**, 714–719.
Gordon, D. (1976). "Health, Sickness and Society," 364. Univ. Queensland Press, St Lucia, Queensland.
"Guinness Book of Superlatives", 155. (1956).
Hackney, J. D., Linn, W. S., Buckley, R. D., Pedersen, E. E., Karuza, S. K., Law, D. C. and Fisher, D. A. (1975a), *Archs environ. Hlth* **30**, 373–378.
Hackney, J. D., Linn, W. S., Mohler, J. G. *et al.* (1975b). *Archs. environ. Hlth* **30**, 379–390.
Hammer, D. I., Hasselblad, V., Portnoy, B., Wehrle, P. F. (1974), *Archs environ. Hlth* **28**, 255–260.
Hickey, R. J. (1971). *In* "Environment Resources, Pollution and Society" (W. Murdoch, Ed.). Sinauer Ass., Sunderland, Mass.
Hirsch, F. (1977). "Social Limits to Growth". Routledge and Kegan Paul, London.
Indiana University Institute for Research in Public Safety. (1973). 'Study to Determine the Relationship Between Vehicle Defects and Failures, and Vehicle Crashes". Final Report, Vol. 1 and 2. DOT-HS-800-850 and 851.
Jamieson, K. G., Duggan, A. W., Tweddell, J., Pope, L. I. and Zvirbulis, V. E. (1971). "Traffic Crashes in Brisbane". Special Report No. 2. Australian Road Research Board.
Jamieson, K. G. and Tait, I. A. (1966). "Traffic Injury in Brisbane". Special Report Series No. 13. National Health and Medical Research Council, Canberra.
Klemer, B. C. and Spengler, J. D. (1976). *J. air Poll. Control Ass.* **26**, 146–149.
Lin Fu, J. S. (1979). *New Engl. J. Med.* **300**, 13, 731–732.
Mackay, G. M. (1966). "Road Accident Research". Report No. 4. Publication No. 17, Department of Transportation and Environmental Planning, Univ. Birmingham.
McMichael, A. J., Andjelkovic, D. A. and Tyroler, H. A. (1976a) *Ann. NY Acad. Sci.* **271**, 125–127.
McMichael, A. J., Gerber, W. S., Gamble, J. F. *et al.* (1976b). *J occup. Med.* **18**, 611–617.
Ministry of Transport. (1967) "Cars for Cities". HMSO, London.
National Academy of Sciences—National Academy of Engineering (1974). "Air Quality and Automobile Emission Control". Report for the Coordinating Committee on Air Quality Studies. Serial No. 93–24. US Government Printing Office, Washington DC.
National Safety Council (1976). "Accident Facts". Chicago, Ill.
Needleman, H. L., Gunnoe, C., Leviton, A., *et al.* (1979). *New Engl. J. Med.* **300**, 13, 689–695.
Nelson, P. G. (1974). "Pattern of Injury Survey of Automobile Accidents, Victoria, Australia. June 1971 – June 1973". Royal Australasian College of Surgeons. Melbourne.

O'Flaherty, C. A. (1973). People, transport systems and the urban scene. An overview – 1. *In* "Wheels of Progress?" (Rose, J. Ed.). Gordon and Breach, London.

Reid, D. D. (1964). *Proc. R. Soc. Med.* **57**, 965.

Robertson, J. S. (1969). *In* "The Management of Road Traffic Casualties". Royal Australasian College of Surgeons, Melbourne.

Robertson, J. S., McLean, A. J. and Ryan, G. A. (1966). "Traffic Accidents in Adelaide, South Australia". Special Report No. 1. Australian Road Research Board.

Rohl, A. N., Langer, A. M., Wolff, M. S. and Weisman, I. (1976). *Environ. Res.* **12**, 110–128.

Rolt, L. T. C. (1956). "Motoring, a Picture History." Hulton Press. London.

Rossi, G. (Ed.) (1976). Urban traffic noise: auditory and extra-auditory effects. *Acta oto-Laryngol.* Supp. 339.

Ryan, G. A. (1967). *New Engl. J. Med.* **276**, 1066–1076.

Ryan, G. A., Douglas-Smith, L. A., Fusinato, L. A. and Youngman, J. H. R. (1978). "Report of the Road Accident Research Unit". Health Commission of Victoria, Melbourne.

Ryan, G. A. and Salter, W. E. (1977). "Blood Alcohol Levels and Drinking Behaviour of Road Crash Victims". Department of Social and Preventive Medicine, Monash University, Melbourne.

Sedgwick, A. W., Davidson, A. H. and Taplin, R. E. (1979). Community Health Studies **111** 1, 13–20.

Selikoff, I. J., Nicholson, W. J., and Langer, A. H. (1972). *Archs environ. Hlth* **25**, 1–13.

Smeed, R. J. and Jeffcoate, G. O. (1969). International comparison of road accident statistics. Paper presented at "Symposium on the Use of Statistical Methods in the Analysis of Road Accidents". Road Research Laboratory, UK.

Stopps, G. J. (1969) *J. air Poll. Control Ass.* **19**, 719–721.

Szalai, A. (Ed.) (1972). "The Use of Time: Daily Activities of Urban and Suburban Populations in Twelve Countries". Mouton, The Hague.

South Australian Government Committee of Enquiry (1970). "Report on Road Safety". Adelaide.

"The News". Wednesday 6 October 1965. Adelaide, South Australia. Quoting an un-named source.

Thomas, H. V., Milmore, B. K., Heidbreder, G. A. and Kogan, B. A. (1967). Archs environ. Hlth **15**, 695–702.

US Department of Transportation (1968). "Alcohol and Highway Safety". Washington DC.

Vulcan, A. P. (1978). Effects of the Victorian child restraint legislation. Paper presented at Royal Australasian College of Surgeons Seminar: "Restraining the Child in a Car". Road Safety and Traffic Authority, Melbourne.

Warnock, M. L. and Churg, A. M. (1975). *Cancer* **35**, 1236–1242.

Whitlock, F. A. (1971). "Death on the Road: a Study in Social Violence". Tavistock, London.

Winkelstein, W. Jr, Kantor, S., Davis, E. W., Maneri, C. S. and Mosher, W. E. (1967). *Archs environ. Hlth* **14**, 162.
Woodruff, P. (1963). *Med. J. Aust.* **11**, 392–400.
World Health Organization. (1977) "World Health Statistics". WHO, Geneva.

27
Overnutrition

B. K. Armstrong and A. J. McMichael
Department of Medicine, University of Western Australia, Perth, Australia and Division of Human Nutrition, Commonwealth Scientific and Industrial Research Organization, Adelaide, Australia

---

The artificiality of much modern food (nutrient imbalances, energy denseness, additives, and micronutrient losses), shored up by political, economic and commercial interests, and presented to an under-informed advertising-saturated, and often behaviourally malconditioned community, comprises a compelling recipe for overnutrition.

I. Introduction

The transition, in recent human history, from lack of close control over the amount and composition of the food supply to, at least in wealthy countries, virtually complete control, has led to the emergence of health problems related to over—rather than under—nutrition.

Until about 10 000 years ago, hunting and gathering were the only means of obtaining food. The result was generally a varied diet, mainly of vegetable origin and adequate in both major and minor nutrients. The effort of collecting it did not permit consumption of excess, and famine was an everpresent possibility.

Only in the most recent 1% of human evolutionary history has hunting and gathering given way, in most populations, to the cultivation of food crops and the domestication of animals for meat. The result has been, until overpopulation developed, a more certain but often less varied food supply. For modern, wealthy man, industrialization and the growth of trade have made all types of food available on virtually a seasonless basis. This, together with the development of food technology and its production of highly refined "energy-dense" foods, has set the scene for overnutrition.

II. Definition of Overnutrition

For our purposes, overnutrition will be defined as an abnormal state resulting from excessive consumption of food or of some specific nutrient. While increased body fatness (estimated by any of a variety of means such as measurement of body weight, body weight adjusted for body height and/or age, skinfold thickness, body density, etc.; will often be associated with overnutrition, it is by no means its only manifestation. Excessive intakes of major nutrients (such as fat) may occur without an overall excess of dietary energy, and excessive consumption of vitamins and minerals, particularly salt, may sometimes lead to disease.

Overnutrition may be a result, therefore, not only of increased availability of all food, but of a relative increase in availability of specific foods and nutrients. Those which are probably most important to current human disease are foods of animal origin (meat and dairy produce), refined carbohydrates (with the associated loss of food fibre), and fat.

III. Trends in Food Consumption with Affluence

Trends in the apparent consumption of various foods in the United States from 1909 to 1975 are summarized in Fig. 1 (Friend *et al.*, 1979). The most dramatic changes were the decline in consumption of potatoes and flour and other cereal products. In parallel, consumption

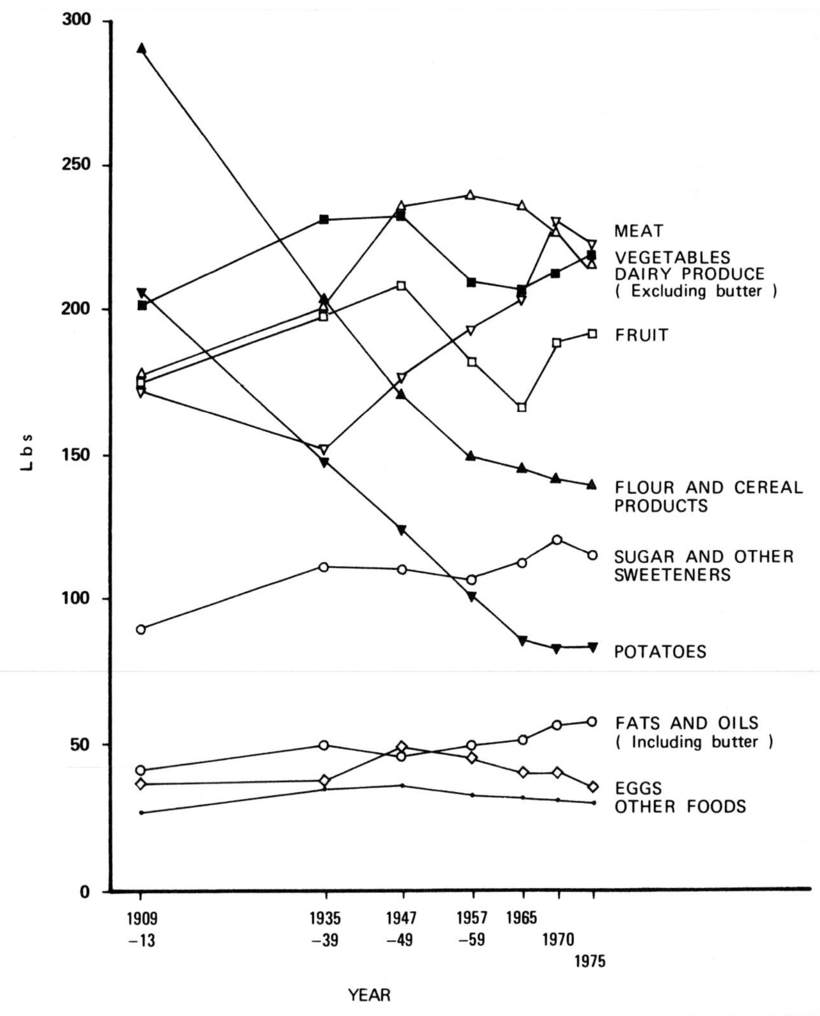

Fig. 1. Changes in consumption of foods in the United States, 1909–13 to 1975 (Friend *et al.*, 1979; dairy produce consumption measured in quarts).

of meat, poultry and fish (predominantly meat and poultry) and dairy products increased. Contrary, perhaps, to expectation these changes in food consumption produced a nett decline in per caput food energy consumption (about 7·5%). A 25% decline in carbohydrate consumption more than balanced a 26% increase in fat consumption. As a result, the proportion of total food energy from carbohydrate fell from 56% to 46% and that from fat rose from 32% to 42%, while that from protein remained relatively constant at 11 to 12%,

Although intake of both meat and dairy products increased, the amount of animal fat consumed declined (from 105·5 g in 1909–13 to 86·8 g in 1975. The overall increase in fat consumption was due, therefore, to increases in the use of vegetable fats, mainly vegetable oils and the vegetable portion of margarine and shortening. The consumption of simple carbohydrates relative to complex carbohydrates increased and the consumption of food fibre decreased (Heller and Hackler, 1978).

Similar trends have been reported from Britain (Greaves and Hollingsworth, 1966), and some earlier data from both countries suggest that the major trends were established at least as early as the second half of the nineteenth century (Antar *et al.*, 1964; Greaves and Hollingsworth, 1966). It is likely, therefore, that these more recent observations on food consumption in Britain and America have come toward the end of the main effects of economic development on dietary patterns. Indeed, the estimated per caput consumption figures in England and Wales during the last 200 years indicate substantial dietary changes—a sixfold increase in sugar consumption, a fivefold increase in fat consumption, a halving of wheat flour consumption, and a tenfold reduction in cereal crude fibre consumption (Trowell, 1975).

Another view of the effects of economic development comes from Japan, whose affluence dates mainly from the Second World War. In this country, between 1949 and 1973, total food energy, total protein and total fat consumption increased, while total carbohydrate intake declined. The major contributors to these changes were tenfold or greater increases in milk, eggs, meat and poultry intake, a 50% increase in fish and shellfish consumption, and increased consumption of refined sugars and visible fats and oils. Intake of the traditional cereal, rice, declined by about one-third (Oiso, 1975).

IV. Trends in Body Height and Weight

It is difficult to relate trends in body height and weight to the changes in dietary patterns described above. This is at least partly because of concomitant declines in energy expenditure. What data are available suggest, at least in Britain, that both average body height and weight increased during the first half of the twentieth century (Boyne and Leitch, 1954; Leitch and Boyne, 1960). Average weight increased relatively more than did average height, thus giving an increase in the weight/height ratio. This strongly suggests that dietary energy intake increased relative to energy expenditure. Similar trends have been observed more recently in Japan with, for example, the average body weight of twelve-year-old girls increasing by 9 kg between 1950 and 1974. At the latter time their average height and weight was essentially identical to that of United States white girls (Kagawa, 1978).

V. The Health Consequences of Overnutrition

The main health consequences of overnutrition are summarized in Table I. The most obvious manifestation is obesity (increased body

TABLE I. *The Major Health Consequences of Overnutrition*

Health consequences	Associated dietary excess[a]
Obesity	Energy
Coronary atherosclerosis	Saturated fat Cholesterol (?)
Hypertension	Salt (?) Meat (?) Fat (?)
Diabetes mellitus	Energy Refined carbohydrate (?)
Cancer	
Endometrium	Energy Fat (?)
Breast	Energy (?) Fat (?)
Colon and rectum	Meat (?) Fat (?) Refined carbohydrate (?)
Other diseases	
Diverticulosis, appendicitis, hiatus hernia, varicose veins, haemorrhoids	Refined carbohydrate (?)

[a] (?) indicates less well-established associations.

fatness) which, in turn, is associated with coronary atherosclerosis, high blood pressure, diabetes mellitus, cancers of the breast and endometrium, and a number of less serious problems such as degenerative arthritis and skin problems (Kannel and Gordon, 1974).

Whether obesity lies directly in the causal chain leading to these disorders, or is simply a parallel consequence of overnutrition, is open to some debate. Reduction in body weight will reduce blood pressure, blood cholesterol levels (a major indicator of risk of coronary atherosclerosis) and render the associated diabetes much easier to control. Weight reduction is, however, nearly always associated with dietary change; therefore these responses do not prove that obesity is a causal factor. Most studies suggest that extreme obesity increases overall mortality rates about twofold, although here again the details of the causal chain are not well understood (Sorensen and Sonne-Holm, 1977; Walker, 1978).

The consequences of coronary atherosclerosis (angina pectoris, acute myocardial infarction, chronic ischaemic heart disease, etc.) are positively associated with obesity (Kannel and Gordon, 1974), elevated levels of blood cholesterol (which is strongly determined by an individual's saturated fat intake) and, at least in populations, the total intake of saturated fat (Stamler, 1979). These conditions have emerged in parallel with economic development and are almost certainly the result of overnutrition, with saturated fat being the nutrient mainly responsible. Insofar as dietary cholesterol contributes to blood cholesterol levels, it may also be a contributory factor.

High blood pressure is closely associated with coronary atherosclerosis and may also be a consequence of overnutrition. It is virtually non-existent in underdeveloped societies. For example, the blood pressures of New Guinea highlanders remain constant throughout life whereas in affluent societies there is a progressive rise with age (Sinnett and Whyte, 1978). The association of increasing salt intake with affluence has long been suspected as explanatory of the association between affluence and blood pressure. High salt intakes may also explain the paradoxically high blood pressures in some Japanese populations. Recent evidence, however, has linked hypertension to excessive consumption of meat and/or fat (Armstrong *et al.*, 1977).

Maturity-onset diabetes mellitus is also associated with obesity and coronary atherosclerosis. It has variously been suggested that the diabetes is a result of insulin resistance due to obesity, to exhaustion of pancreatic islet-cells (the normal source of insulin) following sustained excessive consumption of refined carbohydrate, or to a genetically determined resistance of muscle cells to insulin (Whichelow, 1974).

The incidence of a number of cancers, particularly those listed in Table I, is strongly associated with economic affluence and, therefore, the associated dietary patterns (Armstrong and Doll, 1975). Obesity is a risk factor for cancers of the breast and endometrium, and increased body height may be a risk factor for cancer of the breast (Armstrong, 1977; Staszewski, 1977). Several studies have suggested that excess intake of dietary fat is causally related to breast cancer (Miller *et al.*, 1978; Hirayama, 1978).

Excessive consumption of meat, fat, and refined carbohydrate (or fibre deficiency) have all been suggested to be responsible for the high incidence of cancers of the colon and rectum in developed countries (Wynder *et al.*, 1977). There is some support for each of these possibilities and a unifying hypothesis may be offered. Dietary fat has been shown to alter the nature and concentration of biliary steroids and may thus provide a substrate from which colonic bacteria produce carcinogens. In turn, dietary meat alters the profile of the bacterial flora in the colon, and may produce a more anaerobic bacterial population which is more active in carcinogen production. An associated lack of dietary fibre may, by both a reduced sequestration of biliary steroids and a decrease in the volume of colonic contents, increase the production and concentration, respectively, of these carcinogens.

The deficiency of food fibre associated with increased consumption of refined carbohydrate has been variously blamed for diverticulosis, appendicitis, hiatus hernia, varicose veins, haemorrhoids and a number of other diseases, as well as colorectal cancer (Burkitt, 1973). Fibre deficiency probably does cause diverticulosis, but insufficient data are available to connect it with any certainty to the other conditions listed.

VI. Host–Environment Interactions in Overnutrition

The preceding discussion has considered the role of overnutrition *per se* in producing adverse effects on health. These effects should be seen, however, as the joint product of overnutrition and the genetic constitution of the host individual. Indeed it is not surprising that many people are ill-adapted to the affluent diet, since this diet is vastly different from that which prevailed during 99% of human evolutionary history (Davidson *et al.*, 1975).

On present evidence, obesity and maturity-onset diabetes exemplify best this environmental–constitutional interaction. Their occurrence in certain individuals is thought to reflect some degree of genetic predisposition, deriving from individual variations in the mechanisms of storage, interconversion and retrieval of energy. While there is undoubtedly some truth in the popular notion that obesity is caused by eating too much (or exercising too little), nevertheless, formal studies of food intake usually show that most obese persons eat no more (and often less) than their slim counterparts. This applies in children and adolescents as well as in adults (James and Trayhurn, 1976).

The primary "problem" in persons disposed to develop these closely related conditions may be an above-average metabolic "efficiency" (Miller, 1974). This "efficiency" may be an important adaptive mechanism that has recently become maladaptive under the provocation of year-round dietary abundance.

Obese persons often claim that they have a particular propensity to obesity in contrast to other members of the community who can eat liberally without putting on weight. Review of the experimental and epidemiological evidence, and consideration of the processes of biological evolution, suggests that obesity occurs most readily in metabolically thrifty individuals—that is, those who would be genetically favoured to survive if food supplies were scarce. These individuals may be limited in their ability to produce body heat, because of a reduced metabolic activity in skeletal muscle, or they may be predisposed to convert excess energy into fat, rather than lean, tissue (James and Trayhurn, 1976). This latter characteristic may reflect, at least partially, the "thrifty genotype" with exaggerated insulin response, first proposed by the geneticist J. V. Neel (1969).

In modern-day hunter-gatherer and subsistence agricultural societies, most adults are smaller and eat less food than those in affluent communities. In particular, the pattern of eating is typically "feast-and-fast". The heavy work of out-of-season hunting and gathering, or of cultivating next year's crops, often coincides with reduced food supply. In these circumstances, the ability to store excess energy efficiently, to conserve it, and to release it when needed for physical work would enhance survival. In affluent societies, however, a regular and adequate food supply is guaranteed, and activity is usually both limited and fairly constant throughout the year. The thrifty, survival-enhancing genetic package is, therefore, unnecessary in circumstances of dietary abundance, and may even be detrimental.

Given the genetic basis of natural selection, wherein gene mutation and sexual reproduction ensure continuing genetic diversity within a species, it is not surprising that individuals vary in their energy-handling characteristics. It is this genetic diversity that confers species adaptability in the face of environmental change. Alteration of food availability is one such environmental challenge.

Further, one would expect that, when long-standing environmental selection pressures are reduced, genetic diversity for the relevant biological attribute would increase. It is likely, therefore, that in affluent societies which have been freed from serious food shortages for several centuries at least, the current proportion of "thrifty" genotypes is less than in populations still, or at least recently experiencing intermittent food shortages. That is, there may well have been some recent genetic drift in Western populations towards less metabolic "thriftiness". This could explain, at least partially, the comparatively higher incidence of obesity and diabetes reported in communities only recently exposed to Western-style diets. In Australian Aborigines (Wise *et al.*, 1976), Pima Indians (Bennett *et al.*, 1976) and Pacific Islanders (Zimmet, 1979), unusually high rates of obesity and diabetes now occur.

It is notable also that studies of both the Kalahari bushmen and the Aborigines have shown that adults have a reduced thermogenic (i.e. heat-producing) response to cold, allowing their core temperatures to fall during a cool night, this reducing the temperature gradient and the rate of heat loss (James and Trayhurn, 1976). Recent work suggests that this is achieved at least in some individuals by a reduction in energy-wasting metabolic cycles, initially labelled as "futile cycles" (Katz and Rognstad, 1978). These cycles (now less presumptuously called "substrate cycles") have been demonstrated in muscle, liver and adipose tissue from various animal species. Such cycles can occur along the pathways of protein, fat or carbohydrate metabolism, but share the common feature of ATP wastage—and therefore heat generation. The metabolically efficient genotype with fewer energy-wasting cycles— for which there are clear animal experimental models, but as yet only fragmentary human evidence—apparently has therefore a tendency to conserve caloric fuel.

An alternative metabolic mechanism of energy conservation is variation in the ratio of lean tissue deposition to fat tissue deposition. The efficiency of converting food to fat is about 70%, whereas conversion to protein (lean tissue) is only about 40% efficient (Dugdale and Payne, 1977). Again, the thrifty genotype, whose survival is enhanced in times of food shortage, would be disposed to "run to fat" in circumstances of plenty.

Further, populations such as the Pima Indians and Pacific Islanders seem to be predisposed jointly to both obesity and maturity-onset diabetes. Indeed, these conditions tend to concur in individuals (Zimmet, 1979). The predisposition to diabetes appears to be accompanied by an enhanced insulin response to glucose. In the two abovementioned populations a clear bimodality in glucose tolerance strongly suggests the existence of a diabetic genotype. An enhanced insulin response would increase the efficiency of fat deposition, and may therefore be a major metabolic factor in determining the individual's lean tissue : fat tissue deposition ratio. This would also perhaps partly account for the tendency of obesity and maturity-onset diabetes to co-exist.

These several different, possibly interacting, metabolic mechanisms for the phenotypic manifestation of the "thrifty gene" may eventually be related back to genetically determined variations in sympathetic nervous system response to energy intake (Lansberg and Young, 1978). In general, this sympathetic activity varies in proportion to level of food intake, with high intake triggering high dissipation of energy. It may also explain how individual body weight varies very little despite marked variations in food intake. Perhaps in "thrifty" genotypes the sympathetic nervous system response to excess calorie intake is reduced.

The close associations between obesity and diabetes mellitus and hypertension, hyperlipidaemia and coronary atherosclerosis suggest that genetic predisposition may also underlie the manifestation, in individuals, of these latter conditions when exposed to the relevant dietary excess. Indeed, the development of hypertension and ischaemic heart disease also appear to be exaggerated in Aboriginal populations undergoing rapid Westernization (Bastian, 1979).

VII. The Social Determinants of Overnutrition

While innate characteristics influence the risk of disease in overconsuming individuals, another important consideration is the variation in actual eating behaviour between individuals, groups and populations. A convenient approach is to consider influences upon eating behaviour operating at the societal, group and individual levels. While individual variations in some physiological mechanisms—involving, for example, satiety reflexes or other neurohormonal feedback systems—may affect individual eating behaviour, the purpose of this section is to examine "non-biological" influences.

At the societal level, the major factors are, firstly, the availability and promotion of different foods—reflecting agricultural, food production and marketing practices, and political and economic policies—and, secondly, the prevailing norms of food preference and eating patterns.

The first set of factors influences the prominence of calorie-dense, highly processed foods in the market, and the second affects both personal choice from among those options and the total amount consumed.

The concept of health-oriented national nutrition planning has not yet been established in developed countries. Governments, through their agricultural, economic, and educational policies, have at best usually ignored overnutrition. At worst, they have promoted unhealthy consumption trends. For example, faced with mountains of surplus butter, the EEC's European Commission recently proposed taxing edible oils to make margarine more expensive, thereby encouraging higher consumption of saturated fats. The Congressionally mandated involvement of the US Department of Agriculture, in promoting higher egg consumption in the United States, provides another case in point.

Apart from the direct influence that food manufacturers exert through the range of foods presented for sale, a persuasive indirect influence is exerted through advertising. Since everybody eats, and since many can be enticed to eat more, huge sums of advertising money are spent in an area in which there is a dearth of public education and balanced information. In Australia, it is estimated that more is spent on advertising food than any other consumer commodity (English, 1979). Assessments of advertisements for food and drink reveal a strong imbalance favouring alcoholic beverages, confectionery, soft drinks, sweet biscuits, sweetened cereals and other highly processed and refined foods, while wholegrain cereal products, fresh vegetables and fruits get very little attention. These highly processed foods are those most likely to be high in calories, sugar, fat and salt, the dietary components contributing most to current problems of overnutrition.

With respect to the prevailing sociocultural norms of types and amounts of food eaten, these are inevitably somewhat mobile in a rapidly changing society. For example, the increasing availability, and promotion, of convenient snack foods and fast-food restaurants has enticed us into eating large quantities of high-fat, nutritionally suspect foods, and eating them rapidly, often "on the run", and in an atmosphere of stress. The effects of this all-too-often excessive and imbalanced food intake are compounded by the prevailing practice in Western society of eating the largest meal at the end of the day. The low physical activity between dinner and breakfast maximizes the conversion of dietary substrate and energy into adipose tissue. Animal experimental data have shown that varying the meal pattern, while maintaining constant the total daily energy intake, considerably influences fat deposition (Cohn and Joseph, 1960).

Attitudes to obesity may also be important. In Western society, its prevalence varies considerably with social class. Surveys in Europe and the United States have shown obesity to be most prevalent in middle-aged working class women, and far less common among younger women, and those from the upper social classes whatever their age (Stunkard, 1977). A similar pattern is emerging in children; the less privileged are more likely to be fat (Silverstone, 1974).

These variations in prevalence of obesity are more likely to reflect general social pressures than individual metabolic or psychological disturbances. Thus it is not the tendency to become fat, but the concern with being overweight, that most distinguishes those of upper from those of lower social class. This difference probably not only implies a greater understanding within the upper classes of the causes and consequences of obesity, but also reflects a different set of social expectations. Such differences between groups within a culture reflect the even greater differences that can exist between cultures. For example, certain East African tribes traditionally fatten their girls from the age of eight, with the king's harem containing the fattest women in the tribe. Such cultural patterns are likely to reflect economic as well as aesthetic differences between one society and another.

Recent studies of Australian adolescents emphasize how differences in cognition between sexes, and between subgroups, influence perceptions of the causes of obesity (Worsley, 1979). Girls view obesity more seriously than boys, and attribute more of its causation to emotional and social disturbances. Girls appear to see overeating more as the result of external factors, whereas boys regard lack of self-control as more important. In adult life, this view is probably reinforced by women's magazines, with their interminable publication of "new" dieting strategies for women to combat that remorseless external foe, overeating and overweight.

At the personal level, emotional disturbance has been proposed by some to be all-important in the aetiology of obesity: "Persistence in overeating has its basis in unresolved emotional patterns . . . the overeating serves as a substitute for other satisfactions" (Kiell, 1973). However, comparative studies have not found obese persons to be generally more emotionally reactive (neurotic) than the non-obese Stunkard, 1975). That, of course, is not to deny that a proportion of obese people overeat in response to stress. Certain households are highly preoccupied with the subject of food (Bruch, 1964). Not only is food proffered in abundance, but food, particularly sweets, is seen as a short-term panacea for all emotional distress and minor physical trauma. Within that social environment, the child readily learns to use food as an anxiety reducer. When such conditioning coexists with an emotionally reactive temperament in a stressful environment the risk of adult obesity is high.

Overall, the non-biological causes of overeating, overnutrition and obesity are many and complex. For most people in contemporary Western society, and particularly for some genotypes, the cards are stacked against the maintenance of normal nutritional status and weight. The artificiality of much modern food (nutrient imbalances, energy denseness, additives, and micronutrient losses), shored up by political, economic and commercial interests, and presented to an underinformed, advertising-saturated, and often behaviourally malconditioned community, comprises a compelling recipe for overnutrition.

VIII. The Prevention of Overnutrition

The various factors contributing to overnutrition and its consequences are summarized in Fig. 2. Ultimately the evolutionary pressures on the right may correct our present maladaptation. Many of the factors on the left, however, are subject to human manipulation.

Most often, prominence is given to the role of the individual in controlling his own environment. Thus we are exhorted to eat less, exercise more, and modify our diets in such a way as to reduce our risk of cardiovascular disease and cancer. In practice, and particularly for the less intelligent and/or less well-educated, these educational messages cannot penetrate the screen thrown up by commercial practices and promotion.

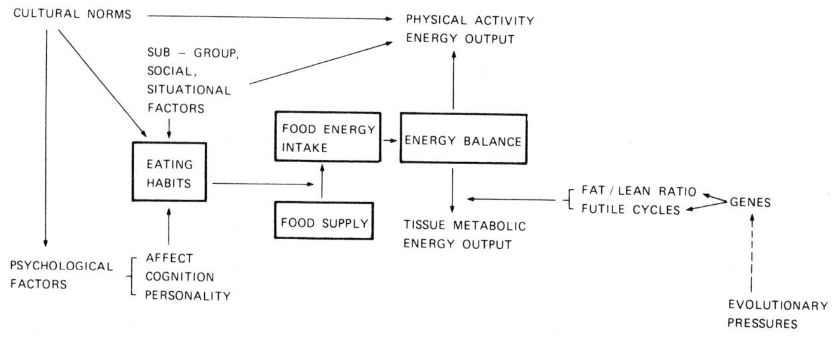

Fig. 2. Determinants of energy balance and overnutrition.

Effective action on overnutrition will, therefore, require government intervention. A national strategy to counter overnutrition would involve a wide range of policies, not all of them directly linked to food and agriculture. The marketplace has its own set of priorities, and health is not one of them. Nutrition planning must include the development of economic incentives and institutions that encourage healthy food-production and consumption patterns. Agricultural research, crop subsidies, taxes, meat-grading, international trade, and medical and general education rank high among the many concerns that a strategy to combat overnutrition must encompass. Since over-nutrition and lack of exercise are part of the same problem, such topics as recreation and transportation are also included. For example, the construction of bicycle paths rather than parking lots for urban commuters would create, among other benefits, the opportunity for regular exercise and could thereby reduce the incidence of obesity and heart disease.

Among the industrial countries, Sweden and Norway stand alone in their recent decisions to integrate modern dietary health concerns into national economic and agricultural planning. Through a vigorous public education programme the Swedish Government has worked to reduce the amount of calories, fats, sugar and alcohol Swedes consume, and to increase the amount of exercise Swedes get. The Norwegian Government has proposed to its legislature a nutrition and food policy aimed at increasing national self-sufficiency in food supplies and at cutting the mounting national toll of cardiovascular and other diet-related diseases (Ringen, 1977).

Such initiatives are inevitable in other affluent societies; it is to be hoped that they are not too much delayed.

References

Antar, M. A., Ohlson, M. A. and Hodges, R. E. (1964). Changes in retail market food supplies in the United States in the last seventy years in relation to the incidence of coronary heart disease, with special reference to dietary carbohydrates and essential fatty acids. *Am. J. clin. Nutr.* **14**, 169–178.

Armstrong, B. K. (1977). "The Role of Diet in Human carcinogenesis with Special Reference to Endometrial Cancer. *In* "Origins of Human Cancer" H. H. Hiatt, J. D. Watson and J. A. Winsten, Eds), 557–565. Cold Spring Harbor Laboratory, New York.

Armstrong, B. and Doll, R. (1975). Evironmental factors and cancer incidence and mortality in different countries with special reference to dietary practices. *Int. J. Cancer* **15**, 617–631.

Armstrong, B., Van Merwyk, A. J. and Coates, H. (1977). Blood pressure in

Seventh-day Adventist vegetarians. *Am. J. Epidemiol.* **105**, 444–449.
Bastian, P. (1979). Coronary heart disease in tribal Aborigines—The West Kimberley Survey. *Aust. N.Z. J. Med.* **9**, 284–292.
Bennett, P. H., Rushforth, N. B., Miller, M. and Lecompte, P. M. (1976). Epidemiological studies of diabetes in the Pima Indians. *Rec. Progr. horm. Res.* **32**, 333–371.
Boyne, A. W. and Leitch, I. (1954). Secular changes in the height of British adults. *Nutr. Abst. Rev.* **24**, 255–269.
Bruch, H. (1964). Psychological aspects of overeating and obesity. *Psychosomatics* **5**, 269–276.
Burkitt, D. P. (1973). Some diseases characteristic of modern Western civilization. *Brit. med. J.* i, 274–278.
Cohn, C. and Joseph, D. (1960). Role of rate of ingestion of diet on regulation of intermediary metabolism ("meal eating" vs. "nibbling"). *Metabolism* **9**, 492–500.
Davidson, S., Passmore, R., Brock, J. F. and Truswell, A. S. (1975). Historical and geographical perspectives. *In* "Human Nutrition and Dietetics". Churchill Livingstone, Edinburgh. 1975.
Dugdale, A. E. and Payne, P. R. (1977). Pattern of lean and fat deposition in adults. *Nature* **266**, 349–351.
English, R. (1979). Nutrition education versus food advertising. *Food Nutr. Notes Rev.* **36**, 117–120.
Friend, B., Page, L. and Marston, R. (1979). Food consumption patterns in the United States: 1909–13 to 1976. *In* "Nutrition, Lipids and Coronary Heart Disease" (R. Levy, B. Rifkind, B. Dennis and N. Ernst, Eds.), 489–522. Raven Press, New York.
Greaves, J. P. and Hollingsworth, D. F. (1966). Trends in food consumption in the United Kingdom. *Wld Rev. Nutr. Diet* **6**, 34–89.
Heller, S. N. and Hackler, L. R. (1978). Changes in the crude fibre content of the American diet. *Am. J. clin Nutr.* **31**, 1510–1514.
Hirayama, T. (1978). Epidemiology of breast cancer with special reference to the role of diet. *Prev. Med.* **7**, 173–195.
James, W. P. T. and Trayhurn, P. (1976). An integrated view of the metabolic and genetic basis for obesity. *Lancet* ii, 770–773.
Kagawa, Y. (1978). Impact of Westernization on the nutrition of Japanese: Changes in physique, cancer, longevity and centenarians. *Prev. Med.* **7**, 205–217.
Kannel, W. B. and Gordon, T. (1974). Obesity and cardiovascular disease. The Framingham study. *In* "Obesity" (W. L. Burland, P. D. Samuel and J. Yudkin, Eds), 24–51. Churchill Livingstone, Edinburgh.
Katz, J. and Rognstad, R. (1978). Futile cycling in glucose metabolism. *Trends Biochem. Sci.* **3**, 171–174.
Kiell, N. (1973). Introduction. *In* "The Psychology of Obesity" (N. Kiell, Ed.), i–xv. Thomas, Springfield.
Lansburg, L. and Young, J. B. (1978). Fasting, feeding and regulation of the sympathetic nervous system. *New Engl. J. Med.* **298**, 1295–1301.

Leitch, I. and Boyne, A. W. (1960). Recent changes in the height and weight of adolescents. *Nutr. Abst. Rev.* **30**, 1173–1186.

Miller, D. S. (1974). Energy balance and obesity. *In* "Obesity" (W. L. Burland, P. D. Samuel and J. Yudkin, Eds), 160–170. Churchill Livingstone, Edinburgh.

Miller, A. B., Kelly, A., Choi, N. W., Matthews, V., Morgan, R. W., Munan, L., Burch, J. D., Feather, J., Howe, G. R. and Jain, M. (1978). A study of diet and breast cancer. *Am. J. Epidemiol.* **107**, 499–509.

Neel, J. V. (1969). Current concepts of the genetic basis of diabetes mellitus and the biological significance of the diabetic predisposition. *In* "Diabetes" (J. Ostman and R. D. G. Milner, Eds), 68–78. Excerpta Medica, Amsterdam.

Oiso, R. (1975). Incidence of stomach cancer and its relation to dietary habits and nutrition in Japan between 1900 and 1975. *Cancer Res.* **35**, 3254–3258.

Ringen, K. (1977). The Norwegian food and nutritional policy. *Am. J. publ. Hlth* **67**, 550–551.

Silverstone, J. T. (1974). Psychological and social factors in the pathogenesis of obesity. "Obesity" (W. L. Burland, P. D. Samuel and J. Yudkin, Eds), 105–111. Churchill Livingstone, Edinburgh.

Sinnett, P. and Whyte, M. (1978). Lifestyle, health and disease: A comparison between Papua New Guinea and Australia. *Med. J. Aust.* **1**, 1–5.

Sorensen, T. I. A. and Sonne-Holm, S. (1977). Mortality in extremely overweight young men. *J. chron. Dis.* **30**, 359–367.

Stamler, J. (1979). Population studies. *In* "Nutrition, Lipids and Coronary Heart Disease" (R. Levy, B. Rifkind, B. Dennis and N. Ernst, Eds), 25–88. Raven Press, New York.

Staszewski, J. (1977). Breast cancer and body build. *Prev. Med.* **6**, 410–415.

Stunkard, A. J. (1975). From explanation to action in psychosomatic medicine: The case of obesity. *Psychosom. Med.* **37**, 195–236.

Stunkard, A. J. (1977). Obesity and the social environment: Current status, future prospects. *Ann. NY Acad, Sci.* **300**, 298–320.

Trowell, H. C. (1975). Dietary changes in modern times. *In* "refined Carbohydrate Foods and Disease" (D. P. Burkitt and H. C. Trowell, Eds), 47–56. Academic Press, London and New York.

Walker, A. R. P. (1978). Does obesity matter? *S. Afr. med. J.* **53**, 918.

Whichelow, M. J. (1974). Peripheral metabolism of carbohydrate in obesity and diabetes. *In* "Obesity" (W. L. Burland, P. D. Samuel and J. Yudkin, Eds), Churchill Livingstone, Edinburgh.

Wise, P. H., Edwards, F. M., Craig, R. J., Evans, B., Murchland, J., Sutherland, B. and Thomas, D. W. (1976). Diabetes and associated variables in the South Australian Aboriginal. *Aust. NZ J. Med.* **6**, 191–196.

Worsley, A. (1979). Adolescents' views of obesity. *Food Nutr. Notes Rev.* **36**, 57–63.

Wynder, E. L., Reddy, B. S., McCoy, G. D. S. *et al.* (1977). Diet and cancer of the gastrointestinal tract. *Adv. intern. Med.* **22**, 397–419.

Zimmet, P. (1979). Epidemiology of diabetes and its macrovascular manifestations in Pacific populations: The medical effects of social progress. *Diabetes Care* **2**, 144–153.

28

Cardiovascular Disease

M. G. McCall

Department of Medicine, University of Western Australia, Perth, Australia

---

Developed, affluent countries have been in the grip of a rising epidemic of cardiovascular disease throughout the course of this century . . . There is now a large body of scientific opinion that changes in food pattern are fundamental to the development of atherosclerotic disease.

I. Introduction

The term cardiovascular disease includes coronary heart disease (CHD), peripheral vascular disease and obstructive cerebrovascular disease. The chief clinical manifestations of CHD are angina, myocardial infarction and sudden death, of peripheral vascular disease claudication and gangrene, and of obstructive cerebrovascular disease, transient ischaemic attacks and thrombotic stroke.

There is much evidence to suggest that developed, affluent countries have been in the grip of a rising epidemic of cardiovascular disease throughout the course of this century. In some countries, USA (Cooper *et al.*, 1978), Australia (Reader, 1975) and more recently in the UK (*British Medical Journal*, 1976; Florey *et al.*, 1978), this epidemic appears to have peaked and is now slowly declining. In other countries cardiovascular disease is still an increasing cause of morbidity and mortality (Guberan, 1979). The magnitude of this epidemic has not been readily recognized because the rise in deaths has been offset by a dramatic fall in deaths from other causes, notably infectious diseases. In the specific area of cerebrovascular disease the beneficial impact of treatment with hypotensive agents on death rates has provided a further ameliorating factor in the past twenty years (Reader, 1975).

Initial reports drawing attention to increasing death rates from CHD were subject to criticism that the rise in deaths within this category was a consequence of greater clinical awareness and of increased diagnostic accuracy, or of changes in coding rubrics under which causes of death were classified (Morris, 1970). Acceptance of the reality of these changes followed detailed epidemiological studies in many countries. Not surprisingly some of these studies also looked for correlations between the presence of cardiovascular disease and other variables such as life-style, diet and physiological and biochemical measurements in affected individuals and population samples. These studies gave rise to the concept of "risk" factors. It has been particularly difficult to establish with accustomed scientific rigour the specific causes of cardiovascular disease. There are intrinsic difficulties in studying, in man himself, diseases with a natural history measured in decades, particularly when pathological change can only be quantitated at autopsy. In consequence the factors identified have been labelled "risk" factors recognizing the strength of their association, but stopping short of implying unequivocal causation. There is increasing acceptance, however, that some of these factors are causative.

The so-called major risk factors include hypercholesterolaemia, hypertension, cigarette smoking, diabetes mellitus, obesity, physical inactivity and a positive family history of premature vascular disease (Stamler, 1967; National Heart Foundation of New Zealand, 1971; Working Group, 1975). These major factors have been implicated in the development of CHD, and also in peripheral vascular disease and obstructive cerebrovascular disease. Minor factors, or factors less certainly associated with cardiovascular disease include personality type, high haematocrit, hyperuricaemia, and a high refined carbohydrate and low fibre intake (Stamler, 1967; National Heart Foundation of New Zealand, 1971; Working Group, 1975).

Epidemiological studies from many parts of the world repeatedly underline the significance of hypercholesterolaemia, hypertension, and cigarette smoking. Relative weighting of risk factors is difficult but the evidence suggests that the influence of various factors may vary at different ages and in different countries for each of CHD, peripheral vascular disease and obstructive cerebrovascular disease (Sturmans *et al.*, 1977). It is clear, however, that the combination of two or more risk factors greatly increases the probability of developing cardiovascular disease (Gordon *et al.*, 1976).

In order to simplify the discussion CHD will, from here on, be used as the exemplar of all forms of cardiovascular disease. This decision is taken in view of the preeminent position of CHD as a cause of death and the predominance of studies relating to this condition as compared to peripheral vascular disease and obstructive cerebrovascular disease. While the balance of risk factors and contributory factors for these latter two diseases will differ (WHO, 1971) it seems unlikely that the overall picture will be misrepresented by confining the subsequent discussion in this way.

Before the further discussion of risk factors it is appropriate to recognize the nature of the primary arterial lesion which underlies cardiovascular disease, namely atheroma.

Atheroma is a lesion affecting the lining of the wall of the larger arteries, and as such may with or without associated thrombus be responsible for progressive occlusion of the lumen of the vessel with consequent reduction of blood flow to the organ concerned. Three types of change have been described (WHO, 1958).

1. *Fatty streaks*—may be observed in the first decade of life and may not be precursors of raised lesions.
2. *Raised lesions*:
   (a) *Fibrous plaques*—are localized fatty or fibrous accumulations associated with a proliferation of smooth muscle cells.

(b) *Complicated lesions*—are derived from fibrous plaques by the additional changes of thrombosis, ulceration and/or haemorrhage.

In the study of risk factors it will be helpful where possible to identify those which are implicated in the development of atheroma from those which contribute in other ways to the clinical manifestations of vascular disease.

II. Risk Factors

The important risk factors are considered below in some detail.

A. Lipid Abnormalities

Epidemiologists have made use of the striking differences in incidence amongst adult populations of the frequency of raised atheromatous lesions and their clinical sequellae, CHD, stroke and peripheral arterial disease. An early and important study, the International Atherosclerosis Project (McGill, 1968), measured according to a standardized protocol the extent of atheroma in subjects autopsied for accidental or traumatic death in twelve different countries, allowing comparisons of nineteen different location–race groups. The prevalence of raised atheroma as measured in the autopsied subgroup correlated closely as would be expected with the prevalence of atheroma related disease.

When the populations were ranked in order of consumption of various dietary components the frequency of advanced atherosclerotic lesions was highly correlated with the percentage of calories derived from fat, and with the level of serum cholesterol. Fat intake in turn was highly correlated with animal protein intake. These findings were mirrored in the Seven Countries Study (Taylor *et al.*, 1970) where for defined population subsamples CHD incidence was measured in a standard way, diets from sample households were analysed and blood lipids were measured in a central laboratory. Populations with high CHD rates were characterized by high serum cholesterol levels and a high level of saturated fat in their diet, i.e. providing in excess of 15% of total calories. Those populations with little CHD had low average serum cholesterol levels and a low intake of saturated fat which provided 10% or less of total calories.

The importance of an elevated serum cholesterol level as a risk factor for raised atheromatous lesions and atheroma-related vascular disease has been supported by a wide variety of population studies and by animal experiments (National Heart Foundation of Australia, 1974). In man the value of the serum cholesterol level as a predictor of future morbidity and mortality from CHD has been confirmed in many studies in a number of different countries. The carefully analysed Framingham Study (Kannel *et al.*, 1971; McGee and Gordon, 1976) may be taken as the paradigm for such investigations and shows that within the range of serum cholesterol values found in a US population increasing serum cholesterol is almost linearly related to an increasing CHD risk.

In animals the induction of atheroma by dietary elevation of the serum cholesterol has been well known for many years, and more recently in rhesus monkeys dietary induced hyperlipidaemia was accompanied by atheroma formation, which subsequently largely regressed when the animals were restored to a normal diet (Armstrong *et al.*, 1970).

The association in epidemiological data between atheroma-caused disease and elevated blood lipids, in particular plasma cholesterol has been taken increasingly to indicate a causal relationship (Mann, 1979). This conclusion has been based upon a number of grounds which include:

1. The observed development of premature and severe atheromatous disease in individuals and families with inherited forms of hypercholesterolaemia.
2. The absence of atheroma in populations with low levels of plasma cholesterol.
3. The presence of atheroma at an early age and an increased frequency in populations with elevated levels of plasma cholesterol.
4. The increased risk of development of atheroma-related diseases in individuals with raised cholesterol levels.
5. The presence of cholesterol in the atheromatous lesion.
6. The observation that atheroma can be induced in the experimental animal by the feeding of cholesterol and in the presence of a consequently raised plasma cholesterol level.
7. Descriptions of reduction in atheromatous deposits in man and primates as a consequence of lowering the plasma cholesterol level by dietary and pharmacological intervention.
8. The pattern of an epidemic of atheroma-induced disease in high risk countries over past 100 years.

The whole question of the relationship of elevated plasma cholesterol levels to the development of atheroma has taken a further step with the demonstration that high density lipoprotein (HDL), a cholesterol carrying specific lipoprotein, has a greater predictive value for CHD risk than total cholesterol concentration (Kannel *et al.*, 1979). There is a strong negative correlation between HDL cholesterol levels and the incidence of CHD (National Heart Foundation, 1979). High levels of HDL are present in women in comparison with men and in persons with high exercise levels, while familial hyperalphalipoproteinaemia (excess HDL) appears to be associated with reduced vascular disease and longevity. Low levels of HDL occur in the obese, cigarette smokers, and diabetics (National Heart Foundation, 1979). It should be noted, however, that the low risk of vascular disease of vegetarians is not associated with high levels of HDL (Simons *et al.*, 1979).

The cumulative evidence that hyperlipidaemia and in particular hypercholesterolaemia, or low HDL levels, are implicated in the development of raised atheroma has led to a plethora of studies of the relationship between diet and the development of lipid abnormality. Cholesterol in the body derives from both *in vivo* synthesis and the diet. Excessive dietary cholesterol intake results in a predictable rise in blood cholesterol, though smaller rises are said to occur in those individuals who can suppress synthesis in these circumstances. The fatty acid pattern of glycerides is however the major dietary influence on the plasma total cholesterol level. Saturated fats are twice as powerful in raising cholesterol as polyunsaturated fats are in lowering the level (Blackburn, 1979). In most unsophisticated diets saturated fats provide some 8–10% of total calories, while total calories provided from all fats is below 15% (Stamler, 1967). In the affluent diet fats may provide up to 35–40% calories and the great preponderance of fats are saturated animal fats. In some countries with low CHD rates the diet includes a significant amount of olive oil which appears to have neither a cholesterol raising or lowering effect. Dietary plant sterols cause competitive inhibition of cholesterol absorption and hence lower the plasma cholesterol (Grundy and Mok, 1976). Other dietary components such as citrus pectins and plant gums also cause significant falls in serum cholesterol (Kay and Truswell, 1977). Fibre as such has not been shown to reduce plasma cholesterol in man (Raymond *et al.*, 1977; Truswell, 1978).

B. Smoking

Cigarette smoking is a potent risk factor for CHD in some countries. In the USA and UK the increase in mortality from CHD for cigarette smokers appears on average to be twofold but is significantly higher (three- to fivefold) for those in their thirties and forties and commensurately low (one and a half times) for those in their fifties and sixties

(Hammond, 1966; Hammond and Garfinkel, 1969; Doll and Peto, 1976). Some studies indicate that for smokers other manifestations of CHD such as angina and non-fatal infarction also increase comparably. The risk relates to the amount smoked and there is an almost linear dose response with those smoking most having the highest risk of CHD morbidity and mortality. Cessation of smoking is accompanied by a loss of risk back to a non-smoking level within a few years (Kannel *et al.*, 1968; Hammond, 1971). In male smokers who have suffered a non-fatal myocardial infarct, cessation of smoking halves future risk of both non-fatal and fatal infarction (Wilhelmsson *et al.*, 1975). In women who smoke less and inhale less the risk of complications are lower (Hammond, 1971).

The effects of cigarette smoking on the heart are thought in part to be mediated through nicotine which causes well described acute circulatory effects and predisposes to tachycardia and arrhythmias (Herxheimer *et al.*, 1967). Smoking also causes elevated free fatty acid levels in the blood (Kershbaum *et al.*, 1962), increased platelet adhesiveness (Mustard and Packham, 1970) and reduced oxygen-carrying capacity due to the presence of carboxyhaemoglobin. Whether or not cigarette smoking is a cause of atheroma is uncertain. The Seven Countries Study (Taylor *et al.*, 1970) found the highest smoking levels in the Japanese who had the lowest CHD mortality rates. In that study the effect of smoking on CHD mortality was not evident in other low risk populations including the Italians and Greeks. In high risk populations, as in USA and Sweden, the effect of smoking is markedly enhanced by the presence of other risk factors notably hypercholesterolaemia; for example, the incidence of CHD is five times higher in a population of smokers with elevated blood cholesterol as compared with normocholesterolaemic smokers (Doyle *et al.*, 1964).

The absence of effect of smoking in populations with an otherwise low risk factor status, in particular with low plasma cholesterol levels, and the relatively rapid loss of risk with cessation of smoking suggest that most of the effect is not through the development of atheroma but through other shorter term effects such as might occur with changes in blood flow, oxygen carriage and electrical stability of the heart.

C. Hypertension

One of the most consistent findings in major prospective epidemiological studies of cardiovascular risk factors has been the significant correlations of increased risk of CHD across a wide range of increase in blood pressure. In both men and women in middle age a two to threefold increase in CDH occurs in hypertensives as compared to normotensives (Kannel *et al.*, 1961; Kannel *et al.*, 1969). As previously indicated the combination with one or more other major risk factors has a marked additional effect on the incidence of morbidity and mortality.

Treatment of hypertension has clear-cut benefit on the incidence of haemorrhagic cerebrovascular accident but has not always been shown to be of benefit in preventing future CHD (Veterans Administration Cooperative Study Group, 1967, 1970). Positive benefit has been described in recent trials in Sweden (Berglund *et al.*, 1978) and Australia (Reader *et al.*, 1979) where reduction of blood pressure has been associated with a reduction in both fatal and non-fatal manifestations of CHD.

In autopsy studies correlations between blood pressure and evidence of atherosclerosis have been established and it seems probable that arterial hypertension accelerates the development of atherosclerosis in larger arteries including the coronary arteries (Evans, 1965). In some populations where hypertension is common such as Japan, atheroma is rare, adding further weight to the hypothesis that hypertension is additive to, rather than causative of, atherosclerosis. The cumulative effect of risk factors has been noted already in man, and in this instance has been confirmed in animal experiments where atherosclerosis has been accelerated in hypertensive rats fed an atherogenic diet in comparison to normotensive control animals (Daley and Deming, 1963).

D. Diabetes Mellitus

As a group, diabetics, including those with mild diabetes, have a higher death rate than age, sex matched controls (Pell and D'Alonzo, 1970). They have a higher incidence of obesity (Welborn *et al.*, 1969b), hypertension (Welborn *et al.*, 1970), hyperlipidaemia (Keen, 1972) and low levels of HDL (Stamler, 1967). At autopsy extensive atherosclerosis is common, and it is the complications of atherosclerosis including CHD which predominate as the cause of mortality in diabetes (Robertson and Strory, 1968).

The outstanding abnormality of diabetes is, of course, the elevated blood glucose. Hyperglycaemia has been suggested as an independent risk factor for CHD. Diabetes is, however, a complex metabolic disturbance and a clear-cut determination of the role of hyperglycaemia is not available.

E. Physical Inactivity

The evidence for an association between physical inactivity and an increased risk of CHD has been reviewed in a number of reports (National Heart Foundation of New Zealand, 1971; Working Group, 1975). The cohort study of longshoremen showed that a high energy expenditure at work reduced the risk of fatal myocardial infarction in males under fifty-four by threefold in comparison to less physically active workers. The combination of low energy output, heavy smoking and high blood pressure increased risk by up to twentyfold (Paffenbarger *et al.*, 1977). These findings are in keeping with earlier reports (Morris *et al.*, 1973; Paffenbarger and Hale, 1975).

Physical exercise seems to make little difference to blood cholesterol levels but is associated with increased levels of HDL (Wood *et al.*, 1976). Triglyceride levels are usually reduced significantly (Carlson and Mossfeldt, 1964). The coagulation characteristics of the blood are also changed by exercise which causes an increase in fibrinolytic activity in many individuals (Berkanda *et al.*, 1971). Exercise is also held to promote vasodilation and collateral vessel formation in the coronary circulation, but direct evidence of this is difficult to obtain. Certainly regular exercise increases the functional capacity of the heart as evidenced by maximal oxygen uptake, but a certain minimum level of exercise is necessary to achieve this response (Siegel *et al.*, 1970). Regular exercise is usually a significant aid to weight control.

The general thesis of the benefits of exercise is difficult to refute and only sporadic observations such as the high incidence of CHD in Finnish lumberjacks have been offered as detracting from the evidence cited above. The overall disadvantageous risk status of the Finns in relation to blood lipids and cigarette smoking has now been extensively documented and the unusual features of timber work in subarctic temperatures may also be relevant.

F. Obesity

The measurement of obesity presents methodological difficulties that have been reviewed elsewhere (National Heart Foundation of New Zealand, 1971; Working Group, 1975). Actuarial data offer extensive documentation of the relationship between excess weight and the risk of dying of cardiovascular disease (Kannel *et al.*, 1967). In men increased weight has been shown to correlate with an increased risk of sudden death (CHD), independent of the associated increase in hypertension and blood cholesterol (Kannel *et al.*, 1967). It must be recognized, however, that obesity is highly correlated in affluent populations with increased blood pressure, lipidaemia and diabetes mellitus (Welborn *et al.*, 1969a). This does not hold for all populations since in the Seven Countries Study (Taylor *et al.*, 1970) Italian and Yugoslav men were fatter as measured by skinfold thickness than US men but had a much lower incidence of CHD. The obesity of the two European populations was not associated with the marked lipidaemia of the US population.

G. Endocrine

(1) Hypothyroidism has been reported as being associated with increased mortality from CHD and an increased prevalence of coronary artery atherosclerosis (Varhaelst *et al.*, 1967). In hypothyroidism the blood cholesterol level is usually elevated.

(2) The pharmacological administration of oestrogens has been recorded as increasing the incidence of CHD in two situations. Firstly, high dose oestrogen when given to men suffering from carcinoma of the prostate was shown to be associated with an increased death rate from CHD (The Coronary Drug Project Research Group, 1970). In premenopausal women the use of oestrogen in the oral contraceptive pill has been shown to increase the frequency of both fatal and non-fatal myocardial infarction (Rosenberg *et al.*, 1976). The usual cumulation with other major risk factors has been observed in this instance.

H. Stress and Personality Type, Social Status

There is a public belief in the role of stress in the causation of CHD. Measurement of stress poses major methodological problems. Wilhelmsen was unable to show any increase in CHD in men suffering from self-perceived stress (L. Wilhelmsen, personal communication).

Personality types have been described which are said to be associated with an increased incidence of CHD. Such at-risk personalities are often found to suffer from other risk factors such as elevated serum cholesterol levels and high blood pressure and to include more cigarette smokers. The role of these factors is uncertain and definitive reviews suggest the need for further studies in this area (Jenkins, 1976).

The risk of CHD now appears to be more closely related to socioeconomic background and educational status than to job stress. While CHD levels were once reported to be highest in professional and white collar workers this is no longer the case. Morris (1970) has recorded the marked decline in deaths from CHD in upper socioeconomic groups in the UK. Current studies now show an excess of risk in the lower social groups, so-called blue collar workers (Pole *et al.*, 1977). This reversal of risk status is an interesting phenomenon of the progress of the epidemic.

I. A Positive Family History of Premature Vascular Disease

Familial aggregation of cardiovascular disease is not surprising. Genetic factors are clearly influential and may rarely be overwhelmingly so as in familial hypercholesterolaemia or familial hyperalphalipoproteinaemia. Other not yet identified genetic influences may also be significant to some degree. On the other hand, because families tend to share a common diet and life-style, the effect of environmental influences will be similar. Studies quoted later, in particular those of migrant groups, suggest that so far as the epidemic appearance of vascular disease is concerned, environmental factors are primarily responsible.

J. Risk Factors—Summary

In simplified form the propositions of the risk factor hypothesis of vascular disease are as follows:

Atheroma is the basic lesion of cardiovascular disease.

Atheroma is a consequence of blood lipid abnormalities and its development is hastened by other physiological and biochemical abnormalities such as are caused by hypertension and possibly cigarette smoking.

The major lipid abnormality causing atheroma is hypercholesterolaemia and/or low HDL levels, and the frequency of these abnormalities in high risk populations is primarily due to extrinsic factors though in a small group of people genetic factors are of major importance.

The factors which cause hypercholesterolaemia are chiefly dietary.

The dietary factors of recognized importance are the total fat intake, the proportion of saturated to unsaturated fats, the total cholesterol intake and possibly the intake of refined carbohydrates.

These factors have come to be major components of the diet of particular affluent societies because of the technological developments of this century.

The clinical complications or manifestations of atheromatous disease are influenced by other factors such as cigarette smoking, lack of exercise and obesity.

The complex web of interactions which finally manifests in overt CHD is shown schematically in Fig. 1. The influence of lipid abnormality is central to the development of atherosclerosis but the onset of consequences of arterial obstruction may be influenced by many factors such as work level of the heart, the presence or absence of collateral vessels, and the influence of nicotine on myocardial electrical stability.

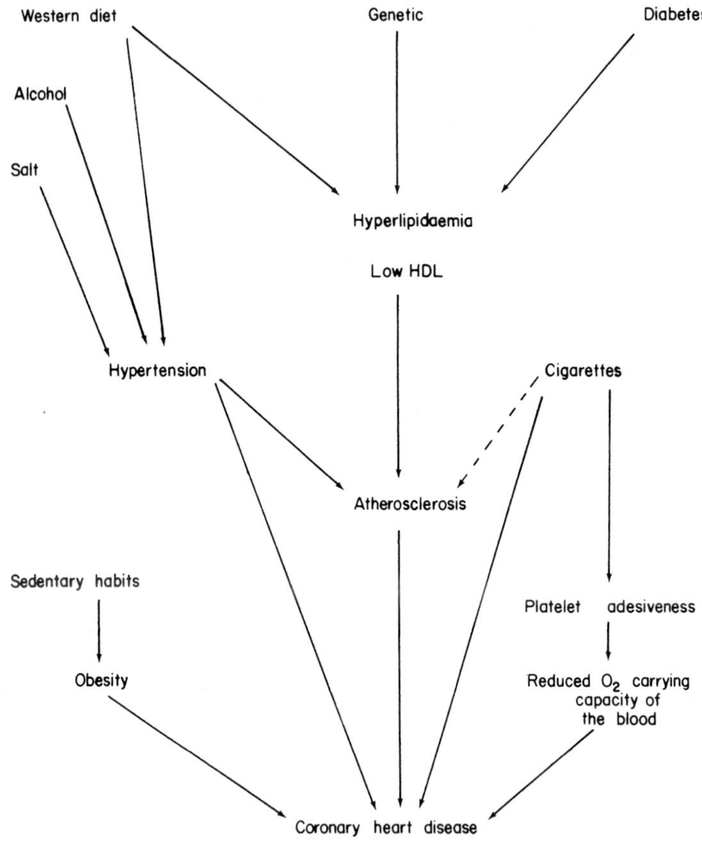

Fig. 1. Illustrates the complexity of the interrelationships between risk factors, the development of primary arterial lesion (atherosclerosis) and the onset of clinical coronary heart disease.

III. Diet, Society and Vascular Disease

The role of risk factors, and in particular lipid abnormality in the causation of atheroma has been reviewed in the preceding section. As already indicated the generally accepted explanation of the current epidemic of vascular disease in affluent countries posits that environmental factors, in particular diet, have been responsible in certain affluent societies for community-wide hyperlipidaemia. Evidence for this has been extensively reviewed elsewhere and the following commentary is consequently brief.

Of the diversity of studies which have addressed this problem, one of the simplest approaches has been the cross-sectional comparison of commodity consumption patterns of countries with differing CHD mortality rates. A frequent finding of such studies is a strong positive correlation between consumption of animal protein, saturated fat and refined carbohydrate and CHD levels. The limitations of such studies have been recently reviewed (Armstrong *et al.*, 1975).

Within a single population changes in commodity consumption with time can be recorded and related to changes in plasma lipid level and vascular mortality. In a recent example of such a study in Belgium (Joosens *et al.*, 1977) a strong association was found between both increasing intakes of polyunsaturated fats and decreasing consumption of saturated fats with falling blood lipid levels and lower CHD mortality. Within-country comparisons can also be made between groups whose diet differs for ethnic religious or other reasons. Seventh-Day Adventists are a vegetarian group who also avoid cigarette and alcohol consumption; as such they have extremely low rates of cardiovascular morbidity and mortality in comparison with other members of affluent communities (Phillips *et al.*, 1975). In both USA (West and Hayes, 1968; Sacks *et al.*, 1975) and Australia (Armstrong *et al.*, 1977) low lipid levels and blood pressure levels have been found in Seventh-Day Adventists in comparison with age–sex matched non-vegetarian controls. Within vegetarian groups, as adherence to absolute vegetarianism decreased, blood pressure and serum cholesteral levels increased (Armstrong *et al.*, 1977). Manipulation of the proportions of saturated and unsaturated fat in the diet of vegetarians causes changes in blood lipids with the cholesterol level falling as the polyunsaturated: saturated fat ratio increases (Walden *et al.*, 1964).

Of particular significance are studies of diet, lipid level and vascular disease frequency in populations migrating from low CHD risk areas to high risk areas (Toore *et al.*, 1957; Stenhouse and McCall, 1970; Abu-zeid *et al.*, 1978). Kagan *et al.* (1974), in serial studies of Japanese living in Japan, Hawaii and California, have confirmed genetic homogeneity of these populations and found strong associations between increasing levels of dietary fat and increasing serum cholesterol levels.

A general pattern of the effect of specific dietary ingredients on blood lipid levels and the incidence of CHD has been built up from a large number of studies, examples of which have been quoted. Where apparently contradictory findings have been investigated, i.e. populations with high fat intakes and a low level of cardiovascular disease, low cholesterol levels have been present. The low cholesterol levels have resulted from particular characteristics of the fats ingested. For example, Eskimos (Dyerberg and Bang, 1979) have a high polyunsaturated fat intake which is associated not only with low cholesterol levels but alteration in platelet function. In the Masei (National Heart Foundation, 1979), despite the preponderance of saturated fats in milk, a variety of factors appear to inhibit the effect of the saturated fats including changes occurring in the souring process of milk. There are then substantial data bodies (Mann, 1979) to support the role of diet in determining blood lipid level at both a population level and in the individual.

Why has a particular diet with such an influence on blood lipids and hence atheroma formation developed in some affluent countries?

The development of the affluent life-style has been the remarkable socioeconomic phenomenon of this century. As a result of technological innovation, systems of food production, processing and marketing have developed which, while adhering to the established tenets of hygiene have never been assessed as to their long-term effects on health. Knowledge about the nutritional aspects of diet, including discovery of trace elements and vitamins largely originated from short-term animal experiments. Relatively few long-term experiments have been conducted and it is understandable that this aspect of the consequences of eating patterns has been hitherto neglected by industry.

The pattern of increasing technology has been the further processing of basic food items to increase appeal and facilitate marketing. There has been a concentration on the extreme taste sensations of sweetness and saltiness, and the achievement of textural characteristics analagous to those resulting from mastication. Another component of this change has been to maximize caloric content. To these ends we have seen grains milled, stripping away the fibre and germinal layers and then pre-treated to render the carbohydrate core more digestible. Fruit bearing plants and vegetables have been progressively selected to achieve greater sweetness often at the expense of more subtle flavour characteristics. The end result of plant breeding and the processing of foods of basically complex carbohydrate construction has been to speed the release of simple carbohydrate constituents to give immediate appeal to the palate. In the alimentary tract digestion continues with unwonted speed. Cleeve (1974) has written convincingly of the likely consequences of the surges of blood sugar which result in these circumstances in contrast to the slow release of sugars which occurs from the digestion of the unprocessed food stuff. In human studies the magnitude of these blood sugar surges are now being measured and the consequences for insulin production and body metabolism are being recognized (Simpson *et al.*, 1979). The remarkable frequency of development of diabetes in Aboriginal people who adopt to excess the worst aspects of the affluent refined carbohydrate diet (namely white flour and sugar) is now a well-described phenomenon (Cleeve, 1974). It appears that they may represent only the extreme end of the spectrum with much of the affluent population in close proximity.

As Blackburn (1979) has indicated the changes wrought by technology on national dietary habits have not been as a consequence of awareness of desirable eating patterns, nor as part of any deliberate overall policy, but have evolved from economic productivity, where availability, cost and marketing have each played significant roles. The particular food products which have come to dominate any particular national dietary have been promoted by "happenstance".

In those countries with highest rates for CHD a major original component in the national dietary was the cow and its products. Technological changes expanded these components of the national diet. Beef production and consumption have risen remarkably in countries such as USA and Australia. At the same time the characteristics of the beef changed to favour higher percentages of intramuscular fat. Breeding programmes favoured those strains which achieved early fat cover while grain feed lots replaced free range grazing, hastening the production of prime "marbled", i.e. fat-infiltrated meat.

The provision of cow's milk for infants and the continuation of milk drinking into adult life was facilitated by the development of pasteurization and then by the increasing availability of cold storage and later refrigeration. Milk purity was judged by its butterfat content and again breeding programmes concentrated upon dairy strains with high butterfat yield. Refrigeration also lead to the mass availability of a new range of dairy products such as icecream in which the fat content of milk is augmented and sugars are added to increase sweetness. Similar factors contributed to increased butter and cheese availability. The role of fat in increasing palatability has not been confined to meat. The fast food industry has produced fat rich, highly salted meat and vegetable products which are playing an increasing role in the national diet of many countries.

The importance of hypertension in the acceleration of atheroma has already been remarked. Hypertension like hyperlipidaemia has a pronounced variation in geographic incidence. Freis (1976) in a substantial review of the relationship of salt intake to hypertension finds evidence to suggest that:

In unaccultured peoples the prevalence of hypertension is inversely correlated with the degree of salt intake.

The extracellular fluid volume is expanded in salt eaters in comparison to non-salt eaters and experimentally chronic hypertension is a response to a sustained increase in extracellular fluid volume.

The blood pressure of hypertensive patients falls with dietary salt restriction.

Elsewhere, Armstrong *et al.* (1977) have published evidence relating the lower blood pressures found in vegetarians of varying strictness not to differences in salt intake but to the intake of non-vegetable protein, higher levels of non-vegetable protein intake being associated with higher blood pressure readings. In other studies elevated blood pressure has been associated with high alcohol intake (Mathews, 1976).

While it is too early to certainly implicate diet as the cause of hypertension in affluent countries the studies noted above are highly suggestive that as with hyperlipidaemia the cause may well lie in the dietary practices of affluent communities.

IV. Conclusion

There is now a large body of scientific opinion supporting the view that changes in food pattern are fundamental to the development of atherosclerotic disease. The effect of the nutritional pattern has been exaggerated by other cultural changes. The provision of cheap mass motorized transportation and the consequent reduction in exercise in work and at leisure has contributed to the high frequency of obesity in adult life. Furthermore, the habit of inhalation of tobacco smoke results in chemical and physiological changes which are particularly deleterious to myocardial function. Looking at these phenomena in the light of human evolution it is not surprising to find that an animal adapted originally to the gathering of fruits, nuts and cereals and which probably obtained animal protein only at the price of severe physical exertion should develop metabolic disorders when confronted with an *ad lib* supply of nutrients which were scarce in its evolutionary history and that addictive habits such as cigarette smoking will have unwanted side effects.

The difficulties of the epidemic of cardiovascular disease stem not from any problem in comprehending its causes, but because whole populations are involved and the economic fabric of their societies is bound up in the established patterns of agriculture and the food industry.

There is evidence that the upper socioeconomic groups were initially the major victims of affluence but that this is no longer the case. Upper socioeconomic groups have changed their patterns of consumption from the norm. They smoke less (Doll and Peto, 1976), take more exercise in leisure time and would appear to be reducing their fat and refined carbohydrate consumption (Macoby and Farquhar, 1975; Gibson *et al.*, 1977). The required changes to life-style do not require intelligence so much as the capacity for self-discipline—the cessation of smoking, continuation of exercise in later life, consumption of food and alcohol in moderation and the replacement of dietary components associated with a high atherosclerosis rate with those which are not. We live in an age where the cult of individual freedom from restraint and inhibition is exalted and self-discipline and self-denial are denigrated. The response of the majority of the population may remain at issue for years to come.

References

Abu-Zeid, H. A. H., Maini, K. K. and Choi, N. W. (1978). *J. chron, Dis.* **31**, 137–146.

Armstrong, M. L., Warner, E. D. and Connor, W. E. (1970). *Circulation Res.* **27**, 59.

Armstrong, B. K., Mann, J. I., Adelstein, A. M. and Eskin, F. (1975). *J. chron. Dis.* **28**, 455–469.

Armstrong, B. K., van Merwyk, A. J. and Coates, H. (1977). *Am. J. Epidemiol.* **105**, 444–449.

Berglund, G., Wilhelmson, L. *et al.* (1978). *Lancet* i, 1–5.

Berkanda, B., Akokan, G. and Derman, U. (1971). *Atherosclerosis* **13**, 85.

Blackburn, H. (1979). *In* "Nutrition, Lipids and Coronary Heart Disease" (R. Levy, B. Refkind, B. Dennis and N. Ernst, Eds). Raven Press, New York.

British Medical Journal (1976). Editorial. *Br. med. J.* i, 58.

Carlson, L. A. and Mossfeldt, F. (1964). *Acta physiol. scand,* **62**, 51.

Cleeve, T. L. (1974). *In* "The Saccharine Disease", Wright, Bristol.

Cooper, R., Stamler, J., Dyer, A. and Garside, D. (1978). *J. chron. Dis.* **31**, 709–720.

Coronary Drug Project Research Group (1970). *J. Am. Med. Ass.* **214**, 1303–1313.

Daley, M. M. and Deming, Q. B. (1963). *J. clin. Invest.* **43**, 1606.

Doll, R. and Peto, R. (1976). *Br. med. J.* ii, 1525–1536.

Doyle, J. T., Dawber, T. R., Kannel, W. B., Kinch, S. H. and Khan, H. A. (1964). *J. Am. med. Ass.* **190**, 886.
Dyerberg, J. and Bang, H. O. (1979). *Lancet* i, 433–435.
Evans, P. H. (1965). *Lancet* i, 516.
Florey, C. du V., Melia, R. J. W. and Darby, S. C. (1978). *Br. med. J.* i, 635–637.
Freis, E. D. (1976). *Circulation* **53**, 589–595.
Gibson, J., Johansen, A., Rawson, G. and Webster, I. (1977). *Med. J. Aust.* **2**, 459–461.
Gordon, T., Sorlie, P. and Kannel, W. B. (1976). "The Framingham Study. An epidemiological investigation of cardiovascular disease", Section 27. Department of Health, Education and Welfare Publ., Washington, DC. US Govt. Printing Office.
Grundy, S. M. and Mok, H. Y. I. (1976). *In* "Lipoprotein Metabolism" (H. Greten, Ed.). Springer-Verlag, Berlin.
Guberan, E. (1979). *J. Epidem. Comm. Hlth* **33**, 114–120.
Hammond, E. C. (1966). *In* "Epidemiological Approaches to the Study of Cancer and Other Diseases". National Cancer Institute Monograph No. 19.
Hammond, E. C. (1971). *In* "The Second World Conference on Smoking and Health".
Hammond, E. C. and Garfinkel, L. (1969). *Archs environ. Hlth* **19**, 167.
Herxheimer, A., Griffiths, R. L., Hamilton, B. and Wakefield, M. (1967). *Lancet* ii, 754.
Jenkins, D. C. (1976). *New Engl. J. Med.* **294**, 987–994 and 1033–1038.
Joosens, J. V., Vuylsteek, K., Bremo-Heyns, E. *et al.* (1977). *Lancet* i, 1069–1072.
Kagan, A., Harris, B. R., Winkelstein, W., Johnson, K. G., Kato, H., Syme, S. L., Rhoads, G.G., Gay M. L., Nickaman, M. Z., Hamilton, H. B. and Tillotson, J. (1974). *J. chron. Dis.* **27**, 345–364.
Kannel, W. B., Dawber, T. R., Kagan, A., Revotskie, N. and Stokes, J. (1961). *Ann. intern. Med.* **55**, 33.
Kannel, W. B., Castelli, W. P. and McNamara, P. M. (1967). *J. occup. Med.* **9**, 611.
Kannel, W. B., Castelli, W. P. and McNamara, P. M. (1968). "Cigarette Smoking and Risk of Coronary Heart Disease. Epidemiologic Clues to Pathogenesis. The Framingham Study". National Cancer Institute Monograph No. 28.
Kannel, W. B., Schwartz, M. J. and McNamara, P. M. (1969). *Dis. Chest* **56**, 43.
Kannel, W. B., Castelli, W. P., Gordon, T. and McNamara, P. M. (1971). *Ann. intern Med.* **74**, 1–12.
Kannel, W. B., Castelli, W. P. and Gordon, T. (1979). *Ann. intern Med.* **90**, 85–91.
Kay, R. M. and Truswell, A. S. (1977). *Am. J. clin. Nutr.* **30**, 171.
Keen, H. (1972). *Proc Nutr. Soc.* **31**, 339–345.

Kershbaum, A., Bellet, S., Caplin, R. F. and Feinberg, L. J. (1962). *Am. J. Cardiol.* **10**, 204.
Macoby, N. and Farquhar, J. W. (1975). *J. Commun.* **25**, 114–126.
Mann, J. I. (1979). *Br. med. J.* i, 732–734.
Mathews, J. D. (1976). *Aust. N.Z. J. Med.* **6**, 393–397.
McGee, D. and Gordon, T. (1976). "The Framingham Study: The Results of the Framingham Study Applied to Four Other US-based Epidemiologic Studies of Cardiovascular Disease", Section 31, 76–1083. Department of Health, Education and Welfare Publ., Washington DC.
McGill, H. C. (1968). *J. Lab. Invest.* **18**, 465–467.
Morris, J. N. (1970). "Uses of Epidemiology". E. and S. Livingstone, Edinburgh.
Morris, J. N., Chave, S. P. W., Adam, C. and Sirey, C. (1973). *Lancet* i, 333–339.
Mustard, J. F. and Packham, M. A. (1970). *Pharmac. Rev.* **22**, 97.
National Heart Foundation of Australia (1974). *Med. J. Aust.* **1**, 575.
National Heart Foundation of Australia (1979). *Med. J. Aust.* **2**, 294–357.
National Heart Foundation of New Zealand (1971). "Coronary Heart Disease, a New Zealand Report". NHF of NZ.
Paffenbarger, R. S. and Hale, W. E. (1975). *New Engl. J. Med.* **292**, 545–550.
Paffenbarger, R. S., Hale, W. E., Brand, R. J. and Hyde, R. T. (1977). *Am. J. Epidem.* **105**, 200–213.
Pell, S. and D'Alonzo, C. A. (1970). *J. Am. med. Ass.* **214**, 1833.
Phillips, R. L., Lemon, F., Hammond, C. and Kuzma, J. (1975). American Public Health Association Meeting, Chicago.
Pole, D. J., McCall, M. G., Reader, R. and Woodings, T. J. (1977). *J. chron. Dis.* **30**, 19–27.
Raymond, T. L., Connor, W. E., Lui, D. S. *et al.* (1977). *J. clin. Invest.* **60**, 1429.
Reader, R. (1975). *In* "Patholphysiology and Management of Arterial Hypertension" (G. Berglund, ed.), Lindgren and Soner, Sweden.
Reader, R. *et al.* (1980). The Australian Therapeutic Trial in Mild Hypertension. *Lancet* i, 1261–1267.
Robertson, W. B. and Strory, J. P. (1968). *Lab. Invest.* **18**, 538.
Rosenberg, L., Armstrong, B. and Jick, H. (1976). *New Engl. J. Med.* **294**, 1256–1259.
Sacks, F. N., Castelli, W. P., Donner, A. and Kass, E. H. (1975). *New Engl. J. Med.* **292**, 1148–1151.
Siegel, W., Blomquist, G. and Mitchell, J. H. (1970). *Circulation* **41**, 19.
Simons, L., Gibson, J., Jones, A. and Bain, D. (1979). *Med. J. Aust.* **2**, 148.
Simpson, R. W., Mann, J. I., Eaton, J., Carter, R. D. and Hockaday, T. D. R. (1979). *Br. med. J.* ii, 523–525.
Stamler, J. (1967). *In* "Lectures on Preventive Cardiology". Grune-Stratton, New York.
Stenhouse, N. S. and McCall, M. G. (1970). *J. chron. Dis.* **23**, 423.
Sturmans, F., Mulder, P. G. H. and Valkenburg, H. A. (1977). *Am. J. Epidem.* **105**, 281–289.

Taylor, H. L., Blackburn, H., Keys, A., Parlin, R. W., Vaquez, C. and Puckness, T. (1970). *Circulation* **41**, Suppl. 1, 1–211.

Toore, M., Katchalsky, A., Agmon, J. and Allouf, D. (1957). *Lancet* i, 1270–1273.

Truswell, A. S. (1978). *Am. J. Nutr.* **31**, 977.

Varhaelst, L., Neve, P., Chailly, P. and Besteine, P. A. (1967). *Lancet* ii, 800.

Veterans Administration Cooperative Study Group (1967). *J. Am. med. Ass.* **202**, 1028–1034.

Veterans Administration Cooperative Study Group (1970). *J. Am. med. Ass.* **213**, 1143–1152.

Walden, R. T., Schaeffer, L. E., Lemon, F. R., Sunshine, A. and Wynder, E. L. (1964). *Am. J. Med.* **36**, 269–276.

Welborn, T. A., Cumpston, G. N., Cullen, K. J., Curnow, D. H., McCall, M. G. and Stenhouse, N. S. (1969a). *Am. J. Epidem.* **89**, 521–536.

Welborn, T. A., Stenhouse, N. S. and Johnstone, C. G. (1969b). *Diabetologia* **5**, 263–266.

Welborn, T. A., Jenkins, D. J. A., Cumpston, N. G., Goff, D. V., Curnow, D. H., Johnstone, C. G., Stenhouse, N. S. and Summers, M. (1970). *In* "Proceedings of the Second International Symposium on Atherosclerosis", 369–374, Chicago.

West, R. O. and Hayes, O. B. (1968). *Am. J. clin. Nutr.* **21**, 853–862.

WHO (1958). Classification of Atherosclerotic Lesions. *Wld Hlth Org. Tech. Rep. Ser.* No. 143.

WHO (1971). Cerebrovascular diseases. *Wld Hlth Org. Tech. Rep. Ser.* No. 469.

Wilhelmsson, C., Vedin, A., Elmfeldt, D., Tibblin, G. and Wilhelmsen, L. (1975). *Lancet* i, 415–419.

Wood, P. D., Haskell, W., Klein, H. *et al.* (1976). *Metabolism* **25**, 1249.

Working Group, Australian Academy of Science (1975). "Report on Diet and Coronary Heart Disease". Griffin Press, South Australia.

29
Medical Care of Elderly Disabled People

R. B. Lefroy*

Department of Medicine, University of Western Australia, Perth, Australia

---

Attention must be given not only to the study of disease but to the essential nature of the ageing process if we are to progress towards a healthy old age.

---

* Associate Professor.

Progress generally refers to beneficial growth and change. Diseases of progress, on the other hand, represent some of the adverse effects of change. Is it reasonable to include old age among them? It cannot be denied that along with the progress made towards higher standards of living in the so-called developed countries old age is more in evidence; moreover, there is a significant group of diseased old people. Although it is misleading to regard old age as a disease, there are some important connections between these three factors—age, disease and progress.

I. Survival and Longevity

The experience of old age by a significant proportion of the population is a relatively new phenomenon. In ancient Rome the mean human life span was twenty-two years (Walford, 1974). There was little change until about three centuries ago and it was not until the first sixty years of this century that a spectacular rise occurred; at the end of that period twenty years had been added to life expectancy at birth. This undeniable progress has been directly associated with industrialization; in particular, it has been due to development of public health measures, better nutrition and the absence of infectious disease. The difference in the survival curve for a population in ancient Rome compared with one of our own time is represented in Fig. 1. Formerly the advent of death was relatively uncontrolled and often happened early in life: it was not predominantly a feature of late life as it is today.

The increase in life expectancy at birth which has led to more people surviving to old age is not an indication of improvement in longevity. The curve, as Fig. 1 illustrates, has altered its shape but not its termination. More people can now expect to survive the vicissitudes of early and middle life; this represents progress but not an increase in life span. "Roman senators lived just as long as our own—and were just as useful" (Walford, 1974).

Longevity, in contradistinction to life expectancy, is concerned with what happens at the right-hand end of the curve; this is where the consequences of the ageing process are to be found. Whatever progress has been achieved in earlier life the chances of survival now lessen while mortality rate increases. Gompertz in 1825 pointed out that after middle life mortality is a logarithmic function of chronological age, with the probability of dying doubling every eight years. Whatever eventually prove to be the actual causes of ageing, this dramatic increase in mortality in the latter part of life is the essence of the process. Comfort (1977) refers to the "rising force of mortality" with the exam-

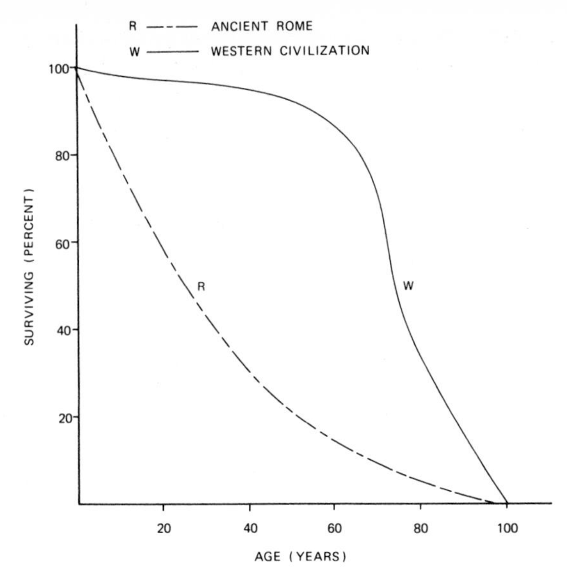

Fig. 1. Survival curves for populations of ancient Rome and Western civilization. (After Walford, 1974.)

ple of a man seventy-one years old who is forty-one times more likely to die that year than his twenty-one year old colleague.

Old age is neither a disease nor a phenomenon of progress. Nevertheless, an increased proportion of the population now survives to the phase of life when ageing becomes manifest as a force of mortality and morbidity. To what extent does this represent progress: or does the increase in numbers of elderly people mean nothing more than increase in disease?

II. Age, Health and Disease

Because of the fundamental association between ageing and mortality it is frequently assumed that there is a similar connection between ageing and disease. This myth has had unfortunate consequences for elderly people. All societies, ancient and modern, have had their biological élite, people who are chronologically old but who display considerable vigour in the absence of disease; they are proof that there is no essential association between age and disease and that these two phenomena must be given separate consideration. An understanding of the so-called diseases of progress—diseases seen in (but not necessarily of) old age—is impossible if this distinction is not made.

The new phenomenon is that death can now be postponed by public health and other measures but not necessarily with retention of vigour and adaptability. Those who have lived through middle life have made the survival curve more square; but this also means that an increased proportion of people are now more susceptible to disease. More of those who have reached old age, by virtue of society's progress, are vulnerable to the conditions known as the diseases of progress.

Experimental gerontologists are often criticized on the grounds that their work will merely increase the period of infirm old age, but this is not their intention. Rather, it is to promote health by increasing the length of adult vigour and thereby decreasing vulnerability to disease. Attention must be given not only to the study of disease but to the essential nature of the ageing process if we are to progress towards a healthy old age. Increase in survival need not result in increase in disease.

III. Characteristics of the Ageing Process

Even though the underlying causes of ageing are obscure, it is possible to describe the nature of the process in general terms. It is an essential part of the developmental life-cycle, beginning in human beings in their twenties and manifest by progressive and irreversible changes eventually leading to death. Compared with the specific names given to many diseases, lethal or otherwise, this terminology is purposely vague. When searching for a description of the effects of the ageing process one relies on general terms such as decline in vigour and increased vulnerability to disease. The lack of specificity and its general effect on mortality is one of the hallmarks of the ageing process. It is, of course, possible to describe certain manifestations of human ageing. There are obvious features such as decline in body height due to degeneration of intervertebral discs, thinning and wrinkling of the skin, some diminution in the energy output of heart and lungs and in the efficiency of eye and ear; changes in the nervous system are represented by less agility in maintaining balance and posture, by difficulty with memory, slowness of perception and by alterations in certain regulatory functions such as temperature and blood pressure. Less obvious are a decrease in lean body mass and changes in the function of endocrine glands and immune reactions. Nevertheless, such a description does not provide a full appreciation of the process of ageing.

An essential part of the ageing concept is that it leads to death. Natural death, if it occurred, would be solely due to ageing; a number of other processes determine the more frequent form of unnatural death. The full force of ageing leading to natural death can rarely be recognized in the wild because of the abundance of predators and other adverse aspects of the environment (Comfort, 1969). Similarly it is often prevented from exerting its full influence in our so-called developed society—for instance, the victims of traffic crashes. Decline in vigour is masked in both these situations; although it does become evident in animals held captive in a protected environment, as well as in the pedestrian who by virtue of his age becomes more vulnerable to the lethal effect of motor vehicles.

It follows from the above that the increased liability of dying can be used as a measurement of the ageing process. Susceptibility to disease and death increases with age in exponential terms; physiological adaptation progressively declines. In this manner longevity is determined.

Walford (1974) draws attention to measurement of the effect of ageing in a different context. In order to obtain the best single statistical parameter of ageing one should seek out the longest living survivors in a population. Being relatively free from disease they are a group whose survival has not been significantly affected by their environment. Probably because of their genetic inheritance they have become the biologic élite.

IV. The Demography of Ageing

Survival into old age is now not only a fact, it is often referred to as a problem because of associated disease. We need to estimate the extent to which this occurs if a rational approach is to be made to the so-called problem; wrong assumptions lead to misguided solutions, to the detriment particularly of old people.

The increasing proportion of elderly people in the population has followed industrialization; consequently, it has only affected the minority of the world's population. The ratio of the less developed to the more developed nations is about 2·5 to 1 (Hendricks and Hendricks, 1978). As this ratio changes so also will the numbers of people who make up the aged section of each society; this is not a change which occurs in isolation but one which must have its effect on those other major sections of the population—the workforce and the young dependant. Nor does it happen simply because of a lowered mortality rate. Countries which have shown the more dramatic increase in life expectancy have been those with the lowest birth rate. Declining fertility rate is the crucial variable in determining the ageing of a society.

A diagrammatic representation (Fig. 2) of these different age groups—the so-called elderly, the workforce and the young dependant—show the changes that have taken place and that are being forecast for the future in Australia and similar countries. At the beginning of the century the shape of the diagram was pyramidal; the diagram became more square with the "middle-aged spread" in the 1950s due to the smaller proportion of children. As life expectancy increases along with the stable or declining birth rate the increased proportion in the over sixty-five age group makes a further change in configuration. Because of the increased life expectancy of women the diagram has become lop-sided. Factors other than fertility rate and mortality rate influence the age grouping of society; migration is one such factor as has been seen in Australia since the Second World War. Between 1966–71 about 50% of the considerable growth rate (12%) of Sydney and Melbourne was attributable to immigration (Borrie, 1977). However, it is the increased number of people surviving to old age which gives the pyramid its top-heavy appearance.

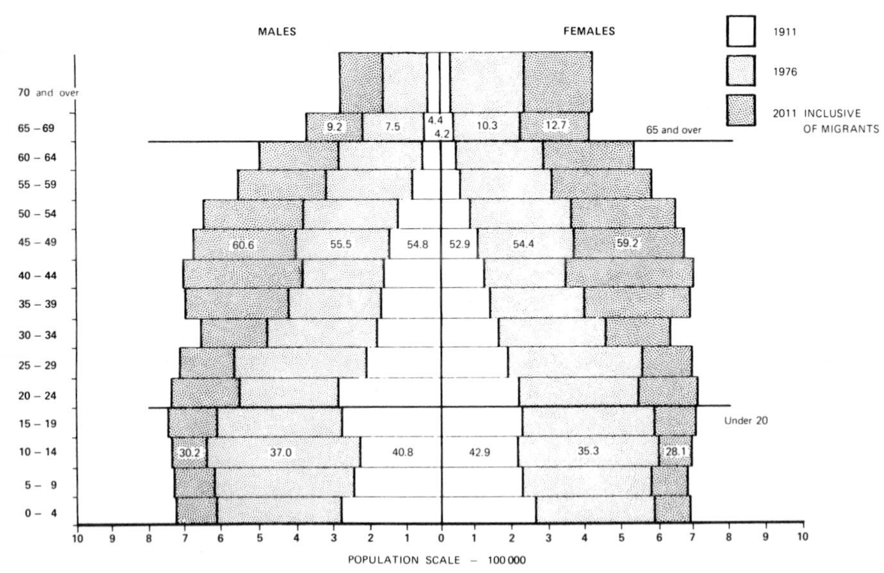

Fig. 2. Past and projected changes in age groups of the Australian population. (Source: Australian Bureau of Census and Statistics.)

It is insufficient merely to note an increase in the proportion of people aged over sixty-five years. Disease in elderly people is much more evident after the middle seventies; and it is this group whose increase is more apparent. In Britain it is expected that during the twenty years after 1976 there will be a fall in the numbers of people between sixty-four and seventy-five years, while a rise of 23% will take place in people over seventy-five years; the expected increase in those over eighty-five years is 42% (Abrams, 1978).

The health and general expectations of people in the older age groups is a compound of a number of events, two of which—increased life expectancy and increased vulnerability to disease—have already been mentioned. The increase in the proportion of elderly people largely determines the magnitude of the problem; however, there are other important features of the so-called ageing society which also stem from the growth of industrialism but which cannot be fully appreciated merely by considering changes in population numbers. There has been a tendency towards relocation leaving the older people in rural areas or in the inner and older urban areas. Retirement from the workforce, with consequent income loss and change in life-style has become an important feature with serious implications in a society bent on adding to the gross national product. Borrie (1977) regards the four features of life in Australia and similar countries—the degree of urbanization, the mobility of people, the degree of affluence, and the expectation of life from birth of around seventy years—as unique in human experience. The effects of these social changes have reached many levels of society; some have directly concerned elderly people while the indirect effect of others has also had widespread consequences. "The apparently simple fact of improved life expectancy implies a complex interweaving of social and biological factors that contribute to the additional years of life and are in turn modified by those years" (Hendricks and Hendricks, 1978). The so-called diseases of progress have a place in this complicated pattern; included among them is a considerable amount of social pathology as well as disease in the more conventional sense. The numbers involved are only one aspect of the "problem" of ageing.

V. The Health Needs of Elderly People

One measure of disease among elderly people is the utilization of health services. In Great Britain the average number of consultations with general practitioners for the whole population is 3·8 per year compared with 6·3 per year for the over sixty-five group. Thirty-three percent of the national health expenditure and an equivalent proportion of the drug bill in Great Britain is consumed by the 12% of the population who are over the age of sixty-five years (Judge and Caird, 1978). Over 40% of all hospital beds are occupied by people in this age group.

Studies of the health care costs in a well-defined community in Busselton, Western Australia, indicate the high proportion consumed by the group of people over the age of sixty-five (Simon *et al.*, 1978). Contacts between general practitioners and their patients showed a striking increase in numbers with respect to people over the age of sixty-five. It was found that the overall prescribing rate of drugs was 2·21 per person for the whole population. However, the over sixty-five age group were clearly the largest users: for males the rate was 4·15 and for females 5·85 drugs per person. A similar trend was evident with regard to radiological and laboratory tests. The escalation in total costs generated by elderly people is seen in Fig. 3.

Although these examples do not prove that resources are being used to the best advantage they are evidence of the disproportionate use of health care facilities by one section of the population, loosely defined as

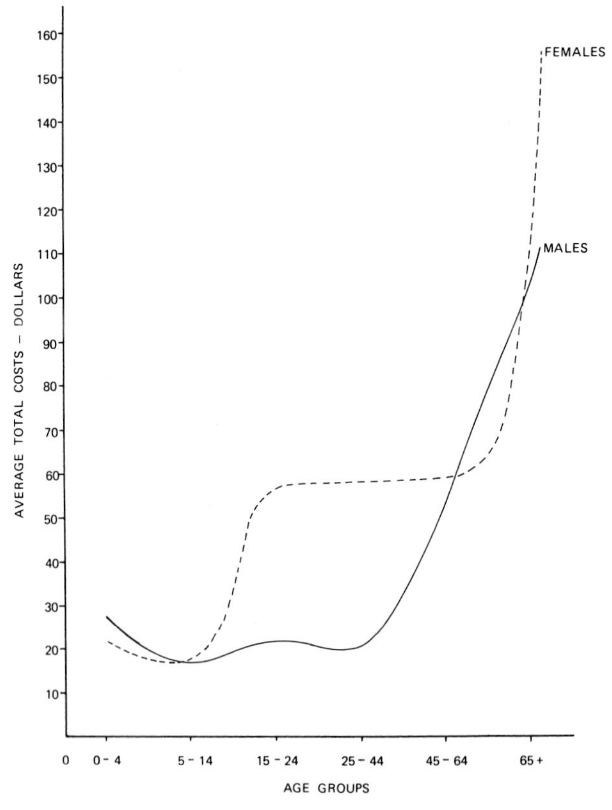

Fig. 3. For six months, the average total health cost per person in Busselton, Western Australia.

"the elderly". However, the indiscriminate use of this blanket term has been misleading and given rise to the idea that all people over a certain age are necessarily afflicted with the diseases of progress. We need to be clear on two aspects: first, it is necessary to be more precise as to description of disease in old people; secondly, we should discover what proportion of this age group is so affected.

VI. Description of Disease

Disease is conventionally described in terms of pathology. Heart disease, stroke and cancer are the three pathological labels heading the causes of death in old people. The manner in which heart disease increases with age as a cause of death is shown in Fig. 4.

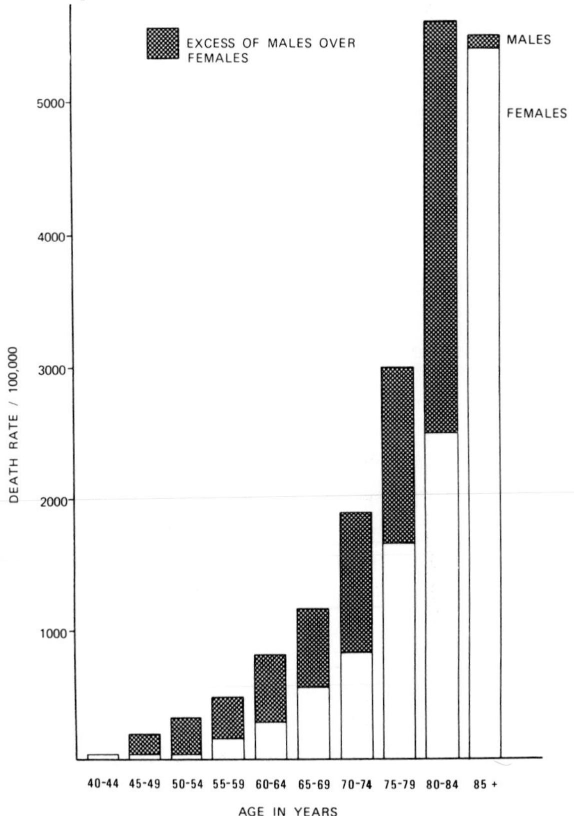

Fig. 4. Mortality from ischaemic heart disease in Western Australia, 1976. (Source: Australian Bureau of Census and Statistics.)

Hospital admission rates give another indication of morbidity in elderly people: the dramatic rise during later life in the proportion of the population admitted with stroke is seen in Fig. 5.

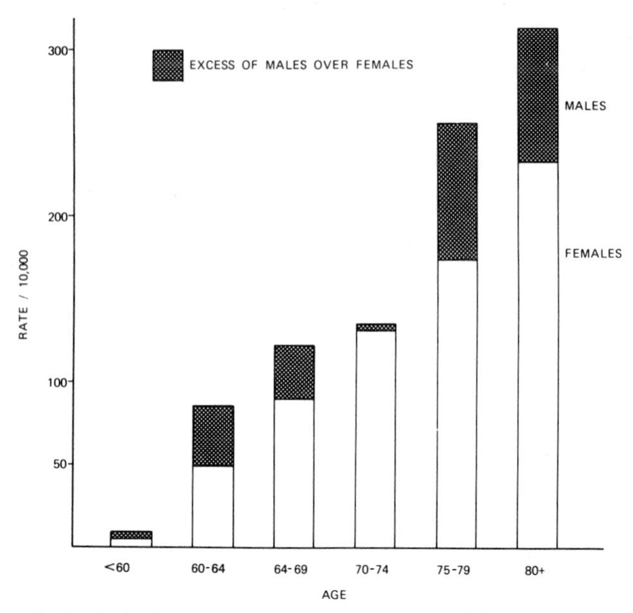

Fig. 5. Hospital admission rates for stroke patients, Western Australia, 1973. (Source: Unit of Clinical Epidemiology, Univ. Western Australia.)

Similarly the admission rate for people with fractured femur is considerably increased in late life. When old people are investigated at home it is found that a higher percentage of people over seventy-five years of age have Alzheimer's disease (senile dementia) than in those under seventy-five. While each of these examples underlines the increase of certain pathological processes in late life, one cannot accept these labels—whether they refer to mortality rates, hospital admissions, or prevalence in the community—as a complete and satisfactory description of the person's disease. One reason for this is that pathology is multiple and not an isolated phenomenon in any one person. It is not uncommon to find evidence of at least four pathological processes in a 75 year-old person. No longer can a single pathological label be expected to describe a person and his disease. A good example of this is the person with a fractured femur. In Fig. 6 the columns on the left represent comparatively young people whose change in structure is generally limited to pathology in bone; but the right-hand columns represent people not only of a different age but with a galaxy of changes which often have little relationship to the fractured bone. The fracture is, in fact, but an incident in a lifetime which has become studded by a number of disorders; some of these can be described in the language of the pathologist while others come within the category of behavioural or social changes. The implications with regard to methods of treatment and to prognosis are obvious.

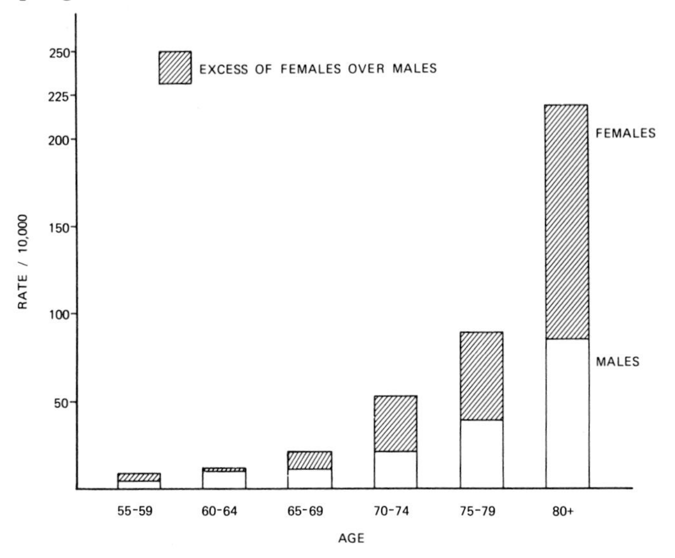

Fig. 6. Hospital admission rates for proximal fracture of the femur, Western Australia, 1971–73. (Source: Unit of Clinical Epidemiology, Univ. Western Australia.)

What other facts need to be added to the pathological label in order to achieve a more complete understanding of diseases in late life? We should regard each individual as having three territories—physical, mental and social. As age advances it is likely that more than one of these is affected at any one time; nor can any of them be regarded in isolation. It has been estimated (Kay *et al.*, 1964) that as many as 40% of elderly people in the community suffer from some form of psychiatric disorder; in 15% of these people symptoms are severe. But mental disorders seldom exist in isolation; not only are physical symptoms present but they are frequently the precipitating cause of a change in mental function. The suicide rate in males rises in late life; both physical disease and the social environment contribute to the mental depression which underlines this event. This complicated pattern of disease cannot be adequately explained if it is merely labelled with the name of one of the several items of pathological change. A combination of physical, mental and social changes is the rule, not the exception; a description of the person's disorder must include all three.

Finally, in order to complete the picture we need a description of function in terms of what he is able or unable to do. A list of disabilities, described in terms of the simple or complex acts of daily living which affect that particular person needs to be made if his problem is to be accurately identified. Pathological labels by themselves are insufficient; a comprehensive understanding of the consequences of disease in an old person only becomes possible when two other features are included—an enquiry into the extent to which the physical, mental or social territories have been invaded and a precise description of the disabilities which have been encountered in each territory. One is then in a position to make a rational plan of care.

VII. The Cause(s) and Extent of Disease in Elderly People

The facts considered so far—the increasing number of elderly survivors, their increasing health needs and the kinds of disease associated with old age—are impressive to the point of being overwhelming. To what extent is it true that survival has led to a new phenomenon—the survival of the unfittest (Isaacs *et al.*, 1972)? Further attention needs to be given to the causes of unfitness; the extent to which this exists in the older section of the population will then be considered.

1 Cause—Ageing or Disease?

If there is difficulty in describing the precise nature of these diseases, there is often more difficulty in nominating the causes. A fallacy, both misleading to the observer and damaging to the old person, is to ascribe old age as the cause. Opportunity to reverse disability and improve function is lost when one assumes that the sole cause is a process which is irreversible. Ageing may make a significant contribution to a person's diseased state, but rarely is it the one responsible agent. It is necessary to search for the contribution not only of ageing but of genetic and environmental influence in the disease state of any one individual; and to disregard the idea of listing diseases of old age in favour of diseases *in* old people (Fig. 7). Not only is multiple pathology the rule but rarely is there an isolated cause in the disorders which accumulate in the survivors of a long lifetime. It is more common for all three factors—genetic, exogenous and ageing—to be found operative.

Accidental hypothermia is an affliction of people whose temperature regulation is less effective due to changes of ageing, whose immediate

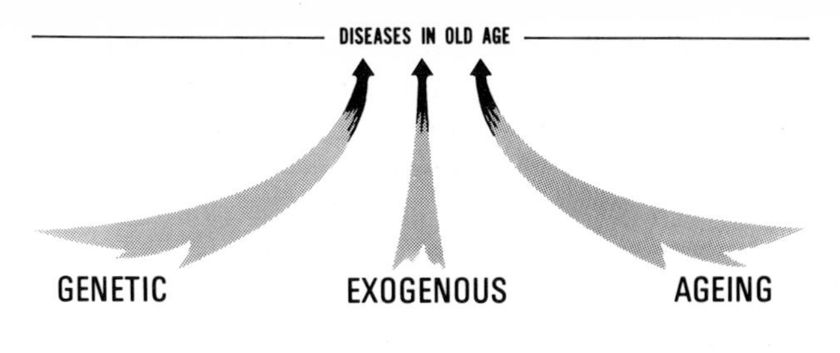

Fig. 7. Factors contributing to age-associated disease.

environment is a cold house generally in poor repair, with insufficient finance for adequate heating, and who are less mobile from some condition such as arthritis or a stroke. The "accident" cannot be ascribed to old age alone, but to a combination of the ageing process and a number of exogenous factors—social, economic and acquired disease. The way an old person walks and his tendency to fall may be a compound of joint disease due to past injury, diabetes affecting his vision and the changes of ageing in his nervous system—or even the effects of a genetically determined neurological disorder.

When attempting to separate disease from ageing one should restrict the former to those pathological processes which occur occasionally in the young and not universally in the old; while ageing is represented by the progression of adult changes characteristic of the species and which should occur in all individuals if they live long enough (Libow, 1963). The disabilities of old people will continue to be misunderstood and will remain unrectified unless this kind of basic approach is made.

2 Longitudinal Studies

The contribution of the ageing process to these disorders is not always easy to assess. In more recent years, however, longitudinal studies of elderly people have been in progress, recognizing the fact that ageing is a process of biological change over a span of fifty years or more in a person's lifetime. The study undertaken by the National Institute of Mental Health in the United States (Granick and Patterson, 1971) is noteworthy in this regard. Their first step was to select a group of elderly men who lived in the community and had no overt evidence of physical disease or psychosis. This selection yielded two subgroups: group 1 revealed no trace of disease after exhaustive investigation, while group 2 had some evidence of asymptomatic and subclinical disorder. The next step was to make comparisons in both biomedical and behavioural parameters between these selected elderly people and younger people. The differences between the young and group 1 were assumed to be due to the ageing process; while the differences from normal exhibited by those in group 2 were regarded as representing disease.

The list of changes considered to be due to ageing, both biomedical and behavioural, is impressive in that the emphasis is on minimal shifts in most parameters rather than on serious decline in function. In the fields of psychiatry and social psychology it was more difficult to separate the effects of ageing from those of disease; but by carefully noting the relationship between variables in the different situations under review these observers were able to make valuable comments on the likely causes of the changes which were recorded. Senile quality, the condition when comprehension, memory, attention and emotional responses are diminished, correlated with the presence of vascular disease, but was not related to social losses experienced in late life; nor did it correlate with advanced chronological age. When psychological testing of intellectual tasks was made there was reduced speed of response; this was regarded as age-related. ". . . But when disease, such as arteriosclerosis, intervened, it became the pacemaker in changes of the brain which superficially appeared as ageing" (Birren *et al.*, 1971).

One of the features of this study, in contrast to many which have previously given rise to theories on the effects of ageing, is that it was performed not on an institutionalized group but on people in the normal community. Disengagement from social activities by older people was not found to be a consequence of ageing, as is often supposed. A significant observation—particularly with regard to psychosocial function—was the effect of the person's immediate environment in contrast to the effect of the process of ageing. Life was less satisfying, less organized and more demanding to those men who had experienced losses involving close relationships. These social losses, not their age, provided the more significant influences on their behaviour.

Twenty-three of the forty-seven men originally selected survived; nineteen were followed up after eleven years. Ten of these were declared free of disease; their changes were generally described as remarkably limited, and were summed up as a gradual erosion of capacities which were regarded as part of normal ageing. In contrast were the changes due to disease; only a few (30%) of the original group 2 were among the eleven-year survivors; these were the people who originally had shown minimal but nonetheless significant evidence of disease.

Several facts of considerable importance emerge from this study. First, it is possible to separate disease from the consequence of the ageing process. Secondly, the changes of ageing are represented by relatively small if progressive decrements of function rather than the catastrophic changes which are popularly imagined. Thirdly, the four key areas "most likely to make substantial contributions to the quality of old age and to longevity" (Granick and Patterson, 1971)—namely, preventing arteriosclerosis, avoiding the harmful effects of cigarette smoking, reducing the detrimental sequelae of psychosocial losses and assisting people to sustain effective goals in late life—these are concerned not with the fundamental process of ageing but with the person's environment. They represent the exogenous factors in the production of diseases in old age; there is no good reason why they should not yield to our manipulation in the future.

3 The Extent of Disability and Disease in Old Age

It is important to attempt to measure the extent of disease in elderly people even if only to correct the unfortunate myth that age is synonymous with disease. Research along these lines in recent years has done much to counteract the ignorance and the unnecessary gloom that surrounds old age. Shanas *et al.* (1968) made an important contribution in this regard. They studied old people in three different industrial societies in order to provide a factual basis upon which to consider future needs. They attempted to estimate function rather than to list disease in terms of pathology. They enquired into physical capacity, means of support both from families and the rest of society, occupation and in particular why people retired and what income they had. Because it was a study of old people in normal society—not in institutions—they endeavoured to discover whether there was integration at a functional level of this group with other sections of society, paying particular attention to family relationships and their place in the workforce.

Their studies confirmed that incapacity increases with age; but their important contribution was to point out that the extent of incapacity was less than generally expected. Ten per cent of those over sixty-five years were either institutionalized or were seriously incapacitated at home, while a further 10–20% were moderately incapacitated. The most seriously incapacitated were elderly women, either single or widowed. Nevertheless, they concluded that in spite of this degree of incapacity, people over sixty-five years were more strongly integrated within society than was generally believed. Disease had not overwhelmed the majority of old people. Integration was particularly noticeable in family relationships; a substantial minority shared households, mobility had not destroyed family proximity for the majority, contacts with their children were described as frequent for most and there was noticeable exchange of family services which was not merely in the direction of parents. Social services, they noted, were a vital factor in complementing rather than smothering endeavours from other informal sources, thus assisting with the important feature of integration within society. Separation of older people from normal society was indeed present to some extent often as "the consequence of formal actions on the part of mass society" rather than as a natural phenomenon. They concluded that "there are serious problems of the elderly in all three societies, but they do not assume dimensions that are inherently unmanageable given imaginative leadership and the accelerated development of social services". Compensation for at least part of the diseases of progress, they would argue, is eminently possible.

VIII. Future Progress

Elderly people have suffered from the erroneous idea that old age is an inevitable disease of progress. An understanding of the process of ageing and its separation from disease, as well as studies similar to those cited above, should pave the way to replacing the unfortunate mythology surrounding this subject. What is likely to be the expectation of elderly people in the future? This will depend on the extent to which society can make three major corrections.

1 Medical Care

The first correction is in the care of those elderly people who are disabled. Their diseases need to be studied in terms of the physical, mental and social disabilities which they cause. It cannot be denied that they represent a considerable burden both to those old people who suffer them, to their families and to the community who become responsible for their care. As far as this section of the population is concerned it would appear that progress has resulted in survival of the unfittest with a large period of dependency at the close of life as well as at the beginning. In concluding their account of unfit old people in Glasgow, Isaacs and his colleagues (1972) pointed out that "man has learned to outlive the vigour of his body and the wisdom of his brain, but he has not yet learned how to provide, from the society which he has created, for the new needs of those who survive unfit".

Although "care" and "cure" were both derived from the same word (*cura*) medical practice has given most attention to the latter. Doctors and their professional colleagues tend to regard the incurable as evidence of their personal failure and thereby a threat to their fundamental purpose. Rehabilitation becomes restricted to getting people home or back to work—not to assisting them to do as much as they can as well as they can for as long as they can, wherever they are. Elderly disabled people have consequently been largely excluded from the mainstream of medicine; a new and often second-class system, frequently relying on motives of profit or charity, has had to be constructed in an attempt to answer their needs. The chairman of a subcommittee in the United States House of Representatives (Biaggi, 1978) remarked on the "appalling lack of commitment" by the American medical profession and related health professions to the training of personnel in geriatric medicine. From a total of 25 000 members of medical school faculties there were fifteen trained geriatricians and only one established chair in geriatric medicine (at the time still vacant). Considerable progress has been made in Great Britain where there are now thirteen professorial departments, but growth of this branch of medicine has been slow, even though its benefits, as well as the reasons why it should be part of the conventional organization of medicine and not some apartheid arrangement, have been proclaimed for the last thirty years (Warren, 1946; Gibson, 1957; Bluestone, 1964; Anderson, 1976). More spectacular has been the rapid expansion in developed countries such as the United States of America and Australia of a private nursing home industry. Reversal of disability with improvement in function, even if the result does not constitute a cure, has been repeatedly demonstrated. Nevertheless, physicians engaged in this field of rapidly increasing proportions have shown the lowest increase in growth in a long list of specialties, many of which belong to areas of comparative obscurity. The medical care of elderly people has yet to be afforded reasonable priority in the mainstream of medicine. What is now needed is a service to include home care, restorative care and permanent institutional care, based on established (acute) medical centres, complementing present medical practice (Lefroy, 1978).

2 Research

In addition to this exercise there needs to be further research. Biologic and Social Gerontology are two studies which are specifically directed towards both an understanding of the process of ageing and the many circumstances responsible for the three territories of disability referred to above. The aim of biologic gerontology is to learn how to retain vigour so that we are less vulnerable to disease and more able to adapt successfully to the tasks of post-maturity; the basic aim is not to increase life span. Comfort (1969) believed that a fundamental interference must be made with the present length of adult vigour; and that this is the only way of making another gain comparable to the increase in survival which has already been made in early adult life. When this is achieved the first of Isaacs' critical comments will be answered.

Nevertheless, research concerned with diseases occurring in the preceding phases of life—vascular disease, cancer, the addictions, traffic accidents—are also relevant to old age. When these omissions have been corrected the numbers who survive to late life as the unfittest will diminish.

3 Ageism

Those elderly people who are disabled by disease—in its conventional sense—are the minority. Nevertheless, the 80% who are not afflicted in this way are in danger of being disabled by the disease of ageism. This is the third and in some aspects the most important correction to be made if elderly people, disabled or otherwise, are to have a reasonable expectation in the future.

Discrimination against elderly people, although it is an established feature of modern society, is not a new phenomenon. Six centuries ago, when the Statute of Labourers was proclaimed in Britain in an attempt by landowners to assure themselves of a supply of labour, a sharp distinction between the capable and the incapable emerged. Legislation later attempted to provide for the latter: ". . . The lame, impotent, old, blind and such other among them being poor and not able to work." Being old became equated with uselessness, along with the other forms of infirmity. With the progress of industrialization this equation became accentuated; and although more people now survive to old age the erroneous idea of uselessness and incapability hovers around them in the form of a conspiracy. We still tend to lump together the "aged and infirm". Present retirement ages reflect conditions of the late nineteenth and early twentieth centuries; even at that time, the health and vigour of elderly people had probably improved to the extent of making these conditions inappropriate (Thane, 1978). But the myth that a particular chronological age is synonymous with disease is kept alive by attitudes which deprecate the esteem and usefulness of people over the age of sixty-five. It seems ironical that we not only fail to appreciate the particular manner in which the 20% are disabled—their disabilities are neither critically assessed nor adequately cared for—but we fail to delineate them from the majority of elderly people who remain relatively fit. The very fact of making a division at a certain chronological age, instead of on the grounds of ability, is artificial. Until it becomes customary to recognize the distinction between such disorders as arteriosclerosis, cancer, the numerous neurological degenerative diseases on the one hand, and the process of ageing on the other, the mythology associated with the latter and the resultant discrimination of ageism will continue to exist.

The cult of ageism has flourished on the idea that old age is necessarily associated with infirmity; it is also connected with theories regarding a person's economic usefulness. Herbert Spencer, anticipating Darwin, stated that the struggle for existence and survival of the fittest were of major importance to the development of society. In his celebrated essay of 1857, "Progress: its law and cause", he proclaimed that the idea of evolution was universally applicable and was the basis of all understanding, whether biological or social (Goldthorpe, 1969). Conflict, particularly in the economic field, was a necessary evolutionary force not to be avoided; even warfare had been important to the formation of societies. The ideas of progress and evolution became fused and the concept of social Darwinism later took shape. The fit were those best able to take advantage of the situation; their social and economic survival was their demonstration of fitness. Such a doctrine eliminates from further consideration those who cease to add to the gross national product.

The proper study of society, by including people over sixty-five years of age instead of separating them, has provided evidence against the nonsense of ageism. But because mobility has increased in modern society the erroneous idea that the extended family has disintegrated still lingers on. Despite evidence to the contrary (Shanas *et al.*, 1968) it is still argued that there is now comparatively little support of older people by their children. Those who hold this belief often imagine that there was once blissful equanimity between generations; historical evidence, however, does not substantiate the idea that pre-industrial society always acted with concern and veneration towards its elders once they had ceased to be economically and socially useful (Laslett, 1977). Problems regarding the care of older people cannot be ascribed to the inevitable consequence of industrialism alone; nor can they be referred to an illusory past for an easy solution.

The prevailing attitude to elderly people—the very fact of nominating them as a separate section of society—had its origin in the distinction between fitness and unfitness for physical labour. This attitude has subsequently become entrenched in the form of a mythology largely depending for its continuation on misinformation and an unwillingness to concede that usefulness still remains even if capacity to add to the gross national product has dwindled.

As well as the fact that an old person is more likely to experience physical and mental disabilities, the combination of ageism and comparative neglect leaves him balancing precariously and with little support on a social tight-rope.

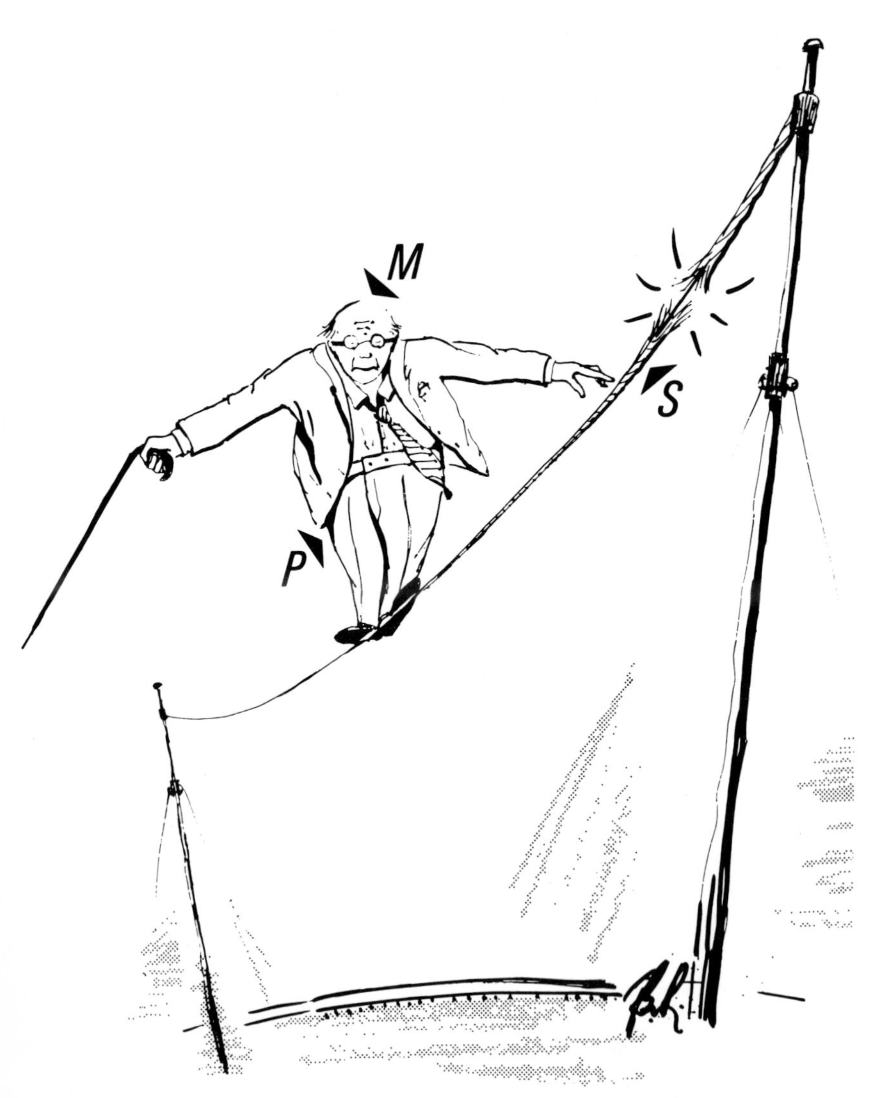

Fig 8. Society—life-line or tight-rope?

IX. Conclusions

Progress has led to an increased proportion of the population surviving to old age. A significant minority (20%) suffer disabilities and warrant a much higher standard of care than they presently receive; nevertheless, it is a fallacy to equate old age with disease. The process of ageing contributes to disease in old people but is only one of the responsible factors. Progress cannot be blamed; the fault is lack of progress. In the first place, we have as yet failed to eliminate such exogenous causes as vascular disease, cigarette addiction, cancer, etc., or to compensate for the serious psychosocial losses experienced in old age. Secondly, gerontologists have yet to determine a method of increasing adult vigour and thereby decreasing susceptibility to disease. If, in addition to those achievements, a proper understanding of the biological and social status of older people can put an end to the existing attitude of discrimination against them future progress will allow an even larger majority of elderly people to look forward to health, not disease.

References

Abrams, M. (1978). "Beyond Three-Score and Ten". Age Concern, Mitcham.

Anderson, W. F. (1976). "Practical Management of the Elderly", 3rd edn. Blackwell Scientific, Oxford.

Borrie, W. D. (1977). "Some Social Aspects of Ageing". Proc. 13th Annual Conf. Aust. Ass. Gerontol. 12–20.

Biaggi, M. (1978). "Future of Health Care and the Elderly". Report to Select Committee on Aging, House of Representatives, Ninety-fifth Congress (Comm. Pub. No. 95–141). US Govt. Printing Office, Washington, DC.

Birren, J. E., Butler, R.N., Greenhouse, S. W., Sokoloff, L. and Yarrow, W. M. (1971). Reflections on human aging. *In* "Human Aging II" (S. Granick and R. D. Patterson, Eds). US. DHEW No. (HSM) 71–9037.

Bluestone, E. M. (1964). Towards a deeper understanding of the geriatric problem. *Gerontologica clinica* **6**, 101–108.

Comfort, A. (1969). "Nature and Human Nature". Pelican Books, Harmondsworth.

Comfort, A. (1977). "A Good Age". Mitchell Beazley, London.

Gibson, R. M. (1957). Domiciliary care in the Newcastle district. *Med. J. Aust.* **ii**, 485–489.

Goldthorpe, J. H. (1969) Herbert Spencer. *In* "The Founding Fathers of Social Science" (T. Raison, Ed.). Penguin Books, Harmondsworth.

Granick, S. and Patterson, R. D. (1971). An eleven year follow-up biomedical and behavioural study. *In* "Human Aging II". US. DHEW No. (HSM) 71–9037.
Hendricks, J. and Hendricks, C. D. (1978). Ageing in advanced industrial societies. *In* "An Ageing Population". (V. Carver, and P. Liddiard, Eds). Hodder and Stoughton, London.
Isaacs, B., Livingstone, M. and Neville, Y. (1972). "Survival of the Unfittest: A Study of Geriatric Patients in Glasgow". Routledge and Kegan Paul, London.
Judge, T. G. and Caird, F. I. (1978). "Drug Treatment of the Elderly Patient". Pitman Medical, Tunbridge Wells.
Kay, D. W. K., Beamish, P. and Roth, M. (1964). Old age mental disorders in Newcastle upon Tyne. Brit. J. Psychiat. 110, 146–158.
Laslett, P. (1977). "The History of Ageing and the Aged in Family Life and Illicit Love in Earlier Generations". Cambridge Univ. Press.
Lefroy, R. B. (1978). Extended care: medical care of the elderly disabled. *Aust. Family Physician* **7**, 259–265.
Libow, L. S. (1963). Medical investigation of the processes of aging. *In* "Human Aging: A Biological and Behavioural Study" (J. E. Birren, *et al.*, Eds). US. DHEW No. (PHS) 986.
Shanas, E., Townsend, P., Wedderburn, D., Friis, H., Milhøj, P. and Stehouwer, J. (1968). "Old People in Three Industrial Societies". Routledge and Kegan Paul, London.
Simon, B., Hobbs, M.S.T. and Cullen, K. (1978). "A Study of General Practice and Its cost in a Rural Community". Report from the Unit of Clinical Epidemiology, University of Western Australia.
Thane, P. (1978). The muddled history of retiring at 60 and 65. *New Society*. Aug. 3, 234.
Walford, R. L. (1974). Immunologic theory of ageing: current status. *Fedn Proc. Fedn Am. Socs exp. Biol.* **33**, 2020–2027.
Warren, M. W. (1946). Care of the chronic aged sick. *Lancet* i, 841–843.

Part V

Epilogue

Introduction

The chapters in this final section are a partial summary of the subjects discussed in detail in the preceding sections, and look forward to the future.

The first one by Professor Joske critically examines medical care during earlier times and reaches the conclusion that physicians have not been greatly effective in modifying the patterns of disease and death during either the pre-urban phase of human existence or the subsequent millenia dominated by infectious diseases. They did, however, play a major part in the development of preventive medicine, and thus, indirectly, achieved results beyond the bounds of curative medicine. (The power and scope of preventive medicine has been strikingly demonstrated in the story of smallpox by Professor Fenner in Chapter 13.) Professor Joske also points out the possible long-term hazards of modern medicine in permitting survival and replication of deleterious genes: this will be of increasing importance in the future.

Two themes are discernible in discussions of medicine in the next decades: increasing technical competence, and more formal and fundamental consideration of the human and ethical problems resulting from advances in medical and biological techniques. The first theme is illustrated by a superb essay on modern immunology by Professor Mitchison. Other examples might have been chosen, but immunology is the "growth subject" of current medical research and offers a cross-disciplinary approach involving advanced technical methods and brilliance of biological thought and ideas. The synthesis of immunology, genetics and epidemiology appears at present the most exciting and potentially productive of the many facets of current medical research.

The second, humanistic, approach to health and well-being is exemplified by the considered, idealistic, chapter by Dr Daisaku Ikeda. This might at first be considered irrelevant or even antithetical to the technical approach, but is in fact complementary to it. Both the scientific and moral-ethical approaches are essential if medicine (used in the broadest sense) is to become a tool for the promotion of human well-being.

Achieving such a synthesis is not easy. Sir Charles Snow has rightly pointed out the differences in these two basic themes of the human mind. The chapters by Dr Farrands and Dr Boyden discuss the necessity and methods for such integration. They are the pointers to the future use of medical (and scientific) thought and techniques.

30
The Physician and Changing Patterns of Human Disease and Death

R. A. Joske
Department of Medicine, University of Western Australia, Perth, Australia

---

. . . *It is difficult to credit the physician with more than a minor role in changing patterns of human morbidity and mortality.*

Patterns of human morbidity and mortality have changed greatly, both qualitatively and quantitatively, over the ages, but the role of the physician in this change is debatable. It appears, on examination, to be of lesser importance than often supposed today by a public accustomed to announcements in the media of a continuing succession of "breakthroughs" in medical research. It may be examined by relating patterns of human illness and death in successive eras to the medical practice of each. For this purpose the most convenient division of human existence is into pre-urban, urban and recent phases. This sequence is not absolute. The change from one phase to another has been gradual, and the various phases co-exist at the same time in different places. However, it summarizes the progression of human development, and at each stage different selective forces act, patterns of health and disease alter, and methods of medical practice change and develop.

I. Demography of Pre-urban Man

The pre-urban phase of human development is characterized by its duration. It spans some millions of years during which the physical form of the species was shaped by natural selection. This long evolution determined not only the external, but also the internal structure of man, including the central nervous system. This clearly means that the potential and limitations of human thought are determined by an evolution during which the species adapted to a way of life very different from the later urban phases of human existence. This fact, often and conveniently overlooked, may well prove to be of increasing importance and even represent the limiting factor in urban development.

The physical conditions of pre-urban man are poorly understood. The thoughts of these ages must remain speculative, although Marshack (1972) has produced strong evidence that they were oriented to time and seasons. It appears that pre-urban peoples lived in small, socially cohesive groups with restricted mobility and a precarious existence based upon hunting and gathering. Population density was necessarily low. The best estimates of the numbers of Neolithic man throughout the world are of the order of five million.

Knowledge of the diseases and mortality of pre-urban groups is gathered from three main sources. These are the study of surviving pre-urban societies such as Australian Aboriginals and African Bushmen, paleopathology, and deduction from the state of subsequent urban society. There is general agreement between the three methods.

The general picture is of a high fecundity balanced by a high mortality affecting especially the years before and during reproduction. These conditions favour rapid adaption and evolution of the species. Life in these ages was certainly short. Over 90% of prehistoric human remains are of individuals below 40 years of age. Most surviving pre-urban peoples have a mortality exceeding 25% before the age of five years (Polunin, 1967). The major causes of death were probably related to childbirth, or due to starvation, infectious disease or injury from accident or conflict. Restricted mobility meant susceptibility to local famine. Low population density prevented major plagues, but the parallel interrelated evolution of man and his pathogens implies the continuing presence of infectious disease. Diseases of plenty such as atherosclerosis must have been rare. Genetic disorders such as diabetes or haemophilia must have been rapidly lethal, and genes for these diseases were maintained at a low frequency by natural selection.

Survival of the species thus depended upon a high birth rate with a correspondingly high mortality, especially of the young. The consequences were a low population density and a relatively rapid biological and social adaption. It is no accident that even today throughout much of the world children are considered a blessing and the aged revered: they were the means and evidence of survival.

The medical practice of pre-urban societies is suggested by studies of some surviving groups. The traditional medicine of the Australian Aboriginals has been recorded by many observers (see Moodie and Pederson, 1971). It is limited to nursing measures, some herbal remedies of uncertain efficacy, and incantations by tribal medicine-men. There is no evidence that it significantly affected morbidity or mortality, although the role of the medicine-man was undoubtedly of the greatest importance in maintaining social cohesion among small groups of nomads, a necessary condition for survival. Similar remarks apply to the traditional medicine of other pre-urban groups such as the Bushmen of South Africa (Bronte-Stewart *et al.*, 1960).

II. Urbanization and Disease

The development and habitation of cities began in the river valleys of Egypt and Mesopotamia and has progressed steadily to the gigantic conurbations of today in a relatively short time, some 400 generations compared to over 100 000 in the pre-urban phase of human development. It has, nevertheless, altered profoundly and irrevocably patterns of human morbidity and mortality, and altered both the nature and severity of selective factors in human evolution.

Urbanization has several factors directly relevant to the present theme. A city is a geographical focus with a high population density related to a hinterland with settled agriculture. There must be a relatively complex technology, effective transport of goods, raw materials, food, water, wastes, and people to and from the city, and achievement of craft specialization and an hierarchical social ogranization, as well as development of literacy and the keeping of records. These latter factors are necessary prerequisites for the development of demography and preventive and curative medicine.

The basic consequences of urbanization for the study of human mortality were three: an increase in the numbers of people, changes in population density with development of local areas of extremely high population density, and movement of people on a large scale for pleasure, war or trade, but predominantly between cities and from the rural areas to the urban fair. These factors are obviously related.

The population increase has been dramatic by biological standards. The Neolithic population estimated at 5 million, had increased by the Roman period to some 200 million, and today is of the order of 4000 million. More important than even this increase in numbers has been a change in the distribution of people. The increase has been disproportionately urban, from small relatively isolated nomadic groups to large agglomerations. Imperial Rome held more people than all North America at that time. These alterations in population density were of major importance in the rise of infectious disease, the major medical consequence of urbanization.

The population increase during the last 400 or so generations of mankind has been due to increased longevity rather than increased fertility. This was already maximal and no evidence of increased human fecundity during this period has been presented except for restricted groups where birth control was a result of religious practice. Rather, of children conceived, more were born safely and survived to reproductive age, while survival beyond this became increasingly frequent. Despite this, morbidity and mortality in early and medieval cities were extremely high by present standards. Brunt (1971) has estimated that in Imperial Rome infant mortality exceeded 200 per 1000 live births and that the expectation of life from birth was about twenty-five years. Corresponding figures for contemporary Western society are an infant mortality below 20 per 1000 live births and a life expectancy from birth of over seventy years.

This high mortality was predominately urban. The new cities were centres of disease and death, and their continued growth was maintained by draining their hinterlands of excess, susceptible population. As late as the seventeenth century, deaths in the city of London exceeded births by some 6000 yearly, over half a million during the century. In Ireland during the nineteenth century the average age of death in the cities was twenty-four years compared to twenty-nine years in the country. The drift to the city is no recent phenomenon.

Information about the causes of death in ancient and medieval cities is not great, although the general outlines seem clear. Lord Amulree (1964) studied the archives of St Bartholomew's Abbey and Hospital in London for the thirteenth and fourteenth centuries and showed that most deaths followed short acute illnesses, presumably due to infection. Other evidence supports this suggestion of such a role of infectious disease.

There is little doubt that both ancient and medieval cities were ideal breeding grounds for infectious disease. Surviving contemporary accounts show them to have been squalid, filthy, poorly sewered, with dubious water supplies, limited means of preserving food, and crowded with horses, cattle, dogs, cats, rats, mice, lice and other insects as well as large numbers of susceptible people with a low standard of personal hygiene. Spread of pathogens from other animals to men and between persons was easy and frequent by direct contact, fomites, air droplets, excreta, unsterile foods and contaminated water. The inevitable result was a massive increase in infectious disease, with a high mortality, especially in infants and children. This selected directly for resistance to these diseases, although the cumulative effect became apparent only after many centuries.

More dramatic than the toll due to endemic infectious disease was the occurrence of epidemics of a severity almost beyond modern comprehension. These were the result of formation of areas of high population density combined with a new movement of people on a large scale. Documentation of these epidemics is extensive and a few examples must suffice. Livy records eleven severe plagues in Rome from 387 B.C. onward, and over 5000 persons died daily in the plague of Rome in 251. The Chinese annals identify over eighty major epidemics from the birth of Christ to 1200. The Black Death is estimated to have killed a third of the people of Europe between 1346 and 1350. In 1575 a third of the people of Venice died of plague. The great epidemic of influenza A in 1919 and 1920 claimed at least 20 million victims.

These major epidemics were a direct consequence of increased human mobility. Travel necessarily meant movement of people with their parasites and pathogens from one place to another and brought infectious diseases from endemic areas to places where the population was still susceptible and the population density high in urban foci. The effects are well seen during the expansion of European peoples from the fourteenth century onwards. Fifty years after Cortez landed in America the native population fell from 30 million to only 3 million. A similar massive mortality of indigenes occurred in the Pacific Islands and Australia. There was a similar high mortality among European migrants to Africa and America. The west coast of equatorial Africa was long known as the white man's graveyard. Mortality from disease among the Spanish, French and English armies in the West Indies in the sixteenth and seventeenth centuries often exceeded 60%, far higher than losses from accidents and war. The building of the Panama Canal was delayed until 1914 by the effects of malaria and yellow fever upon the workforce. Notably, however, the Caucasian settlers of Australia, moving to a place with a low Aboriginal population density and without cities, met no "new" diseases and their patterns of morbidity and mortality continued to mirror those of their countries of origin (Joske and Joske, 1979).

Famine and malnutrition were also frequent causes of death in cities. Cities were (and are) dependent upon their hinterlands for production of food and upon transport and storage for its delivery. Until the last century, transport was limited to the speed of a man, or a horse and dray, or a ship with sails or oars. Local droughts, floods or plant pestilences could thus produce severe local famines and many records of such catastrophes are documented by writers such as Malthus. Despite their local importance, however, famines were probably of little selective importance, since the first victims of famine are usually those already infirm, or aged beyond the time of reproduction.

Warfare and judicial execution were also significant causes of death. Apart from the spread of infection by movement of armies, their biological significance is debatable. It will probably ultimately be found to be considerable. Until the development of "total warfare" and decreasing use of capital punishment, war and execution were the methods by which genes related to aggression and antisocial behaviour were associated with a significant excess mortality. It may be that progressive elimination of these genes has been a factor in the progression of civilization. In developed societies today, the excess mortality from motor vehicles in young males with criminal records may be exerting a similar selective effect.

The biological consequences of urbanization can now be summarized. The era of formation of cities has been associated with an increase in population due more to increased longevity than increased fertility, and by development of areas of high population density growing by migration from more sparsely settled rural areas. Accompanying this process and resulting from it, has been a massive increase in endemic and epidemic infectious disease with a high mortality concentrated in children and those of reproductive age. Famine and other natural or man-made catastrophes played a significant but lesser role in determining patterns of mortality.

Formal curative medicine was of little if any avail during the centuries dominated by infectious disease. The changing and evolving practice of therapeutic medicine can fairly be assessed from the many surviving texts, although it must be emphasized that they present an often idealized picture of medical practice. Such works include the Chinese Neiching (*c.* 2700 B.C.), Hammurabi (*c.* 2250 B.C.), the Rig Veda (*c.* 1500 B.C.), the Edwin Smith and Ebers papyri (*c.* 1500 B.C.) the Hippocratic corpus (*c.* 350 B.C.), the works of Galen and Oribasius, and the better-known medieval and renaissance treatises. The general picture is one of compassion and endeavour. Some effective traditional medicines undoubtedly existed (see World Health Organization, 1978), but there is no significant evidence that curative medicine was of more than minimal value, especially in the field of infectious disease. It is improbable that ancient and medieval physicians were able to alleviate in any positive fashion sufferers from infectious disease.

Considerable progress was, however, made in preventive medicine, despite the absence of any realistic theories of the causes or mechanisms of disease.

The relations between disease and poor living conditions, water and food supplies, and the fact (although not the theory) of contagion, were realized early and correctly, and steps were taken to reduce the incidence of some diseases. Hippodamus in the fifth century B.C. established rules for the selection of town sites that show concern for public health, and many Hellenic sites selected according to his criteria remain inhabited today. Great attention was paid to the water supply, and penalties for fouling this were severe. Baths, gymnasia and public lavatories were constructed. The efficient Romans carried these principles further. Aediles (sanitary police) were first appointed in 494 B.C. and followed later by the aquarium curatores with a permanent labour force of 240 slaves by Augustus. The construction of the Roman aqueducts began with the Aqua Appia in 312 B.C. and the Anio Vetus in 272 B.C. Later measures included regular filtration and inspection of water. Similar care for food supplies included regulation of importation, storage and organized distribution and retailing in market places. The Cloaca Maxima, still in use, was constructed in 590 B.C., probably following an earlier Etruscan canal.

Construction of hospitals was a later development, largely under the influence of Christian monasticism. Justinian founded the Hospital of St Basil at Caesarea in 369 A.D., and many others followed in later centuries. Despite their humanistic motives, it is doubtful if they were effective. More probably, the majority were foci of infectious disease and admission was often a sentence of death. In the late nineteenth century. Florence Nightingale wrote:

> It may seem a strange principle to enunciate as the very first requirement in a Hospital that it should do the sick no harm. It is quite necessary nevertheless to lay down such a principle, because the actual mortality in hospitals . . . is very much higher than any calculation founded on the same class of patients treated *out* of hospital would lead us to expect.

This gloomy appreciation survives even today, in some cases not without reason. Hospital mortality dropped significantly only late in the nineteenth century, following the work of pioneers such as Semmelweis and Miss Nightingale herself.

Attempts to prevent the spread of infectious disease began early and were of greater importance. Migration of lepers was interdicted by the Council of Lyons in 583, and Rotharus, King of Lombardy, formally segregated them in 644, although a special hospital for lepers was founded in Ireland in the seventh century. By the fourteenth century sufferers from a number of diseases were not permitted in Christendom, to enter cities or to sell food or drink. These diseases included plague, tuberculosis, epilepsy, anthrax, trachoma and leprosy. The Black Death reached Europe by the trade routes from Asia in 1348, and its fearsome mortality led to formal efforts to contain it. The Republic of Venice appointed public health officials in 1348, excluded possibly infected ships in 1374, and imposed a quarantine of 40 days on arrivals in 1403. This followed the example of Marseilles in 1383. Important as these various measures were, the evident history of plague and other epidemics is itself evidence of their failure.

In summary therefore, there is no great evidence that medical theory or practice played more than a minor role in altering patterns of disease or death during the early millenia of human urban existence. Measures directed towards hygiene—provision of water and food supplies—were sufficiently efficacious to make urbanization possible, but not to contain its inevitable biological consequences. The role of cities has been to select from the human gene pool for resistance to infection. This selection has been intense and prolonged, over 400 generations. Its ultimate effect has become apparent only in recent times. The physician played only an insignificant part in this process, although the steady growth of medical science during these years was to bear later fruit.

III. Decline of Infectious Disease

During the last 150 years there has been in many countries a dramatic change in the pattern of human disease. It is characterized by a precipitous decline in morbidity and mortality from infectious disease, and an increase in mortality from vascular and neoplastic causes, and has been accompanied by changes in the age at death, with significantly increased longevity.

These changes may be documented from many sources. They are illustrated in this essay by comparisons of the causes and ages of death in Western Australia between 1829–55 and in 1970. These are shown in Fig. 1 and Table I, although allowance must be made for difficulties in transcribing nineteenth-century diagnoses into modern terms.

Figure 1 compares the ages at death in the two series. Differences are both obvious and striking. In the early series 42·7% of deaths occurred in infants and children below the age of reproduction, compared to only 8·4% in the recent series. Conversely, in the early series only 6·4% of deaths were in persons over fifty-four years of age, compared to 76·0% in the later series. These changes have important consequences, notably an increase in longevity and a change in the age structure of the

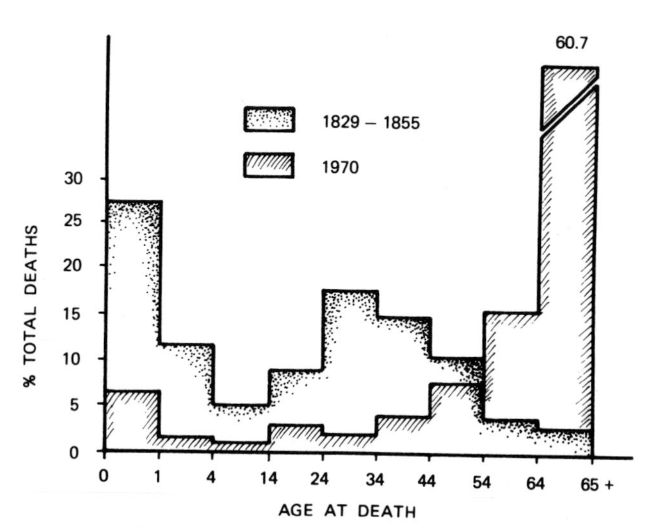

Fig. 1. Comparison of ages at death in Western Australia 1829–55 and 1970. (Data from Joske and Joske (1979), and Western Australian Year Book No. 11–1972.)

TABLE I. *Percentage Frequencies of Causes of Death, Western Australia, 1829–55 and 1970*

Disease classification	% frequency 1829–55	1970
Infective and parasitic disease		
Respiratory tuberculosis	6·2	0·1
Other infective and parasitic diseases	18·4	1·2
Neoplasms	0·5	18·0
Endocrine, nutritional, metabolic	1·3	2·0
Diseases of blood and blood forming organs	0·3	0·3
Mental disorders	1·3	1·1
Disease of nervous system	4·8	1·0
Disease of circulatory system incl. cerebral vascular disease	6·2	49·0
Diseases of respiratory system	4·4	7·2
Diseases of digestive system	4·1	2·6
Diseases of genitourinary system	1·0	1·5
Complications of pregnancy, childbirth and puerperium	1·4	(3cases)
Disease of skin and subcutaneous tissue	0·0	0·1
Diseases of musculoskeletal system and connective tissue	0·0	0·4
Congenital anomalies	0·3	1·8
Perinatal morbidity and mortality	11·0	3·0
Ill-defined conditions	22·9	1·7
Accidents, poisonings and violence	15·9	9·0
	100·0	100·0
Absolute numbers	1067	7543

Data from Western Australia Year Book (1972) and Joske and Joske (1979), modified according to the International Classification of Causes of Death.

population. The decreased infant and childhood mortality means lessening of selection pressures. The increased number of elderly and relatively non-productive persons means increased political and economic pressures. The changes are similar in kind although vastly different in degree to those associated with urbanization, when population increase was due also to prolongation of life rather than greater fecundity.

The changes in the age of death result from changes in the causes of death, notably a decline in the numbers and proportion of persons dying from infectious disease. These are shown in Table I. Deaths from infectious disease exceeded 25% in the early series and were less than 2% in the later series. The mortality from pulmonary tuberculosis fell from 6·2% to 0·1%, and perinatal morbidity and mortality from 11·0% to 3·0%. Similar decreases are seen in other identifiable infectious diseases.

The coincidence in time of the decline in infectious disease and the use of scientific medicine, including development of the germ theory of infectious disease, the establishment of aseptic surgery and the use of antibiotics, led to the suggestion that these were related, and that advances in scientific medicine were the cause of the decline in infectious disease. There are, however, cogent reasons for rejecting this convenient if simplistic hypothesis.

In the first instance, the decline in infectious disease has been essentially a local and not a general phenomenon. It has occurred in Europe, North America, Australasia and some other areas, but not throughout most of Africa, Asia and South America. In these places a high mortality from infectious disease has continued until the present. Two explanations are possible. The first possibility is that the predominantly Caucasian populations of the areas with diminished infectious disease have lived in cities for longer periods and acquired by natural selection increased resistance to these diseases. The second is that the decline of infectious disease is related to altered standards of nutrition, hygiene and public health, with increased host resistance to infection.

These possibilities can best be examined by considering some individual diseases in more detail. It becomes apparent that there is no single or simple explanation applicable to all infectious diseases.

Tuberculosis in England and Wales has been studied in detail by Hart and Wright (1939). There has been a steady and linear decline in the annual death rate from about 3000 per million in 1850 to only 14·6 per million in 1975, although the tubercle bacillus was identified only in 1882, specific chemotherapy discovered only in 1945, and BCG vaccine introduced a decade later. This time sequence clearly shows that the fall in mortality preceded and was little influenced by advances in formal medicine. It is most reasonable to ascribe it to improvements in living standards, especially as tuberculosis remains a serious health problem in some undeveloped countries.

Leprosy is a chronic disease caused by an organism related to the tubercle bacillus. The disease is associated with great emotional overtones because of its long incubation period, steady progression, and the grotesque deformities that it may cause, although in fact it is of very low

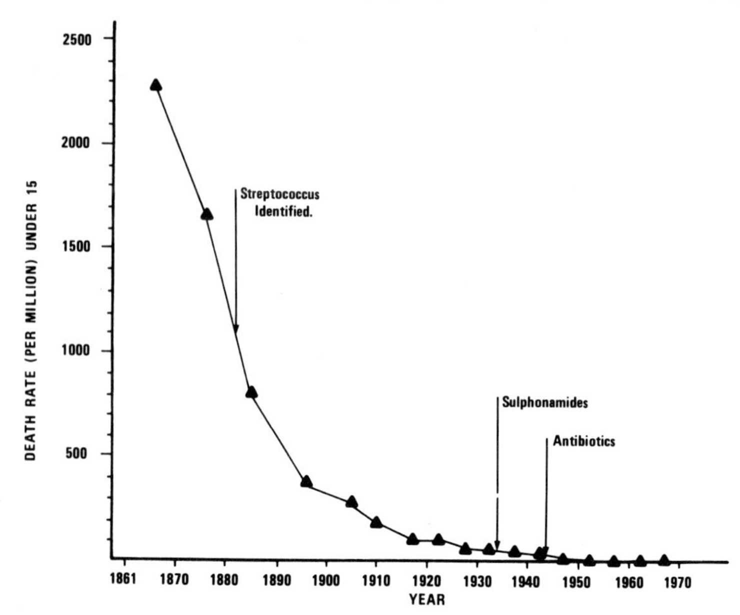

Fig. 2. Death rate from scarlet fever in England and Wales, 1870 to 1970. (Modified after McKeown and Lowe (1974), with permission.)

infectivity. Leprosy was endemic in the Middle East and spread to Europe in the sixth century, a process accelerated by the Crusades and reaching a climax in the thirteenth century. Attempts to contain the disease by quarantine measures have already been described, and were augmented by the establishment of leprosaria, of which there were over 2000 in France alone in the late medieval times. From this time the disease declined, and was rare in most of Europe after the sixteenth century, although it persisted in Scandinavia for another 300 years and remains endemic in some other parts of the world. These changes were not due to advances in diagnosis or treatment. The leprosy bacillus was identified in 1874 by Hansen, and chemotherapy became available only in this century. The long incubation period and prolonged course of leprosy means that death rarely occurs before the age of reproduction, so that biological selection for resistance to the disease is slight. Two factors seem to have been important: containment of the disease by segregation of lepers, and improved standards of nutrition and hygiene. Both are aspects of preventive medicine, but were due to fear and economic circumstance rather than formal medical decision.

Medical action does however appear to have played a part in the decline and ultimate disappearance of smallpox. The introduction of vaccination by Jenner in 1796 has beyond doubt been the direct cause of the eradication of smallpox. Nevertheless, the ravages of smallpox among the indigenes of America after its introduction in the sixteenth century show that natural selection for resistance to the virus had taken place in Europe.

In a further group of diseases, neither preventive nor curative medical action nor improved living standards seem to have been of great moment, and changes in their incidence appear to have been dependent upon biological factors, including evolutionary interaction between host and pathogen resulting in a change from a serious to a more benign condition. Diseases in this class include scarlet fever (Fig. 2) and syphilis.

Syphilis was probably introduced to Europe from Central America in the sixteenth century and spread throughout the continent as an acute, florid, progressive and often fatal disease. The clinical picture changed over the years to that of a chronic condition with a natural history measured in decades. During this time there were little changes in either sexual behaviour or curative medical science, except for the introduction of mercurial ointment in the late sixteenth century. Biological selection of both parasite and host appear to be responsible for this change, especially as syphilis is associated with both abortion and neonatal death, complications making for rapid elimination of susceptibles.

In summary, therefore, the last 150 years have seen a steady decline in the incidence and mortality from infectious disease in many parts of the world. This has coincided in time and place with the development and use of effective scientific curative medicine. However, examination in detail of specific infectious diseases suggests that in most cases medical advances have not been the cause of the change in mortality from infectious disease. Three factors seem to be of greater importance. The first is altered standards of hygiene and nutrition, a view strongly advocated by McKeown *et al.*, (1972) and supported by demographic data showing the relative limitation of this change to developed countries, and by the precise timing of the change. The second factor is an indirect effect of the role of the physician in public health and preventive medicine, seen most evidently in diseases such as smallpox and malaria. The third factor has received little study or emphasis, but will probably prove to be of even greater ultimate significance. This is Darwinian selection and biological adaption of human hosts and their pathogens and parasites, most clearly seen in diseases such as scarlet fever and syphilis. It may be significant that the developed countries with the greatest decline in infectious diseases are also those with the longest history of urbanization. In any instance, it is difficult to credit the physician with more than a minor direct role to date in changing patterns of human morbidity and mortality.

IV. Medicine and the Future of Man

The decline of infectious disease has had two main consequences: an increase in longevity and hence in number of people, and replacement of infectious diseases as causes of death by other conditions, notably vascular disease and malignancies. These are discussed elsewhere in this volume.

Advances in living standards and widespread use of preventive and therapeutic medicine lead, however, to further problems of great potential gravity.

Improved standards of hygiene mean that more individuals contract endemic infectious diseases later in life. For some conditions, notably those due to picorna viruses such as poliomyelitis and hepatitis A, an older age of infection is associated with a higher morbidity and mortality. The paradoxical result is that as the incidence of these diseases decreases, subclinical immunizing infections become less common and the overt mortality is increased.

Control of infectious disease by public health measures and immunization does in many instances lead to decreases in the incidence of these diseases, but leads also to increases in the number and proportion of susceptible individuals in the population. This is not of great immediate moment if these measures can be maintained or the agent responsible totally eliminated. But apparent "success" in control of a disease leads in time to public pressures to decrease the severity of control measures. The proportion of children immunized against tetanus, diphtheria and poliomyelitis is already falling in developed countries. The ultimate result is a "virgin population", so that reappearance of the disease from an external reservoir or by mutation of the organism, may lead to a major epidemic with high mortality. This is already a theme of science fiction, but may well become science fact in the future should social upheaval or complacency cause relaxation of measures for the control of infectious disease. A protected population is dependent for continuing survival upon continuance of protection.

The final problem, potentially the most serious, is a change in the human gene pool. Preventive measures and use of antibiotics have greatly reduced selection pressures favouring genetic resistance to infectious disease. Advances in therapy are reducing also mortality from non-infectious diseases with a genetic component. Examples are numerous and include juvenile diabetes, haemophilia, and phenyl pyruvic oligophrenia. Treatment of genetic disorders affecting resistance to infection also comes in this category, and have led to the ultimate inhumanity of the "bubble baby" leading a restricted life devoid of hope or human contact in a sterile plastic chamber. These conditions were once lethal before the age of reproduction; carriers of such genes now survive and pass the gene to their children.

These processes imply a slow change in the human gene pool, with slow increase in the numbers of carriers of once-lethal genes, and increasing numbers in the community depending for their existence upon continuing medical treatment. Such a population can survive only if this treatment is available, and includes an increasing number of biological cripples of low economic productivity.

This is ultimately an ethical rather than a medical problem, but (assuming the human species survives nuclear holocaust) must become of increasing concern. It may be that the Judaic–Christian ethic that each human life is to be preserved at all costs will require re-examination. Certainly eugenics will become a central social, political and scientific problem. Medicine has already reached the point of no return.

References

Amulree, Lord (1964). *In* "The Evolution of Hospitals in Britain" (F. N. L. Poynter, Ed.), 11–26. Pitman, London.

Bronte-Stewart, B., Budtz-Olsen, O. E., Hickley, J. M. and Brock, J. F. (1960). *S. Afr. J. lab. clin. Med.* **6**, 188–216.

Brunt, P. A. (1971). "Italian Manpower 225BC–AD14". Clarendon Press, Oxford.

Hart, P. D'A. and Wright, G. P. (1939). "Tuberculosis and Social Conditions in England". National Association for the Prevention of Tuberculosis, London.

Joske, R. A. and Joske, E. J. P. (1979). *Med. J. Aust.* **1**, 508–510.

Marshack, A. (1972). "The Roots of Civilization". McGraw-Hill, New York.

McKeown, T., Brown, R. G. and Record, R. G. (1972). *Population Studies* **27**, 354–382.

McKeown, T. and Lowe, C. R. (1974). "An Introduction to Social Medicine", 2nd edn. Blackwell, Oxford.

Moodie, P. M. and Pederson, E. B. (1971). "The Health of Australian Aborigines: An Annotated Bibliography". Australian Government Publishing Service, Canberra.

Polunin, I. V. (1967). *In* "Disease in Antiquity" (D. Bruthwell and A. T. Sanderson, Eds), 69–97. C. C. Thomas, Springfield, Ill.
World Health Organization (1978). The Promotion and Development of Traditional Medicine. *Wld Hlth Org. Tech. Rep. Ser.* No. 622.

31

The Impact of Immunology

N. A. Mitchison

Department of Zoology, University College London, London, England

---

Immunology is like coming upon a game of chess which clever opponents have been playing against one another for a million years.

I. Introduction

Immunology occupies a unique place among the medical sciences. It is generally agreed that the immunological approach to infectious disease is in the long run likely to prove the most effective, the most complete, the most easily applied, the least damaging, and the cheapest. In comparison with antibiotics, immunology perturbs the balance of nature to a lesser extent, and offers hope of really long term protection. Much the same can be said of the immunological approach to cancer in comparison to treatment with surgery or radiation. Yet for all this, the science of immunology is as repulsive as it is lovable. The main building has an intellectual framework which creates and bends. The walls are papered with baffling jargon. Every now and then a whole wing collapses. (Whatever happened to immunological surveillance of cancer? Or to that T cell receptor which was encoded within the major histocompatibility complex?) The practical men inhabit a row of outhouses more or less fully detached from the main edifice, perhaps wisely considering its shaky condition. Let no one enter immunology who is not endowed with patience, curiosity and a long memory.

That this should be the case is not surprising. Immunology is like coming upon a game of chess which clever opponents have been playing against one another for a million years. Host and parasite have each sifted through a multitude of ingenious strategies. He who thinks he knows what they are up to, and can help the game along with a nudge or two, is likely to be in for a surprise. So the difficult, unpredictable, and often paradoxical nature of the subject needs no excuse.

We shall begin with a brief visit to the immune system, with the aim of trying to get clear about what is known definitely, and what is likely to remain uncertain for the time being. We shall then examine the impact which immunology is likely to have on infectious diseases. Next comes organ transplantation, the area in which immunology has had its greatest triumph in the last few years. We shall also consider how the immune system plays traitor by acting to the detriment of the body. Then comes fields which immunology is even now trying to enter, particularly cancer and fertility control. Finally, we shall see how immunological methods are changing other branches of science, such as biochemistry and genetics.

Useful short textbooks of basic immunology are available (Eisen, 1974; Golub, 1977; Hobart and McConnell, 1978; Roitt, 1978) as are longer texts on clinical immunology (Lachmann and Peters, 1980). A more detailed text on cellular immunology (Loor and Roelants, 1977) is already getting out of date, a reflection of the speed with which the subject moves.

II. The Immune System

In man the immune system has about a million million cells. This is much the same as the number of nerve cells. The immune system is second only to the nervous system in its degree of complexity and integration, and much can be learned from comparing them. Both show a very high degree of precision. Vernier acuity—the ability of the visual system to distinguish verniers set apart by less than the diameter of a retinal cone cell—may be compared with the spatial acuity of antibody combining sites, which can distinguish between antigens which differ from one another by less than the radius of an atom. Both show memory. Both are highly adaptive, in the sense that the environment moulds both systems as they develop, so that at the end of its life an individual is uniquely suited to the environment in which it lives. Both, in the course of becoming more integrated, have turned a larger and larger proportion of their cells towards purely internal activities. These cells are the interneurones and regulatory lymphocytes, as distinct from the motor neurones and effector lymphocytes. Yet, great as these similarities are, the underlying mechanisms are really quite different. The immune system integrates through transient as distinct from stable contacts, relies on a far greater range of different molecules (although the number of types of molecule may actually be smaller), and utilizes selection (i.e. the discarding of useless molecules and cells) to a far greater extent. Occasionally immunologists and neurobiologists underestimate these differences, and in a fit of enthusiasm try to force their principles down one another's throats.

A. Range, Precision and Sensitivity

The outstanding features of the immune system are its range, precision, sensitivity and flexibility. Almost any macromolecule can arouse an immune response. This includes not only all the diverse structures which are found on microorganisms and parasites, with which it is the business of the system to deal, but also entirely new compounds which chemists have synthesized for the first time. This is as it should be, for it is the business of the system to deal with microorganisms, and they can evolve new structures rapidly in an endeavour to escape its attention. The exceptions are interesting. During the Second World War an urgent search was made for plasma extenders, macromolecules which could be dissolved in saline for use in place of blood for transfusion. Many polysaccharides were tried but turned out to arouse an immune response. Eventually straight-chain dextrans were adopted for use. Nevertheless, we now know that the immune system itself is perfectly capable of making antibodies which can fit; what is missing in these molecules is the triggering action which initiates a response (Kabat, 1976). Much the same probably applies to the "inert" plastics and metals which are used in surgical prostheses, and to the inert coats of multicellular parasites.

A feature of the range is its extraordinary sharp cut-off where self begins (Howard and Mitchison, 1975; Mitchison, 1978). This also is as it should be, in order to prevent an immune attack upon self cells. Many years ago, Burnet proposed that cells of the same body as the immune system carry self-markers, by which they are recognized and which prevent immune attack. The theory implies that there is active recognition of self combined with a mechanism of suppression. The truth as we understand it now is rather different. The first thing which happens is that the immune system loses the ability to react with the cells of its own body, probably by losing certain cells of its own. After that there is no active recognition of self, but simply an absence of recognition. However, if through some mischance this first stage does not work properly, a second fail-safe mechanism comes into operation, in which recognition of self does occur and which does generate suppression of the response. Experiments in animals suggest that this is how autoimmune diseases go spontaneously into remission.

The extreme precision of the immune response is shown in many ways (Kabat, 1976). Landsteiner found that structurally similar small chemicals could be distinguished from one another with great precision if they were attached to macromolecules to act as antigens. The A and B blood groups are sugars which differ little from one another. Single amino acid substitutions in proteins can readily be recognized, as has best been shown by the reaction of rabbits to human haemoglobins. In all these instances the actual difference is much smaller than the entire cavity of the antibody combining site. What does the recognizing is no more than a wrinkle on the wall of the cavity.

Even more impressive is the precision with which the immune response is tailored to need. There is economy of effort both in size and duration. The larger the antigenic stimulus, the larger the amount of antibody which is made in response. And the response continues for just so long as antigen remains present in the body. This can be a long while, for the immune system has devised ingenious strategies for latching onto and retaining antigens (Unanue, 1978). This serves the purpose of eliminating the last traces of an invader and building up immunological memory against any subsequent invasion. Responses usually cover a certain range, as a result of the simultaneous activation of cells which differ slightly from one another. This ensures that minor variations among invaders can be dealt with; it also enables the response to explore the surface of invading antigens and come to fit it more and more closely—"maturation" of the response. Tailoring to need can also be seen when exceptionally large quantities of antigen confront the immune system. Then special mechanisms come into play which ensure that the system does not become entirely preoccupied, but reserves some potential to deal with other antigenic contingencies.

The system is exquisitely sensitive to foreign molecules provided that they are concentrated together, as on the surface of a bacterium or virus (Feldmann, 1976). One of the reasons why bacterial toxins are dangerous is because they are so dispersed. The system has accessory cells whose function is to concentrate antigen on their surfaces, as well as to retain it, and helper lymphocytes probably serve the same function. In fact much of the regulation of the immune response can best be understood in terms of antigen-concentrating mechanisms. As a result of the activation of antigen-concentrating lymphocytes, someone who has once been exposed to an antigen becomes as much as a 1000 fold more sensitive to a subsequent exposure. These concentrating cells have another effect: having recognized one part of an antigen, which may be a molecule or even a structure as large as a foreign cell, other parts of that antigen get dragged into the response (Lake and Mitchison, 1977). Consequently a response which may start against a dispensable part of an invader tends to spread and attack the vital parts.

All this has not been accomplished without a measure of waste, or so it seems. A substantial fraction of the antibodies and effector cells which are generated by an antigenic stimulus do not seen to be directed at that stimulus. Some of them react with self molecules. One should be a little cautious in accepting this simply as unavoidable overspill. Perhaps these concomitant autoantibodies and self-reactive cells serve a useful function in mopping up damage done by invaders. Much the same applies to the hypersensitivities: maybe hay fever is the price which we pay for being able to slough off Nippostrongylus and other worms of the intestinal wall.

B. Selection at Three Levels

The mechanism of the immune system which is best understood is clonal selection (Jerne, 1967). Clonal selection operates in a simple way. Lymphocytes occur as clones: each clone is a little family, descended from a single ancestor, and each member of the family bears on its surface a single kind of antibody molecule. This is the only kind of antibody that this cell will ever make, unless (as happens very occasionally) it switches. Even then it makes antibodies which differ in other parts of the molecule, but not in the antigen-combining site itself. Lymphocytes spend most of their lives at rest, if a ceaseless circulation in and out of the blood system can be so described. At any rate, they do not divide and they do not secrete much, until they encounter their own particular antigen. When that happens their surface antibody molecules come into action and trigger the cell to divide; some of the cells among the progeny then start secreting antibody, others go on to become memory cells. The important point is that any antigen which enters the body selectively stimulates those lymphocytes with receptors which fit.

This theory took a long time to become established. One difficulty was to imagine how the diversity of antibody molecules could be generated, and another the amount of waste. These inspired two famous jokes: abbreviating the Generator Of Diversity to its initials, to show that something had to do the job even if we do not understand how it works, and pointing out that Nature wastes more spermatozoa than lymphocytes (Lennox and Cohn, 1967).

By now the advance of molecular biology has largely solved the GOD problem (Tonegawa *et al.*, 1977; Seidman *et al.*, 1978). DNA hybridization techniques show that most of our cells have a string of DNA sequences coding for the variable regions of antibodies, which are the part of an antibody which contains the antigen combining site. Nearby, but separate, are the DNA sequences which code for the antibody constant region. This arrangement is repeated at least six times, to code for the various protein chains which make up the antibody molecule. Sometime during the early development of a lymphocyte, long before antibody receptors have appeared, something unique occurs. Most of the DNA which separates the variable and constant regions is excised, so that one of the variable regions genes becomes placed next to one of the constant regions. This fixes the antibody gene for that cell, and for all its descendants unless switching occurs.

Many of the details have not yet been worked out, such as the nature of switching, or what goes on in T cells, the lymphocytes which do not secrete antibodies. One would very much like to know more about the enzymes responsible for the crucial event of DNA excision. Perhaps they are cousins of the enzymes which cleave and rejoin the other important nucleic acid, RNA, in all cells. But at any rate, what happens is now clear in outline: one among a range of inherited DNA sequences is selected at random by an excision enzyme. This is what generates diversity. To this is added some further mutational drift, which produces even greater diversity. This then represents the first level at which selection occurs.

In between this level and the final level of clonal selection by antigen during an immune response, there occurs at least one intermediate level of selection (Marshall-Clarke and Playfair, 1979). Just what happens at this point is still uncertain, but its effect is important: it regulates the lymphocyte repertoire, i.e. the range and relative frequency of lymphocyte receptors which are actually present in the body, as distinct from the range and relative frequency which is generated to begin with by the GOD. In fact, the repertoire seems to be regulated in at least three ways, and it is not clear whether or not these three forms of regulation are imposed at the same time. One of them is the deletion of clones which react with self-molecules, something which has already been mentioned. Another is the dictation of restriction elements in the thymus, something which probably occurs only for T cells, and which will be further discussed in the next section. A third form of regulation seems to occur when young lymphocytes first encounter antigen. For B cells (the lymphocytes which can generate antibody-secreting cells) this is just after they leave the fetal liver or bone marrow. For T cells, if the same occurs for them, it would be either just before or just after leaving the thymus. These young cells are short-lived and do not recirculate through the blood, unless they encounter antigen. At this stage, an encounter with antigen causes a further step in differentiation, as a result of which the clone becomes immortal. This intermediate level of selection is adaptive: it has the effect of filling the final pool of mature lymphocytes with those cells which are best suited to deal with antigens of the local environment.

C. The Major Histocompatibility Complex and Immune Regulation

Interest in the major histocompatibility complex (MHC) grew out of transplantation biology, but as we shall see this was a matter of chance: work on immune responsiveness, or on antigen presentation, might equally well have led to its discovery (Schreffler and David, 1975; Festenstein and Dement, 1978). Until a few years ago what was known about the MHC seemed oddly assorted, and can be summarized as follows: (i) the MHC codes for three classes of protein, one a single chain of 45 000 Daltons which occurs on the cell surface in association with a small protein β_2 microglobulin coded for elsewhere, another a cell surface dimer with 28 000 and 32 000 Dalton chains, and the third a group of complement components which are secreted. Each class has several representatives encoded within the complex. The first, the K/D molecules have four, and the second, the Ia class, eight. These numbers and nomenclature are for the diploid set of the mouse, and the numbers may well be an underestimate. The complex is about 1 cM long, which in theory leaves plenty of room for encoding other molecules. (ii) The arrangement is stable in evolution, dating back at least to the common ancestor of birds and mammals, and probably into the fish. (iii) The K/D and Ia classes of molecule are exceptionally polymorphic. (iv) Both these classes are strong alloantigens (i.e. antigens as tested in other members of the same animal species); paradoxically they may be stronger as alloantigens than when tested as antigens in other species. As alloantigens they arouse different responses, K/D molecules arousing mainly cytotoxic cells (T_C cells) and Ia molecules stimulating mainly helper or factor-secreting cells (T_H cells). Neither of these are antibody-secreting cells, and the lymphocytes which upon arousal do secrete antibodies (B cells) are not particularly responsive to MHC alloantigens. (v) The Ia molecules behave as strong immune response (IR) genes for antibody production. In breeding experiments certain alleles in the Ia region associate with responsiveness to certain antigens, others with non-responsiveness, although no allele can make a mouse a universal responder or non-responder. The K/D molecules behave in the same way for cytotoxic cell responses, although this was only found out later and causes some confusion in the nomenclature. The term Ir-1, as applied to IR genes which map in the Ia region is best avoided. Other IR genes map elsewhere in the genome, and the total umber of IR genes must be enormous. (vi) The molecules have an odd distribution. K/D molecules occur on all cells except trophoblast and erythrocytes (where they do occur in small amounts in some species). Ia molecules occur on lymphocytes, dendritic cells, and to a variable extent on macrophages.

So matters stood, and nobody could quite tie all this together. Benacerraf and his colleagues tried once and missed, with the proposal that Ia molecules code for the antigen receptor on T cells (Benacerraf and McDevitt, 1972). Jerne also tried and missed, with the proposal that MHC molecules within the thymus generate diversity in receptors of T cells and control the T cell repertoire (Jerne, 1971). This proposal has an element of truth, insofar as the thymus does indeed affect the T cell repertoire, but it probably does so in an indirect fashion. What was missing was one more clue, one which was provided by Zinkernagel and Doherty (1974) for T_C cells and by Katz and his colleagues (1973) for T_H cells.

Their crucial discovery was that T cells recognize not only antigen, but also an MHC molecule with which the antigen must be associated (Zinkernagel and Doherty, 1977). This MHC molecule is called a restriction element, and we do not know quite how it works. Probably T cells have two receptors, one for the antigen and one for the restriction element. Probably also the antigen must bind to the MHC molecule on the surface of an antigen presenting cell. T cells receive their instructions about which restriction element to recognize within the thymus, and it has been possible in chimaeric mice to programme these cells so that they do not even recognize MHC molecules identical to their own as restriction elements.

Now it was possible for Zinkernagel to build a general theory (Zinkernagel, 1977). It starts from the fact that lymphocytes occur in parallel sets, each of which contains a more or less complete repertoire of binding sites. This is well known for B cells, where there are parallel sets of B cells for IgA antibodies, IgM, IgE, etc. Their counterpart among T cells are T_C, T_H, and suppressor cells (T_S), sets which will probably be further subdivided sometime in the future. This arrangement into parallel sets gives the immune system an element of flexibility, which it needs in order to cope with the multitude of types of infection. In this theory the response to infection occupies its proper place at the centre of the evolutionary stage. Antigens which associate with K/D molecules arouse a T_C cell response, appropriately for example if the antigen is a budding virus and the T_C cell succeeds in destroying its host cell. Antigens which associate with Ia molecules on the surface of macrophages arouse a T_H cell response. These cells release macrophage-activating factor, again appropriately if the antigen is from an intracellular parasite which the macrophage harbours. The theory was vindicated by experiments which showed that when immunity was transferred from one mouse to another by means of lymphocytes, for the budding virus of lymphocytic choriomeningitis the mice had to match at K/D, while for the bacterial parasite *Listeria monocytogenes* they had to match at Ia. This has now become a standard procedure for identifying the type of T cell responsible for protective immunity to an infective agent (Howes *et al.*, 1979a).

The genetics now fall into line. The IR gene effect operates at the level of antigen presentation, where it controls the ability of MHC molecules acting as restriction elements to associate with particular antigens. Naturally this affects the T cell repertoire, but it does so only indirectly by determining which T cell clones receive stimulation. Viruses and other infective agents will try to avoid stimulating T cells, and so they will tend to evolve forms which do not associate with restriction elements. This in turn will drive the MHC towards polymorphism and gene duplication. It is deeply significant that all ordinary mice (as distinct from specially bred ones) possess at least one responder-type MHC molecule for all viruses which have so far been tested, although they often have other non-responder-type MHC molecules as well for these viruses. Evolutionary strategies may become more complex, without altering the general trend towards polymorphism. Thus some viruses, exemplified by Semliki Forrest Virus, take advantage of physical association to use the K/D molecules as receptors for entering cells (Helenius *et al.*, 1978). And the optimal evolutionary strategy of viruses is certainly not to make all hosts completely defenceless.

It should be emphasized that our understanding of how the T cell part of the immune system works is much less complete than it is for B cells. Important regulatory mechanisms may operate through T cells in addition to those that we have discussed. For example, in several experimental systems regulatory T cells work by recognizing receptors carrying specific binding sites (idiotypes); this may or may not be a general mechanism (Jerne, 1974). Furthermore, T cells can operate through longer pathways than have been mentioned here, involving three of more cells regulating one another in series (Eardley *et al.*, 1978). Such pathways can give rise to feedback circuits, with their own regulatory properties. T cells may release their receptors in the form of soluble factors, which they use to regulate other cells; this does not alter the principles which we have been discussing, but it does remove the difficulty of rare clones having to encounter one another. MHC molecules may occur as part of these factors, which is puzzling (Feldmann *et al.*, 1977). So the picture is not yet complete. Yet it is pleasant to contemplate T cells at a time when one large and important area has been largely brought to order.

D. Mathematical Models

Immunology has begun to attract the interest of systems engineers as a subject ripe for the application of mathematical models (Bell *et al.*, 1978). Computer models are penetrating biology, particularly in areas of applied biology where decisions have to be based on complex factors and where there may be very large amounts of data to evaluate. One would not want nowadays, for example, to advise on fishery policy in North Atlantic waters without a proper demographic model, and much the same is true of insect parasites on crops. Immunology offers the same order of complexity. The main aim of the models so far has been to predict quantity and goodness-of-fit of antibody which will be made in response to various schedules of antigen administrations. The first primitive models were based simply on clonal selection among B cells. More sophisticated models are now being run which take account of regulatory T cells and antigen-presenting cells. Both types of model, but particularly the second, match experimental data quite well.

So far these models have attracted attention mainly among experimentalists. Surely this is the wrong audience, for what experimentalists really enjoy is demolishing models. One hopes that these models will find their main use among clinicians. It is in the nature of clinical work to generate the repetitive data which models can best handle, and it is there that short-term predictions are most needed.

Immunology is also important for mathematical models of another kind (Conway, 1977; Anderson and May, 1979). Starting from the classical Ross equations, elaborate models have been erected of the population dynamics of host–parasite relationships. Immunology necessarily enters these models as a factor affecting not only mortality and morbidity after infection, but also the parasite density which in turn affects transmission rate. As these models develop and find wider application, they will need better immunological inputs.

III. The Control of Infection

Immunology has always found its principal application in the control of infection, and this is likely to remain so in the future. Far the most important form of immunological intervention in diseases both of man and animals has been vaccination: the prevention, partial or complete, of a disease by the administration of the infectious agent in the form of an attenuated or killed organism or a purified antigenic component. Over the last few decades immunological intervention has taken second place to the use of antibiotics, but these will lose some of their value as resistance spreads. To an extent, the discovery of new antibiotics will compensate but this will prove progressively more difficult and expensive. Just where equilibrium will be reached nobody knows, but it is likely that over the next decade immunology will grow rather than decline in importance. This decade has probably, though not certainly, seen the greatest triumph of vaccination, the eradication of smallpox. At the time of writing the last case of smallpox not due to laboratory infection had been reported in October 1977 (Arita, 1979). The danger still remains that fresh cases may yet arise either from unreported pockets of infection in man, or by genetic change from related animal viruses; that danger will increase as the unvaccinated proportion of the human population increases (see Fenner, this volume).

The case for the development of vaccines rests primarily on the direct benefits to the individual vaccinated, in terms of decreased mortality and morbidity from disease. Then there are the benefits which accrue to the entire population at risk from the disease, in terms of lower transmission rates and reduced epidemics. There are obvious economic benefits when the burdens of a debilitating disease are lifted: this applies particularly to endemic parasites. The economic benefits which would accrue from the development of veterinary vaccines are equally obvious, particularly for trypanosomiasis and East Coast fever (Theileria) in Africa. But there are other major benefits which are less obvious. For example, infectious disease imposes genetic burdens on the population at risk. These include (i) the cost of maintaining immune response gene polymorphisms (ii) the cost of maintaining polymorphisms not directly associated with immunity, but which could be dispensed with if the diseases responsible could be eradicated by immunological intervention; (iii) the cost of maintaining in the population non-polymorphic genes which fall into either of these categories, and which are otherwise disadvantageous; and (iv) the cost of spreading resistance genes for new diseases, which are often in fact old diseases introduced into previously unexposed populations. Often these costs are attributable to many diseases, as must be the case with the HLA polymorphisms (Festenstein and Dement, 1978). But sometimes they can fairly clearly be attributable to a single disease, as is the case with sickling, thalassaemia, and glucose-6-phosphate dehydrogenase deficiency in relation to malaria (Brown, 1976). All these costs are proper targets for saving by adequate immunological intervention.

A. Immune Prophylaxis

When considering future prospects in vaccination, we can start with the course of progress as it should ideally go. At any time in history the vaccines which are in use should be a window in the range of what is possible. At one end vaccines go out of use, as their infectious agent is eradicated: smallpox at the present time would be an example of this. At the other, candidate vaccines are being chosen for general use, on the basis of their effectiveness, the size of threat from the disease, and their hazards: cytomegalovirus, Herpesvirus simplex type II, and gonococci, would be examples of such candidates at the present time.

This would be accompanied by a progressive refinement of vaccines designed to increase their effectiveness, diminish their hazards, and lower their cost; at the same time more effective vehicles, adjuvants, and modes of administration would be sought. Examples at the present time would be the fractionation of viral vaccines into their component proteins, and eventually, as is now possible with some adenoviruses, the use of crystalline coat proteins. Indeed, at the present moment it would be technically possible to manufacture a flu vaccine based on synthetic peptide fragments of spike protein: the current price would be around $25 000 per gram, which is not yet competitive with egg-grown vaccine (see Mackenzie, this volume). However, genetic engineering offers another approach to the large-scale production of defined peptides which is likely to prove cheaper. In the meanwhile, hazards from contaminants can be reduced by growing viruses in human diploid cell lines rather than in animal cells. Such cell lines were first introduced for the production of poliovirus, where any possible risk from human oncogenic viruses now seems smaller than the known risk of viruses from monkey cells. This sort of programme aims ultimately at treating all vaccines in the way in which meningococcal vaccines are treated at present: instead of being handled as biologicals, with all the uncertainties which that implies, they will be handled as chemicals, and dosed out in micrograms.

Why then has this programme not achieved more? For there is little reason to fear that the capacity of the immune system has yet been overstretched. Part of the problem is scientific. For malaria and trypanosomiasis the main problem is antigenic variation of the parasites during the course of infection (Terry, 1976). For influenza, antigenic variation occurs from year to another. Perhaps this variation can be predicted: Fazekas's theory of senior and junior antigens must surely have at least a grain of truth, although the practical men are not impressed by its application (Fazekas, 1977). For tuberculosis, although BCG vaccine proves moderately effective in developed countries, in India the level of natural exposure to related antigens is too high for it to have much effect. Not much can be expected of cholera vaccines since the disease itself arouses little long-term immunity.

The biggest problem in developing vaccines lies in arranging for them to arouse a response which is appropriate in the sense defined above. The problem is essentially one of arousing activity in an appropriate lymphocyte parallel set, or rather of choosing an appropriately balanced selection of such sets. Take cholera, for example (Holmgren and Svennerholm, 1977). So far as B cells are concerned, the appropriate set would presumably be the IgA-secreting cells which recirculate through gut tissue. Conventional vaccination, given intramuscularly in the arm, is not calculated to arouse a response in this set. But the lesson which basic studies in cellular immunology surely teach us is that what matters most are the regulatory T cell sets. Their science is still very young. We hardly know how to start measuring activity among T cell parallel sets in man. For some time to come we shall certainly have to rely on very blunt procedures, such as the use of selected adjuvants and live versus dead organisms in vaccines.

A major part of the problem with vaccine development is social rather than scientific. Why spend energy on developing a trypanosomiasis vaccine, for example, when better husbandry and vector control could already do so much to expand the area in which cattle could graze? Or to take another example, a recent trial of flu vaccine in British post-office workers showed that the benefits of vaccination were smaller than expected. Many of those who take sick-leave during flu epidemics, particularly around Christmas, do not as it turns out actually suffer from infection!

The possibility of non-specific immunoprophylaxis is worth a mention (Allison, 1978). This has been proposed for use in controlling haemoparasite infections in cattle. Experiments in mice suggest that infection with the Babesias can be controlled by administering agents which stimulate macrophages. Agricultural animals might be treated with these agents at the crucial time when they are losing maternally transmitted immunity while being bitten by infected mosquitoes. A strategy of this sort would be well worth testing in these and perhaps other diseases.

B. Immunotherapy

Immunotherapy is the treatment of disease by immunological methods after infection has occured. Except in rabies, it is little used. When the reverse transcriptase assay for the virus of serum hepatitis was first intoduced, it was said that although one could predict who was going to come down with the disease some weeks ahead, all that could then be done was to study the benefit of staying in bed. That is not quite fair. But nearly all the interest in immunotherapy in man has focused on two agents, transfer factor and interferon. Both have been available for more than a decade, and neither one is of more than doubtful value. This is partly because they have both been hard to come by, but this is not the only reason.

Interferon—or the interferons, as is now known—is an agent which arouses in mammalian cells a form of resistance to viruses at large (Burke, 1979). Because it is non-specific in its action it does not really fall within the scope of this discussion, except insofar as anything which delays the course of viral infection will tend to help the specific immune defences. Our understanding of the biochemical action of interferon is improving steadily, as are methods of production in bulk, and clinical trials are getting underway.

Unfortunately, the same cannot be said of transfer factor (Spitler, 1978). This is a mysterious agent which is prepared from blood leukocytes, and which transfers certain forms of immunity to recipients. Research has been held up by the absence of convincing animal or *in vitro* models. From a scientific point of view, transfer factor hovers unhappily between two extremes. It may be a form of processed antigen, perhaps something like the complexes of Ia molecules with antigenic fragments that antigen-processing cells may release. Or it may be a messenger RNA, a concept which is clouded by much utterly uncritical work.

In the next stage one hopes that agents which are much more firmly based on modern cellular immunology will come into use. Antibodies directed at surface markers on lymphocytes are one obvious possibility, for antibodies directed at various Ia molecules have already been used successfully in the mouse to perturb the immune response. Antisera directed at factors which mediate cell–cell interactions in the immune system offer another possibility; indeed certain antibodies which were first thought to act directly on cell surfaces may in fact act principally on soluble products released by cells. Antibodies of animal origin are unsatisfactory as therapeutic agents, and it stretches the imagination to suppose that human autoimmune anti-lymphocyte antibodies will ever be manufactured in bulk, even using the latest cloning techniques *in vitro*. One is left for the time being with the hope of finding highly selective immunopharmacological agents: some super-subtle version of cyclophosphamide, perhaps. Nothing of the sort has yet turned up, but then the necessary screening procedures are only just becoming available. If such agents can exist then microorganisms in their age-old game with their hosts should have hit on them, so perhaps new light will come from the study of infection.

C. Immunodiagnosis and Immunological Typing

Immunology will continue to find a useful if humdrum place in clinical tests. Advances can be expected in the typing of microorganisms and metazoan parasites, particularly in the sorting out of closely related types through the use of monoclonal antibodies. More information about *Herpes simplex* type-specific antigens would be valuable for instance, not only for the very practical purpose of tracking venereal disease but also from a theoretical standpoint in understanding the evolution of the complex and ubiquitous Herpesvirus group (Howes *et al.*, 1979b).

Cell-based tests are likely to grow in importance. Proliferation assays provide a straightforward method of assessing a specific state of cellular immunity; this will become even more valuable when the populations of T cells engaged in proliferation can be sorted out. Cytotoxic assays have been difficult to handle and interpret, but recent work with influenza virus shows that the well-tried animal technique of restimulating *in vitro* lymphocytes isolated from blood may help (McMichael *et al.*, 1977). Dare one hope that these *in vitro* tests will form the basis of some future therapy: for instance that autologous cytomegalovirus-specific cytotoxic T cells, grown up *in vitro*, will be used to protect autologous bone marrow transplant patients against this virus which is at present their greatest scourge?

D. Immunodeficiencies

Alert paediatricians made an important contribution to the immunology of resistance to infection when they began to study the diseases of congenitally immunodeficient children (Good and Hansen, 1976). These diseases conform to a pattern which is related to the nature of the deficiency. Thus congenitally athymic infants tend to suffer from infections with budding viruses, whereas infants who lack the ability to produce antibodies often suffer from pyogenic infections. This is the kind of information upon which our earliest knowledge of the functions of different lymphocyte sets was based. When inquiries are being pursued about any disease it is still well worth finding out about its incidence in the various types of immunodeficiences.

Although rare, these deficiences have contributed an enormous amount of useful information about the working of the immune system (Cooper *et al.*, 1975; Waldmann *et al.*, 1978). Much of what we know about lymphocyte subpopulations in man has been learned from the peripheral blood of immunodeficient individuals. Patients suffering from partial agammaglobulinaemia have proved particularly revealing: practically every defect which could be imagined does in fact occur, ranging from an excess of suppressor T cell activity to an inability of normally responsive B cells to secrete antibody. Leukocytes from these individuals offer an arena in which new theories of immunology can be tested.

IV. Organ and Tissue Transplantation

Tissue transplantation occupies a curious position in the history of immunology. Many, perhaps most, of the advances in cellular immunology made over the last forty years have had their origin in studies on tissue transplantation: immunological tolerance, cell transfers in inbred animals, the discovery of the major histocompatibility complex are but a few examples. And transplantation of the kidney has been one of the major advances in clinical medicine, and certainly the major scientific advance in surgery. Yet the major histocompatibility complex is now seen as related to infectious disease rather then transplant surgery, and even a question whether it should be rechristened as the "T cell activation complex" has been raised (Mitchison, 1979). Studies on self-tolerance have contributed little to the practice of organ transplantation, where immunosuppression is still carried out on a largely empirical basis. And transplantation, jointly with open heart surgery, has been denounced on grounds of cost.

Now that much of the early drama has blown over, organ transplantation has found a limited but definite role in surgical practice (Merrill, 1978). In comparison with dialysis which is the normal alternative to kidney transplantation in a developed country, transplantation comes ahead in a proportion of cases not only in terms of patient preference but also in terms of cost. The results of kidney transplantation are steadily improving, more because of better patient selection and milder immunosuppression than because of technical advances; reducing immunosuppression decreases the chances of survival for the graft, but increases them for the patient.

On the scientific side, there is no question that the enormous investment in mouse immunogenetics has amply paid off. Over a million mice have been bred in order to find out about their transplantation antigens. As a result of this effort we have a unique body of information plus a unique collection of genetically defined strains. So powerful are these that most of immunology in other animals has been reduced to a side-show: if it cannot be done in man or the mouse, it is not worth doing. Much of the information described in the first section of this chapter was acquired in the mouse, and for the time being there is no reason to expect this pattern of scientific investment to change.

V. Cancer

Medawar describes the immunology of cancer as a subject where the goods have long been invoiced but not yet delivered. Certainly the practical rewards from a very great deal of effort have been meagre. What, at the present time, are we left with?

First, immunology makes a small but useful contribution to the diagnosis and monitoring of cancer. The carcinoembryonic antigen (CEA) test and the alpha-feto-protein (AFP) test are useful for this purpose respectively in carcinoma of the gut and the liver (Burtin, 1978; Phillips *et al.*, 1977). Both have a false positive rate which is high enough to make their use as screening procedures doubtful, although this has been advocated. It is a matter of interest that by far the largest experience with the AFP test has been acquired in China, where well over half a million individuals have been examined (reported at the XI International Cancer Congress, Florence, 1974). But, even our Chinese colleagues have for the time being given up their test as a mass screening procedure.

Antigens on the surface of leukaemic cells provide valuable guidance to the nature and course of this group of diseases (Greaves *et al.*, 1977). Antigens are one among a battery of leukaemia markers that include lectin and virus receptors, and intracellular enzymes. Together these markers now provide a means of rationally classifying the leukaemias so that the course of disease can be predicted, and appropriate treatment selected. The fluorescence-activated cell sorter, a sophisticated instrument which assays surface antigens quantitatively, is useful in this work. With its aid, leukaemic cells can be detected at frequencies of $<10^{-4}$, enough to improve the prediction and early treatment of relapse.

Of the two main areas of progress in experimental systems, one has been with cancer viruses. Cancer cells which have been induced by viruses usually retain part of the viral genome, which is expressed on the cell surface in the form of viral proteins. With appropriate immunization these can cause rejection of the cancer cells. One important practical example of this is in the prevention of Marek's disease, a leukosis of chickens caused by a herpesvirus, through immunization with a viral vaccine in the form of a cross-reactive turkey herpesvirus (Biggs, 1975). It is likely that another herpesvirus, Epstein-Barr virus (EBV) plays a part in causing two human cancers, Burkitt's lymphoma and nasopharyngeal cancer. A case can be made on this basis for developing a vaccine against EBV for use in man (Epstein, 1978).

Immunology has made a useful contribution to the molecular biology of the retroviruses, the C-type viruses which cause leukaemia and mammary cancer in mice and other animals (Shellam *et al.*, 1975). It had been hoped that the cell surface antigens, which alone can provoke protective immunity, might include a molecule which would be directly responsible for the cell being neoplastic. A molecule which may indeed be responsible in this way has now been found by the use of immunological techniques, but unfortunately it is located only within cancer cells. It is the product of the src gene, and is an enzyme with the remarkable property of phosphorylating antibody which binds to it (Purchio *et al*., 1978).

The other main area of progress in experimental systems has been with chemically and physically induced tumours. Some of these have quite strong rejection antigens which are unique to each tumour. Perhaps the most interesting system is the ultraviolet light-induced tumours of mice which have been worked out in some detail (Kripke, 1974; Fisher and Kripke, 1978). Many of these are so strongly antigenic that they cannot be transplanted in unconditioned compatible hosts. They can grow in their mouse of origin probably only because the UV light which induced the tumour also induced suppressor T cells; these cells recognize an antigen shared among the tumours of this type, which is surprising since each tumour's rejection antigen is unique. These tumours are the only non-viral animal tumours where there is convincing evidence of immune surveillance against cancer. It is significant that in man the only convincing evidence of surveillance is for a comparable group of skin tumours: these are tumours with a raised incidence in immunosuppressed individuals. High exposure to sunlight raises their incidence in white people, and they respond well to surgical treatment.

The unique rejection antigens are a challenge to molecular biology. Their isolation and characterization should be the next step forward in cancer immunology.

VI. Autoimmune Diseases and Hypersensitivity

In these diseases and conditions the immune system is working to the detriment of the body, and treatment aims at suppressing the immune response and its consequences. We can include here one of the triumphs of immunology, haemolytic disease of the newborn, where history went the way it should (Mollison, 1973). First the causation was worked out; the disease occurs when a mother responds to fetal Rh antigens and transmits damaging antibodies back across the placenta. Next a treatment was worked out, consisting of removing the target of these antibodies by exchange-transfusing the newborn with Rh-negative blood. Finally a way of preventing the disease was found, by giving the mothers at risk a small amount of anti-Rh antibody to inhibit their own responses. Desensitization in allergy probably works in much the same way through antibody feedback inhibition of a deleterious response.

Treatment of most autoimmune diseases and hypersensitivities is far less specific, and relies at present mainly on non-specific anti-lymphocyte and anti-inflammatory agents. Some hypersensitivities can be controlled through the unique pharmacology of the mast cell. But otherwise, the main hope lies in pinning down what has gone wrong within the immune system (Ishizaka and Ishizaka, 1979; Ovary *et al*., 1979). Probably any step can fault, including antigen sequestration, processing by antigen-processing cells, lymphocyte receptor repertoires, and the balance of regulatory cells. If and when these faults can be diagnosed it may be possible to repair them by precise immunological engineering. In doing so, we shall look for guidance to transplantation immunology with its wealth of experience in manipulating responses to alloantigens.

Only rare diseases have autoimmunity as an unequivocal cause. A much more important group of diseases may have autoimmunity as at least a partial cause, but all that we know for certain is that patients often have autoantibodies or that their tissues seem to suffer from autoimmune attack. Here we can learn something important by looking for associations between the disease and particular MHC genes. The existence of an association would strongly suggest that immunology is involved, although not necessarily through autoimmunity. This kind of evidence has been found for certain types of diabetes (Suciu-Foca *et al*., 1977), rheumatic disease (Kemple and Bluestone, 1976) and multiple sclerosis (Sachs, 1977).

VII. Fertility Control

Immunization against pregnancy may become an important application. Vaccination should in principle be reliable, easy to administer, long-lasting, safe and cheap. For these reasons a fair amount of research into the possibility is under way, much of it with the support of the Human Reproduction Programme of the World Health Organization (Kessler and Standley, 1976). The work is still at an early stage, and it is too soon to know what vaccine will be chosen. The range of possible antigens is extensive: it includes the spermatozoan surface, acrosomal enzymes, zona pelucida, placental proteins, and the peptide hormones associated with menstrual cycling and pregnancy. Some reasonable selection criteria are (1) that the chosen immunogen should not be a normal component of the body undergoing immunization, in order to reduce the hazards of autoimmunization, (2) the immunogen should be available either immediately or in the near future as a well-defined molecule, and (3) immunization should not interfere with menstrual cycling. Needless to say, a candidate vaccine would have to pass stringent tests of efficacy, safety and reversibility in animals including primates, before it could be judged ready for clinical trial (WHO Task Force, 1978).

Possibilities which have been explored in a preliminary way include acrosomal enzymes and placental proteins. Immunity to luteotrophic hormone (LH) has a well documented anti-fertility effect, but is not thought suitable for general contraception because it inhibits cycling. This would not exclude passively administered antibody to LH from use as an abortive agent as part of a larger contraceptive package. A sperm-based vaccine is attractive because (a) the risks of autoimmunity should be small, and (b) anti-sperm antibodies are known to be associated with naturally occurring infertility. It is for the latter reason that WHO has arranged to bank human sera containing anti-sperm antibodies. Lactic dehydrogenase-X, an enzyme thought to occur only in the midpiece of spermatozoa, is particularly attractive as a candidate vaccine of the sperm-based variety.

The most advanced potential vaccines are based on human chorionic gonadotrophin (hCG) (Talwar *et al.*, 1976; Hearn, 1979). This is a peptide hormone which is secreted in large amounts only by the placenta, although the pituitary releases enough of a similar or identical peptide to cause some concern. Immunity to hCG is known to prevent completion of pregnancy in experiments with primates. Several problems remain at present. These include (i) a cross-reaction which may occur with pituitary hormones, particularly LH; (ii) availability of the peptide; (iii) reversability of immunity, and (iv) the fact that in certain animal experiments, during the time when the level of antibody falls, unacceptably late abortions occur. Progress with these matters has been impeded by our lack of information about the counterpart of hCG within the baboon, the best species for this kind of research. In order to circumvent the first two of these problems, the WHO programme has concentrated on the use of synthetic peptides, similar to that part of the hCG molecule which is most different in structure to LH (Stevens, 1978). Thus far vaccines based on these peptides, in the form of conjugates to proteins, have proved moderately effective as contraceptive agents in baboons. The time for clinical trials is near.

It is not difficult to imagine the worldwide use of such a vaccine. If so, it would be by far the largest experiment ever made with immunological intervention. The problems of safety are enormous: it is a very different matter testing a vaccine in animals, even to the most rigorous accepted standards, and employing it in a large human population. This problem is most formidable if one calculates the benefits only for a woman able to use existing methods of fertility control. Judgement changes according to the weight which is put on the benefits to society. One thing is certain: premature experimentation in humans could do far more damage to the progress of these vaccines than delays for proper testing.

In considering the benefits and detriments to society, the genetic consequences of such a programme are worth considering (Mitchison, 1975). Depending on the efficacy of the vaccine and the way it is administered, they might be small. The danger is that fertility control based on immunity may grossly distort selection pressure on immune response genes. It the extreme case, only immunological cripples would reproduce freely.

VIII. The Penetration of Other Sciences by Immunology

Immunology has the habit of penetrating other sciences. Its impact has been biggest on its neighbours pathology, biochemistry and genetics. Nobody nowadays would think of trying to characterize a cell, isolate a protein, or analyse the action of a gene without considering the use of immunology. This is the sort of intermingling of the sciences which makes timetabling for students a nightmare. The impact of immunology is ramifying out into the applied sciences. To take a few examples: in forensic science immunology is used to type body products; in entomology to identify the hosts of bloodsucking insects; in forestry to sort out proteins of sap; and in clinical chemistry to assay hormones. Applications of these sorts are likely to grow as progress continues in three areas of immunological technology: miniaturization and automation, surface immunochemistry, and the use of monoclonal antibodies.

Over the last few years immunological laboratories have passed through two revolutions. First came isotopes. Suddenly one felt naked without a gamma counter for ^{131}I and ^{51}Cr. Then disposable plasticware took over. What before took rack upon rack of little glass tubes could be done in a few multi-well plates. And now these plates are bringing in their own special tools: multi-dispensers, multi-diluters, multi-samplers and so on. Just a few pennies worth of plastic one might think . . . but let no one assume that miniaturization and automation bring economy! These revolutions spread very widely the use of microcytotoxicity assays and radioimmunoassays (RIA). The former, as their name implies involve the use of antibodies or immune cells to kill a population of labelled cells. In this way immunity to cell surface antigens can be measured precisely. In RIA a labelled antigen reacts with a limited amount of antibody: the procedure can be used in innumerable ways to measure small amounts of antigen and antibodies. Another effect has been to make lymphocytes far easier to manipulate in culture. In the last few years immunology has become largely an *in vitro* science (but again, do not assume that expenditure on inbred mice will decline).

The second major area of progress has been in surface immunochemistry. Immunologists had been interested in cell agglutination and lysis from the very beginning, but a new wave started twenty years ago with the introduction of fluorescent antibodies as probes of cell surface structures. Then isotopes came into use, to label antigens either metabolically or by chemical reactions from outside the cell. It is now possible to determine the amino acid sequence of a cell surface protein without having to isolate it first (Silver *et al.*, 1977). So chemistry can now be done on a range of proteins which before were too insoluble or too dilute to handle.

The third important progress has been in finding a solution to the problem of antibody heterogeneity (Melchers *et al.*, 1978). Antibodies come out of an animal as a mixture of related but different molecules, and one which never exactly repeats from one animal to another. In 1974 Kohler and Milstein discovered a solution: they fused antibody-producing cells with a line of myeloma cells growing in culture. From these fused cells they isolated clones, which secrete a single kind of antibody molecule and will continue to do so indefinitely. The method has been widely applied in virology and cell biology, where it has enormous resolving power. By its use, for example, the spike protein of influenza has been shown to have well over a hundred distinguishable antigenic sites. One of its most promising applications is in the sorting out of cells from the nervous system (Raff *et al.*, 1979). Markers have just been found for the five main cell types, and it should be a straightforward matter to pick out more varieties. Groups of scientists all over the world have confidently begun to assemble libraries of antibodies which will pick out all molecules on the surface of this cell or that parasite. This is the technique which for the time being will do most for immunology in other sciences.

References

Allison, A. C. (1978). *Int. Rev. exp. Pathl.* **18**, 303–346.
Anderson, R. M. and May, R. M. (1979). *Nature, Lond.* **280**, 361–367.
Arita, I. (1979). *Nature, Lond.* **279**, 293–298.
Bell, G. I., Perelson, A. S. and Pimbley, G. H. (1978). "Theoretical Immunology". Decker, New York.
Benacerraf, B. and McDevitt, H. O. (1972). *Science, NY* **175**, 273–279.
Biggs, P. M. (1975). *IARC Sci. Publi.* **11**, 317–327.
Brown, K. N. (1976). *In* "Immunology of Parasitic Infections" (S. Cohen and E. Sadun, Eds), 268–295. Blackwell, Oxford.
Burke, D. C. (1979). *Behring Institute Mitteilungen* **63**, 113–122.
Burtin, P. (1978). *Ann. Immunol.* **192**, 185–198.
Conway, G. R. (1977). *Nature, Lond.* **269**, 291–292.
Cooper, M. D., Keightley, R. G. and Lawton, A. R. (1975). *In* "Membrane Receptors of Lymphocytes" (M. Seligmann, J. L. Preud'homme and F. M. Kourilsky, Eds), 403–414. North-Holland, Amsterdam.
Eardley, D. D., Hugenberger, J., McVay-Boudreau, L., Shen, F. W., Gershon, R. K. and Cantor, H. (1978) *J. exp. Med.* **147**, 1106–1115.
Eisen, H. N. (1974). "Immunology: An Introduction to the Molecular and Cellular Principles of the Immune Response". Harper and Row, Haggerstown.
Epstein, M. A. (1978). *Nature, Lond.* **274**, 740–741.
Fazekas de St Groth, S. (1977). *Arb. Paul Ehrlich Inst.* **71**, 21–34.
Feldmann, M. (1976). *In* "Immunology of Parasitic Infections" (S. Cohen and E. Sadun, Eds), 1–18. Blackwell, Oxford.
Feldmann, M., Baltz, M., Erb, P., Howie, S., Kontiainen, S., Woody, J. and Zvaifler, N. (1977). *Progr. Immunol.* **3**, 331–337.
Festenstein, H. and Dement, P. (Eds) (1978). *In* "HLA and H-2: Basic Immunogenetics, Biology and Clinical Relevance", 215. Edward Arnold, London.
Fisher, M. S. and Kripke, M. L. (1978). *J. Immunol.* **121**, 1139–1144.
Golub, E. S. (1977). "The Cellular Basis of the Immune Response". Sinauer, Sunderland, USA.
Good, R. A. and Hansen, M. A. (1976). *Adv. exp. Med. Biol.* **73**, 155–178.
Greaves, M. F., Janossy, G., Roberts, M., Rapson, N. T., Ellis, R. B., Chessels, J., Lister, T. A. and Catovsky, D. (1977). *Haematol. Blood Transfus.* **20**, 61–75.
Hearn, J. P. (1979). *Ciba Foundation Series* **64**, 353–375.
Helenius, A., Morein, B., Fries, E., Simons, K., Robinson, P., Schirrmacher, V., Terhorst, C. and Strominger, J. L. (1978). *Proc. natn. Acad. Sci. USA* **75**, 3846–3850.
Hobart, M. J. and McConnell, I. (1978). "The Immune System: A Course on the Molecular and Cellular Basis of Immunity". Blackwell, Oxford.

Holmgren, J. and Svennerholm, A. M. (1977). *J. infect. Dis.* **136** (suppl.), 105–112.
Howard, J. and Mitchison, N. A. (1975). *Progr. Allergy* **18**, 43–96.
Howes, E., Taylor, W., Mitchison, N. A. and Simpson, E. (1979a). *Nature, Lond.* **277**, 67–68.
Howes, E., Clark, E. A., Smith, E. and Mitchison, N. A. (1979b). *J. gen. Virol.* in press.
Ishizaka, K. and Ishizaka, T. (1979). *Immunol. Rev.* **41**, 109–148.
Jerne, N. K. (1967). *Cold Spring Harb. Symp. quant. Biol.* **32**, 591–603.
Jerne, N. K. (1971). *Eur. J. Immunol.* **1**, 1–61.
Jerne, N. K. (1974). *Ann. Immunol.* **125**, 373–389.
Kabat, E. A. (1976). *In* "Structural Concepts in Immunology and Immunochemistry", 547. Holt, Rinehart and Winston, New York.
Katz, D., Hamaoka, T., Dorf, M. E. and Benacerraf, B. (1973). *Proc. natn. Acad. Sci. USA* **70**, 2624–2628.
Kemple, K. and Bluestone, R. (1976). *Pathobiol. Ann.* **7**, 305–326.
Kessler, A. and Standley, C. C. (1976). *Proc. Ry. Soc. Lond.* **195**, 129–136.
Kripke, M. L. (1974). *J. natn. Cancer Inst.* **53**, 1333–1336.
Lachmann, P. and Peters, K. (Eds) (1980). "Clinical Aspects of Immunology", 4th edn. Blackwell, Oxford. in press.
Lake, P. and Mitchison, N. A. (1977). *Cold Spring Harb. Symp. quant. Biol* **41**, 589–595.
Lennox, E. and Cohn, M. (1967). *Ann. Rev. Biochem.* **36**, 365–406.
Loor, F. and Roelants, G. (Eds) (1977). "B and T Cells in Immune Recognition". Wiley, Chichester.
Marshall-Clarke, S. and Playfair, J. H. L. (1979). *Immunol. Rev.* **43**, 109–141.
McMichael, A. J., Ting, A., Zweerink, H. J. and Askonas, B. A. (1977). *Nature, Lond.* **270**, 524–526.
Melchers, F., Potter, M. and Warner, N. (Eds) (1978). Lymphocyte hybridomas. *Curr. Topics Microbiol. Immun.* **81**, 1–202.
Merrill, J. P. (1978). *Ann. Immunol.* **129**, 347–352.
Mitchison, N. A. (1975). *In* "Proc. VII Karolinska Symposium on Immunobiological Approaches to Fertility Control" (E. Diczfalusy, Ed.) 405–418. Bogtrykkeriet Forum, Copenhagen.
Mitchison, N. A. (1978). *Clin. rheum. Dis.* **4**, 539–548.
Mitchison, N. A. (1979). *Clin. exp. Dermatol.* in press.
Mollison, P. L. (1973). *Am. J. clin. Pathol.* **60**, 287–301.
Ovary, Z., Itaya, T., Watanabe, N. and Kojima, S. (1979). *Immunol. Rev.* **41**, 26–51.
Phillips, P. J., Rowland, R., Reid, D. P. and Coles, M. E. (1977). *J. clin. Pathol.* **30**, 1129–1133.
Purchio, A. F., Erikson, E., Brugge, J. S. and Erikson, R. L. (1978). *Proc. natn. Acad. Sci. USA* **75**, 1567–1571.
Raff, M. C., Fields, K. L., Hakomori, S., Mirsky, R., Prus, R. M. and Winter, J. (1979). *Brain Res.* in press.
Roitt, I. (1978). "Basic Immunology". Blackwell, Oxford.

Sachs, J. A. (1977). *Proc. Ry. Soc. Med.* **70**, 689–691.
Seidman, J. G., Leder, A., Nau, M., Norman, B. and Leder, P. (1978). *Science, NY* **202**, 11–17.
Shellam, G. R., Knight, R. A., Mitchison, N. A., Gorczynski, R. and Maoz, A. (1975). *Transplant. Rev.* **29**, 249–276.
Shreffler, D. C. and David, C. S. (1975). *Adv. Immunol.* **20**, 125–195.
Silver, J., Cecka, J. M., McMillan, M. and Hood, L. (1977). *Cold Spring Harb. Symp. quant. Biol.* **41**, 368–377.
Spitler, L. E. (1978). *Int. J. Dermatol.* **17**, 445–458.
Stevens, V. C. (1978). *Bull, Wld Hlth Org.* **55**, 179–192.
Sucio-Foca, N., Nicholson, J. F., Reemstman, K. and Rubinstein, P. (1977). *Diabet. Metab.* **3**, 193–198.
Talwar, G. P., Dubey, S. K., Salahuddin, M., Dass, C., Ramakrishman, S., Kumar, S. and Hingorani, V. (1976). *Proc. natn. Acad. Sci. USA* **73**, 218–222.
Terry, R. J. (1976). *In* "Immunology of Parasitic Infections" (S. Cohen and E. Sadun, Eds), 203–221. Blackwell, Oxford.
Tonegawa, S., Brack, C., Hozumi, N., Matthyssens, G. and Schuller, R. (1977). *Immunol. Rev.* **36**, 73–97.
Unanue, E. R. (1978). *Immunol. Rev.* **40**, 227–255.
Waldmann, T. A., Blaese, R. M., Broders, S. and Krakauer, R. (1978). *Ann. intern. Med.* **88**, 226–238.
WHO Task Force (1978). *Clin. exp. Immunol.* **33**, 360–375.
Zinkernagel, R. M. and Doherty, P. C. (1974). *Nature, Lond.* **248**, 701–702.
Zinkernagel, R. M. (1977). *Transplant. Proc.* **9**, 1835–1838.
Zinkernagel, R. M. and Doherty, P. C. (1977). *Contemp. Topics Immunobiol.* **7**, 179–220.

32

Ethics and Medical Science

Daisaku Ikeda
Honorary President

The Soka Gakkai, Tokyo, Japan

Medical science [must] be a fusion of scholarly research, practical application, and morality in the most lofty sense.

I. The Demands Made of Medical Science

Medicine is a unique field of study. While founded on the strictest scientific technology, it must respond directly to certain ethical demands. Medicine must encompass science, but it must also rise above science; it must utilize technology, but it must also go beyond the realm of technology. Its mission is to exercise the highest degree of human ethics.

We demand of medical science that it be a fusion of scholarly research, practical application, and morality in the most lofty sense. If any of these three demands is lacking, the meaning of medicine is not fulfilled. The nuclear feature of the three is ethical practice; medical science without ethics is not worthy of its name.

The reason why ethics is necessary in the study of medicine and in medical treatment is simply that they involve the lives of human beings. Medicine exists for the purpose of changing people from one state to another. It operates upon life itself.

Since ancient times it has been said in the Orient that "medicine is the art of benevolence". It is philanthropy in the root meaning of the word. The implication is clear: medicine must not degenerate into a form of technology. Technology is a tool that people use in dealing with natural objects. Medical treatment, on the other hand, is founded on the relationship between man and man. Man's life must not be converted into a tool. It must be treated with compassion, with true philanthropy.

One reason for insisting that medicine be benevolent is that it contains certain elements that are essentially unethical. In particular, it involves human relations—specifically that of the doctor to the patient—that are unequal. The doctor is a specialist who employs high-level technology to safeguard people's health. The patient is an amateur whose health has in some way been damaged to the extent that he must rely on medical science for a cure. Instead of a normal man-to-man relationship, there exists a state in which one person takes an active role and the other a passive role. All medical treatment is based on this fundamental inequality.

Many other phases of medicine lie outside the sphere of ordinary ethics. One is based on the fact that the doctor must have information of a secret or private nature. His patient must reveal to him facts about his body or his private life that he would normally keep to himself. At times, the doctor must, in order to carry out an effective treatment, be in possession of physiological secrets that he does not wish the patient himself to know.

The doctor is allowed to insert knives into living human beings and to introduce foreign substances, such as drugs, into their bodies. In some instances, he assumes control of their minds and their conduct. Outside the field of medicine, such practices would not be condoned.

Doctors are permitted to perform acts that would ordinarily be regarded as unethical because these acts are calculated to cure patients of illnesses, and because people believe that doctors possess a high standard of professional ethics. For this very reason, the slightest lowering of ethical standards is bound to be taken as gross immorality. Without ethics, medical treatment becomes a form of butchery. As more and more giant strides are made in the field of medical technology, and as medical knowledge becomes more and more recondite, the danger to human life that might result from ethical lapses becomes all the more frightening. Herein lies the peculiarity of medical ethics, which does not fall within the realm of ordinary ethics. Herein, too, lies the reason why we must insist on high ethical standards in the medical science of the future.

II. The Doctor's Responsibility

According to Buddhism, man's four fundamental sorrows are birth, old age, sickness, and death. No human being can escape the suffering that comes from being born, from growing old, from becoming ill, or from dying.

The sick person, with whom the medical profession is directly concerned, suffers not only from his illness, but from the threat of other sorrows. To the healthy person, the extent to which an invalid must struggle against the four sorrows is difficult to imagine. The science of medicine is a sacred science because it employs technical methods to rid people of human suffering and cause the light of good health to shine upon them.

All men are born with various hereditary proclivities. Some people are prone to particular illnesses; others come into the world with inherited diseases. Aside from physical characteristics, people receive a wide variety of psychological traits from their ancestors.

Old age is a form of suffering. Senility upsets the body's rhythm, disturbs the harmony of its functioning organs, and frequently leads to mental pain resulting from loss of memory or will-power.

Sickness both causes and aggravates the sorrows of birth and old age.

The invalid fears childbirth, dreads senility, feels himself to be in the shadow of death. If he is seriously ill, the anxiety caused by pain and the thought of death is always in the back of his mind. There is terror in his eyes as he contemplates the malady that is eating away at his life.

Nor does the sorrow that comes from illness end with physical or mental suffering. If the invalid has a family, his family must suffer with him; if he works, illness may damage his position in society. There are medical fees, worries about living expenses, fears as to what will happen to the invalid's family after he dies. These show in the stricken facial expressions of ailing persons.

It is the doctor's responsibility to provide medical treatment for people who are struggling against these various forms of anguish. The doctor must therefore have the ability, the courage, and the humanity needed to cope with a wide range of problems.

What powers does a doctor require?

First of all, a superior knowledge of medical technology. He must be a walking storehouse of knowledge concerning the natural sciences. He must be acquainted with physics and chemistry, biology, and physiology. These sciences are the weapons he requires to attack the physical and biological aspects of disease. A knowledge of psychiatry and depth psychology is also helpful, for it has been amply demonstrated in modern times that many physical illnesses have mental causes. In addition to all these fields of knowledge, the modern doctor must recognize the importance of environmental factors; he should be able to deal with problems having to do with sanitation and public health.

Yet a technical knowledge of various scientific fields and an ability to put this knowledge to practical use are not enough, for the purely scientific eye sees only phenomena of a particular order within the vast totality of elements that constitute human life. To view human life as though it were controlled entirely by physical or chemical laws is to reduce it to the level of matter. This results ultimately in conceiving of human beings as mere things. Similarly, to regard life as a purely physiological phenomenon is to reduce it to the biological level; this is the sort of thinking that has led some medical men to use human beings as guinea pigs. Even to consider life from the purely psychological viewpoint is to ignore many important features of human character and actual existence. Science objectifies whatever it examines. When viewed in a scientific light, even the human spirit becomes an object of sorts—a concatenation of psychological factors devoid of the warmth and sensibility of real human beings.

Medical treatment involves the application of ethical principles; it is related, not to objects, but to real people, who have character and personality. Technical knowledge is necessary, but ethical conduct is even more important. Without it, the science of medicine converts human beings into unfeeling tools, animalizes them, treats their spirits as though they were some sort of solid matter. This is why we demand that doctors be humanistic. We cannot allow them to surrender to scientific theory. They must not be cold-blooded technicians. They must be people full of sympathy and kindness and compassion for their fellow beings.

As was stated earlier, the practice of medicine is from the beginning unethical in certain respects. It happens, unfortunately, that technology has a natural affinity with "unethicality." Doctors can become so absorbed with the purely scientific aspect of what they are doing that they forget to ask themselves whether they ought morally to be doing it or not. When they do, they are apt to regard their patients as test tubes rather than living men and women. To avoid this, they must have the spiritual energy needed to restrain their intellectual or scientific curiosity and prevent them from being lured into paths that are essentially immoral. Only when the doctor's life is enriched by the warm milk of human kindness can he overcome the inherent inequality between himself and his patients.

The way for a doctor to convert the active–passive imbalance between himself and his patients is for him to recognize that he is indebted to them for much of his knowledge. His attitude should be one of humility. Aside from information and medical techniques, the doctor receives from those who suffer an enormously valuable store of knowledge concerning life and people. The very phenomenon of the patient's life furnishes the clues to diagnosis and the proper method of treatment.

To the doctor, the patient is a living reality. No two patients have exactly the same symptoms, even if they are afflicted with the same disease. A thousand patients reveal to the doctor a thousand different varieties of symptoms and a thousand different examples of the way in which a disease might progress. Furthermore each patient's life phenomenon changes by the hour and minute.

III. The Ethical Code

The Hippocratic oath represents one of the high points of human intelligence. Though stated in simple language, it embodies the essence of medical ethics and has served as a spiritual bulwark for physicians throughout the ages. Even today many doctors take it as their principal motto.

Medicine itself has of course changed drastically in the two thousand years since the oath was written. Contemporary doctors have scientific methods not dreamed of by the ancient Greeks. Yet the philosophy and the ethical code reflected in the Hippocratic oath have survived over the centuries and still exercise a powerful spiritual influence on medical practitioners. This is because the code epitomizes the fundamental spirit of the science of healing—a spirit that is not altered by the passage of time.

The core of medical ethics is a love for mankind. That the Hippocratic oath forbids doctors to put their training and their art to evil use, that it enjoins them to maintain a clean and pure attitude toward life, that it clearly enunciates the principle of not revealing patients' secrets, and that it emphasizes the need for treating all men equally is due to Hippocrates' warm, benign love for the human race. By refusing to kill upon request, to practice euthanasia, or to perform abortions, he sought to establish an absolute safeguard for the sanctity of life itself. Love not only for human life but for all life flowed in the veins of the author of this code. If the doctor does not adopt the humble attitude that he is learning from his patients, he cannot accumulate valuable clinical experience or receive hints as to the medicine of the future.

A second important point is that the doctor must, from observing his patients' struggles against the four sorrows, learn about life's rigors, life's beauty, and the sanctity of the human being. The patient is the doctor's instructor in the business of living. In the clinic or hospital, the patient's emotions, be they joy or anger or pleasure or sorrow, are exposed to the doctor's view. The patient is a great turbulent sea of hopes and passions. The doctor is privileged to witness the lamentation of men weeping over their fate, the fear of men who are about to die, the triumphant spirit of men who have challenged death and won, the whole moving drama of life and love. In the troubled lives of the sick, the doctor can catch a glimpse of the beauty of human love and the profundity of the religious spirit.

Apathy toward life and death completely disqualifies a doctor. To look unfeelingly upon the death of a human being, as though it were merely a scientific happening, is the ultimate blasphemy against life itself. The doctor should stand in reverence before the life-and-death struggle of the sick, because from it he can learn both a philosphy of life and the means of coping with death. It is by doing this that he develops genuine humanity. A doctor who respects his patients and is able to learn from them is worthy of the complete trust they place in him. The struggle against the sorrow of illness can be won only when doctor and patient collaborate in a spirit of compassion, mutual confidence, and personal warmth.

Does not love for life in general transcend the level of ethics and soar to the heights of the philosophical and religious spirit?

In the Orient, the teachings of the Buddha have served as the ethical support for the medical profession. Shakyamuni was a religious leader, but he studied medicine himself, received counsel from the famous physician Jīvaka, and stated plain rules for the practice of medicine. His teachings on ethics, which are spread throughout the vast Bhuddist canon, shine like precious jewels. Shakyamuni demanded that doctors not only have a clear-headed command of medical theory and practice, but also be full of love and affection for the sick. A passage in the *Suvarnaprabhāśa-sūtra* states, for example, that doctors must exercise compassion in dealing with the sick, and that they must not be covetous or greedy. In the *Mahāprajñāpāramito-padeśa*, said to have been composed by Nāgārjuna, the Buddhist law is likened to medicine, and it is stated: "If one takes medicine, the main point is to cure illness; it makes no difference whether the patient is great or ordinary, rich or poor." One is reminded by this of the Hippocratic oath.

According to Shakyamuni's teachings, the basic spirit of the medical science is compassion—the compassion for life that overflows from the religious heart. Shakyamuni did not neglect to lay down rules to be followed by nurses and patients. According to him, in order for medical treatment to be effective, it is essential for the ethics of the nurse and the patient to agree with the ethics of the physician. It is a distinctive feature of Buddhist medical ethics that emphasis is placed on harmony between the rules for the doctor and the rules for nurses and patients. The doctor is admonished to treat the sick compassionately; nurses are commanded to understand the patients' feelings and give them spiritual support; patients are instructed to trust their doctors, to remain calm, and to do the best they can to cure themselves. That the Buddha's teachings in this respect are timeless is evident from the modern medical emphasis on natural healing processes and on the need for co-operation between patient and paramedical staff.

The common basic principle between the highest medical ethics of the Occident and those of the Orient is love for the life of all beings and things, which is elevated to the religious level in the form of a moral love for humanity. Love of life and love for human beings form the eternal spiritual basis for the practice of the way of the doctor. They are a heritage that all doctors today must guard and maintain.

In medical treatment, love for mankind, which aims at respect for the dignity of all human life is not itself sufficient. The modern doctor, while setting the highest absolute value on the dignity of man, must also cope with the flood of scientific and technological developments taking place in the medical profession.

At a more profound level, love for humanity must be founded on an absolute respect for all forms of life. This must be a pious love for life itself and at the same time a feeling of humility before the natural healing powers set into motion by life-existence. The feeling intended here is akin to what Dr Albert Schweitzer referred to as awe and reverence for life.

In "Choose Life", Dr Toynbee said, very trenchantly, "I believe that love is the ultimate spiritual reality of the universe." The love for life fuses at the profoundest depths with the ultimate existence that pulsates within every living being or thing.

Fusion with the cosmic life itself—this is the profoundest level of a love for life, and this love must be founded on an indestructible respect for life. It is the source that generates compassion on the religious plane.

Because of the prodigious development of medicine and the life sciences in modern times, there have arisen a host of new problems that involve ethical values. Among these are the question of mercy killing and "vegetable" invalids; of the propriety of warning patients of approaching death; of organ transplants and standards for determining at what point death takes place; of abortion; of artificial insemination; of experiments involving the alteration of genes; of brain surgery and the development of drugs affecting the mental framework. I should like to state my own opinions concerning a few problems that are connected directly with medical science.

The first is the question of mercy killing, particularly in the case of invalids who have ceased to have anything more than a vegetable existence. Those who approve of mercy killing base their arguments on the idea that the will of the invalid should be accorded maximum respect. The theory is that if the patient has signified his wish to die in certain circumstances, this wish ought to be granted. This is what is called voluntary euthanasia.

One is prepared to admit that from the viewpoint of medical ethics, in which the dignity and sanctity of the human being are taken as standards, a body that is alive only in the brain stem is difficult to regard as a genuine living organism, possessed of the dignity of man. There is something to be said, too, for the idea that, as free agents, human beings have the right to choose death if they wish to.

The difficult point is in determining whether the patient's wish to die is really voluntary or not. There is no guarantee that a decision arrived at by an invalid when he is sound of mind remains his volition at the moment when he is put to death. At the moment of death, it may happen that the instinctive urge to remain alive will alter his previous decision, but by this time the patient has normally lost all means of expressing his will.

A second point that needs to be considered, and one in which Buddhists have a special interest, is the question of whether a voluntary choice of death is actually voluntary or not. There are many instances when such a choice appears to have been forced upon a person by social or spiritual pressures. I believe that what makes life is a natural urge to go on living under any circumstances that might arise. This inborn urge should be given the greatest possible encouragement by the families and friends of sick people, and particularly by doctors.

In the third place, to regard as dead a person whose brain stem is still functioning is to deprive "vegetable" patients, along with seriously handicapped persons and the mentally infirm, of their ultimate right to existence. This involves a philosophical problem as to the value of life.

A fourth consideration is that to approve of mercy killing tends to destroy the bonds of mutual trust linking the doctor with the patient and thus to weaken the whole foundation of medical treatment.

A fifth point is that at the point when the doctor decides that the patient is incurable, there is a distinct danger that he will relax his effort to achieve a cure. He is apt to leave off studying possible means of treatment or to cease trying to arrive at prompt diagnoses of new symptoms.

Because of the above factors, I believe we must take a negative attitude toward voluntary euthanasia and instead adopt the definite stand that there is still life so long as the brain stem is functioning.

The brain stem is the seat of life. It is the place where the body lovingly maintains and clings to life, regardless of differences in the individual's physical or spiritual condition. It performs functions that are common to all forms of life, whether human or otherwise, and it is the organism that generates the love of life that derives ultimately from the cosmic life force. The concrete physiological foundation for the dignity and sanctity of life lies within the brain stem. All people can mutually recognize the importance of the workings of the brain stem, which are the same for all human beings regardless of racial, political, or economic differences and conflicts. Within all human lives, there exists an inner impulse that seeks life and shuns death. The minimal operations necessary to life are the functions of the brain stem. Only when all people recognize the sanctity of the life within the brain stem and learn to love and cherish it can we achieve a consensus favouring peace for all mankind; only then can we change the principle of the sanctity of life from ideal into fact.

After recognizing that there is life so long as the brain stem lives, doctors can then pour their energies into the discovery of clinical means of relieving pain. With respect to mental anguish brought on by uncertainty and fear of death, medical men should rely on their own philosophies and their own views of life in trying to help patients form a sound concept of life and death. Special problems are encountered in dealing with invalids in the "vegetable" state; economic or social difficulties will eventually have to be settled by a general elevation of ethics within society as a whole. The medical profession must develop a stronger sense of social responsibility.

The next question concerns the propriety of warning victims of cancer or other fatal diseases that they are on the verge of death. In cases where the invalid has the spiritual strength to face death calmly, I see no reason why he should not be told the truth. There are, however, instances in which the mental shock brought on by the knowledge of impending death can cause the patient to die even sooner. When this is true, the physician must proceed with the utmost caution and discretion, making sure not to break the news at the wrong time. Today, of course, knowledge of medicine is so widespread that there are many cases in which the truth cannot be concealed.

My third point has to do with transplants of organs and with the standards for pronouncing a person dead. As things stand now, one method of deciding whether a patient is still alive or not is to measure his brain waves, but it is said that this method cannot detect minute changes deep within the brain. In short, it does not indicate whether the brain stem has ceased completely to function. If the life of the brain stem is taken as the criterion, the brain wave method cannot be regarded as final. It appears that stoppage of the heartbeat will continue to be a necessary condition, as it has been in the past. As research into brain waves advances, it may well be shown that the death of the brain is directly connected with the stoppage of the heart.

As for transplants, there seems little objection to grafts of the cornea or skin or blood vessels, but I think that the wishes of the patient ought always to be given full consideration in the case of kidney transplants. Furthermore, I believe that heart transplants which do not take cognizance of the functioning of the brain stem should not be carried out, because they go against the basic spirit of respect for the sanctity of life.

A fourth subject for concern is the termination of pregnancy by artificial means. In the code of medical ethics adopted in 1949 at

Geneva, it is stated as a basic principle that, even under threat, doctors will hold human life in the highest respect from the moment of conception. Since the fetus in the womb has a heartbeat, as well as the basic form of the brain, it must be regarded as a living human being. To abort it can only be termed a form of murder. Population control should be carried out, not by abortion, but by limiting conception.

Finally, there is the question of carrying out medical experiments on living human beings, which is related both to artificial insemination and to the use of psychological drugs. Further progress in medical research will probably necessitate experiments on living human subjects, but the greatest caution must be exercised in this field.

Although the Helsinki Declaration, adopted in 1964 by an international conference of medical men, outlines a basic policy, its application depends to a large extent on a doctor's personal sense of ethics. For practical purposes, the doctor alone is free to decide on such important questions as whether human volunteers have been properly informed as to what is in store for them, whether psychological pressures have been applied to prevent them from dropping out of the experiment midway, or whether sufficient experimentation with animals has taken place prior to the use of human volunteers.

As for artificial insemination, even doctors disagree as to whether the principles stated in the Helsinki Declaration have been scrupulously carried out in the intervening years.

It seems to me that only doctors who have a passionate love for human beings and for human life—doctors who have the deepest consideration for the humans on whom they experiment—can be expected to perform such experiments in a perfectly ethical fashion. It is only when medical men have this higher sense of humanitarianism that they can use scientific technique for the betterment of mankind's condition.

The same principle is applicable in the case of experiments with genes and hereditary characteristics. The progress of the life sciences has always had two aspects. The absence of ethics from the study of science is fatal; it leads, as we have seen, to the use of scientific knowledge for such evil and mistaken purposes as the development of bacteriological weaponry, which could eventually cause the destruction of the human race.

Progress in medicine and the life sciences contains quite a few elements of an irreversible nature. If for that reason only, the doctors and scientists of our time must have the spiritual strength and energy to sublate scientific theory. They must have reverent love for all living beings. They must abide by the principle of infinite love and infinite respect for the life of the brain stem, which is the common property of all living existence.

I pray that these men of science and medicine will, for the sake of mankind's existence and peaceful well-being, search humbly and reverently for the spirit of philanthropy and for the love of life that is the basis of ethics.

33

Decision Making in a Rapidly Changing Technological Environment

John L. Farrands
Department of Science and the Environment, Canberra, ACT, Australia

---

"Practitioners of [government and of science] are inadequately equipped to deal alone with the complex interplay of social and technical issues which face modern communities."

I. Introduction

Political and commercial decision makers are now required to take greater account of technical matters than formerly. This obligation stems from the qualitative changes in society in which wealth and health are determined less by natural forces and more by man's technological achievements. Since the practice of government or management is no less a full-time occupation than the practice of science or engineering, it follows that practitioners of either are inadequately equipped to deal alone with the complex interplay of social and technical issues which face modern communities. A new degree of indecision has arisen (or has been exposed) which can be resolved only by greater consultation of the decision makers with the scientific and technical community. Not the least of the problems is the selection of an effective means of obtaining objective advice; a plethora of techniques is being developed which require evaluation.

In community decisions concerned with human and environmental welfare, technological aspects are often seen as mere perturbations, and their importance underrated. Technological factors may be closely connected and highly visible, or they may be loosely connected, distant in discipline and time and even invisible. Techniques are required to make available to decision makers as far as possible the hidden implications of technological developments on social futures.

Decisions involving technology must take account of uncertainties of both technological and non-technological kind; sometimes technological decisions have consequences which are predictable with near certainty, but sometimes a high degree of uncertainty is involved; there are matters apparently lying within the realm of technology in which future consequences may be in principle unknowable. Other uncertainties arise in social consequences of technology, deriving from possible non-deterministic or otherwise unpredictable human behaviour.

In decisions in which a technical component is significant, there may be even greater difficulties generated by the technology itself. Although the introduction or development of a new technology may be the result of a decision at high political level, the technology may acquire a technical momentum of its own in ways which were unlikely to have been foreseen.

Science has its own decision-making problems in regard, for example, to research topic choices and corporate submissions to governments. Such decisions are different in nature from those concerning technology, even though they are sometimes justified in terms of their impact on technology.

This chapter will examine the interaction of science and technology with community decisions directed to development or conservation. It will seek to expose the difficulties; it will refer to some of the techniques being developed to remove where possible, or otherwise to make explicit, the uncertainties facing decision makers. It will expose the need for science and scientists to recognize and admit their limitations. Some guidelines for recognition of these limitations will be given.

II. Technical and Political Decisions Confused

The technological component of the considerations in a public decision-making event may often obscure or be used to obscure the real (political) issues. Public debate may be diverted, or divert itself to the question of means, ignoring by and large the ends. In other cases technical issues may be decided on grounds which are purely political.

Courts of justice and parliaments rely on the presumption that truth and justice will be revealed as a result of vigorous adversary presentations. It is common for public reviews, commissions and the like to operate with such a methodology. There is a growing tendency to use scientists and technologists to support particular points of view in many issues involving major developments (power stations, dams, etc.) with a significant and easily recognizable impact on the local or global quality of life. The use of scientists and technologists in such adversary situations presents difficulties for the scientists and creates confusion in the community. Great care is required if the standards and acceptance of science and technology are to be retained (Nelkin, 1975).

Science is only one instrument amongst many available to the body politic to achieve its ends, and thus "utility" is the measuring rod of the community's interest in scientific research. The philosophical nature of science is not understood by the political community, where it is evaluated as a technique, new practical knowledge, or a source of power. Science thus, with its inner values related to truth and its outer values related to utility, acquires an ambivalence very similar to that of the law which is divided between its zeal for justice and its zeal for the success of its client (Saloman, 1973).

In some circumstances it is possible for governments to achieve political and social objectives which would not be otherwise acceptable for constitutional reasons, through scientific programmes which are presented as unexceptionable. Price (1964) refers to health and rural research programmes in the USA which enabled the Federal Government to intrude into state affairs. Political or corporate ambitions may be disguised as technical adventures. Fishlock (1975) offers as an example the development of (civil) supersonic transports which he alleges are in reality not an expression of technical or commercial adventure but are in fact a disguised attempt to keep in being an advanced military technology.

The community appreciation of science as a form of power and no longer as a philosophical and cultural activity places an obligation on the corporate body of scientists to be aware of the ways in which this power might be misused.

In matters of health, technology or development we are primarily concerned with the future consequences of present decisions. Difficult enough for single decisions in an otherwise unchanging world, it is infinitely more difficult in a world in which multiple, near simultaneous, nearly independent decisions are being made. Recognition of the nature of the uncertainties is at the basis of political wisdom. Attempts to identify the uncertainties have led to a number of forecasting techniques.

Immediate forecasting and distant forecasting have different degrees of uncertainty. There are, however, some issues with a qualitatively different degree of uncertainty which we shall call trans-science issues because they may not yield to scientific analysis or interpretation.

III. Problems Requiring Immediate Information

Very frequently there is required in the process of government immediate technical advice which might reasonably be expected to be available but is in fact not. One interesting example arose in the atmospheric nuclear testing debate, namely the effects of low levels of fall-out on large dispersed communities.

Prediction of fall-out will involve many uncertainties about the explosion itself and atmospheric motions; at the core of the problem, however, resides the scientific question as to whether somatic damage is linearly related to radiation exposure or whether there exists some threshold of dosage below which damage is almost independent of dosage and may even be zero. It might be expected that several decades of radiation biology studies would have produced an adequate data base. This is not the case. Hence the prediction of the effect of an additional load of radiation on a community is fraught with difficulty. Nevertheless, governments have been required to make a decision urgently based on the best scientific advice available.

The matter is succinctly traversed by Burnet (1978). In the end scientists adopted the criterion of the "worst possible" case, but could not resist adding that they could not exclude the possibility that the effect might be very much smaller. Even now the question, although an important one, is not yet resolved. More recent fundamental work has suggested the existence of repair enzymes which would certainly favour the threshold concept. Nevertheless government decisions and community attitudes were developed on the "worst case", because of the absence of a data base.

Many decisions in government face this difficulty of an inadequate data base. Frequently the time scale does not permit the necessary research; most environmental issues are resolved in a context of great uncertainty for this reason. It seems impossible to prepare an adequate environmental data base for future decisions; present decisions must be made on the basis of available (incomplete) knowledge.

IV. Problems Requiring Long-term Data

Longer time forecasts are naturally the more difficult but the degree of difficulty expands in a more than linear way. Decisions made at the present time with long-term consequences may be affected by interacting but unco-ordinated decisions and by technological change in ways that are not immediately obvious.

A. Forecasting

It has therefore been found necessary to attempt to develop techniques to forecast future technological activities and the consequences of present technologies. Such techniques are based on the premise that we can study the future rationally or scientifically and that allowances can be made for free will situations in some way which will become evident to the decision maker. A number of techniques have been generated, often having a great deal in common, but being subtly different in many ways in their application to special situations. Miller (1977) listed no fewer than seventy-three forecasting techniques, and several of the more general of these were described in "The Futures of Europe" (Kennet, 1976), together with examples and suggested areas of applications. Some examples of the genre are Technological Forecasting, Technology Assessment, Environmental Impact Studies, Quality of Life Studies and Risk Analysis.

Most of those techniques are applied to national or local situations.

There exists another class of studies in aid of decision making with global and international pretensions. Among these are the studies of the Club of Rome and the Systems Dynamics Research Project at MIT, the Hudson Institute Project called "The Corporate Environment 1975–1985", and the "Europe 2000" Project.

There are essential differences between these two classes but they do have in common the need for data, analysis, quantification and model building. Both classes are derived to a very large extent from what was called "operations research" in the Second World War and the post-war "systems analysis" of the military technocracy.

Forecasting is fraught with considerable difficulties. Men of imagination may guess at the nature of future technology (Vassiliev and Gouschev, 1961; Gabor, 1963), but the central problem of technological forecasting will always be the prediction of "discontinuities" in technology or science. They are almost always not foreseen. From time to time events occur where the innovation is of such a quality that the consequent social and technical change is so rapid and significant that it appears to create a social discontinuity. Such changes might well be alluded to as quantum jumps. They are not all modern. The development of accurate navigation several centuries ago led to rapid changes in patterns of trade, but more importantly to expansionist, imperial policies which in a short time disturbed the international balances. More modern examples are the invention of the transistor and microprocessor which is transforming science, business, engineering, and social structures at a very rapid rate. It is possible sometimes to guess with confidence at areas where a quantum jump may occur, but this is not always helpful. For example just such a jump may be expected in the technology of controlled fusion for power, but it seems pointless at this time to speculate on the nature of the development. Since the form of the development will determine the nature of the future power source (size, cost, safety) forecasting its consequences has only limited value.

B. Technology Assessment

Efforts to predict the outcome to society of present technology or even of some current scientific research, while still difficult, have some prospects of success. In this decade the method known as "technology assessment" has been found to be valuable. Hetman (1973) has defined the technique in the following way:

> Technology assessment is a systems analysis approach providing a whole conceptual framework, complete both in scope and time, for decisions about the appropriate utilization of technology for social purposes.

The concept is further amplified in the definition offered by the Library of Congress (quoted by Carpenter 1972 namely):

> Technology Assessment is the process of taking a powerful look at the consequences of technological change. It includes the primary cost benefit balance of short-term and localized market-place economics, but particularly goes beyond these to identify affected parties and unanticipated impacts in as broad and long fashion as possible. It is neutral and objective, seeking to enrich the information for management decisions. Both 'good' and 'bad' side effects are investigated since a missed opportunity for benefit may be detrimental to society just as is an unexpected hazard.

Both definitions make reference to social purposes. Note, however, "cost-benefit" requires careful definition and recognition that both its components may sometimes not be amenable to quantification.

Despite the Library of Congress claim, in any forecasting technique the result depends at root on individual, generally subjective, judgements about changing probabilities of interrelated future events. This is as true of the quantified "computer model" as of any individual predictions. The problem is to find techniques with a multidisciplinary mix which will smooth out the impact of the individual judgements. It is not quite clear how much improvement can be obtained by different techniques. Nevertheless, it is claimed that the modern technology assessment techniques including, for example, the cross-impact matrix method, enables a better interaction of disciplines and makes experts aware of the larger context in which their opinions are sought. It makes them appreciate the difficulty of the overall prediction (Gibbons and Voyer 1974).

Technology assessment is highly regarded as a technique, but the method of its integration into a national planning process requires careful consideration of a given society's peculiar needs and constitutional arrangements. That it should be useful is clear; it does not follow that institutional models can be transferred from one country to another without amendment.

C. Futures Research

The exponents of technological assessment would see themselves engaged in an essentially different activity from what is known as futures research (for example, Delphic modelling—Kennet, 1976). Futures research has been examined in a critical fashion by Hoos (1977a, b). Criticism was directed towards three components, namely the information base, cost benefit calculations and the analysis of complex systems. Turning to the latter first, Hoos quoted Zadeh (1972) as saying that the conventional quantitative techniques of systems analysis are intrinsically unsuited for dealing with social problems because, as the complexity of the system increases, our ability to make precise and yet significant statements about its behaviour diminishes until the threshold is reached beyond which precision and significance (or relevance) become almost mutually exclusive characteristics. This is taken further by Von Forerster (1977), who makes the point that the traditional reductionist approach is to chop a large system into smaller and smaller pieces until these pieces are small enough to understand; at this point one knows a great deal about nothing and nothing about the interrelationship of the smaller pieces. Holism, on the other hand, says Von Forerster, leads to knowing nothing about everything.

An interesting example of the difficulties of achieving an analysis by subdivision of the problem on the one hand or by the holistic approach was given by Holling (1977) in which he discussed the problem of stability criteria in ecological systems. His particular example is concerned with fishing criteria in the Great Lakes of America. It is a good example of situations in which linear approaches are clearly invalid and underlines the difficulties of categorizing the kind, intensity and duration of disturbances on any large system and how to classify and compress variables that are insanely multidimensional.

D. Data Selection

Obviously any predictive process will only be as good as its data base. The problem of availability of data has already been mentioned, but the problem of data selection is also important. In any multidisciplinary interactive study there will always be a selection of data; the very process of selection of relevant data must always cast an air of doubt on the conclusions. This is seen clearly in matters of environmental contention where quite unconnected lists of "facts" are selected by the antagonists. It is important then to be aware of the motivations of the analyst and his sources. In public debate, supporters of opposite lines of action are too often able to produce allegedly objective and apparently convincing results derived selectively from different data bases.

The form of presentation of the results and identification of the data base is a most difficult problem for the analysts. Evaluation of the analytical method used and its data base present a very difficult problem for decision makers.

A major difficulty is the proper public use of the results. Too often the analysis acquires an aura of authority not justified by either the data base or the methodology, both of which are often not understood, forgotten or obscured. Nowhere is this more apparent than in the public acceptance of "computer results".

In spite of the difficulties, the use of formalized techniques for forecasting and evaluation is very valuable to decisions makers. Well-presented analyses will serve to reveal the nature of the data bases and the methodology: more importantly they will reveal the hidden assumptions. Since they should also reveal the hidden assumptions in the statement of the problem, public expenditure on them is highly justified.

V. Trans-science Issues

It has been proposed by Weinberg (1972) that there exist problems where questions apparently can reasonably be asked of science but cannot be answered by science. He proposed the term "trans-scientific" for these questions because they transcend science. Some problems may be called trans-science because they are so incredibly difficult that no reasonable effort will illuminate them. Some problems on the other hand may be in principle unsolvable; others may be problems in which the definition of the advice is impossible.

As an example of the first kind, Weinberg adverts to a radiation biology problem similar to that referred to earlier. The example is of some practical public importance, relating as it does to public standards of acceptable doses of radiation to the human population. Given that a dose of 30 roentgen will double the spontaneous mutation rate in mice one would expect, on a linear model, that a dose of 150 millirem would increase the mutation rate by 0·5%. If we wish to test that 150 millirem will indeed increase the mutation rate by 0·5% with, say, a confidence level of 60%, says Weinberg, we would require an experiment utilizing 195 million mice. If, however, a confidence level of 95% were desired then the number would be 8000 million. In either case, the number is so staggeringly large, as a practical matter, that the question is unanswerable by direct scientific investigation.

Trans-scientific questions also arise in the probabilities of extremely unlikely events. One example can be seen in assessment of catastrophic reactor accidents. Accident trees may be constructed and the reliabilities of each component and interactive failures may be calculated. While the results of such calculations may be suspect because not every conceivable mode of failure may have been included, this is not important here. It is the smallness of the probability itself which creates major conceptual difficulty. The number quoted is usually of the order of 10^{-7} per reactor per year. The precise value is unimportant for our consideration so long as it is postulated to be a very small number. There is no practical possibility of determining such a failure rate directly as, for example, by building 1000 reactors and operating them for 10 000 years. Indeed, if the number is as low as suggested, even this experiment would not yield a significant result. As in the previous example the matter is trans-scientific because the numbers of protocols required for validation of the calculation are ridiculously large.

The problem has, however, another trans-scientific dimension in that it is impossible to convert into reasonable judgemental terms for social decision making, the consequences of a statement that the probability of failure of a reactor is say 10^{-7} per reactor per year. Of what consequence, what conclusion should a community make about such a number? Given that there might be a significant number of reactors in a certain community, the probability of the failure of one of them might be calculated. For any individual proposal the community can only be aware in a general way that the risk of a catastrophic accident is low, and the penalty for a catastrophic accident is high. It is impossible to put in communicable and universally acceptable terms to the community a suitable basis for judgement. To those used to dealing in probabilities, such numbers as have been used in this example can be given some intuitive meaning. To the community at large the numbers have no meaning.

The propositions put in earlier paragraphs of this section highlight a peculiar responsibility of the scientist in social matters. The scientist must recognize his similar status in trans-scientific questions to that of other intellectual authorities. It is encumbent upon him to recognize and declare:

(a) when questions belong clearly within the established caucus of knowledge of *his* subject and that he speaks from authority in this area;
(b) when he is speaking within the realm of a subject which is not his;
(c) when the matter is trans-scientific, i.e. either not knowable in principle or not knowable without an impossibly large expenditure of effort or money; and
(d) when the issues are essentially those of value rather then technological content.

It should not be assumed, however, that the scientist has no part to play in debates involving trans-scientific issues. It would be unfortunate indeed if the capabilities of the scientist were excluded while non-professionals and other professions were free to participate. The scientist has, however, a particular responsibility to define and make clear when the topic has transcended scientific issues.

VI. Public Expectations and Scientific Involvement

Public expectations of science and scientists are a curious mixture of fear and confidence. The fear is shown in the statement by Dwight Eisenhower that "public policy could itself become the captive of a scientific technological elite" (Quoted in the *New York Times*, 22 January 1961). Such fear shows confusion between advice and decision. That there is another side can be seen by a statement attributed to Bethe by Wood (1964), namely:

> For instance, when one testifies before a Congressional committee one often has the impression that the purpose of the Hearing is not to search out the facts and then reason a solution, but that the solution has been determined and the Hearing will now put such facts on the record as will support the solution.

Such a view may be justified from time to time but the importance of the scientist to the decision-making process is considerable. While other advisers can speak to decision making in strategic or procedural terms and can even suggest alternative courses of action, only the scientist is likely to be able to propose courses based on changing nature itself or of discovering more about it. Thus while science's value judgement may be questioned, its technical judgement cannot be ignored. The community believes that once objectives are set it should be possible to use science and technology to achieve those objectives, that by massive national effort it can achieve any technological goal once the basic facts are known. It has attempted to erect institutional mechanisms to assist in the use of science to achieve its goals.

A. Advisory Committees and Advisers

The scientific community after 1945 was disturbed at its inability to participate at the highest levels in the decision-making process. It was aware of the enormous contribution it had made during that war and was conscious of the potential for good or evil from its future work. It felt that judgements made without including the scientists themselves might well be unbalanced. Almost everywhere now, however, the process of scientific involvement has been accelerated; there now exists a complex structure of scientific advisers in government departments, scientific advisers to heads of government and everywhere there are numerous scientific advisory committees. In these committees, the higher the level the more political, the lower the level the more technical is the consideration. Their general function is:

(i) analysis and interpretation of the technical aspects of policy issues;
(ii) evaluation of specific scientific and technical programmes for advice with budgetary, welfare and safety aspects;
(iii) identification of new opportunities for research and development;
(iv) advice on organizational matters affecting science; and
(v) advice in the selection of individual research proposals.

To some extent, these contentions are in conflict with the undefined but nevertheless real organizational and institutional forms of the pure science body itself. Participation of scientists in such committees has become a significant part of their workload.

It would seem that the wish of the scientific community and perhaps of the general community to see scientists involved more and more in high-level decision making carries with it certain penalities; only those whose research work can give them sufficient free time will be able to continue to participate in the process and remain active scientists. By and large a new "pseudo-bureaucracy" of non-governmental scientists, apparently objective, apparently uncommitted, has been established. Satisfaction with this involvement may not continue amongst the junior scientists who are still fully engaged in their creative work.

Public expectation that the scientist would leave the ivory tower and participate in the decision-making process has been fulfilled. Other expectations of the community are perhaps less well filled. In the chapter headed "Where are they now?", Fishlock (1975) deals with a number of promises which appear to have been made to the British community by science which have not been carried out.

Fishlock is mainly concerned with commercial success; the general community has other expectations of science. It expects science to provide it with titillation and new forms of entertainment; it expects it to solve particularly its health problems. The community is at the one time entertained by the prospects of major organ transplants and, at the other, frustrated by the inability of science to solve its more common problems of the common cold and cancer. The community may well be disconcerted that the scientific effort is so highly concentrated on problems which affect so few, whereas the real problems of disease and motor accidents and mental health which affect so many neither receive the attention they deserve nor earn for the few workers in these fields the accolades which they deserve.

It is important that the community understand that science is not a mere collection of facts, but it is a system of interpretations based on those facts. Failing this understanding public intrusion into decisions on funding and support distort rather than support the process of the advancement of science.

B. Political Judgements

When all analyses have been completed and scientific, technological, economic and statistical data have been made available, there will remain a need for a human intuitive element to be included in political decision making. This element will attempt to evaluate aspects of proposals which are not quantitative. Political judgement may, on occasions, with good reason, tip the balance against the weight of cognitive evidence. Ashby (1976) refers to "the utility value of the unquantifiable", and uses the example of the value of nightingales. In all environmental issues, when the detailed numerical analyses have been completed, there will remain aspects of aesthetics, of "amenity", and of political feasibility which have to be balanced against the more mechanical aspects.

There are, however, other issues which may appear to be capable of quantification but in reality have to be left, in the end, to judgement. Among these are the costs of pollution abatement, in which eventually community decisions have to be made as to the definite level of pollution which is bearable against the cost which must also be bearable. Zero pollution for example would either be impossible or out of the economic range of any community engaged in obtaining its livelihood by industrial technology. The extreme steepness of the curve which will relate cost to degree of pollution abatement must be appreciated.

It is evident that in many analyses a statistical approach is about all that can be achieved as advice. To individual citizens, however, statistics are not convincing and a degree of concern of the individual members for the existence of a new risk will not be tempered by discussions on the probability of that risk when it concerns, for example, the possible effects on the health of children. A balanced judgement is required in the contention between various groups on the degree of atmospheric pollution which is permissible from motor cars. It is possible to argue that a certain cost might be placed on the motor driver in the way of anti-pollution devices with increased fuel consumption to achieve some specified cleanliness of the air in our cities. If the level of pollution could be restrained to the extent that photochemical smog in cities could be removed completely, then some particular cost (even a high one) would be acceptable to the driver. If pollution control, however, would merely reduce the probability of the instance of photochemical smog then another judgement would be made. However, if the reduction in this pollution is obtained at such cost that the time at which fuel for private motoring will be no longer available is visibly reduced, an entirely different set of judgements is likely to be made.

The major difficulty for the decision makers in dealing with public health matters and environmental issues is the assessment of the true public wishes. The problem is exacerbated by the activities of pressure groups whose audibility is not necessarily related to their size, representativeness or wisdom. Public judgement is also clouded by the behaviour of sections of the news media in selecting certain issues for saturation treatment for a brief time. Depending on the electoral state of the community this may have a very large effect or a very limited effect.

Further difficulty is generated by judgements made on the relative significance of hazards; road accident injury and death have attained an acceptability which matches ill the passion with which other more limited but more interesting hazards are addressed. Public assessment of a hazard and the public risk-benefit impression of it are important factors in any decision-making process in a modern democracy. Edmund Burke wrote: "The public interest requires doing today those things that men of intelligence and goodwill would wish five or ten years hence had been done."

There are facing us today a number of problems which might well suggest that five or ten years is not sufficient. In questions of nuclear waste some would say that we should be thinking in terms of 500 years. In energy matters we must be thinking in terms of fifty years. It would seem evident from earlier sections that we are unlikely to have quantitative data which would justify our having confidence that men of intelligence and goodwill will agree in 100 years or 500 years time that we have done what they would have wanted to have done.

In this period of rapidly changing technology, simple extrapolation is not a sufficient basis for decision, nor is hunch. The techniques of forecasting and assessment, imperfect though they may be, do provide us with a means to ensure that a maximum degree of rationality is included in our decision making. At the same time it is important to realize that balanced judgements of a technical, quantitative kind must be combined with balanced judgements of a subjective and political kind, to allow for proper assessment of values not easily quantified.

VII. Collective Responsibility of Scientists, Politicians and the Lay Community

Much of our present state of development is due to scientific research or to invention. Further progress and the solution of outstanding social problems can be assisted by continuation of this historical process. Community demands on science must, however, be tempered by an understanding of the subtle processes of scientific advancement. Undue interference in the processes of pure science are likely to be counterproductive.

At the same time, there appears to be justification for community involvement in decisions affecting technology:

Despite the complexities and uncertainties society will need to improve its decision-making capabilities and this area should be given increased support as far as studies are concerned.

The institutional links between private, corporate, and government decision makers on the one hand and the scientific community on the other must be maintained and indeed developed further if we are to meet the challenge of the future.

There is a chance that knowledge about the effects and influences of technology is being left for interpretation to those whose role it is to have knowledge about science and technology. Society cannot abdicate its functions by leaving that task to the scientists and technologists, rather it must take action to ensure that knowledge about effects and influences is diffused as broadly as possible.

Decision making about issues involving science and technology very often is done against the background of public opinion and public aspirations for the future. The decision maker at the political level will, in a democratic society at least, be significantly influenced by the existence of an informed society. There is an inescapable duty on the part of the scientists to ensure this level of information and to participate at all levels in the decision-making process.

References

Ashby, The Rt Hon. Lord (1976). *Proc. R. Soc. Med.* **69**, 721.
Burnet, F. M. (1978). "Endurance of Life", 34. Melbourne Univ. Press.
Carpenter, R. A. (1972). "The Scope and Limits of Technology Assessment". OECD Seminar on Technology Assessment, Paris.

Fishlock, D. (1975). "The Risks and Rewards of Research and Development". Associated Business Programmes, London.
Gabor, D. (1963). "Inventing the Future". Pelican Books, London.
Gibbons, M. and Voyer, R. (1974). *In* "A Technology Assessment System—A case Study of East Coast Off-Shore Petroleum Exploration". Science Council of Canada, Cat. SS21–1/30.
Hetman, F. (1973). "Society and the Assessment of Technology". Organization for Economic Co-operation and Development, Paris.
Holling, C. S. (1977). *In* "Futures Research. New Directions" (H. A. Linstone and W. H. Clive Simmonds, Eds). Addison-Wesley, Massachusetts.
Hoos, I. R. (1977a). *J. tech. Forecasting soc. Change* **10**, 335.
Hoos, I. R. (1977b). "Handbook of Futures Research" (J. Fowles, Ed.). Greenwood Press, London.
Kennet, W. (1976). "The Futures of Europe". Cambridge Univ. Press.
Miller, D. C. (1977). *In* "Methodology of Social Impact Assessment: Community Development Series" (Finsterbuch and Wolf, Eds). Dowden Hutchinson, Strandsberg, Pa.
Nelkin, D. (1975). *Soc. Studies Sci.* **5**, 35–54.
Price, D. K. (1964). "Scientists and National Policy Making", 26. Columbia Univ. Press, New York.
Saloman, J. J. (1973). "Science and Politics". MIT Press, Cambridge, Mass.
Vassiliev, M. and Gouschev, S. (1959 (Russia), 1961). "Life in the Twenty-first Century". Penguin Books, Harmondsworth.
Von Forerster, H. (1977). *In* "Futures Research. New Directions" (H. A. Linstone and W. H. Clive Simmonds, Eds). Addison-Wesley, Massachusetts.
Weinberg, A. M. (1972). *Minerva* **10**, 209.
Wood, R. C. (1964). *In* "Scientists and National Policy Making". (R. G. Gilpin and C. Wright, Eds). Columbia Univ. Press, New York.
Zadeh, I. A. (1972). "Outline of a New Approach to the Analyses of Complex Systems and Decision Processes", 2. Memo No. ERL-M342. Electronics Research Laboratory, Berkeley.

34

The Need for An Holistic Approach to Human Health and Well-being

Stephen Boyden

Human Ecology Programme, Centre for Resource and Environmental Studies, Australian National University, Canberra, ACT, Australia

---

Intangibles . . . are almost totally ignored in political rhetoric and in the formation of societal policies for the future.

I. The Hippocratic Postulate

The state of health and well-being of individuals and of populations is largely a function of the environment in which they live and of their life-style or patterns of behaviour within that environment. This simple truth was recognized by Hippocrates and it is so important a principle, if also an obvious one, that it deserves a name. I shall therefore refer to it here as the "Hippocratic postulate".

In this paper I will discuss the interrelationships between environment, behaviour and health and well-being in terms of a conceptual model which some of my colleagues and I have found useful in the study of human ecosystems (Boyden, 1977; Boyden and Millar, 1978; Boyden, 1979; Boyden *et al.*, 1979). This model is introduced in Fig. 1, which depicts the Hippocratic postulate diagrammatically. In this diagram, the term *biopsychic state* refers to the actual state, biological and psychological, that the individual is in at any given time. It incorporates all aspects of the individual, including the genotype and such anthropometric and physiological variables as height, weight, blood pressure, state of lungs and other organs, as well as the individual's knowledge, values, mood and feelings. The biopsychic state thus includes all "health and well-being" variables; conversely, the health and well-being of an individual is an aspect of his or her biopsychic state.

Figure 1 draws attention to a point of great importance in our efforts to comprehend the interrelationships between environment, life-style and health, in that it distinguishes between the *personal environment* of the individual—that is, the environment which the individual personally experiences*—and the *total environment*, or the system as a whole, which includes everything else that exists in the settlement or region in which the individual finds himself or herself.† Clearly only a part of the total environment impinges directly on the individual, who can be said to be separated from it by a series of filters—the socioenconomic, cultural and geographic factors which determine the personal environment of the individual. Thus the personal environment of the individual and hence the individual's state of health and well-being are influenced by

* The personal environment in this model corresponds to the "milieu extérieur" of Claude Bernard (Corson, 1971). His "milieu intérieur" is equivalent to our biopsychic state.

† For some purposes it is useful to recognize different levels of the total environment, ranging from a certain human settlement, through the region in which it exists, to the biosphere as a whole (see Boyden, 1979).

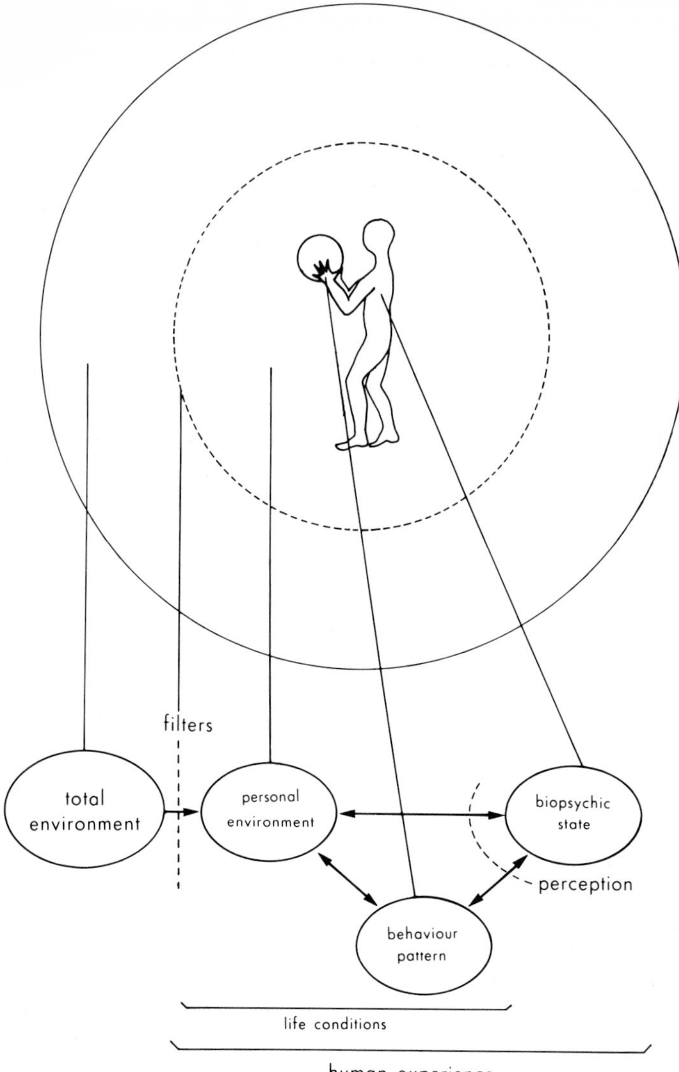

Fig. 1. Conceptual Model, version 1.

the filters and by such aspects of the total environment as the hierarchical structure of society, the economic system, the educational system, the applications of technology and uses of machines, land-use patterns, the design of the built environment and the general pattern of energy use.

The diagram takes account of the fact that human experience also incorporates a behavioural component. The behaviour pattern of an individual is influenced by the personal environment and the biopsychic state, and in turn is itself an influence on the biopsychic state. It is useful for some purposes to include personal environment and behaviour pattern together under the single term *life conditions*.

In the terminology of this diagram, the Hippocratic postulate can be restated as follows: the state of health and well-being (i.e. an aspect of the biopsychic state) of an individual is largely a function of his or her personal environment and behaviour pattern, that is, of his or her life conditions. I shall refer to the concept that the life conditions of individuals and hence also their health and well-being are, in turn, influenced by properties of the total environment as the "extended Hippocratic postulate".

It is well known that the biopsychic state of an individual and also the biopsychic responses to life conditions at any given time are influenced by his or her previous life conditions, such as diet in infancy and socialization experience and also, of course, by the individual's genotype. This refinement of the Hippocratic postulate is depicted in Fig. 2.

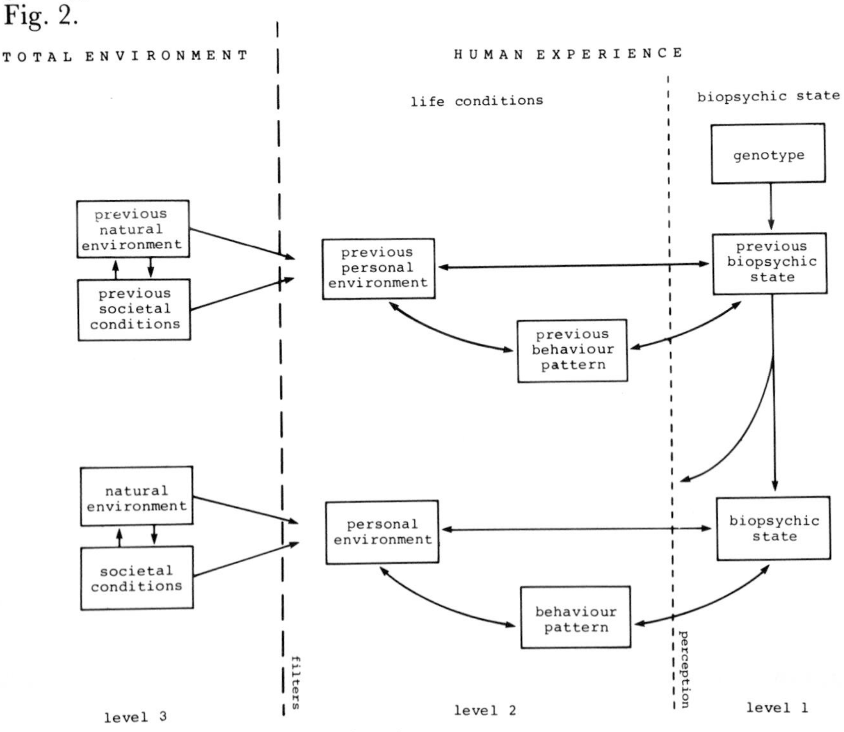

Fig. 2. Conceptual Model, version 2.

This diagram differs from Fig. 1 in that the total environment has been divided into two sets of variables: *societal conditions*, which include human society itself and all its "trappings", such as the built environment, the machines used by society, and all other man-made components of the environment. It also includes human culture (beliefs, knowledge, laws, etc.) and the activities of people and their machines.* It is within the sphere of societal conditions that options exist with respect to change in the future—options which have an important bearing on the quality of human experience. The *natural environment* includes all other components and processes of the total environment, such as the atmosphere, water, soil, flora, fauna, and biogeochemical cycles. These components of the total environment are shown in a third version of the conceptual model in Fig. 3.

Although the life conditions and biopsychic state of any single individual are unique and different in detail from those of any other individual, the model which has just been presented can also be applied to groupings of individuals—such as occupational, ethnic or socioeconomic groupings—which tend to share certain life conditions and hence, in accordance with the Hippocratic postulate, certain health and disease patterns.

The aspect of the model which I wish particularly to emphasize is the fact that it recognizes three levels of reality relating to human health and well-being: level 1—the biopsychic state of individuals or groups of individuals; level 2—the life conditions of individuals or groups of individuals; level 3—the total environment. We consider the distinctions between these three levels to be conceptually important, and suggest that a great deal of the confusion which has characterized work on "social indicators" has been due to failure to take proper account of these distinctions (Boyden, 1976). It follows from the concept of the three levels that we can broadly recognize two sets of interrelationships relevant to human health and well-being. First, there are the interrelationships between life conditions and biopsychic state; and second, there are the interrelationships between the total environment and the life conditions of individuals. (There are also, of course, interactive relationships among the components within each level.)

II. The Importance of Intangibles

I now wish to draw attention to the self evident but all too frequently

* The various components of the total environment are discussed more fully elsewhere (Boyden, 1979).

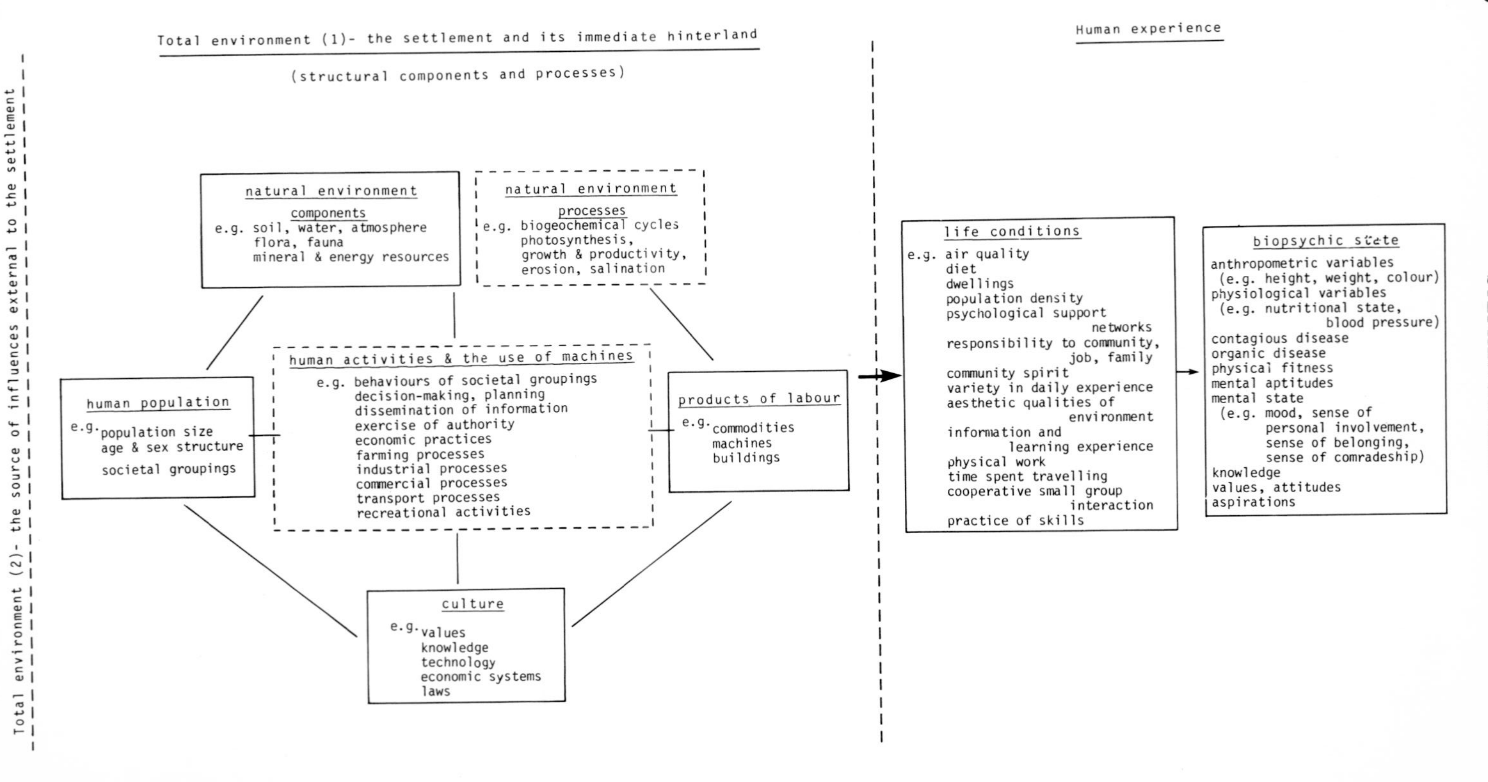

Fig. 3. Conceptual Model, version 3.

neglected fact that, at all three levels of reality, the important variables relevant to human health and well-being range from those which are relatively easy to measure and to describe, to others which cannot be quantified and which are difficult to describe in precise terms. I shall refer to these two kinds of variables as the tangibles and the intangibles,* bearing in mind that the division between these two categories is not a sharp one, in that some variables are intermediate in their "tangibility".

On the level of the biopsychic state the tangibles include, for instance, blood pressure, nutritional state, amount of subcutaneous fat and the presence or absence of lesions in various organs. The intangibles include the individual's knowledge, values and wants, and his or her mental state, mood, and such feelings as a sense of personal involvement, of comradeship, of security, of belonging, of disappointment or frustration. On the level of life conditions the tangible variables include the quality of the air and water and of foodstuffs in the individual's personal environment, noise levels, physical population density in the home, and contact with potentially pathogenic microorganisms. The intangibles on this level include the expectations of friends and relatives (with respect to obligations, etc.), the degree of creative behaviour experienced by the individual and the degree of variety in his or her daily experience. On the level of the total environment, the tangibles include buildings, patterns of energy use, machines, and societal groupings, while the intangibles include the society's value system, legislation and technology (in the strict sense of "knowledge of how to make and how to use tools and machines").

III. The Causes of Ill Health—the Interrelational or Holistic Approach

The concept that the relationship between life conditions and health is often complex and that disease can seldom be explained sufficiently in terms of a single cause is an ancient one (Dubos, 1965). However, despite its antiquity and the fact that it is probably widely accepted on

* The words "tangible" and "intangible" are used in a broad sense in this chapter. "Intangible" is used for that general class of variables which are difficult or impossible to quantify or which are difficult to describe in precise terms (e.g. the Western Idea of Progress, variety in daily experience, sense of purpose). "Tangible" variables are those which are easy to measure and easy to describe—including, for example, energy which, although quantifiable, is admittedly hardly "tangible" in the more strict sense of the term.

the theoretical level, the multifactorial approach can hardly be said to dominate the practice of medicine today.

A classic example of a situation in which a wide range of environmental and life-style factors appear to influence a specific form of physiological maladjustment is the case of coronary thrombosis. Correlations, positive or negative, have been found between the incidence of coronary heart disease and such factors as the intake of coffee, smoking, the consumption of saturated fats, the consumption of calories, levels of physical exercise, the consumption of dietary fibre and the experience of stress (Epstein, 1979). Of course, the acceptance of the idea of a multifactorial contribution to a specific form of ill health, such as coronary thrombosis, must not blind us to the possibility that a substantial increase in the incidence of the condition over a certain period of time might be due to a single change in environment or life-style. The other factors found to correlate with the incidence of the condition might simply reflect states which influence the individual's susceptibility to the effects of the "causal" change.

The proponents of a holistic approach to the understanding of health will appreciate that both tangible and intangible factors are important—not only as influences on, but also as components of health and well-being. Indeed, some authors go so far to suggest that, once survival needs are satisfied, intangible factors are more important in health than tangible ones. Hipsley (1971), for example, has written: "A man is in a far healthier state as a total man when he is half-starved and stunted, and having the opportunity to work at something he likes doing, than when he is well nourished and yet chronically unemployed or working at something that gives no satisfaction."

It will be a theme of this chapter that, despite the widespread general acceptance of the notion that intangible aspects of experience are important influences on, or components of human health and well-being, they are in fact largely ignored in societal policy formulation. We need to examine why this is so, and to work to develop a better theoretical framework and improved methods which will ensure that proper consideration will be given to intangibles in the future.

IV. Coming to Grips with Intangibles

The relative neglect of intangibles in planning for the future is not difficult to understand. Human beings find it much easier to deal with "concrete" measurable variables than with the qualitative aspects of reality, which are not easy to describe and which are difficult or impossible to quantify. Nevertheless, it is imperative that we appreciate the truth of the dictum that there is no relationship in human affairs between quantifiability or tangibility on the one hand and importance on the other. If our aim is to understand human problems and situations, it is surely unscientific to ignore those components or aspects which cannot be easily described and measured—for to do so results in an incomplete, and consequently untrue picture. The fact that the intangibles are more difficult to deal with than the tangibles calls for special intellectual effort to be directed to their study. We must work to develop ways and means which will help us to come to grips with them, to identify them, to communicate effectively about them, and to ensure that they are properly taken into account in our analysis of human situations and in our planning for the future.

There are several ways of approaching the study of the intangible aspects of interrelationships relevant to health and well-being. We will now briefly consider these under three headings: the evolutionary approach; the medical and epidemiological approach; the humanistic approach.

V. The Evolutionary Approach

The evolutionary approach which I shall briefly describe involves concepts and hypotheses which some of my colleagues and I have found attractive in our work on the interrelationships between environment, life style and health and well-being (Boyden, 1972; Boyden and Millar, 1978; Boyden *et al.*, 1979). It is based on what we consider to be a fundamental biological principle which derives from Darwinian theory. According to this theory, animal species are the product of the processes of evolution through natural selection, as a result of which they have acquired genetic characteristics which render them well suited to the conditions of life prevailing in the environment in which this evolution has taken place. The fundamental principle which derives from this theory can be described as follows. If the conditions of life of an animal population suddenly deviate from those of the natural habitat (to which the species has become adapted through natural selection), it is likely that the individual animals will be less well-suited to the changed conditions than to the original conditions, and consequently some signs of maladjustment—physiological, behavioural or both—may be anticipated. We refer to this as the "principle of evodeviance", and to the conditions of life which are different from those of the animal's natural habitat as "evodeviations". Disturbances in physiology or behaviour which result from evodeviations are referred to as examples of "phylogenetic maladjustment" because they are due fundamentally to the fact that the phylogenetic characteristics of the species are not suited to the new conditions.*

People tend to take this fundamental biological principle for granted in the case of animals. If a wild animal is captured and placed in a zoo and begins to show signs of maladjustment, the first question the zoo authorities ask is, "What are we doing wrong?" They look to the animal's life conditions in its natural habitat and ask, for example, whether they are feeding it with the "wrong" diet, or whether it is being provided with the "wrong" environment, in terms for instance, of cover, shade or branches to climb on.

In view of the clear relevance of this principle to problems of human health, it is odd that it should receive so little attention in the medical literature. An exception is a book by T. L. Cleave and G. D. Campbell (1966), in which the authors suggest that much ill-health in human beings is due to diets which, in certain important ways, deviate from that to which our species became adapted through natural selection. In fact, the principle of evodeviance applies as much to *Homo sapiens* as to any other species. The phylogenetic characteristics of the human species were determined by the selection pressures operating in, and before the "primeval" or hunter-gatherer phase of human existence. With respect particularly to urban life conditions, there are several reasons why we can rule out the possibility of major genetic adaptation of human populations to the new situation. In the first place, the first cities came into existence little more than 200 generations ago, and since that time only a very small minority of the human population has actually lived in cities. Moreover, many of the important evodeviations associated with urban living today have been introduced within the last one or two generations. Even over the longer period, appreciable change in the genetic constitution of urban populations in response to new selection pressures would be anticipated only in cases where the selective advantage of a given genotype was strong.

It is necessary to explain, however, that this simple and, to us, rather obvious principle, as it applies to the human species, is not universally accepted. For some people, especially sociologists, it smacks too much of biological determinism. Others misunderstand the principle, imagining, for example, that it implies that animals in natural envi-

* The converse of this principle also applies: "Mutations that give rise to substantial changes in the physical characteristics of the organism . . . are unlikely to be advantageous. Since a population is usually well adapted to its environment, major changes [in genetic constitution] are usually maladaptive . . ." (Ayala, 1978).

ronments always live in a state of "perfect" health (e.g. Geist, 1979). Of course, animals in their wild state sometimes suffer from disease. Nevertheless, natural selection operates to favour phylogenetic characteristics which render individuals likely to survive and to successfully reproduce in their particular and typical ecological niche—in other words, which render individuals healthy in that environment. Similarly, hunter-gatherers may suffer from disease—indeed they all die at one time or another and their average life span is considerably less than that of modern Western people. However, we also know that, with respect to our own primeval ancestors, they were at least healthy enough to survive to reproductive age and to successfully reproduce in an environment which was very much more demanding and rigorous than that which we experience today, and which did not offer the mollycoddling benefits of modern civilization. The view that most hunter-gatherers were, most of the time, in a state of good physical and mental health is supported by the data available on recent hunter-gatherer societies (e.g. Black, this volume).

Another cause for reaction against the idea that the health needs of human beings are phylogenetically determined and that, consequently, consideration should be given to the conditions which prevailed when the phylogenetic characteristics of the species were determined through natural selection, is the false assumption that anyone who accepts this principle as valid advocates a return to the hunter-gatherer way of life. Understandably, this notion elicits a very vigorous response in many people. For example, Alvin Toffler (1970) has written:

> We cannot and must not turn off the switch of technological progress. Only romantic fools babble about returning to a "state of nature". A state of nature is one in which infants shrivel and die for lack of elementary medical care, in which malnutrition stultifies the brain, in which, as Hobbes reminded us, the typical life is "poor, nasty, brutish and short". To turn our back on technology would be not only stupid but immoral.

Incidentally, this commonly held picture of life before the advent of civilization is totally inconsistent with the findings of anthropologists who have studied recent hunter-gatherer societies and it is also inconsistent with basic biological principles. The evolutionary process does not produce species which, in the environment in which they evolve, are constantly in such a state of malnutrition that the brain is stultified, and in fact malnutrition is rare in hunter-gatherers (Dunn, 1968). Moreover, very high infant mortality rates are much more characteristic of agricultural and early urban societies than they are of hunter-gatherers.

In my own view, there can be little argument about the applicability of the principle of evodeviance to material aspects of life conditions. The principle is well illustrated by the findings of nutritional science which, through a great deal of painstaking and excellent research, is effectively showing that there is really no diet better for human kind than that which appears to have been most characteristic of people living under the conditions prevailing during the emergence in evolution of our species. That is to say, there is no diet better for human beings than a wide range of different fresh vegetables and fruit and a certain proportion of lean, cooked meat. If we modify this diet by removing, for example, essential amino acids or vitamins, signs of maladjustment are likely; and experience has shown that we have to be very cautious in adding novel substances, such as lead, pesticides or colouring agents, to our diet. Quite recently nutritional science has determined that it is desirable to restore to the diet the non-digestible fibre which is removed by technological processes from the food of people in modern Western society (Burkitt and Trowell, 1975; Tudge, 1979).

Certainly the main causes of ill health and death in urban communities up until this century, namely specific nutritional deficiency diseases (Drummond and Wilbraham, 1939) and contagious diseases (Fenner, 1970; Black, this volume), were diseases of civilization; that is to say, they are examples of phylogenetic maladjustment. Through the processes of cultural adaptation we have largely overcome these particular causes of ill-health of civilization (Boyden, 1970), only to have them replaced by others. It is generally accepted today that the main killing diseases in modern Western society, namely cardiovascular disease (Epstein, 1979) and cancer (Cairns, 1975; Higginson, 1976; Doll, 1977), are both unnecessary, in the sense that they are mainly the consequence of particular life conditions associated with modern Western society.

It must be stressed that human beings do not all respond alike to biologically novel influences in life conditions. Differences in previous experience and in individual genetic constitution account for variability in susceptibility to potentially detrimental environmental agents and experiences. For example, genetic factors have been shown to affect individuals' reactions to refined carbohydrates in the diet (Steinberg, 1959; Cleave and Campbell, 1966), novel chemical agents in the environment and synthetic drugs (Motulsky, 1977) and unnaturally high intake of salt (Brody, 1979).

The principle of evodeviation is, then, a useful guide to what is likely to be good for people and what is not. If our early urban ancestors had been aware of the principle and had possessed knowledge of the life conditions of hunter-gatherers, a great deal of suffering from specific nutritional deficiency diseases could have been avoided, without any knowledge of the chemistry or even the existence of specific nutrients.

In my view, the evidence that the principle of evodeviance is valid with respect to the material or tangible aspects of life conditions is overwhelming. Returning, however, to the question of intangibles, our working hypothesis is that the principle also applies to intangible aspects of human experience (Boyden and Millar, 1978; Boyden *et al.*, 1979). In other words, we postulate that those psychosocial and behavioural aspects of life experience which were, or are, characteristic of the life experience of hunter-gatherers are likely to be conducive to health, and that major deviations from the characteristic pattern might be suspected of being detrimental.

My own reading of the socioanthropological literature on recent hunter-gatherers leads me to suggest that the life conditions of most of our hunter-gatherer ancestors are likely to have been characterized, for example, by the following intangibles: a fairly extensive emotional support network of family or close acquaintances; a close intimate relationship between infants and their mothers from the moment of birth; considerable "community interaction" and exercise of responsibility towards other members of the community; co-operative small group interaction; incentives and opportunity for creative behaviour and the practice of learned manual skills; emphasis on active (e.g. dancing, singing, music making) rather than passive entertainment; short-term goal-achievement cycles (i.e. goals set and achieved usually in 24 hours or less); an environment which was full of interest; considerable variety in daily experience.

On the level of the biopsychic state, I suggest that it is reasonable to suspect that hunter-gatherers usually experienced a sense of personal involvement, a sense of purpose, a sense of belonging, a sense of interest in their surroundings and in their activities, a sense a comradeship, a sense of challenge and a sense of identity, and that their aspirations were of a kind likely to be fulfilled.

On the basis, then, of our hypothesis, we would suggest that these aspects of life conditions and of biopsychic state would tend to be conducive to health and well-being in members of the human species.

VI. The Medical and Epidemiological Approach

Some people find the evolutionary approach unpalatable, perhaps because it may be too reminiscent of Jean Jacques Rousseau, whose ideas are unfashionable in the social sciences these days. For the scientifically minded, the medical and epidemiological approach to the study of intangible influences on health and well-being may be more acceptable.

During the past two decades, an increasing number of epidemiological studies have shown clearly the importance of intangibles as influences on health and well-being (for a review of much of the relevant literature, see Cox, 1978; Hordern, 1978). The results of fieldwork are entirely consistent, for example, with the view that the emotional support of relatives and close friends contributes importantly to health and well-being, by assisting individuals to cope with stressful situations (Henderson, 1974; Cobb, 1976; Henderson *et al.*, 1978). With respect to work experience, there is an accumulating body of data which suggests that a degree of variety in daily experience, of challenge, of personal interest in work and of responsibility with respect to the quality of the end-product all contribute to the well-being of the worker (Herzberg, 1966; Mackay and Cox, 1978).

Another example of the relevance of intangible experience in relation to health and well-being is provided by the studies of J. Bowlby (1953), who concludes that "mother love in infancy and childhood is as important for mental health as are vitamins and proteins for physical health". He suggests that the infant needs to experience "the warm intimate and continuous relationship with his mother (or permanent mother-substitute—one person who steadily mothers him) in which both find satisfaction and enjoyment", in order to attain a state of mental health and well-being in later life. Thus Bowlby's work, as well as that of other investigators, strongly emphasizes the importance of intangible aspects of early experience on subsequent health and well-being.

There are numerous studies, many of them of an epidemiological nature, which support the view that intangible aspects of life experience, such as the feelings which follow bereavement, and other major upheavals in life experience, have a marked effect on health (Hinkle and Wolff, 1957, 1958). Excessive change *per se* in life experience tends to be associated with ill-health, either physical or mental (Rahe, 1968, 1969). On the other hand, it is also well known that very low levels of environmental change are also detrimental to health (Solomon *et al.*, 1961). As in the case of many other variables in life conditions, both tangible and intangible, there appears to be an optimal range of experience.

With respect to community experience, field studies by N. M. Bradburn and D. Caplowitz (1965) suggest that "positive mental health" relates to levels of environmental participation. C. Leroy has argued that there is a positive relationship between health and potential for local decision making, and that local responsibility for community affairs effectively reduces the sense of alienation (see Freeman, 1978).

VII. The Humanistic Approach

This third approach to the study of intangibles consists of taking note of what people say, or have said, in the light of their own personal experience of life, about what they consider to be important determinants of health and well-being. We can examine, for example, the writings of authors from the humanistic or non-scientific tradition, who are concerned about the human condition. There is, indeed, no shortage of material of this kind. In the last century Karl Marx (1844), assumed that "alienation" is a bad thing (that is, alienation from the process of work, alienation from the products of one's work, alienation of the worker from himself and alienation of the worker from others), and he thus inferred that a sense of personal involvement and of belonging is a good thing. Many other authors have accepted this assumption, and it is rare to come across disagreement on this point (but see Kaufmann, 1973). Also in the nineteenth century, William Morris emphasized the value of creative behaviour and the exercise of learned manual skills (Morris, 1878). Although his arguments seemed to have had little influence on the direction of societal change, no one, to my knowledge, has contradicted his basic assertion, and numerous other writers have expressed the same view.

In the present century, countless authors have alluded to the intangible factors which they personally believe to be important either in contributing to, or in detracting from the quality of life. The names of Aldous Huxley, Lewis Mumford, Abraham Maslow, Arnold Toynbee, Theodore Roszak, Herbert Marcuse and Ivan Illich come to mind, among many others.

It is clearly not feasible in this chapter to attempt an analytical review of this vast literature. However, I would like to make a few brief comments on what I suspect we would find if we did make such a review.

Considering first human experience on the level of *life conditions* (Figs. 1–3), and allowing for the different patterns of words selected by various authors to communicate their meaning, I suspect that we would find that essentially the same basic ideas are expressed again and again. We would find, in essence, a relatively simple and easily recognizable core of intangible aspects of life conditions considered to be important for human well-being. I suggest that, especially prominent among these, we would find the following:

an effective emotional support network;

an environment which offers opportunities and incentives for creative behaviour and the exercise of learned manual skills;

an environment which encourages co-operative small-group interaction;

a social and built environment which encourages community interaction and a feeling of responsibility in the local setting;

job opportunities which offer a degree of responsibility, co-operative small-group interaction, variety in work experience, and the exercise of learned skills;

an environment which has interest value for the individual and which offers considerable opportunity for spontaneity in behaviour.

If we were to attempt the same thing with respect to the intangible aspects of the biopsychic state which are important in health and well-being, the situation would certainly be more complicated. Numerous lists have been drawn up by different authors of the biopsychic "needs" of human beings, and many of these lists are very long. Even so, I suspect that we would find that a few items would be found to be more in evidence than others. I suggest that the more important ones would include, on the positive side, sense of personal involvement, sense of purpose, sense of belonging, sense of comradeship, sense of being needed and loved, sense of being interested, and aspirations of a kind which are likely to be fulfilled. On the negative side, the list would include sense of alienation, sense of anomie, sense of chronic frustration, sense of loneliness, sense of boredom, and sense of being unwanted.

The disturbing fact to which we ought surely to react is that, although numerous individuals have drawn attention to the very real importance of intangible factors in human experience and are more or less agreed as to what the important intangibles are, society seems to have almost totally ignored them in its policy formulation and decision making. This neglect of intangibles may be leading to a state which Heilbroner has called "the civilizational malaise". He writes: "The civilizational malaise, in a word, reflects the inability of a civilization directed to material improvement—higher incomes, better diets, miracles of medicine, triumphs of applied physics and chemistry—to satisfy the human spirit" (Heilbroner, 1975, p. 33).

The insidious and progressive "dehumanization" of which so many people complain in modern society must now be taken very seriously. It is time that we made a deliberate effort to bring the intangibles out into the open, to study them systematically, to improve our language for discussing them, and, on the basis of the various approaches which are available to us, to see whether we can reach a degree of consensus, with respect to their relative importance for the quality of life.

VIII. The Melior–Stressor Concept

The importance of intangible variables becomes especially clear when we consider the problem of stress. Since the pioneer work of Hans Selye (1956), the reality of the stress phenomenon has become widely accepted, and it is generally appreciated that a chronic, unmitigated state of stress is a bad thing, leading to a variety of undesirable outcomes, some physiological and some behavioural. Much attention has been paid to environmental and experiential stressors—that is, those factors which tend to induce a state of stress (Levi, 1971; Cox, 1978).

Following our fieldwork in Hong Kong, my colleagues and I have come to appreciate the importance of the various kinds of experience which produce the opposite effect to that of stressors. We consider that these other kinds of influences are so important that they deserve a name, and we have called them "meliors" (Boyden and Millar, 1978; Boyden *et al.*, 1979). It is useful to suppose that every individual is, at any particular time, at some point on a continuum which ranges from a state of stress at one extreme to a state of non-stress or homeostasis at the other. The position of the individual on this continuum is a function of the balance, in his or her experience, of stressors versus meliors. It is our view that, in Hong Kong for example, certain intangible aspects of life conditions play an extremely important melioric role in maintaining the general level of health in the community and in protecting people from the effects of environmental stressors. For instance, despite the beginning of trends to the contrary, a high proportion of the labour force in that city still works in relatively small-scale enterprises, involving considerable co-operative small-group interaction, and the exercise of personal responsibility. Many people still practise learned manual skills and the nature of the manufacturing industries is such that many factory workers are required to exercise considerable skill. There are also traditional customs, such as the ubiquitous game of mah-jong, which are associated with small group interaction; and networks of psychological support are, despite the growing emphasis on the nuclear family, still very strong. We suggest that, for many people in Hong Kong, such aspects of life conditions as these contribute effectively to well-being by eliciting, for instance, a sense of personal involvement, a sense of purpose, a sense of belonging (to an in-group), a sense of interest and a sense of enjoyment.

The idea that positive experiences are important in health is not new. Referring to the inhabitants of his Utopia, Thomas More (1516) writes: "mere feedom from pain, without positive health, they would call not pleasure but anaesthesia"; and he goes on to discuss various pleasurable experiences which contribute to health and which "give a sort of relish to life". The idea is also implied in much of the humanistic literature referred to above. N. M. Bradburn (1969), in his book "The Structure of Psychological Well-being", discusses the concept and describes a scale of ten questions which he and his colleagues have devised, five of them aimed at measuring negative, and five of them positive influences on well-being. Although I am personally unconvinced of the usefulness of attempts to quantify these intangible variables, I fully support Bradburn's emphasis on the importance of positive as well as negative experiences as determinants of human well-being.

The fact that most meliors are so intangible highlights, in my view, a serious problem confronting human communities today. Because they are difficult or impossible to describe and measure, the very real risk exists that important meliors can be insidiously eroded in a society, much to the detriment of the health and well-being of the people, without any resistance being offered by the community or the government. I am not aware that meliors are taken seriously by any of the major political parties in Western democracies.

IX. The Extended Hippocratic Postulate

Some readers of this paper may feel inclined to make the criticism that what has been said about intangibles is nothing more than common sense. After all, every good general practitioner knows that the family situation, personal relationships and work experience are important influences on his patient's health and well-being, and health workers are well aware of the therapeutic value in convalescence of creative behaviour and the practice of manual skills. It is certainly true that some members of the medical profession, especially those who take a more holistic view of health and disease, not only recognize that the Hippocratic postulate applies to intangibles as well as to tangibles, but take this principle into account in the treatment of their patients.

However, a truly holistic view also recognizes that the life conditions of individuals, in both their tangible and intangible aspects, are determined largely by the properties of the total environment and, in particular, by the set of variables which we have called societal conditions. I referred above to this relationship as the "extended Hippocratic postulate".

The serious cause for concern is the fact that, although intangibles in human experience have been declared to be very important by numerous authors—scientific and humanistic—they are almost totally ignored in political rhetoric and in the formulation of societal policies for the future. Intangibles do not feature in the political platforms of any of the major political parties in, for example, Australia or Britain, which assume that a standard of living as measured in purely material or dollar terms is the only criterion worth taking into account. And yet there is absolutely no doubt that the intangible aspects of life experience which we have discussed are influenced by such aspects of societal conditions as patterns of industrialization, of energy use, of the use of resources, of the use of machines, by the design of the built environment, the educational system, the hierarchical structure of society, the residential distribution of the work force in relation to place of work, land use, community structure, and the size and scale of organizations (Freeman, 1978; Boyden *et al.*, 1979).

An apparent exception to this generalization about the neglect of intangibles on the societal level is the recent expression of concern about the impact of future technological developments on the quality of life. Some governments have recently set up committees, task forces or working groups, to consider this problem. However, the approach so far taken can hardly be said to be a truly holistic or comprehensive one, and the emphasis seems always to be on the ways and means of assisting people to adjust as rapidly as possible to technological change. The implicit assumption seems to be that such change is necessarily good for humanity or that it is inevitable. For example, a leading scientist in Australia is reported to have said recently:

> There is no question that the rapid rate of change makes life uncomfortable or difficult for many people who are unable to change with technological development. This inability may be due to the disappearance of jobs or inability to change skills and attitudes. The solution, I believe, is to change social systems and attitudes, not to inhibit developments (see Juddery, 1979).

The other alternative, namely the idea that we should be selective in our applications of technology, taking the quality of human experience, in the broadest sense of the term, as our criterion for selecting and controlling technological development is much less often mentioned. However, A. Toffler (1970), in his important book "Future Shock", while putting most emphasis on the need for society to prepare people to cope with rapid change, also writes: "One powerful strategy in the battle to prevent mass future shock . . . involves the conscious regulation of technological advance".

More forcefully, R. G. Wilkinson (1973), has written:

> . . . whatever our views, we must expunge the fatalist belief that the great unplanned forces and unintended pressures which shape our society and technology have been, and will remain, magically benevolent. Too often they command our unthinking but reluctant compliance; instead we must make conscious planning decisions about the quality of our lives, hopefully gaining the initiative needed to make man the master of change rather than change the master of man.

It is nonsense to advocate that there should be a blanket encouragement of all technological development regardless of its implications either for the quality of human life or for the integrity of the biosphere. The key word is surely "selective". We must be selective in the application of technology that we introduce into our society. Moreover, we must not discount the possibility that, in the interests of humanity, a selective return to earlier patterns may be desirable in some instances. We often hear dogmatic statements to the effect that it is impossible, or at least unthinkable, for society to "go backwards". But there is nothing impossible or unthinkable about this prospect. Society has, to the great benefit of humankind, selectively gone backwards in the past—for example, by reintroducing vitamins into the diets of human populations. Another example of a selective return to earlier ways is seen in the efforts of many people today to reintroduce relatively high levels of vigorous physical exercise into their life experience.

It is the theme of this essay that the intangible factors influencing human health and well-being should take their place alongside other considerations among the criteria for selective change, "backwards or forwards", in the future.

Before concluding, I would like to link the problem of intangibles with the ecological predicament in which humankind finds itself at the present time. There is no doubt that the developed world today is in an ecological state of disequilibrium with the biosphere—a state which cannot possibly persist *ad infinitum*. Without any question, human society, if it is to survive, has eventually to move into a new ecological phase in which balance is restored between human society and the natural environment (Odum, 1971; Goldsmith *et al*., 1972; Heilbroner, 1975; Boyden *et al*., 1979). The challenge of finding ways and means of bringing the present rampant processes of growth in the consumption of resources and use of energy under control and making a smooth transition into a humanly acceptable new ecological phase may well represent, along with the control of nuclear arms, the greatest challenge that the human species has ever had to face. I suggest that, along with the control of pollution and of energy and resource utilization, a heightened concern about the intangible factors which influence human health and well-being must be an integral part of the processes of reform that will bring about this transition.

X. Conclusions

This chapter has emphasized the need for an holistic approach to human health and well-being. It has been pointed out that such an approach demands that we take full account of the intangible, as well as the tangible factors which influence the quality of human life.

It is not suggested that we devote extra effort to attempts to quantify intangible aspects of life experience. To do so would not only be difficult—it could also lead to false conclusions. Rather, this is an area where our computers are not really of much use, and where we must fall back on our human intelligence and potential for wisdom.

The time has come to make a deliberate effort to overcome the innate difficulties which we experience in dealing with intangibles and our reluctance to discuss them in the open. It is imperative, if life is to be worth living in the future, that the intangibles find their place along with the materialistic variables, as factors to be taken seriously in the consideration of societal options for the future.

It is suggested that we are already in a position to reach a consensus concerning a core of intangible factors important in human health and well-being.

Finally, I would like to comment on the role of the medical profession. With respect to intangibles, physicians have, up to the present, been mainly concerned with the interrelationships between biopsychic state (level 1 in our conceptual model) and life conditions (level 2). In my view, it would be an excellent thing if the profession were to take a very much more active interest in the interrelationships between societal conditions (level 3) and the intangible aspects of human experience. The medical profession played such a role very effectively with respect to certain tangible aspects of reality in the public health movement in the last century (Flinn, 1965). In the present situation, physicians could become a very important force in alerting decision makers and the community at large to the importance of giving full consideration to the intangible components of human experience when formulating policies for societal and technological change.

References

Ayala, J. (1978). *Scient. Am.* Sept., 48–61

Bowlby, J. (1953). *Quoted in* "Tranquility Denied: Stress and Its Impact Today" (A. Horden), 116. Rigby, Sydney.

Boyden, S. (1970). Cultural adaptation to ecological maladjustment. *In* "The Impact of Civilization on the Biology of Man" (S. Boyden, Ed.), 190–218. Australian National Univ. Press, Canberra.

Boyden, S. (1972). Biological determinants of optimum health. *In* "The Human biology of Environmental Change" (D. J. M. Vorster, Ed.), 3–11. International Biological Programme, London.

Boyden, S. (1976). *Urban Ecology* **1**, 413–415.

Boyden, S. (1977). Integrated ecological studies of human settlements. *Impact of Science on Society, Unesco* **27**, 159–169.

Boyden, S. (1979). "An Integrated Ecological Approach to the Study of Human Settlements". MAB Technical Note No. 12. UNESCO, Paris.

Boyden, S. and Millar, S. (1978). *Urban Ecology* **3**, 263–289.

Boyden, S., Millar, S., Newcombe, K. and O'Neill, B. (1979). The ecology of a city and its people—the case of Hong Kong. (submitted for publication).

Bradburn, N. M. (1969). "The Structure of Psychological Well-being". Aldine, Chicago.

Bradburn, N. M. and Caplovitz, D. (1965). "Reports on Happiness: A Pilot Study of Behaviour Related to Mental Health". Aldine, Chicago.

Brody, J. E. (1979). *Canberra Times* 15 July.

Burkitt, D. P. and Trowell, H. C. (Eds) (1975). "Refined Carbohydrate Foods and Disease: Some Implications of Dietary Fibre". Academic Press, London and New York.

Cairns, J. (1975). *Scient. Am.* **233**, 64–78.

Cleave, T. L. and Campbell, G. D. (1966). "Diabetes, Coronary Thrombosis, and the Saccharine Disease". John Wright, Bristol.

Cobb, S. (1976). *Psychosom. Med.* **38**, 301–314.

Corson, S. A. (1971). The lack of feedback in today's societies—a psychosocial stressor. *In* "Society, Stress and Disease". Vol. 1: "The Psychosocial Environment and Psychosomatic Diseases" (Levi, L. Ed.), 181–189. London Univ. Press.

Cox, T. (1978). "Stress". Macmillan, London.

Doll, R. (1977). *Nature, Lond.* **265**, 589–596.

Drummond, J. C. and Wilbraham, A. (1939). "The Englishman's Food". Jonathan Cape, London.

Dubos, R. (1965). "Man Adapting", Chapters 12 and 16. Yale Univ. Press, New Haven, Conn.

Dunn, F. L. (1968). Epidemiological factors: health and disease in hunter-gatherers. *In* "Man the Hunter" (R. B. Lee and I. DeVore, Eds), 221–228. Aldine, Chicago.

Epstein, F. H. (1979). *Mod. Concepts cardiovasc. Dis.* **48**, 7–12.

Fenner, F. (1970). The effects of changing social organization on the infectious diseases of man, *In* "The impact of civilization on the biology of man" (S. Boyden, Ed.), 48–76. Australian National Univ. Press, Canberra.
Flinn, M. N. (1965). "Introduction to Report on the Sanitary Conditions of the Labouring Population of Great Britain. E. Chadwick (1842)", 1–73. Edinburgh Univ. Press.
Freeman, H. (1978). *Br. J. Psychiat.* **132**, 113–124.
Geist, V. (1979). *New Scientist* 22 Feb., 580–582.
Goldsmith, E., Allen, R., Allaby, M., Davull, J. and Lawrence, S. (1972). "A Blueprint for Survival". Tom Stacey, London.
Heilbroner, R. L. (1975). "An Inquiry into the Human Prospect". Calder and Boyars, London.
Henderson, A. S. (1974). *J. nerv. ment. Dis.* **159**, 172–181.
Henderson, S., Byrne, D. G., Duncan-Jones, P., Adcock, S., Scott, R. and Steele, G. P. (1978). *Br. J. Psychiat.* **132**, 463–466.
Herzberg, F. (1966). "Work and the Nature of Man". Staples, London.
Higginson, J. (1976). *Am. J. publ. Hlth* **66**, 359–366.
Hinkle, L. E. and Wolfe, H. G. (1957). *Archs intern. Med.* **99**, 442–460.
Hinkle, L. E. and Wolfe, H. G. (1958). *Ann. intern. Med.* **49**, 1373–1388.
Hipsley, E. (1971). *Med. J. Aust.* **1**, 864–868.
Hordern, A. (1978). "Tranquility Denied". Rigby, Sydney.
Juddery, B. (1979). *Canberra Times* 5 July.
Kaufmann, W. (1973). "Without Guilt and Justice". Peter H. Wyden, New York.
Levi, L. (1971). "Society, Stress and Disease". Vol. 1: "The Psychosocial Environment and Psychosomatic Disease". Oxford Univ. Press.
Mackay, C. and Cox, T. (1978). Stress at work. *In* "Stress", 147–173. Macmillan, London.
Marx, K. (1844). Economic and philosophic manuscripts. *In* "Writings of the Young Marx on Philosophy and Society" (Edited and translated by L. D. Easton and K. H. Guddat, 1967). Anchor Books, New York.
More, T. (1516). "Utopia" (Translated by P. Turner, 1965), 96–98. Penguin Books, Harmondsworth.
Morris, W. (1878). Innate socialism. *In* "William Morris in Selected Writings and Designs" (A. Briggs, Ed., 1962). Penguin Books, Harmondsworth.
Motulsky, A. G. (1977). Ecogenetics: genetic variation in susceptibility to environmental agents. *In* "Human Genetics" (S. Armendares and R. Lisker, Eds), 375–385. Excerpta Medica, Amsterdam.
Odum, E. P. (1971). "The Fundamentals of Ecology", 3rd edn. Saunders, Philadelphia.
Rahe, R. H. (1968). *Proc. R. Soc. Med.* **61**, 44–46.
Rahe, R. H. (1969). *J. psychosocial Res.* **13**, 191–195.
Selye, H. (1956). "The Stress of Life". McGraw-Hill, New York.
Solomon, P., Kubzansky, P. E., Leiderman, P. H., Mendelson, J. H., Trumbull, R. and Wexler, D. (1961). "Sensory deprivation". Harvard Univ. Press, Cambridge, Mass.

Steinberg, A. G. (1959). *Ann. NY Acad. Sci.* **82**, 197–207.
Toffler, A. (1970). "Future Shock", 379. Random House, New York.
Tudge, C. (1979). *New Scientist* **82**, 988–990.
Wilkinson, R. G. (1973). "Poverty and Progress: An Ecological Model of Economic Development". Methuen, London.

Editorial Perspective

The course of this book has meandered gently from side to side, but there has been a consistent general direction: that man and his diseases are like two sides of a coin, each a different aspect of the other. It is not possible to study man without taking cognizance of his diseases and it is not possible to study medicine or human disease without a knowledge of man and his biological and social background.

This simple truth has been at times obscured by lack of knowledge, by disagreements on fact and theory, and by ideological needs to accommodate thoughts and usage. It remains, however, the central theme of social, clinical and experimental medicine.

The corollary of this theme which has been examined in this work is that as man and society have evolved, there have been resulting changes in human disease, qualitatively and quantitatively. Urbanization was accompanied by a rise in infectious disease, and by mental and moral pressures on traditional societies and mores. There were also changes in the distribution of disease, with infectious agents spreading to communities not genetically conditioned to resist them, and the morbidity and mortality were at first extreme. This still occurs in parts of the world, but in the developed countries infectious disease is declining, though not in most cases by deliberate human action. Smallpox is a notable exception.

There have been consequent rises in two other types of disease—the diseases of affluence and overnutrition such as heart disease and obesity, and diseases more often found in the ageing, such as many forms of cancer. The lesson here is clear: disease and death are and always will be part of human existence. For man, being alive is itself a fatal disease.

These changes in "physical" disease have been associated with changes in "mental" disease. Many men expect, as their right, a long, healthy, pain-free life irrespective of external conditions and their own life-style. This is biological nonsense, as Illich and others have pointed out. It leads to "health neurosis", a new and disabling form of hypochondriasis which may cut sufferers off from normal human emotion and activity.

Genetics is another theme which has run through this book. Man is an animal genetically conditioned to life in small groups in a subtropical savannah, an image which still dominates artists' pictures of paradise, as Dubos has pointed out. How such an animal will react to life in the concrete bareness and concentrated pollution of a megapolis is still undetermined. Certainly there will be a major shift in genetic selection pressures. Equally certainly, genetic factors limit the egalitarianism professed by most modern societies: equality of opportunity cannot mean equality of achievement. Genetics, too, is clearly linked with population control, another major health issue but one beyond the scope of this volume.

Man, his world and his health are thus interdependent and promotion of health means not only prevention of disease, but also maintenance of physical environment and solution (or at least partial solution) of social problems. This means political action on a global scale. It has been so far achieved only once— the eradication of smallpox.

Health and disease are public matters requiring open debate. It is our hope that the essays in this book will contribute helpfully to this.

Subject Index

F

G

Q

R